W9-DHV-580

Evaluation of Orthopedic and Athletic Injuries

Evaluation of Orthopedic and Athletic Injuries

Chad Starkey, PhD, ATC
Athletic Training Program Director
Associate Professor
Northeastern University
Bouvé College of Pharmacy and Health Sciences
Boston, Massachusetts

Jeffrey L. Ryan, PT, ATC
Director of Rehabilitation
Department of Orthopaedics and Sports Medicine
Temple University Hospital
Philadelphia

Adjunct Professor
Undergraduate Athletic Training Curriculum
Temple University
Philadelphia

Adjunct Assistant Professor
Program in Physical Therapy
Medical College of PA/Hahnemann University
Philadelphia, Pennsylvania

 F. A. DAVIS COMPANY • Philadelphia

F. A. Davis Company
1915 Arch Street
Philadelphia, PA 19103

Printed in the United States of America

Last digit indicates print number: 10 9 8 7 6 5 4 3 2 1

Publisher: Jean-François Vilain
Developmental Editor: Crystal McNichol
Production Editor: Roberta Massey
Cover Designer: Louis J. Forgione

As new scientific information becomes available through basic and clinical research, recommended treatments and drug therapies undergo changes. The authors and publisher have done everything possible to make this book accurate, up to date, and in accord with accepted standards at the time of publication. The authors, editors, and publisher are not responsible for errors or omissions or for consequences from application of the book, and make no warranty, expressed or implied, in regard to the contents of the book. Any practice described in this book should be applied by the reader in accordance with professional standards of care used in regard to the unique circumstances that may apply in each situation. The reader is advised always to check product information (package inserts) for changes and new information regarding dose and contraindications before administering any drug. Caution is especially urged when using new or infrequently ordered drugs.

Library of Congress Cataloging-in-Publication Data

Starkey, Chad, 1959–
    Evaluation of orthopedic and athletic injuries   / Chad Starkey, Jeffrey L. Ryan.
      p. cm.
    Includes bibliographical references and index.
    ISBN 0-8036-0048-8
    1. Sports injuries. I. Ryan, Jeffrey L., 1962– . II. Title.
  RD97.S83 1995
  617.1'027—dc20
                                  95-24692
                                    CIP

To Eleanor "Rusty" Feather, who taught me my multiplication tables.
And the rest is So Like Candy. . .

Chad Starkey

To my parents, who instilled the foundation for learning and teaching. To my teachers and mentors, who taught me that a thorough evaluation forms the basis of a successful treatment approach. And to my wife, Nancy, for her unending love and support.

Jeff Ryan

Preface

As students we have all faced the dreaded essay question that reads something like, "Explain the rise and fall of the industrial age, drawing parallels to commercial transportation giving way to the information age. Give your response in no more than two pages." This was basically the same type of task we faced in the development of this text. Entire textbooks have been dedicated to the same material that appears as mere sections within our chapters. A plethora of tests exists for determining the stability of the knee. The knowledge of anatomy and biomechanics needed to accurately perform orthopedic evaluations would fill several volumes.

So, as authors, our task was clear: Simply take knowledge needed to conduct a thorough and accurate evaluation of the injuries that are experienced by athletes; formulate it in a clear, concise, and consistent manner; use photographs and illustrations to reinforce these points; and keep the text to fewer than 600 pages.

Understanding the physical evaluation process is a cognitive as well as a psychomotor task. We have focused on the understanding of the anatomy, physiology, and pathophysiology involved so that the user of this text has a clear idea of what is entailed as he or she progresses through an evaluation.

Based on these limitations, we decided that, because of the knowledge of anatomy needed to identify the pathology, each chapter should begin with a review of the pertinent anatomy. This section is not intended to be an all-encompassing treatise of the anatomical features of the particular body part but, rather, to serve as a refresher for the student's knowledge of anatomy and as a resource for the chapter. Depending on the particular skills of the students, some instructors will choose to forgo this section.

We have attempted to adhere to a standardized evaluation model as the format for this material. The model's component parts, history, inspection, palpation, functional testing, ligamentous and capsular testing, neurological tests, and special tests for specific pathology, are modular in nature. Therefore, instructors who use different evaluation formats will still find this text a useful teaching tool.

The text attempts to focus on techniques that are clinically proven and applicable. Early in the student's development, it is far better that he or she use one reliable test than muddle through several less reliable ones. We have attempted to scrutinize the tests described here, although this task has not always been entirely possible. We have, however, attempted to provide evaluative techniques that are founded in logical, reliable science.

The similarities and differences between "clinical" evaluations and "on-field" evaluations are addressed throughout this text. The evaluation of each body area, with the exceptions of cardiopulmonary injuries and environmental injuries, is composed of clinical and on-field evaluation techniques. Each chapter concludes with an on-field management section. Although these sections are not to be construed as the definitive works in this area, the student must recognize that much of the long-term disposition of the athlete and the injury is determined by how the situation is managed in the first few minutes.

The first two chapters introduce the student to the concept and process of evaluating orthopedic and athletic injuries. Chapter 2 defines the general types of injuries addressed in this text and provides standardized evaluative findings for each. From here we proceed through the body sequentially from the feet to the head and then expand into systemic injuries.

We rely heavily on the use of tables and figures to reinforce the information presented in the text and to present an encapsulated version of the textual matter. Words that may be new to the student are defined on the page on which they appear. We believe that the standardized evaluation tables will assist students in developing critical thinking as they progress through the learning curve. Each chapter has an "outline" of the specific steps of the evaluation, which we believe will prove to be a valuable study tool.

Several conventions were used during the assembly of this text. The authors referred to the following texts when describing biomechanics, range of motion, muscle action and nerve supply, muscle testing procedures, and joint end-feel:

Daniels, L, and Worthingham, C: Muscle Testing: Techniques of Manual Examination, ed 5. WB Saunders, Philadelphia, 1986.

Kendall, FP, and McCreary, EK: Muscles: Testing and Function, ed 3. Williams & Wilkins, Baltimore, 1983.

Norkin, CC, and Levangie, PK: Joint Structure and Function: A Comprehensive Analysis, ed 2. FA Davis, Philadelphia, 1992.

Norkin, CC, and White, DJ: Measurement of Joint Motion: A Guide to Goniometry, ed 2. FA Davis, Philadelphia, 1995.

The authors encourage the reader and instructor to refer to these texts for an in-depth description of those topics that fall beyond the realm of this book.

Chad Starkey
Jeff Ryan

Contributors

Peter S. Zulia, PT, ATC
Director
Oxford Physical Therapy and Rehabilitation, Inc.
Oxford

Instructor
Athletic Training Curriculum
Department of Physical Evaluation,
    Health and Sports Studies
Miami University
Oxford, Ohio

Acknowledgments

No work of this magnitude is accomplished in solitude. The following pages represent the combined efforts of numerous athletic trainers, physical therapists, and physicians who, in the spirit of the sports medicine team described in the text, contributed immeasurable hours of their time seeing this project to fruition. We would like to thank the following:

Marcia K. Anderson, PhD, LATC; Gary Ball, EdD, ATC; Sara D. Brown, MS, ATC; Scott T. Doberstein, MS, ATAC/R, CSCS; Francis X. Feld, MEd, RN, ATC, NREMT-P; Richard D. Griswold, MS, ATC; Glen Johnson, MD; Ky Edward Kugler, EdD, ATC; Cynthia Norkin, EdD, PT; Richard Riehl, MS, ATC; Charles M. Rozanski, Jr., MEd; Kim S. Terrell, MS, ATC; and Bruce M. Zagelbaum, MD.

However, to simply thank Sara Brown for her contributions would be an understatement of monumental proportions. She often shoveled through the first drafts of chapters that were otherwise unfit for human consumption. Peter S. Zulia, PT, ATC, contributed his expertise on gait and gait analysis by writing Chapter 8. Extra thanks also goes out to Kim Terrell, who not only served as a reviewer but also took many of the photographs. Additional photographs were taken by Jodie Healy, PT, ATC.

The staff, students, and athletes at Northeastern University, The University of Oregon, Harvard University, Brandeis University, Temple University Sports Medicine, and The Temple University Sports Medicine and Orthopaedic Physical Therapy Center contributed their time in modeling for the photographs.

We couldn't let the opportunity pass to acknowledge the contribution that Steve Bair, MS, ATC, has played in not only our professional development but also in the development of the profession as a whole.

And, as always, we must thank Jean-François Vilain, who, after his cameo role in "Monty Python and the Holy Grail" (he was the guy with the outrageous accent in the castle), encouraged us in pursuing this project and became only slightly irritated when it was late.

Contents

1

The Injury Evaluation Process

The successful management and rehabilitation of injuries depends on the accurate initial assessment of the condition. Although the evaluation process is often thought of in terms of an acute injury, it is in fact an ongoing process throughout all phases of recovery. The determination of the effectiveness of treatment and rehabilitation protocols and the subsequent modification of these regimens require that the athlete's functional status be re-evaluated at regular intervals. Regardless of whether the evaluation is an on-field *triage* of the injury or a re-evaluation of an existing condition, a thorough knowledge of the evaluation process is required so that the correct assessment may be obtained.

An individual's skill in evaluating injuries is based not only on the accuracy of the conclusion reached but also on the efficiency in which it was performed. To perform a thorough and timely evaluation, a standard evaluation model should be adopted. The use of a standardized model leads to efficiency and consistency in the evaluation procedures and assists in developing proficiency in the special skills needed to achieve an optimal outcome.

This chapter presents the evaluation model used throughout this text and introduces the members of the health care team. This model is only one of many that could possibly be used (Fig. 1–1). The number of evaluation models are limited only by the number of health care professionals who are practicing the evaluation and rehabilitation of athletic injuries. Any model may be used, as long as it meets two important criteria: (1) that each step of the model be justified and (2) that the model be followed at all times, with any changes made only with sufficient reason.

PREREQUISITES FOR A THOROUGH EVALUATION

It is said that structure governs function. In the human body, anatomy is the structure and physiology and **biomechanics** are the functions. A proper understanding of the structure and function of the human body is essential for a competent evaluation. Because the body is an integrated machine, the knowledge of the specific structure and function of individual body parts must be expanded to include the relationship between these parts in producing normal movement (biomechanics) and when injured, abnormal movement (**pathomechanics**). It is assumed that the user of this text is versed in anatomy, physiology, and biomechanics.

The evaluation process is nothing more than a search for dysfunctional anatomy, physiology, or biomechanics. Only with a full understanding of the evaluative techniques and the implications of their results can a correct conclusion regarding the injury be made and a successful treatment plan be subsequently formulated.

SYSTEMATIC APPROACH TO THE EVALUATION OF ATHLETIC INJURIES

Arriving at the correct conclusion of an athlete's condition requires that the evaluation process remain focused and thorough. To maintain this focus it is recommended that a standard *systematic* approach be followed using a model from which the evaluation is performed. Any alterations that are needed to meet the specific task at hand can be

---

Triage: The process of determining the priority of treatment.
Biomechanics: The effect of muscular forces, joint axes, and resistance on the quality and quantity of human movement.
Pathomechanics: Abnormal motion and forces produced by the body, most often occurring secondary to trauma.
Systematic: Orderly, based on a specific sequence of events.

History

Determine the mechanism of injury and onset of the symptoms, and question the athlete about any associated sounds or sensations at the time of injury. Ascertain any relevant history of prior injury to the involved and uninvolved sides. The history continues throughout the evaluation based on subsequent findings.

Inspection

Compare the involved and uninvolved sides for signs of swelling, deformity, differences in skin color and texture, muscle tone, and other bilateral differences. The inspection process begins during, or prior to, history taking and continues throughout the evaluation.

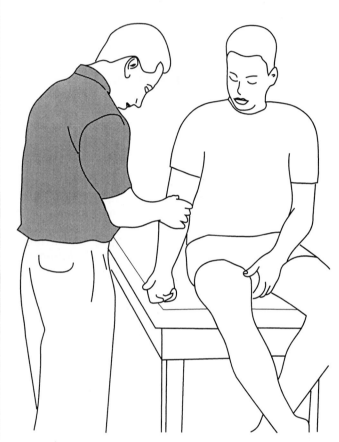

Palpation

Identify areas of point tenderness, crepitus, swelling, malalignment of a joint or bone, or other types of deformity.

Functional Tests

Determine a joint's ability to move actively and passively through a range of motion and its ability to generate tension.

Ligamentous Tests

Apply a stress in one of the cardinal planes to a joint's ligaments and/or capsule.

Special Tests

Apply a stress (often in multiple planes) to isolate a specific anatomical structure or function.

Neurological Tests

Assess motor and sensory nerve function. Identify normal reflex loops. Not required for all evaluations.

Figure 1–1. Injury evaluation model used in this text. History and inspection are performed throughout the examination process. Note that several evaluation models may be used.

made with little changes to the overall model. **Objective data** should be obtained whenever possible and recorded in the athlete's medical file. The use of objective data assists in organizing and setting priorities for the athlete's problems so that the rehabilitation goals and a treatment plan can be formed. **Baseline measurements** obtained during the initial evaluation are referenced and recorded during subsequent re-evaluations to document the athlete's progress and identify the need for changes in the athlete's treatment and rehabilitation regimen.

Description of the Evaluative Model

The evaluation model used in this text is a seven-step process, with each step designed to obtain specific information. For the purposes of this text, the

---

Objective data: Finite measures that are readily reproducible regardless of the individual collecting the information.

Baseline measurements: The initial physical findings, usually performed while the athlete is in a healthy state.

individual steps, as well as the components of each step, are presented sequentially, with one task completed before another is begun. Once the student becomes familiar with the evaluation process, tasks can be combined and the sequence altered, such as inspecting the injured area while conducting the history.

The Importance of the Noninjured Limb

A common flaw when learning to evaluate injuries is to neglect the opposite, or noninjured, limb. Although this section refers to the opposite limb, its content is also applicable in the case of injury to a paired organ.

The importance of the uninvolved limb's role in the evaluation process cannot be understated, as it provides an immediate reference to the relative dysfunction of the injured body part. Also, the individual may use this limb to demonstrate the mechanism of injury or the movements that produce pain.

Table 1–1. Role of the Noninjured Limb in the Evaluation Process

Segment	Relevance
History	Is used to ascertain whether the noninjured limb has a history of injury or a pre-existing condition that can alter the findings (athlete may demonstrate the mechanism of injury using the noninjured limb)
Inspection	Provides a reference for symmetry and color of the superficial tissues
Palpation	Is used to compare bilateral symmetry of bones, alignment, tissue temperature, or other deformity
Functional tests	Provide reference for range of motion, strength, and painful arcs
Ligamentous tests	Determine end-feel, relative laxity, and pain
Special tests	Act as reference points for laxity of individual ligaments, joint capsules, and other articular components
Neurological tests	Act as reference points for bilateral sensory and motor function

Table 1–1 describes the role of the noninjured limb in each element of the evaluation model. Because of the importance of the uninvolved limb, a portion of the history process should be dedicated to identifying a prior or existing injury to this limb, which may influence the bilateral comparison.

There is debate among clinicians regarding sequencing when comparing the noninjured and injured limbs. One school of thought is to first perform each task on the noninjured limb before involving the injured side. The rationale for this is that the athlete's apprehension will be decreased if the evaluation is first performed on the noninjured limb. The other school of thought suggests that this practice may actually increase the athlete's apprehension and therefore increase muscle *guarding* because of the anticipation of pain resulting from the technique.

CLINICAL EVALUATIONS

Clinical evaluations, whether in an athletic training room, physical therapy facility, or physician's office, are performed in a relatively controlled environment compared with evaluations performed on the playing field. In the clinic the evaluator has luxuries that are not available on the field, including evaluation tools (e.g., tape measures, *goniometers*), references, medical records, and, perhaps most importantly, time.

History

The most important portion of an evaluation is the history. In many instances the history itself informs the examiner about the structures involved and the extent of the tissue damage. Perhaps the single most important piece of information obtained during the history-taking process is the injury mechanism, which describes the forces that were placed on the body and potentially identifies the injured tissues.

Questions posed to the athlete during the history-taking process should be open-ended. For instance, rather than asking a closed-ended question such as "Does it hurt when you raise your arm?" which can be answered simply by "yes" or "no," an open-ended question such as "What movement causes you pain?" allows the athlete to describe in detail those motions causing discomfort.

The athlete's medical file is a valuable resource for establishing the previous history of injury, providing documentation regarding the rehabilitation program

Guarding: Voluntarily or involuntarily assuming a posture to protect an injured body area, often through muscular spasm.

Goniometer: A device used to measure the motion, in degrees, that a joint is capable of producing around its axis.

in use and identifying any factors that may predispose the athlete to further injury. The athlete's medical file is often one of the best resources for identifying circumstances that predispose the athlete to injury. The National Collegiate Athletic Association (NCAA) has identified the primary components of the athlete's medical record (Table 1–2).

An additional resource when dealing with athletes is the use of practice or game videos. These films may allow the medical team to actually view the mechanism and circumstances surrounding the injury.

The following information should be obtained during the history-taking process:

• **Location of the pain:** Where does the athlete perceive the pain? In many cases the location of the pain correlates with the damaged tissue. However, pain may also be referred from another source, so the evaluator must be familiar with *referred pain* patterns, which are discussed in the appropriate chapters of this text. It is often useful to ask the athlete to point to the area of pain. An athlete who uses one finger to isolate the area of pain is more likely to pinpoint the involved structure(s), as opposed to an athlete who describes the painful by waiving the hand over a general area, indicating *diffuse* pain.

• **Mechanism of the injury:** How did the injury occur? Through the athlete's description of the mechanism of the injury (e.g., "I rolled my ankle in"), the involved structures and the forces placed on them may be visualized. The onset of the injury must also be ascertained. Was it due to a single traumatic force (*macrotrauma*) or was it the accumulation of repeated forces, resulting in an *insidious* onset of the symptoms (*microtrauma*)?

• **Duration of symptoms:** When did this problem start? With macrotrauma, the *signs* and *symptoms* tend to present themselves immediately. The signs and symptoms associated with microtrauma, such as *overuse syndromes*, tend to progressively worsen with time and continued

Table 1–2. NCAA Guideline 1B: Medical Evaluations, Immunizations, and Records

- History of injury, illness, pregnancy, and surgery of both athletic and nonathletic origin
- Physician referrals and subsequent feedback regarding treatment, rehabilitation, and disposition
- Preparticipation and preseason medical questionnaire detailing the following items:
  - Illnesses suffered (acute and chronic)
  - Surgery and/or hospitalization
  - Allergies
  - Medications taken on a regular basis
  - Conditioning status
  - Injuries suffered (acute and chronic; athletic and nonathletic)
    - Cerebral concussions sustained
    - Episodes involving the loss of consciousness
    - *Syncope*
    - Exercised-induced asthma or bronchospasm
    - Loss of paired organs
    - Heat-related injury
    - Cardiac conditions, including those involving the immediate family
      - *Sudden death* in a family member under age 50
      - Family history of *Marfan syndrome*
- Immunization records
  - Measles
  - Mumps
  - Rubella
  - Hepatitis B
  - Diphtheria
  - Tetanus
- Other documentation, signed by the athlete and parent if the athlete is under 18 years of age
  - Release of medical records
  - Consent to treatment

Adapted from Benson, MT,[1] p 8.

stresses. The severity of overuse conditions may be graded based on the duration of time since the onset of symptoms and the amount of associated dysfunction to the body part (Table 1–3).

Referred pain: Pain at a site other than the actual location of trauma. Referred pain tends to be projected outward from the torso and distally along the extremities.

Diffuse: Scattered; widespread.

Macrotrauma: A single force resulting in trauma to the body's tissues.

Insidious: Of gradual onset; with respect to symptoms of an injury or disease having no apparent cause.

Microtrauma: Small, repetitive injurious forces.

Sign: An observable condition that indicates the existence of a disease or injury. Signs are usually apparent during the inspection process.

Symptom: A condition not visually apparent to the examiner, indicating the existence of a disease or injury. Symptoms are usually obtained during the history-taking process.

Overuse syndrome: Injury caused by accumulated microtraumatic stress placed on a structure or body area.

Syncope: Fainting caused by a transient loss of oxygen supply to the brain.

Sudden death: Unexpected and instantaneous death occurring within 1 hour of the onset of symptoms; most often used to describe death caused secondary to cardiac failure.

Marfan syndrome: A hereditary condition of the connective tissue, bones, muscles, and ligaments. Over time, this condition results in degeneration of brain function and in cardiac failure.

Table 1–3. Classification System for Overuse Injuries

Stage	Presentation of Symptoms	Functional Ability
I	Pain following activity	Little dysfunction initially, pain with movement increases as the athlete nears stage II
II	Pain during and following activity	Pain with movement of the body part, with associated decreased performance. In the latter stages dysfunction of the body part may make the athlete ineffective
III	Constant pain	Great loss of function

- **Description of symptoms:** How does the athlete describe the pain? Is it sharp, dull, or achy? Is it intermittent or constant? Does the athlete have other symptoms such as weakness or paresthesia?

- **Relevant sounds or sensations at the time of injury:** Did the athlete experience any sensations or hear any sounds such as a "pop" that could be associated with a tearing ligament or a bone fracturing?

- **Previous history:** Does the athlete have any history of previous injury to this body area? Are there any possible sources of weakness from a previous injury? If there is a history of injury to this body part, the athlete should be asked to describe and compare this injury with the previous injury. Were the mechanisms similar? Do the present symptoms duplicate the previous symptoms?

    If the athlete's injury appears to be a chronic condition or if there was previous injury to this body part, any prior medical referral and subsequent treatment and rehabilitation protocol must be determined:
    - By whom was this injury previously evaluated and treated?
    - What diagnosis or evaluation was made?
    - What was the course of treatment and rehabilitation? Was surgery performed or medication administered?
    - Did the previous treatment plan decrease the symptoms?

- **Related history to the opposite body part:** Much of what is deduced during the examination of an injury is based on the findings of the injured limb compared with those of the uninjured side. Any previous injury to the uninvolved side that may affect the findings of any bilateral comparison must be determined.

- **General medical health:** Athletes are often assumed to be in prime physical health. Unfortunately, this is not always correct. Anyone undergoing a preparticipation physical examination and subsequent update should be reviewed for the presence of any **congenital** abnormality or disease that may affect the evaluation and treatment of the injury.

At the conclusion of the history-taking process, the examiner should have a good understanding of the events causing the injury, predisposing conditions that may have led to its occurrence, and the activities and motions increasing the symptoms. This portion of the evaluation is a dialogue between the examiner and the athlete. The clinician should not hesitate to "follow leads" to fully ascertain all the facts regarding the athlete's condition. The history may be expanded upon during the remainder of the evaluation, with the clinician backtracking or asking further questions relevant to the athlete's condition.

Although the physical aspect of the evaluation takes priority, the athlete's psychological and emotional state must also be considered. Individual athletes react to an injury differently, each with varying levels of pain tolerance, apprehension, fear, and desire to return to competition.

The information gained and the impression formed from the athlete's history should be confirmed or denied during the rest of the examination. However, the clinician should keep an open mind about the injury and not overlook the actual tissue damage.

Inspection

The inspection process begins when the injured athlete first comes into the evaluator's view. During the clinical evaluation, the inspection begins as soon as the athlete enters the facility. At this time **gait** and posture can be assessed. Also, the athlete can be candidly observed for normal and abnormal movement patterns. Any guarding or "carrying" postures in which the athlete splints the body part in a protective position can be noted. Assessing movement patterns throughout the course of the evaluation is also valuable.

One should visually inspect the athlete to assess any **gross deformity** or obvious injury, including serious bleeding, signs of fracture, or swelling. Signs of joint displacement or bony fracture warrant the termination of the evaluation and the immediate referral to a physician. Careful bilateral inspection may reveal subtle differences in otherwise healthy-

---

Congenital: A condition existing at or before birth.
Gait: The sequential movements of the spine, pelvis, knee, ankle, and foot when walking or running.
Gross deformity: An abnormality that is visible to the unaided eye.

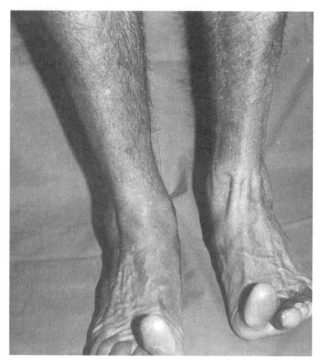

Figure 1–2. What's wrong with this picture? The athlete has few functional complaints other than decreased strength during dorsiflexion of the right ankle. There is no history of trauma to the body area. Carefully examine both ankles to determine the cause of these complaints. The answer is given in the legend of Figure 1–3.

looking body parts. The two ankles shown in Figure 1–2 should be inspected to determine any abnormality.

The clinician should inspect the injured body part and compare the results with the opposite extremity for:

- **Gross deformity:** Are there signs of fracture or joint **dislocation**? These may manifest themselves through disrupted contour of long bones, unequal symmetry, or malalignment of joints. If one of these conditions is suspected, the presence of any other significant trauma must be ruled out, the evaluation terminated, emergency management procedures implemented (e.g., splinting, checking for a **distal** pulse), and the athlete transported to a medical facility.

- **Swelling:** Does the involved body part show signs of swelling? Is the swelling localized or diffuse? The amount of swelling and the elapsed time since the onset of the injury should be ascertained.

- **Bilateral symmetry:** Bilateral body parts should normally be mirror images of each other. Inspect the problematic area and compare it with its counterpart, noting any discrepancy between the two.

- **Discoloration:** Does the area show redness that may be associated with inflammation? Is a contusion present, indicating direct impact?

- **Infection:** If an open wound is being examined, does it show signs of infection (e.g., redness, swelling, pus, or red streaks)?

The inspection of the athlete and the injury continues throughout the entire evaluation process. The athlete may become less apprehensive during the course of the evaluation and begin to move the limb more freely.

Palpation

This step may be considered an extension of the inspection process because the fingers are used to "see" what the eyes cannot. Palpation, the process of touching and feeling the tissues, allows the examiner to detect tissue damage that cannot be observed by comparing the findings of one body part with those of the opposite one and to identify areas of point tenderness.

Palpation should be performed in a specific sequence, beginning with structures away from the site of pain and progressively moving toward the damaged tissues. This allows the different causes of the athlete's pain to be ruled out and helps identify any secondary structures that may be involved.

One form of sequencing is to first palpate the bones and ligaments, then to palpate the muscles and tendons, and then to locate any other items such as pulses. The second form of sequencing is to palpate all structures (e.g., bones, muscles, ligaments) farthest from the suspected injury and to continue to palpate toward the injured site. Regardless of the palpation strategy that is used, the clinician must ensure that all pertinent structures are palpated.

During the palpation phase of the evaluation, the clinician should make note of any of the following findings:

- **Point tenderness:** Palpate toward the injured area, visualizing the structures that lie beneath the fingers. The ability to accurately identify the structure being palpated greatly assists in the identification of the traumatized tissues.

- **Crepitus:** A crunching or grinding of the tissues, crepitus is indicative of fractures when felt over bone or of inflammation when felt over tendon, bursa, or joint capsule.

- **Symmetry:** Muscle tone, joint surfaces, and bony prominences should be compared bilaterally.

Dislocation: The displacement of the articular surfaces of two joints.
Distal: Away from the midline of the body moving toward the periphery; the opposite of proximal.

• **Increased tissue temperature:** Increased temperature of the injured area relative to the surrounding sites is indicative of an active inflammatory process.

Some clinicians prefer to delay the palpation process until the end of the evaluation, as this is often the most painful aspect of the evaluation. Excess pain caused by palpation can lead the athlete to guard the area and alter the rest of the evaluation.

Functional Tests

Assessment of the athlete's functional status identifies the athlete's ability to move the limb through the range of motion actively, passively, and against resistance. As with all evaluation tools, comparisons should be made bilaterally and, when possible, against established **normative data**. Tests for a particular body part must include all the motions allowed by the joint. Additionally, the findings may necessitate the evaluation of the **proximal** and distal joints. Although a motion may be common to many joints (e.g., **flexion**), some motions, such as ankle **inversion**, are found in only one joint. Those motions found in only one joint are most often overlooked during an assessment.

The evaluation of active and passive range of motion may be made grossly by observation of the evaluator or, more precisely, objectively measured with the use of a goniometer (Fig. 1–3).

Active Range of Motion

Active range of motion (AROM) should always be evaluated first, as long as it is not **contraindicated**

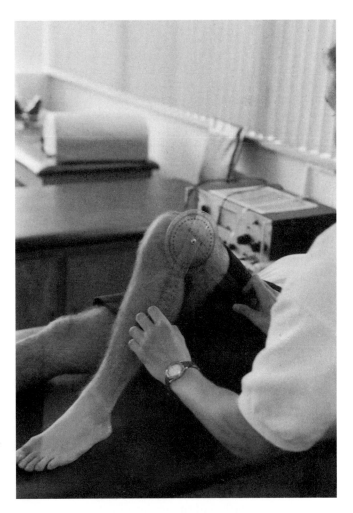

Figure 1–3. Use of a goniometer to measure a joint's range of motion. Refer to Norkin, CC, and White, DJ,[1a] for a complete explanation of the use of a goniometer. Answer to Figure 1–2: The right ankle is missing the tibialis anterior muscle. Note the absence of its tendon as it crosses the joint line.

Normative data: Normal ranges of data collected for comparison during the evaluation of an athlete. Athletes have norms different from the general population on most measures.

Proximal: Near the midline of the body; the opposite of distal.

Flexion: The act of bending a joint, decreasing its angle.

Inversion: The movement of the plantar aspect of the calcaneus toward the midline of the body.

Contraindication: Procedure that may prove harmful given the athlete's current condition.

by immature fracture sites or recently repaired *soft tissues*. Active range of motion is evaluated first so that the athlete's willingness and ability to move the body part through the range of motion can be determined. An unwillingness to move the extremity could signify an extreme degree of pain, neurological deficit, or possible *malingering*.

While the athlete actively moves the joint through all the possible motions in the *cardinal planes*, the ease with which the movement is made as well as the total range of motion produced should be observed. Any compensation or abnormal movement in the surrounding structures should also be noted. The athlete may verbally or nonverbally describe a *painful arc* within the range of motion.

Passive Range of Motion

Passive range of motion (PROM) should be evaluated following active range of motion and is evaluated not only for the quantity of available movement but for the *end-feel* of the tissues as they reach the limit of the available range of motion. The different end-feels as established by Cyrax are listed in Table 1–4.[1a] Certain movements have particular normal end-feels (e.g., elbow *extension* should have a hard or bony end-feel), and the clinician must be familiar with these end-feels so that pathological limits to range of motion are identified (Table 1–5).

Useful information can be obtained by comparing the range of movement obtained for active range of motion with that obtained for passive range of motion. Values for active motion that approximate the values of passive motion signify a capsular or joint tightness causing the restriction of the range of motion. Active motion that is less than the passive motion signifies a muscular weakness or a lesion within the active *contractile tissue* that is causing pain and inhibiting motion.

Resistive Range of Motion

Resistive range of motion (RROM) testing can be performed through the joint's entire range of motion or, more commonly, tested isometrically through

Table 1–4. Physiological (Normal) End-Feels

End-Feel	Structure	Example
Soft	Soft tissue approximation	Knee flexion (contact between soft issue of the posterior leg and posterior thigh)
Firm	Muscular stretch	Hip flexion with the knee extended (passive elastic tension of hamstring muscles)
	Capsular stretch	Extension of the metacarpophalangeal joints of the fingers (tension in the anterior capsule)
	Ligamentous stretch	Forearm supination (tension in the palmar radioulnar ligament of the inferior radioulnar joint, interosseous membrane, oblique cord)
Hard	Bone contacting bone	Elbow extension (contact between the olecranon process of the ulna and the olecranon *fossa* of the humerus)

From Norkin, CC, and White, DJ,[1a] p 9, with permission.

the use of a *break test*, in which the amount of strength available within a muscle or muscle group is determined by trying to break the contraction exhibited by the athlete. Contraindications to resistive testing are similar to those for active range of motion.

Resistive testing of contractile tissues can be assessed with various grading scales, but the results are negated if the contraction causes pain (Table 1–6). With the exception of neurological involvement, the use of these grading scales is rarely of benefit in the athletic population. Resistive testing is particularly useful in determining any lesion that may be causing pain in a contractile tissue (Table

---

Soft tissue: Structures other than bone, including muscle, tendon, ligament, capsule, bursa, and skin.

Malingering: Faking or exaggerating the symptoms of an injury or illness.

Cardinal planes: Imaginary lines dividing the body into upper and lower (transverse planes), anterior and posterior (frontal plane), and left and right (sagittal plane) relative to the anatomical position.

Painful arc: An area within a joint's range of motion that causes pain, representing compression, impingement, or abrasion of the underlying tissues.

End-feel: The specific quality of movement felt by an examiner moving a joint to the end of its range of motion.

Extension: The act of straightening a joint, increasing its angle.

Contractile tissue: Tissue that is capable of shortening and subsequently elongating; muscular tissue.

Break test: An isometric contraction against manual resistance provided by the examiner; used to determine the athlete's ability to generate a static force within a muscle or muscle group.

Fossa: A depression on a bone.

Table 1–5. Pathological (Abnormal) End-Feels

End-Feel	Description	Example
Soft	Occurs sooner or later in the ROM than is usual, or occurs in a joint that normally has a firm or hard end-feel; feels boggy	Soft tissue edema Synovitis
Firm	Occurs sooner or later in the ROM than is usual, or occurs in a joint that normally has a soft or hard end-feel	Increased muscular tonus Capsular, muscular, ligamentous shortening
Hard	Occurs sooner or later in the ROM than is usual, or occurs in a joint that normally has a soft or firm end-feel; feels like a bony block	Chondromalacia Osteoarthritis Loose bodies in joint Myositis ossificans Fracture
Empty	Has no real end-feel because end of ROM is never reached, owing to pain; no resistance felt except for patient's protective muscle splinting or muscle spasm	Acute joint inflammation Bursitis Abscess Fracture Psychogenic origin

From Norkin, CC, and White, DJ,[1a] p 9, with permission.

1–7). During the evaluation of an acute injury, resisted range of motion is used to establish the presence of pain or weakness during the contraction.

During manual resistance, the limb is stabilized proximally to prevent other motions from compensating for weakness of the involved muscle. Resistance is provided distally on the bone to which the muscle or muscle group attaches and should not be distal to a second joint (Fig. 1–4).

Ligamentous and Capsular Testing

Ligamentous and capsular testing evaluates the structural integrity of the **noncontractile tissues** surrounding a joint. **Sprains** of ligamentous tissue are generally graded on a three-degree scale (Table 1–8). Ligamentous and capsular tests can also help to confirm an injury history that is suggestive of **subluxation** as well as the predisposition for dislo-

Table 1–6. Grading Systems for Manual Muscle Tests in an Athletic Population

Verbal	Numerical	Clinical Finding
Normal	5/5	The athlete can resist against maximal pressure. The examiner is unable to break the athlete's resistance.
Good	4/5	The athlete can resist against moderate pressure.
Fair	3/5	The athlete can move the body part against gravity through the full range of motion.
Poor	2/5	The athlete can move the body part in a gravity-eliminated position through the full range of motion.
Trace	1/5	The athlete cannot produce movement, but a muscle contraction is palpable.
Gone	0/5	No contraction is felt.

cation. Testing involves the application of a specific stress to a tissue to test its laxity, but a distinction must be made between laxity and instability. **Laxity** describes the amount of "give" within a joint's supportive tissue. An athlete may have congenital laxity throughout all of the joints, which may be determined by generalized measures such as having the athlete attempt to pull the thumb to the forearm (Fig. 1–5). **Instability** is a joint's inability to function under the stresses encountered during functional activities. The amount of joint laxity does not always correlate with the degree of instability that an athlete experiences. During ligament stress tests, the relative difference in laxity between joints is often a more important finding than the absolute difference.[2]

All ligamentous testing should be evaluated bilaterally and, whenever possible, compared with baseline measures. Using the proper joint angle while stressing a particular tissue is essential because a

Table 1–7. Findings of Resisted Range of Motion Tests

Strength	Pain	Clinical Indication
Good	None	Normal
Good	Present	Minor soft tissue injury
Weak	Present	Significant soft tissue injury
Weak	None	Neurological deficit

Noncontractile tissue: Ligamentous and capsular tissue surrounding a joint.
Sprain: The stretching or tearing of ligamentous or capsular tissue.
Subluxation: The partial or incomplete dislocation of a joint, usually transient in nature; the joint surfaces relocate as the forces causing the joint displacement are relieved.

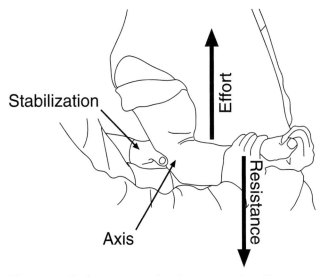

Figure 1–4. Performing manual resistance exercises. The extremity is stabilized proximal to the joint being tested while resistance is provided distal to the joint.

seemingly insignificant change in the joint angle can significantly alter the laxity of the tissue being stressed.

Special Tests

Special tests are specific procedures applied to a joint in order to determine the presence of pathomechanics and therefore are unique to each structure,

Table 1–8. Grading System for Ligamentous Laxity

Grade	Ligamentous End-Feel	Damage
I	Firm (normal)	Slight stretching of the ligament with little, if any, tearing of the fibers. Pain is present, but the degree of stability roughly compares with that of the opposite extremity.
II	Soft	Partial tearing of the fibers. The joint line "opens up" significantly when compared with the opposite side.
III	Empty	Complete tearing of the ligament. The motion is restricted by other joint structures, such as tendons.

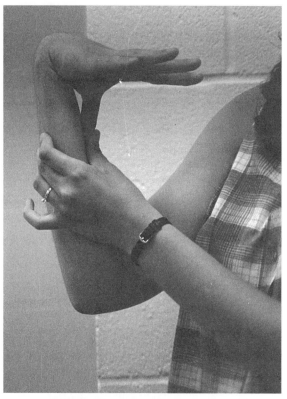

Figure 1–5. Determining systemic laxity. Some athletes may be naturally lax in all of their joints. A simple test to determine laxity is to have the athlete try to pull the thumb to the forearm. If this can be accomplished, it may be assumed that all of the athlete's joints are lax.

joint, or body part. Care must be taken to perform the test precisely as described to properly stress the involved tissue. As with all tests, a bilateral comparison must be performed. Examples of special tests are the impingement test in the shoulder or Lachman's test for laxity of the anterior cruciate ligament.

Neurological Testing

Neurological testing of the athlete involves an ***upper and lower quarter screen*** of sensation, motor function, and ***deep tendon reflexes***. Proper neurological testing is of vital importance in the clinical evaluation of the athlete suffering from nerve root impingement or peripheral nerve damage. Any true neurological signs in the spine-injured athlete must be determined so that proper management techniques may be performed.

Upper and lower quarter screens: Assessments of the neurological status of the peripheral nervous system of the upper and lower extremities, respectively, through the evaluation of sensation, motor function, and deep tendon reflexes.

Deep tendon reflex: An involuntary muscle contraction caused by a reflex arc in the spinal cord, initiated by the stretching of receptors within a tendon.

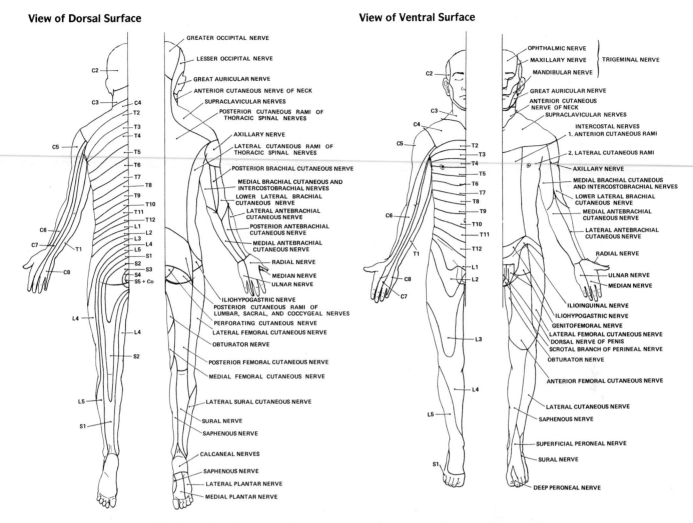

View of Dorsal Surface

Cutaneous innervation of the back of the body. Dermatomes are on the left, and peripheral nerves are on the right.

View of Ventral Surface

Cutaneous innervation of the front of the body. Dermatomes are on the left, and peripheral nerves are on the right.

Figure 1–6. The body's dermatomes. These charts describe the area of skin receiving sensory input from each of the nerve roots. Note that there are many different dermatome references, thus explaining the inconsistencies from text to text. (From Rothstein, JM, Roy, SH, and Wolf, SL,[1b] pp 208–209, with permission.)

Sensory testing can usually be performed with a bilateral comparison of light touch discrimination. The clinician should attempt to maintain a light stroke within the central portion of the **dermatome** to avoid overlap (Fig. 1–6). The athlete's response indicating whether the stroke was felt to the same extent on each side is usually sufficient. Sensory tests using sharp and dull discrimination, hot and cold discrimination, and two-point discrimination are less frequently used in the athlete except in the case of peripheral nerve injury (Fig. 1–7).

Manual muscle tests are used to test the **motor neurons** that are innervating the upper and lower extremities. In the case of manual muscle testing to determine neurological involvement, it is valid to use manual muscle grades (see Table 1–6). Although all muscles tend to have overlap of innervation, some muscles are more commonly tested for each nerve root. Whichever muscles are chosen, the clinician should be consistent in the use of these muscles and should develop a standard pattern.

Sensation: The ability of the athlete to perceive sensory stimuli such as touch discrimination or temperature.

Dermatome: An area of skin innervated by a single nerve root.

Motor neurons: Those neurons that send signals from the central nervous system to the muscular system.

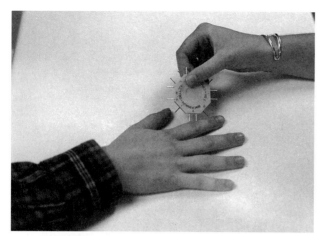

Figure 1–7. Two-point discrimination test. This evaluative procedure is used to determine the degree of sensory loss. A negative test results in the athlete's feeling both points touching the skin; a positive result is the athlete's feeling only one.

Deep tendon reflexes (DTR) provide further information as to the integrity of the nerve roots emanating from the cervical and lumbar spine. One limitation of testing the deep tendon reflexes is that not all nerve roots have a DTR. In the athlete it is suitable to test DTRs on a three-point scale: 0 = no response, 1 = weakened response, 2 = normal response. The DTR should always be compared with this scale and assessed bilaterally. If an athlete has a diminished response for a specific DTR and further testing demonstrates that all DTRs are diminished, this may be normal for this particular athlete. Appendix A describes the reflex tests commonly used in the evaluation of athletic injuries. Increased response to a reflex test is indicative of an **upper motor neuron lesion,** whereas decreased responses could signify a **lower motor neuron lesion.**

Neurological testing is not required for all injuries. During the clinical evaluation of orthopedic injuries, neurological examination is indicated when the athlete complains of numbness or **paresthesia** or suffers from unexplained muscular weakness.

Sport-Specific Functional Testing

For the last 25 years clinicians dealing with athletes have been researching and using devices such as the **isokinetic dynamometer** to help determine the rehabilitating athlete's readiness to return to full activity (Fig. 1–8). Although methods such as isoki-

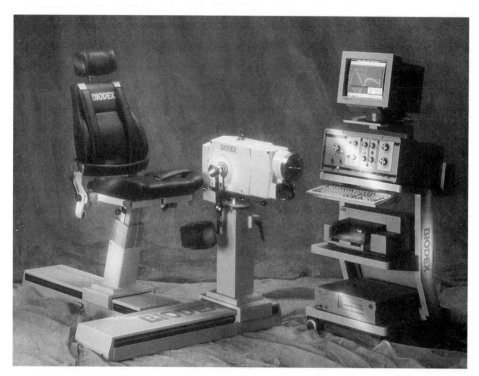

Figure 1–8. Isokinetic dynamometer used in determining muscular strength, power, and endurance. (Courtesy of the Biodex Medical Systems, Inc, Shirley, NY.)

Upper motor neuron lesion: A spinal cord lesion that results in paralysis, loss of voluntary movement, spasticity, sensory loss, and pathological reflexes.

Lower motor neuron lesion: A spinal cord lesion resulting in decreased reflexes, flaccid paralysis, and atrophy.

Paresthesia: The sensation of numbness or tingling, often described as a "pins and needles" sensation, caused by peripheral nerve lesions.

Isokinetic dynamometer: A device that quantitatively measures muscular strength through a preset speed of movement.

netic testing are still valuable, the clinician must have a working knowledge of the functional sport-specific demands of the athlete. As the body of knowledge on *proprioceptive* and objective functional tests increases, the clinician dealing with the athlete must stay abreast of these developments.

ON-FIELD EVALUATION

On-field injuries may be divided into two categories: ambulatory and athlete-down. Because ambulatory conditions are marked by the athlete's coming to the clinician to be evaluated, there is little difference between ambulatory evaluation and clinical evaluation. Athlete-down conditions are signified by the athletic trainer's responding to the athlete and the situation.

In order of their importance, the on-field evaluation must rule out:

• Inhibition of the cardiovascular and respiratory systems

• Life-threatening trauma to the head or spinal column

• Profuse bleeding

• Fractures

• Joint dislocations

• Other soft tissue trauma

Based on the findings of this triage, the athletic trainer must determine the immediate *disposition* of the condition. This includes the on-field management of the injury, the safest method of removing the athlete from the field, and the urgency of referring the athlete to a physician for further medical care.

On-field evaluations are best performed with two responders. In cases of head or spine trauma, one responder is responsible for stabilizing the spine while the other performs the needed tests. For non-catastrophic conditions, one responder conducts the on-field evaluation while the other responder calms and communicates with the athlete (Fig. 1–9).

When one athletic trainer is responsible for the on-field evaluation of an injury, a clear communication and evaluation protocol must be established (Fig. 1–10). In all instances, the coaching staff and other personnel must receive regular CPR training and be prepared to lend assistance in the event of a *catas-trophic injury*.

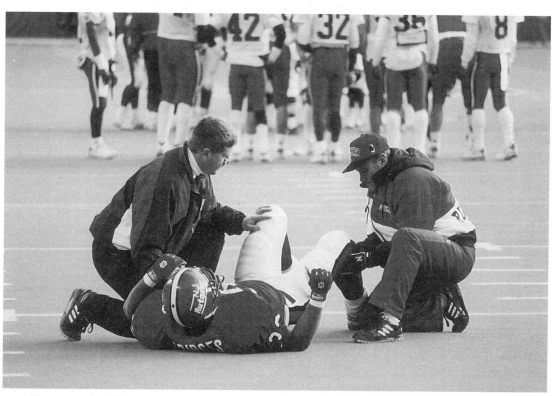

Figure 1–9. On-field evaluation performed by two responders. One responder calms and communicates with the athlete while the second performs the tests. This method is considered to be the optimal method for handling on-field injuries, especially in emergency situations.

Proprioception: The athlete's ability to sense the position of one or more joints.
Disposition: The immediate and long-term management of an injury or illness.
Catastrophic injury: An injury that causes permanent disability or death.

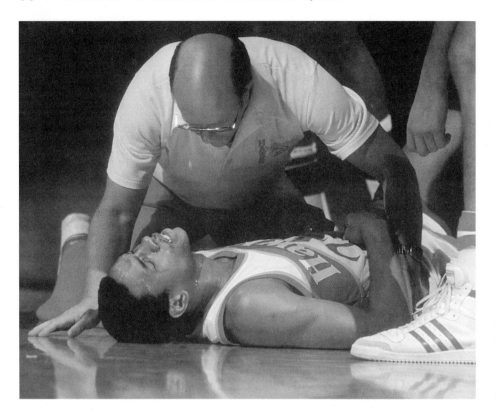

Figure 1-10. One examiner responding to an on-field injury. This method requires that the individual perform the evaluation, communicate with the athlete, and, if necessary, summon emergency personnel.

A communication plan must be established for game-day on-field injuries. The use of pre-established hand signals or walkie-talkies allows the individuals conducting the on-field evaluation to communicate with the sideline. In this manner the need for emergency equipment, special response equipment, the team physician, other emergency personnel, and transport squad can be quickly relayed.

Each sport at each level of competition has rules governing the on-field evaluation of athletic injuries during sanctioned competition. In most cases, the official must summon assistance onto the field or court and in some cases, such as wrestling, the evaluation must be completed and the disposition of the athlete determined in a limited period of time; otherwise, the athlete is disqualified from competition. It is the responsibility of the medical staff to be familiar with the pertinent rules governing the administration of medical assistance. Before each contest the athletic trainer should meet with the head official and clarify these points. It is also necessary to discuss procedures with on-site emergency personnel to facilitate communication if a need arises.

On-Field History

The injury history can be obtained from the athlete as well as from bystanders who witnessed the injury. However, if the athlete is unconscious, it is extremely important to obtain as much information as possible from those who witnessed the episode.

The history portion of the on-field evaluation is relatively brief as compared with the clinical evaluation. The primary information to be gained includes:

- **Location of the pain:** The site of pain should be identified as closely as possible. Although the athlete may be holding an area, one should not assume that this is the only site of trauma, as more than one body areas may be injured.

- **Mechanism of the injury:** The athlete should be asked about the force that caused the injury (e.g., contact-related injuries or tearing of the tissues while running, jumping, or throwing).

- **Associated sounds and symptoms:** A "snap" or "pop" at the time of injury may indicate a tearing of ligaments or tendons or may be related to the fracture of a bone.

In cases when the injury is apparent, such as an obvious fracture or dislocation, the history of the injury may become irrelevant. The responder should then rule out head or spinal trauma, attempt to calm the athlete, rule out injury to other body areas while initiating appropriate management of the condition, and, if appropriate, treat the athlete for shock.

On-Field Inspection

In an athlete-down situation, the observation process begins as soon as the individual is in the responder's sight. Therefore, much of this process occurs before history-taking. During this time the following should be observed:

- **Is the athlete moving?** An athlete moving, holding the injured body part, or writhing in pain indicates consciousness, an intact central nervous system (CNS), and cardiovascular function. Far more critical are those athletes who show no signs of movement or are seizing, indicating possible CNS trauma. Unconscious athletes should not be moved unless cardiopulmonary resuscitation is to be started, the athlete is to be transported to the hospital via an emergency squad, or the athlete regains consciousness (see Chapter 16).

- **What is the position of the athlete?** Is the athlete prone, supine, or side-lying? Is a body part in an awkward position? Is any gross deformity evident? These factors take on added importance if the athlete is unconscious and must be moved to begin cardiopulmonary resuscitation.

- **Is the athlete conscious?** If the athlete is not moving when the responder arrives at the scene, the level of consciousness must be determined. This is most easily accomplished by speaking to the athlete and attempting to gain some type of verbal feedback or gesture.

- **Primary survey:** If the athlete is unconscious, the inspection process takes the form of a primary survey. This employs the ABC technique of checking for an open **A**irway, checking for **B**reathing, and checking for **C**irculation.

- **Inspection of the injured area:** This process is an abbreviated version of the steps presented during the clinical evaluation section. Here, the primary task is to observe for:
  - Signs of fractures
  - Joint alignment
  - Swelling
  - Discoloration

- **Secondary survey:** The responder should observe the athlete and note the presence of any bleeding, gross deformity, or other signs of trauma to other parts of the body.

Inspecting the injured body part is a method of determining injury by comparing one side with the opposite side. Many times, simply looking at the injured site provides enough information to obtain a correct evaluation (e.g., a dislocated finger). The clinician should compare and contrast the findings of the inspection and history phases of the examination and be prepared to correlate these findings throughout the remainder of the evaluation.

On-Field Palpation

During the assessment of the injured athlete on the field, palpation is performed after a quick but thorough inspection, allowing the evaluation to focus on specific areas and triage the athlete's injuries. Often it must be decided immediately whether to move the athlete at all, to move the athlete using special care such as with a spine board or stretcher, or to move the athlete only after further assessment. Palpation helps to focus the evaluation at a time when it may not be appropriate to undertake all possible assessment tools.

The following should be determined during on-field palpation:

- Palpation of the bony structures
  - **Bony alignment:** The length of the injured bone is palpated to identify any discontinuity. Although fractures of large bones (e.g., femur, humerus) are often accompanied by gross deformity, those of smaller bones may present no outward signs.
  - **Crepitus:** *Crepitus* is associated with fractures, swelling, or inflammation.
  - **Joint alignment:** If the injury involves a joint, the clinician should palpate along the joint line to determine whether the joint is assuming its normal alignment.
- Palpation of the soft tissues
  - **Swelling:** Swelling immediately after the injury is often associated with a major disruption of the tissues. The exception to this is trauma to bursae, which tend to swell disproportionately to the severity of the injury.
  - **Hypersensitive areas:** One should note areas that, when palpated, result in pain, indicating trauma to underlying tissue.
  - **Deficit in the muscles or tendons:** Severe tearing of a muscle or tendon can result in a palpable defect.

On-Field Functional Testing

While evaluating acute injuries, functional testing should identify the athlete's ability and willingness to move the involved extremity. If the athlete's injury involves the lower extremity, functional testing should be expanded to include the body part's ability to bear weight. On-field functional testing should not be performed in the presence of a suspected fracture, dislocation, and/or muscle or tendon rupture.

Crepitus: Repeated crackling sensations or sound emanating from a joint or tissue.

• Active range of motion: The athlete is asked to move the limb through the range of motion, while the quality and quantity of movement are noted.

• Passive range of motion: This is used to determine the degree of muscular damage by placing the muscle on stretch.

• Resisted range of motion: Break pressure is used to determine the involved muscles' ability to sustain a forceful contraction.

• Weight-bearing status (lower extremity injuries): If the athlete is able to complete the active, passive, and resisted range of motion tests, he or she can be permitted to walk off the field, with assistance if necessary. If the athlete is unable to perform these tests or signs and symptoms of a potential fracture or dislocation exist, the athlete should be removed from the field in a non–weight-bearing manner.

On-Field Ligamentous Testing

The purpose of on-field ligamentous tests is to gain an immediate impression of the integrity of the ligaments involved in the injury before muscle guarding or swelling masks the degree of instability. Often, on-field ligamentous tests involve only the single-plane tests, which are then compared with the opposite side.

On-Field Neurological Testing

Neurological testing becomes particularly important in the on-field evaluation of the head-injured and/or spine-injured athlete. A thorough evaluation of the spine-injured athlete can ensure the proper management of this potentially catastrophic injury. When responding to acute on-field neurological injuries, a strong background in the tests for cranial nerve and cervical nerve root involvement as well as Babinski's test for upper motor neuron lesions are needed. These tests are described in Chapters 9 and 16.

Following the dislocation of a major joint or the fracture of a large bone, the integrity of the distal *neurovascular* structures must be determined. Bony displacement may impinge on or lacerate the nerves, arteries, and veins supplying the distal portion of the extremity. The specific processes for

identifying these deficits are described in the appropriate chapters of this text.

Removing the Athlete from the Field

A decision must be made regarding how and when to remove the athlete from the playing area and how to do so in the safest manner possible. If a fracture, dislocation, gross joint instability, or other significant musculoskeletal trauma is suspected, the involved body part must be splinted so that the injured area, and the joints proximal and distal to it, are immobilized (Fig. 1–11).

Several methods may be used to assist the athlete from the field (Fig. 1–12). The type of extraction method should be commensurate with the severity and type of injury being managed. With most upper extremity injuries, the body part may be immobilized and the athlete then walked off the field. With cases of lower extremity injuries, in which the athlete is unable to bear weight or upright posturing is contraindicated, several types of stretchers may be used. Injury to the spine requires the use of a spine board and cervical collar.

TERMINATION OF THE EVALUATION

During an evaluation a clinical finding may be so profound that no other information need be collected; management procedures are implemented and the athlete is immediately referred to an appropriate medical facility. Such findings include but are not limited to obvious fractures or dislocations, gross joint instability, and neurovascular deficits (Table 1–9). The clinician's discretion must be used on a case-by-case basis to determine when to terminate the evaluation and refer the athlete to a physician. It is always best to err on the side of caution.

UNIVERSAL PRECAUTIONS AGAINST BLOODBORNE PATHOGENS

Blood, synovial fluid, saliva, and other bodily fluids can potentially transmit bloodborne pathogens such as the *hepatitis B virus (HBV)* and the *human immunodeficiency virus (HIV)*.[3] All bodily fluids,

---

Neurovascular: Pertaining to a bundle formed by nerves, arteries, and veins.

Hepatitis B virus (HBV): A virus resulting in inflammation of the liver. Following a 2- to 6-week incubation period symptoms develop, including gastrointestinal and respiratory disturbances, jaundice, enlarged liver, muscle pain, and weight loss.

Human immunodeficiency virus (HIV): The virus that causes acquired immune deficiency syndrome (AIDS).

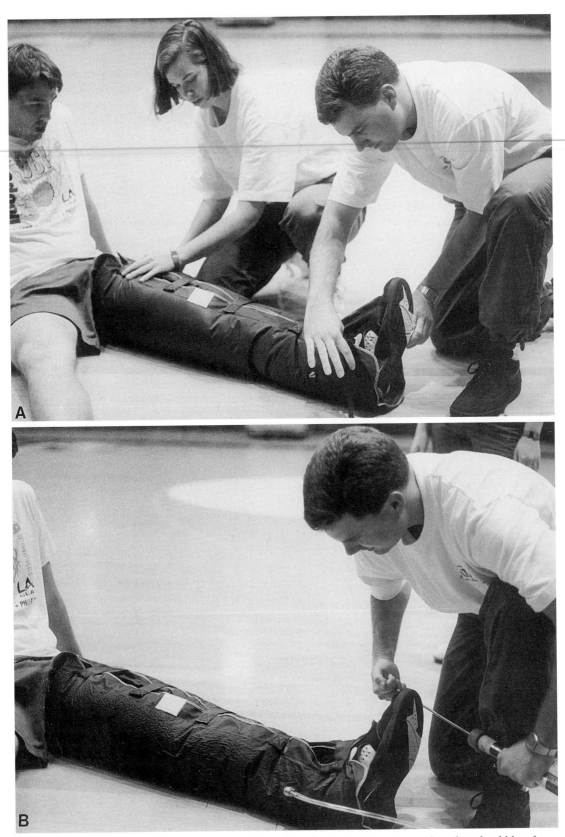

Figure 1–11 (*A* and *B*). Use of a vacuum splint to immobilize the injured area. The splint should be of sufficient size to immobilize the joints proximal and distal to the injured area.

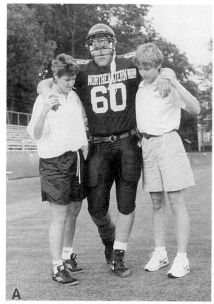

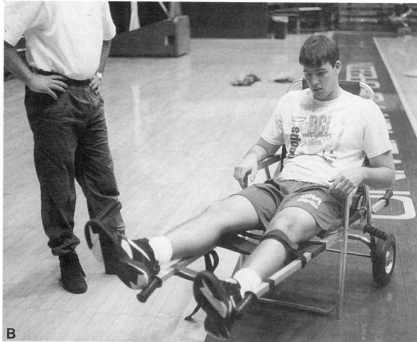

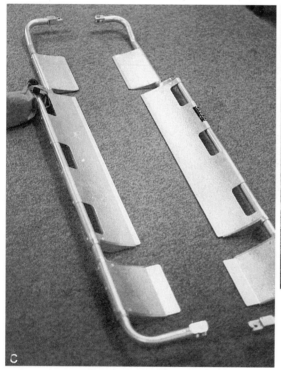

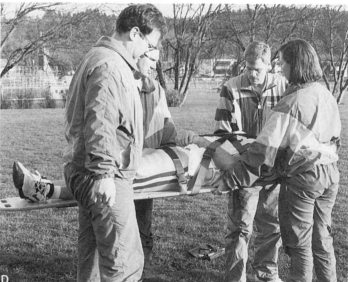

Figure 1–12. Various athlete extraction techniques: (*A*) assisted walking, (*B*) pull cart, (*C*) scoop stretcher, (*D*) full spine board.

with the exception of perspiration, must be treated as though they contain these viruses. The treatment of acute injuries and postsurgical wounds, along with the handling of mouthpieces and soiled dressings and instruments, must all be managed with caution (Fig. 1–13).

The use of **universal precautions against blood-borne pathogens** serves to reduce the possibility of accidental exposure to these pathogens (Table 1–10). These methods of protecting against accidental exposure include using *biohazard* disposal containers and washing soiled towels, uniforms,

---

Biohazard: A substance that is toxic to humans, animals, or the environment.

Table 1–9. Conditions Warranting Evaluation Termination and Physician Referral

Segment	Findings to Warrant Immediate Physician Referral
History	
Inspection	• Obvious fracture • Obvious joint dislocation
Palpation	• Disruption in the contour of bone, indicating a fracture or joint dislocation • Gross joint instability • Malalignment of joint structures
Functional tests	• Gross joint instability • Neurological dysfunction • Third-degree muscle tears
Special tests	• Gross joint instability • Ñeurological dysfunction

and other material separately, using the appropriate guidelines. Each institution must conduct an annual in-service defining the steps used in protecting employees from exposure to bloodborne pathogens.

THE ROLES OF DIFFERENT HEALTH CARE PROFESSIONALS

An athlete may become involved with health care providers who assume various roles in the evaluation, treatment, and rehabilitation of an injury. Such cooperation between health care professionals and a synthesis of their different areas of expertise have been thought to best benefit the injured athlete. The goal of providing a comprehensive team approach to the rehabilitation of athletes led to the formation of the first *sports medicine* centers in the United States. Approximately a quarter century later there is proof that the team approach is effective, as athletes return to sports after suffering what were once considered debilitating injuries.

As with the players on an athletic team, many areas of knowledge and skills overlap with others on the athletic health care team. It is essential that roles and duties be established before the first injury is sustained in a season. Members of the health care team must be aware of their position and must be willing to relinquish control and refer the athlete whenever necessary. Four key players on the health care team that may become involved in the evaluation of the injured athlete are the athletic trainer, physical therapist, emergency medical technician, and physician. The following is a description of the possible roles that the team members may play.

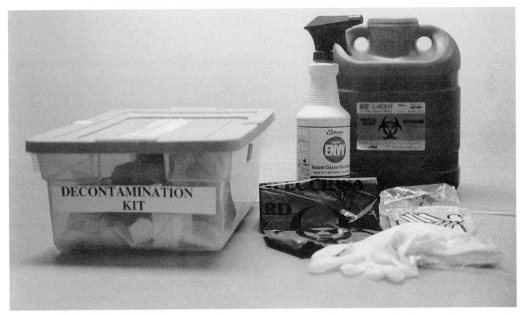

Figure 1–13. Use of universal precautions in the management of open wounds. Appropriate personal safeguards include the use of rubber gloves to protect the hands from blood, a disinfectant to clean up blood, and proper methods of disposing of soiled dressings and instruments.

Sports medicine: The application of medical and scientific knowledge to the prevention (including training methods and practices), care, and rehabilitation of injuries suffered by individuals participating in athletics.

Table 1–10. Universal Precautions
Against Bloodborne Pathogens

Skin and mucous membranes should be protected against blood and other fluids through the use of a barrier membrane, such as rubber gloves.

Skin coming into contact with a potential carrying agent should be washed immediately with soap and water.

Contaminated surfaces, such as tables and countertops, should be cleansed with a 1:10 mixture of household bleach and water.

All used needles, scalpels, and so on should be disposed of in a proper manner using a biohazard container.

Staff members who have open, draining sores or skin lesions should refrain from direct patient care until the condition clears.

Soiled linen or uniforms should be bagged and washed separately from other items in hot water and detergent.

Adapted from Bloodborne pathogens.[3]

Each team must develop its own specific roles within the legal guidelines of its state and work cooperatively for care to be successful.

The Athletic Trainer

The certified athletic trainer has been educated in the domains of athletic training as established by the **Role Delineation** Study of the National Athletic Trainers' Association Board of Certification, Inc. (Table 1–11). The athletic trainer has the knowledge base to take the athlete from the time of initial injury through evaluation, treatment, rehabilitation, and on to full return to activity.

The athletic trainer is the logical selection for coordinator of the health care team when the injured athlete is a member of an organized institution (e.g., high school, college, or professional teams). Usually the athletic trainer is the only health care team member to be a full-time employee of the institution, placing the athletic trainer in a medical, legal, ethical, and fiscal position of responsibility for the health care of the athlete. This is a perceived benefit to the hiring of an athletic trainer as a full-time staff member versus contracting such services from a sports medicine clinic or hospital. Both the athlete and the organization benefit from the athletic trainer's being a full-time staff member whose duties and responsibilities are solely those of meeting the needs of the injured athlete.

Athletic trainers do not diagnose an athlete's condition. Rather, they perform a primary screen, or evaluation, of an athlete's condition and subsequently determine the disposition of the case. Athletic trainers are required by national certification standards and state licensure laws to work under the direction and supervision of a physician.

The Physical Therapist

The physical therapist can be a vital member of the evaluation and rehabilitation team of the injured athlete. The physical therapist has a broad base of evaluation skills for orthopedic and nonorthopedic injuries and illnesses. Certain physical therapists have refined their evaluation and rehabilitation skills specifically for athletic injuries through either continuing education or specialization and competence in sports physical therapy as established by the Sports Physical Therapy Section of the American Physical Therapy Association.

It is more common to find the physical therapist as a member of the athlete's health care team when the athlete is a recreational athlete or a member of an institution that does not employ a full-time athletic trainer. In these cases the physical therapist is vital to the overall rehabilitation process. Because of the lack of education in the emergency management of athletic injuries, the physical therapist should refrain from situations in which such duties are performed. In these situations it is prudent to defer to the athletic trainer or emergency medical technician.

The Emergency Medical Technician

The emergency medical technician (EMT) possesses many valuable skills to be offered as a member of the athletic health care team. The EMT is fully competent in the emergency management of injury and illness, but the type of care provided is dependent on the qualifications of the individual EMT (Table 1–12). The roles and responsibilities of the EMT squad should be determined and communicated before the start of each season. This planning process eliminates many questions that may arise during the most inopportune moments during the management of an acute injury.

One of the primary concerns in the transportation of injured athletes is that of equipment. Management of the athlete who wears equipment that may interfere with normal practices of emergency care must be established prior to the time of the injury. Many pieces of equipment, such as the football helmet and facemask, are designed to allow access to the athlete's face if needed. Guidelines such as the management of facemask and/or helmet as well as

---

Role delineation: The determination of the tasks and functions particular to a profession.

Table 1–11. Role Delineation Matrix of the Athletic Training Profession

Universal Competencies	Performance Domains				
	Prevention of Athletic Injuries	Recognition, Evaluation, and Immediate Care of Athletic Injuries	Rehabilitation and Reconditioning of Athletic Injuries	Health Care Administration	Professional Development and Responsibility
Domain-specific content		Knowledge and skills particular to each performance domain			
Athletic training evaluation	Determination of an athlete's readiness to participate	Identification of underlying trauma	Ongoing evaluation of an athlete's progress through various stages of rehabilitation	Documentation of injury status and rehabilitation	Remains up to date with current evaluation skills, techniques, and knowledge
Human anatomy	Normal anatomical structure and function	Recognition of signs and symptoms of athletic injury and illness	Normal anatomical structure and function		Remains up to date in current human anatomical research and trends
Human physiology	Normal physiological function	Recognition of signs and symptoms of athletic injury and illness	Stages of injury response		Remains up to date in current human physiology research and trends
Exercise physiology	Physiological demand and response to exercise	Recognition of systemic and local metabolic failure	Musculoskeletal and cardiovascular demands placed on the injured athlete		Remains up to date with current exercise physiology research and trends
Biomechanics	Normal biomechanical demands of exercise	Identification of pathomechanics	Resolution of pathomechanical motion		Remains up to date with current biomechanical research and trends
Psychology/counseling	Educational programs for the healthy and injured athlete (i.e., alcohol and other drug abuse, performance anxiety)	Recognition of the psychological signs and symptoms of athletic injury and illness	Psychological implications of injury	Communication with, and referral to, the appropriate health care provider	Continues to develop interpersonal and communication skills

continued

Table 1–11. Role Delineation Matrix of the Athletic Training Profession—*Continued*

Performance Domains

Universal Competencies	Prevention of Athletic Injuries	Recognition, Evaluation, and Immediate Care of Athletic Injuries	Rehabilitation and Reconditioning of Athletic Injuries	Health Care Administration	Professional Development and Responsibility
Nutrition	Nutritional demands of the athlete	Recognition of the effects of improper nutritional needs of the competing athlete (i.e., fluid replacement, diabetic shock)	Nutritional demands placed on the injured athlete	Referral to the appropriate health care provider	Remains up to date with current nutritional research
Pharmacology	Contraindications and side effects of prescription and nonprescription medications	The role of prescription and nonprescription medication in the immediate/emergency care of athletic injury and illness	The role of prescription and nonprescription medications in the stages of injury response	Proper maintenance and documentation of records for the administration of prescription and nonprescription medication	Remains up to date with current pharmacological research and trends
Physics	Absorption, dissipation, and transmission of energy of varying materials	The effect of stress loads on the human body (i.e., shear, tensile, compressive forces)	Physiological response to various energies imposed on the body		Remains up to date with current knowledge of physics as it relates to athletic training
Organization and administration	Legal requirements and rules of the sport	Planning, documentation, and communication of appropriate rehabilitation strategies to the necessary parties	Planning, documentation, and communication of appropriate rehabilitation strategies to the necessary parties	Development of operational policies and procedures	Remains up to date with current standards of professional practice

From The National Athletic Trainers' Association Board of Certification, Inc., with permission.

Table 1–12. Classification of Emergency Medical Technicians

Level	Skills
EMT-A	Trained for basic ambulance service
EMT-D	Trained for defibrillation
EMT-I	Trained for defibrillation, intravenous infusion administration, and endotracheal intubation
EMT-P	Paramedic; provides the highest level of prehospital care

Table 1–13. Medical Specialties

Specialty	Description
Family (primary care)	Provides comprehensive, continuing care that is not limited by the patient's age, gender, or particular body area
Internal medicine	Treats diseases to, and injuries of, the internal organs by means other than surgery
Gynecology	Specializes in the care and treatment of the female reproductive system
Ophthalmology	Specializes in the treatment of eye injuries and disorders
Orthopedics	Specializes in the treatment of the skeletal, articular, and muscular systems
Pediatrics	Specializes in the medical care of children
Radiology	Specializes in diagnosis of x rays and other imaging techniques
Resident	Member of the hospital staff who is gaining clinical training after an internship

any piece of equipment should be jointly established by the athletic trainer, EMTs, and team physicians before the start of the season rather than debating about it in the midst of a crisis situation.

The Physician

Ideally, a physician would be present at all athletic practices and games; in reality this seldom occurs, and recreational athletes are usually without the immediate services of a physician during competition. In either case it is essential that the injured athlete have access to a physician trained in the evaluation and care of athletic injuries or illnesses (Medical Doctor or Doctor of Osteopathy).[4]

One physician directs the athlete's health care team and is responsible for the overall medical care provided to the athlete. Historically this has been an orthopedic surgeon or general practitioner who is aided by specialists in internal medicine, dentistry, cardiology, psychology, and so on (Table 1–13).

Other health care team members must recognize when to refer an athlete to the physician, and the physician needs to understand the proper role of the other health care team members.

DOCUMENTATION

The findings of the initial and follow-up evaluations and any subsequent referrals must be documented in the athlete's medical record. In addition to their strong legal function, medical records have an important practical purpose. Through the use of clear, concise terminology and objective findings, the medical record can serve as a method of communicating the athlete's current medical disposition to all who read it.

The initial injury report serves as the baseline when planning an athlete's treatment and rehabilitation program. Through re-evaluating the athlete's condition and comparing it with the initial findings, the athlete's progress may be monitored and subsequent adjustments made in the rehabilitation plan.

REFERENCES

1. Benson, MT: 1994–1995 NCAA Sports Medicine Handbook, ed 7. The National Collegiate Athletic Association, Overland Park, KS, 1994.
1a. Norkin, CC, and White, DJ: Measurement of Joint Motion: A Guide to Goniometry, ed 2. FA Davis, Philadelphia, 1995, p 9.
1b. Rothstein, JM, Roy, SH, and Wolf, SL: The Rehabilitation Specialist's Handbook. FA Davis, Phildelphia, 1991.
2. Harter, RA, et al: A comparison of instrumented and manual Lachman test results in anterior cruciate ligament-reconstructed knees. Athletic Training: Journal of the National Athletic Trainers Association 25:330, 1990.
3. Bloodborne pathogens: Rules and regulations. Federal Register 56:64175, 1991.
4. Rich, BSE: "All physicians are not created equal." Understanding the education background of the sports medicine professional. Journal of Athletic Training 28:177, 1993.

2

Injury Nomenclature

Effective communication between members of the medical team is imperative and relies on the use of standardized terminology. Each member of the team must be able to accurately describe an athlete's condition and the examination findings. In turn, the receiver of this information must accurately interpret the structures involved and the type of damage that has occurred. Additionally, this information must be communicated in an understandable manner to the athlete, the athlete's parent(s), and the coaching staff.

Knowledge of the defining characteristics of injury classification is an extremely valuable tool for the clinician. During an evaluation, the characteristics of an injury allow the clinician to differentiate between injuries that seem similar. In some cases this distinction may be the deciding factor between causing harm and a successful treatment and rehabilitation outcome. For instance, the treatment of an athlete complaining of lower leg pain would be much different if the pain were caused by stress fractures than if it were caused by muscle strain.

SOFT TISSUE INJURY

Soft tissues are the most often injured tissues in athletics. Soft tissue injuries include trauma to the muscles and their tendons, skin, joint capsules, ligaments, and **bursae**. These injuries affect performance by hindering the motion at one or more joints, either by causing inability of a muscle to generate force or joint instability or by mechanically limiting the amount of motion available to the joint.

Musculotendinous Injuries

Injuries to a muscle belly or tendon adversely affect the muscle's ability to contract fully because of a mechanical insufficiency or because of pain. If the *musculotendinous unit* has been mechanically altered through partial or complete tears, the unit can no longer produce the forces required to perform simple movements or meet the demands required by athletic activity. Partial tears may create decreased force production secondary to pain elicited during the contraction. Complete tears of the unit results in the muscle's inability to produce any motion.

Strains

Strains are an indirect injury to muscles and tendons caused by excessive stretch or tension within the fibers.[1] **Tensile forces** are produced when the muscle is stretched beyond its normal range of motion, causing the fibers to tear. Muscle fibers can also be traumatized by **dynamic overload**, which occurs when the muscle generates more force than its fibers can withstand. The amount of tension produced during dynamic overload, as occurs during an *eccentric muscle contraction*, is an elongating force exerted distal to a muscle's attachment.

The grading of the severity of the strain is based on the number and extent of the fibers that have been traumatized and is usually graded on a three-degree scale.[2]

First-degree strains involve stretching and limited tearing of the fibers. Pain increases as the muscle contracts, especially against resistance, and the site of injury is point tender. Swelling may be present as well.

Second-degree strains involve the actual tearing of some of the muscle fibers and result in *ecchymosis*. These injuries present the same findings as a first-degree strain but are more severe.

Third-degree strains involve the complete rupture of the muscle, resulting in a complete loss of function and a palpable defect in the muscle. Pain, swelling, and ecchymosis are also present.

Bursa (pl. *bursae*): A fluid-filled sac that decreases friction between adjoining soft tissues or between soft tissue and bones.

Musculotendinous unit: The group formed by a muscle and its tendons.

Eccentric muscle contraction: A contraction in which the elongation of the muscle is voluntarily controlled. Lowering a weight is an example of an eccentric contraction.

Ecchymosis: A blue or purple area of skin caused by the movement of blood into the skin.

Muscle strains tend to occur at the junction between the muscle's belly and its tendon and most frequently involve the distal junction.[3-6] With first- and second-degree strains, there is local tenderness over the site of the injury; that is, pain is elicited when the muscle is either actively shortened or passively elongated. Resisted range of motion results in decreased muscular strength secondary to pain and/or the muscle's mechanical inability to produce force. In third-degree strains the muscle is incapable of producing force, and the athlete attempts to compensate through the use of other muscles and body position. No tension is felt with passive elongation and, after the initial pain has subsided, pain may be minimal to nonexistent.

Depending on the depth of the muscle relative to the skin, swelling and ecchymosis may be visible, but the force of gravity may cause these fluids to accumulate distal to the actual site of the injury (Fig. 2–1). The muscular defect is often palpable in second-degree strains and may be visible as well as palpable in third-degree strains.

Examination Segment	Clinical Findings of Muscle Strains	
History	Onset:	Acute.
	Location of pain:	Pain is located at the site of the injury, which tends to be at, or near, the junction between the muscle belly and tendon. The distal musculotendinous junction is most often involved, regardless of whether the muscle was strained from its proximal or distal end.
	Mechanism:	Strains usually result from a single episode of overstretching or overloading of the muscle but is more likely to result from eccentric loading.[7]
Inspection	Ecchymosis is evident in cases of severe muscle strains. Gravity causes the blood to pool distal to the site of trauma. Swelling may be present over the involved area. In severe cases, a defect may be visible in the muscle or tendon. If the strain involves a muscle of the lower extremity, the athlete may walk with a limp.	
Palpation	Point tenderness exists over the site of the injury, with the degree of pain increasing with the severity of the injury. A defect or spasm may be palpable at the injury site.	
Functional tests	AROM:	Pain is elicited at the injury site. In the case of second- or third-degree strains, the athlete may be unable to complete the movement.
	PROM:	Pain is elicited at the injury site during passive motion in the direction opposite that of the muscle, placing it on stretch.
	RROM:	Muscle strength is reduced. Pain increases as the amount of resistance is increased. Third-degree strains result in a loss of function.

Tendinitis

As indicated by the "-itis" suffix, tendinitis is inflammation of the muscle tendon. Although tendinitis may result from a single traumatic force, it most commonly arises from smaller repetitive forces, or **microtrauma,** being placed on the structure. This insult to the tendon activates an inflammatory process (Table 2–1). In chronic inflammation, the tendon thickens.

Tendinitis is used to describe the inflammation of the structures encased within the tendon's outer layering.[8] **Tenosynovitis,** an inflammation of the synovial sheath surrounding a tendon, tends to be more common in the hands and feet because of the relatively smaller size of the tendon. Over time adhesions can develop, causing restricted movement of the tendon within its sheath. Not all tendons are encased by a synovial sheath, however; some are encased by a peritendinous layering of thick tissue. Such inflammation is termed **peritendinitis.**[9]

The signs and symptoms of tenosynovitis are similar to those of tendinitis, except that the pain tends to be more localized and crepitus more pronounced. The clinical grading of tendinitis is based on when symptoms occur:

First-degree tendinitis is marked by pain and slight dysfunction during activity.
Second-degree tendinitis results in decreased function and pain after activity.
Third-degree tendinitis is characterized by constant pain that prohibits activity.

Prolonged tendinitis can result in tearing of the tendon's outer sheath, a **partial-thickness tear.** Most often occurring in the tendons of the glenohumeral joint, continued stress to the tendon can result in a **full-thickness tear.** Another potential complication of tendinitis with an extended duration is the development of calcium deposits within the tendon, **calcific tendinitis.** The calcium build-up within the

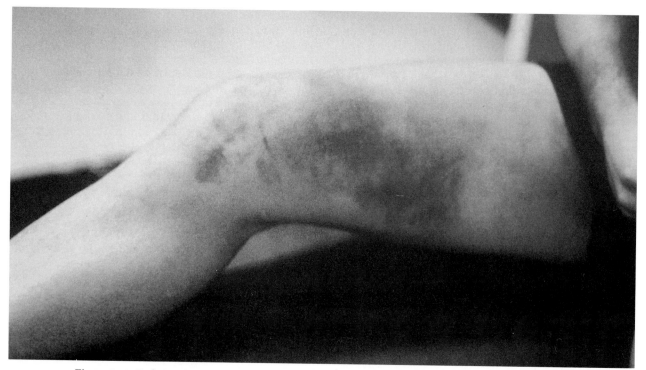

Figure 2–1. Ecchymosis associated with a muscular strain. Gravity causes blood that has seeped into the tissues to drift inferiorly.

Table 2–1. Mechanisms Leading to Tendinitis

Mechanism	Implications
Microtrauma	Repetitive tensile loading, compression, and abrasion of the working tendons. Insufficient rest periods allow for the accumulation of the microtrauma, possibly leading to tendon failure.
Macrotrauma	A single force is placed on the muscle, causing discrete tearing within the tendon or at the musculotendinous junction. This area becomes the weak link when the forces of otherwise normal walking or running are sufficient to cause further inflammation.
Biomechanical alteration	The alteration of otherwise normal motion redistributes the forces around a joint, resulting in new tensile loads, compressive forces, or abrasion of the tendons. Examples of this include running on uneven terrain or using improper sporting equipment such as a tennis racquet.

Adapted from Gross, MT,[8] 1992.

substance of the tendon causes pain with active contraction, as well as a decreased range of motion.

Active range of motion may produce pain at the end of the range of motion, especially if the tendon meets a bony structure. Passive motion in the muscle's **antagonistic** direction results in pain as the tendon is stretched. The dynamic tension produced during resisted range of motion testing results in pain, decreasing the amount of force produced (see top of page 27).

Myositis Ossificans

Myositis ossificans is the formation of bone within the belly of a muscle (Fig. 2–2). It is important to understand that myositis ossificans does not involve the muscle itself but, rather, the connective tissue of the **fascia** and its intramuscular extensions.[10] The **etiology** of myositis ossificans can be traced to the genetic formation of abnormal tissue (myositis ossificans progressiva), neurological disease, bloodborne disease (myositis ossificans circumscripta), or trauma (myositis ossificans traumatica). This text deals with myositis ossificans traumatica.

Antagonistic: In the opposite direction of movement (e.g., the antagonistic motion of extension is flexion).
Fascia: A fibrous membrane that supports and separates muscles and unites the skin with the underlying tissues.
Etiology: The cause of a disease (also the study of the causes of disease).

Examination Segment	Clinical Findings of Tendinitis		
History	Onset:	Location of pain:	Gradual or chronic. Pain exists throughout the tendon. Tendinitis results from microtraumatic forces applied to the tendon.
		Mechanism:	
Inspection	Swelling may be noted. If the inflammation involves a tendon of the lower extremity, the athlete may walk with a limp or demonstrate some other compensatory gait. Inflammation involving the upper extremity results in abnormal movement patterns. Many tendons are not directly visible or palpable.		
Palpation	The tendon is tender to the touch. Crepitus or thickening of the tendon may be noted.		
Functional tests	AROM:	Pain in the tendon is possible at the extremes of the range of motion as force is generated within the tendon.	
	PROM:	Pain is elicited during the extremes of the range of motion as the tendon is stretched. Pain can be elicited earlier in the ROM in more severe cases.	
	RROM:	Strength is decreased by pain. Pain is increased when the joint is isometrically stressed in its open-packed position.[8]	

In athletes, myositis ossificans occurs secondary to a traumatic injury such as a deep contusion or muscle strain and most commonly afflicts the quadriceps femoris, hip adductor group, or biceps brachii muscles. The formation of the ossified area can be traced to an error in the body's healing process.[11] Following the injury, fibroblasts begin to transform into ***osteoblasts*** and ***chondroblasts***, giving rise to the formation of immature bone.

Calcification appears on x-ray examination approximately 3 weeks after the injury. As the size of the mass continues to expand, it becomes palpable, and the joint's range of motion is affected as the bony mass impedes the muscle's ability to function.

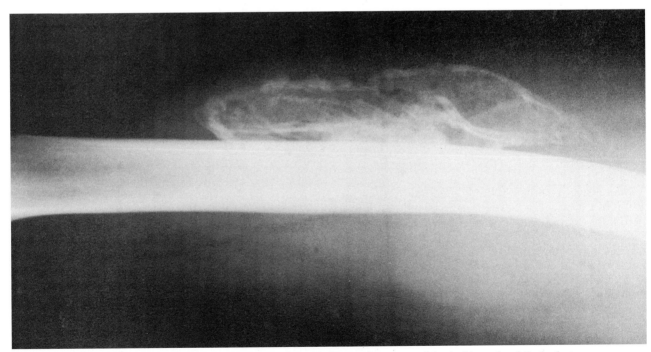

Figure 2–2. X ray of myositis ossificans. This calcification has occurred in the biceps brachii of a football lineman who sustained multiple blows to the muscle during the act of blocking.

Osteoblasts: Cells concerned with the formation of new bone.
Chondroblast: A cell that forms cartilage.

Examination Segment	Clinical Findings of Myositis Ossificans		
History	Onset:		The initial trauma is a **hematoma** caused by a single acute or repeated blows to the muscle. The ossification occurs gradually.
	Location of pain:		Pain occurs at the site of ossification, usually the site of a large muscle mass that is exposed to blows (e.g., the quadriceps femoris or biceps brachii muscles).
	Mechanism:		Myositis ossifications is caused by single or multiple direct blows to a single area.
Inspection	A superficial bruise may be noted. Effusion of the distal joint closest to the site injury occurs. Ecchymosis may be present.		
Palpation	Acutely, the muscle is tender. As the ossification develops, it may become palpable within the muscle mass. Swelling may be felt at the site of injury.		
Functional tests	AROM:		This is limited by pain. As the ossification grows, the number of contractile units available to the muscle decreases. Antagonist motion is painful secondary to decreased flexibility.
	PROM:		This is decreased secondary to pain and adhesions within the muscle.
	RROM:		This is decreased secondary to pain. The ossification does not allow the muscle to contract normally.
Special tests	X-ray examination shows the ossification as it matures. A bone scan may be positive in the earlier stages.		

Bursitis

Bursae are fluid-filled sacs that serve to buffer muscles, tendons, and ligaments from other friction-causing structures and to facilitate smooth motion. Although there are common sites of bursa formation, such as over the patella and olecranon process, these structures spontaneously develop over areas in which they are needed. Normally, bursae cannot be specifically palpated unless they are inflamed. The triggering event causing bursitis is the irritation of the bursal sac secondary to a disease state, increased stress, friction, or a single traumatic force that activates the inflammatory process.

The clinical findings of bursitis depend on the location of the involved structure. Bursae that are immediately subcutaneous can enlarge to enormous sizes, but the swelling remains localized within the sac, and often the joint can be moved in a relatively pain-free manner. Bursae separating tendinous, bony, and/or ligamentous tissues often cause exquisite pain during all forms of joint movements, which may limit the degree of motion available to the joint.

Bursal inflammation can also be the result of local or systemic infection. Lacerations, abrasions, or puncture wounds entering a bursa can introduce an infectious agent, resulting in the subsequent enlargement of the bursa. A **staphylococcal infection** can localize within a bursa, producing symptoms resembling an overuse syndrome. Often, bursal infections are accompanied by red streaks along the extremity and enlarged proximal **lymph nodes**. An analysis of the bursal fluid is required to determine the etiology of the bursitis[12] (see top of page 29).

Injury to the Joint Structures

Although soft tissue injuries are the most common injuries found in athletes, the most prevalent of these are injuries to the capsular and ligamentous tissues, with the ligaments of the ankle being the most frequently involved.[13,14] Ligamentous injury to the knee, elbow, and shoulder are also quite prevalent. These injuries directly affect the ability of the joint to function in a stable manner during movement.

Hematoma: A collection of clotted blood within a confined space (*hemat,* blood; *oma* tumor).
Staphylococcal infection: An infection caused by the *Staphylococcus* bacteria.
Lymph nodes: Nodules located in the cervical, axillary, and inguinal regions, producing white blood cells and filtering bacteria from the bloodstream. Lymph nodes become enlarged secondary to an infection.

Examination Segment	Clinical Findings of Bursitis	
History	Onset:	Acute in the case of direct trauma to the bursa; insidious in the case of overuse or infection.
	Location of pain:	Pain occurs at the site of the bursal sac.
	Mechanism:	Acute: A direct blow to the bursa, causing its rupture or active inflammatory process.
		Overuse: Repetitive rubbing of the soft tissue over a bony prominence; may be related to improper biomechanics.
		Infection: Viral or bacterial invasion of the bursa.
Inspection	Local swelling of bursae can be very pronounced, especially those located over the olecranon process and patella.	
Palpation	Point tenderness is noted over the site of the bursa. Localized heat and swelling may be noted.	
Functional tests	AROM:	Pain may be noted.
	PROM:	Pain is produced if the motion causes the tendon or other structure to rub across the inflamed bursa.
	RROM:	This is limited by pain. As the muscle contracts it compresses the bursal sac.

Sprains

Sprains occur when a joint is stretched beyond its normal anatomical limits, resulting in the stretching or tearing of the ligaments and/or joint capsule. Although ligaments are commonly thought of and presented as discrete structures, they are often simply thickened areas within the joint capsule. When torn, those ligaments that are continuous with the joint capsule produce more swelling because of the associated disruption of the capsule than those ligaments that are *extracapsular*.

The three degrees of sprains are based on the amount of laxity produced by the injury relative to the opposite limb (see also Table 1–8):

First-degree sprain: The ligament is stretched with little or no tearing of its fibers. No abnormal motion is produced when the joint is stressed, and a firm *end-point* is felt. There is local pain, mild point tenderness, and slight swelling of the joint.

Second-degree sprain: Partial tearing of the ligament's fibers has occurred, resulting in joint laxity when the ligament is stressed, but a definite end-point is present. Moderate pain and swelling occur and a loss of the joint's function is noted.

Third-degree sprain: The ligament has been completely ruptured, causing gross joint instability and an empty or absent end-point. Swelling is marked, but pain may be limited secondary to tearing of the local nerves. A complete loss of function of the joint is usually noted (see top of page 30).

Joint Subluxation

A subluxation involves the partial or complete disassociation of the joint's articulating surfaces, which may or may not spontaneously return to their normal alignments. The amount of force required to displace the bones is often sufficient to cause soft tissue or bony injury. Tearing of the joint capsule and/or ligaments, as well as bony fractures, must be suspected following a reported subluxation.

Subluxating joints are a progressive condition, in which each subluxation predisposes the joint to subsequent episodes by stretching the supporting structures. All first-time subluxations must be evaluated by a physician, who must clearly indicate how subsequent subluxations of the joint should be managed.

Clinically, joint subluxations are determined by the athlete's describing a history of the "joint went out and then popped back in." The joint's range of motion is limited by pain and instability. Chronically, the joint displays instability during ligamentous and capsular testing. In each case these tests may produce an **apprehension response**, meaning that the athlete displays anxiety that a specific test will cause the joint to again subluxate (see bottom of page 30).

Joint Dislocation

Dislocations involve the complete disassociation of the joint's articulating surfaces. The forces causing the dislocation are usually sufficient to rupture many of the joint's soft tissue constraints. Joint

---

Extracapsular: Outside of the joint capsule.
End-point: The quality and quantity of a ligament's ability to limit movement.

Examination Segment	Clinical Findings of Ligament Sprains		
History	Onset: Location of pain: Mechanism:	Acute. Pain is localized to the site of injury with first-degree sprains. As the severity of the sprain increases, the pain is radiated throughout the joint. A "popping" sensation or sound may be reported by the athlete. Sprains result from tensile forces caused by the stretching of the ligament.	
Inspection	Swelling of the joint is evident. Ecchymosis will form at, and distal to, the site of injury.		
Palpation	Point tenderness is noted over the ligament. The entire joint may be tender.		
Functional tests	AROM: PROM: RROM:	This is limited by pain in the direction that stresses the involved ligament(s). This is limited by pain, especially in the direction that stresses the involved ligament(s). Manual resistance throughout the range of motion is painful. Isometric contractions may not produce as intense pain.	
Ligamentous tests	The ligament can be stressed by producing a force through the joint that causes the ligament to stretch. The examiner should note the amount of increased laxity as compared with the opposite side, as well as the quality of the end-point. The end-point should be distinct and crisp. A soft, "mushy," or absent end-point is a sign of ligamentous rupture.		
Special tests	These are determined by the particular joint being examined.		

dislocations result in obvious deformity and therefore normally do not require any evaluative tests (Fig. 2–3). In some instances the dislocation may cause the joint surfaces to protrude through the skin, especially when the fingers are involved (Fig. 2–4).

Because of the inherent risk of injury to bony, vascular, neurological, or other soft tissue structures, reduction of the dislocation should not be attempted prior to an x-ray examination, and the reduction procedure should be performed only by a physician. When a major joint (e.g., shoulder, knee,

Examination Segment	Clinical Findings of Joint Subluxations		
History	Onset: Location of pain: Mechanism:	Acute. Chronic subluxation can occur as the joint's supportive structures are progressively stretched. Pain occurs throughout the involved joint. Associated muscle spasm may involve the muscles proximal and distal to the joint. Joint subluxation results from a stress that takes the joint beyond its normal anatomical limits.	
Inspection	Swelling is usually present. No gross deformity is noted because the joint relocates.		
Palpation	Pain along the tissues that have been stretched or compressed.		
Functional tests	AROM: PROM: RROM:	This is limited owing to pain and possible instability. This is limited owing to pain and possible instability. Muscular strength is decreased secondary to pain and joint instability.	
Ligamentous tests	Pain is elicited during stress testing of the involved ligament(s). Laxity of the tissues is present, particularly postacutely. The athlete may note instability and react to guard against this by contracting the surrounding musculature or pulling away, an apprehension response.		
Special tests	These vary according to the body part being tested.		

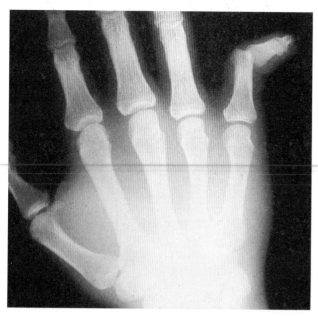

Figure 2–3. X ray of a dislocation of the fifth proximal interphalangeal joint (PIP joint).

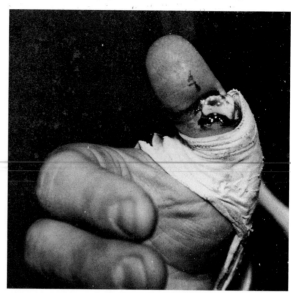

Figure 2–4. Open dislocation of the thumb's interphalangeal joint. Note the glossy appearance of the proximal articular surface. There appears to be a defect of the hyaline cartilage on the ulnar side of the bone.

ankle) is dislocated, the presence of the distal pulse and the normal sensory distribution of the involved extremity must be established. Dislocations of these joints are inherently considered medical emergencies, and the possible involvement of the neurovascular structures increases the urgency for prompt medical treatment.

Synovitis

The inflammation of a joint's capsule often occurs secondary to the presence of existing inflammation in or around the joint that spreads to the **synovial membrane** (Fig. 2–5). The athlete complains of "bogginess" within the joint and tends to hold it in

Examination Segment	Clinical Findings of Joint Subluxations		
History	Onset:		Acute. Chronic dislocation can occur as the joint's supportive structures are progressively stretched.
	Location of pain:		At the involved joint.
	Mechanism:		Dislocation is caused by a stress that takes the joint beyond its normal anatomical limits.
Inspection	Gross joint deformity may be present and swelling is observed.		
Palpation	Pain is elicited throughout the joint.		
Functional tests	Range of motion is not possible because of the disruption of the joint's alignment.		
Ligamentous tests	These are contraindicated at this time.		
Neurological tests	Sensory distribution distal to the dislocated joint should be established.		
Special tests	Except for checking neurovascular injury, these are contraindicated at this time.		
Comments	Dislocations of the major joints represent a medical emergency. The presence of the distal pulse must be established. A lack of circulation to the distal extremity threatens the viability of the body part.		

Synovial membrane: The membrane lining a fluid-filled joint.

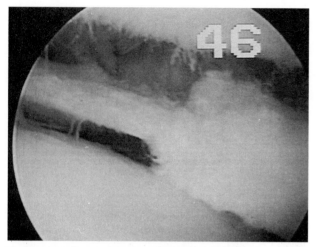

Figure 2–5. Illustration of synovitis of the knee joint capsule. The hairlike strands emerging from the top border of the joint represent inflammation of the synovial capsule.

a position that applies the least amount of stress on the capsule's fibers (usually a position between the extremes of the joint's range of motion). The remaining signs and symptoms of synovitis are similar to those of bursitis, but the swelling is more diffuse and less localized.

Articular Surface Injuries

The **hyaline cartilage** lining a bone's articular surface is commonly injured acutely in young athletes and may be damaged as the result of degenerative changes in older athletes. Most of these injuries are irreversible and result in chronic joint pain and/or dysfunction.

Osteochondral Defects

Fractures of a bone's articular cartilage and the progressive softening of this cartilage are collec-

Examination Segment	Clinical Findings of Capsular Synovitis		
History	Onset:		Insidious; often subsequent to a previous injury to the joint.
	Location of pain:		Pain occurs throughout the entire joint, causing aching at rest and with activity.
	Mechanism:		The synovial lining becomes inflamed, often following an injury to the joint. The resulting inflammatory reaction triggers inflammation within the synovium.
Inspection	The joint may appear swollen. The athlete may move the joint in a guarded manner.		
Palpation	Warmth may be felt. A boggy swelling is present. No distinct area of point tenderness is usually present.		
Functional tests	AROM:	Limitations exist within the **capsular pattern** of the joint.	
	PROM:	Normally, this is greater than active range of motion but is still limited by pain.	
	RROM:	Weakness is present owing to muscular contraction.	
Ligamentous tests	In the absence of underlying **pathology** to the ligaments, the ligamentous test result is negative. Pain may be elicited by stretching the inflamed tissues.		
Special tests	Same findings are produced as for ligamentous testing.		
Comments	The signs and symptoms of synovitis may mimic those of an infected joint. A history of overuse or closed trauma to the involved joint is needed to identify synovitis.		

Hyaline cartilage: Cartilage found on the articular surface of bones. It is especially suited to withstand compressive and shearing forces.

Capsular pattern: A line of decreased motion associated with injury of joint's capsular tissue. Capsular patterns are specific to each joint.

Pathology: A condition produced by an injury or disease.

tively referred to as osteochondral defects (OCDs). The severity of an OCD is based on its depth. Partial-thickness OCDs involve the outer layering of the articular cartilage, whereas full-thickness OCDs expose the underlying bone (Fig. 2−6).

As the depth of the defect increases, the stresses that are applied to the underlying bone are increased, resulting in pain during activity. The amount of disability found following an OCD is also dependent on the location of the defect on the articular surface. If the area containing the defect is located in an area of high joint forces, the disability secondary to pain is increased.

Osteochondritis Dissecans

Characterized by dislodged fragments of bone within the joint space, osteochondritis dissecans is a lesion of the bone and articular cartilage that results in the delamination of the subchondral bone. The piece of bone may be stable within the joint or it may be free floating within the joint space, where it is capable of creating greater problems of pain and decreased function (Fig. 2−7). Most frequently occurring in the knee and elbow, the underlying cause resulting in the destruction of bone has been proposed to be *ischemia*, trauma, and degenerative changes.[15−17]

Typically, the athlete complains of increasing pain, episodes of the joint "locking," and an inabil-

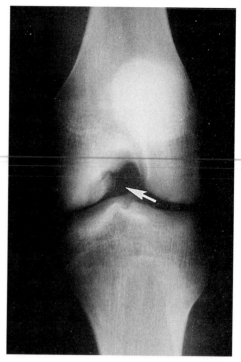

Figure 2−6. X ray of an osteochondral defect. Note the small fracture line on the medial portion of the trochanteric groove.

Examination Segment	Clinical Findings of an Osteochondral Defect	
History	Onset: Location of pain: Mechanism:	Acute or insidious. The athlete usually complains of pain in the joint during weight-bearing activities, depending on the site of the defect. The entire joint may be painful secondary to a synovial reaction (see Synovitis). Acute: A rotational and/or axial load placed on two opposing joint surfaces. The resulting friction results in a tearing away of the cartilage. Chronic: A progressive degeneration of the articular cartilage.
Inspection	Effusion is present.	
Palpation	The joint line may be tender from the defect, although the defect itself is usually not palpable. Tenderness may also be caused by synovitis.	
Functional tests	AROM: PROM: RROM:	This is limited owing to pain and swelling. This is increased relative to the active range of motion but is still limited by pain and swelling. Decreased strength occurs, secondary to pain.
Special tests	The defect may be present on a standard x-ray examination. Better imaging is obtained through the use of magnetic resonance imaging (MRI) or bone scan.	

Ischemia: Decrease in local blood flow secondary to the obstruction of the blood vessels.

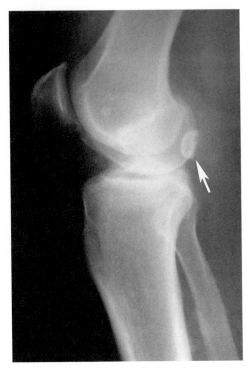

Figure 2–7. X ray of a free-floating body in the joint space.

gresses, the function of the joint becomes limited as the range of motion decreases and the ability to produce forceful contractions of the surrounding muscles declines.

Osteoarthritis

Although there are many types of arthritis, the degeneration of a joint's articular surface, the most common type found in athletes is osteoarthritis. This chronic condition most often affects the body's weight-bearing joints, especially the knees. With time the articular surfaces begin to degenerate, and the regenerative process causes bony outgrowths on what should be an otherwise smooth surface (Fig. 2–8). This degeneration of the articular cartilage of the knee can eventually lead to the complete destruction of the cartilage and the exposure of the subchondral bone. Flaking pieces of bone can result in loose bodies.

The outward signs and symptoms of osteoarthritis depend on the duration of the condition. In acute cases the athlete may have minimal swelling and redness, with the chief complaint of pain during movement when the joint surfaces are compressed. Chronically, the affected area is marked by obvious deformity and pain during joint movement.

Athletes may also suffer from rheumatoid arthritis, a systemic condition that affects the articular cartilages of multiple joints. As this condition worsens, the joints appear to be hard and nodular, with

ity to function. The onset is usually not related to any specific trauma and is typically from overuse. The complaints of pain are usually specific to the area of the affected joint. As the condition pro-

Examination Segment	Clinical Findings of Osteochondritis Dissecans	
History	Onset:	Insidious or acute.
	Location of pain:	Pain occurs within the joint, increasing with motion and possibly absent when the joint is at rest.
	Mechanism:	Insidious: Progressive degeneration of the joint structures.
		Acute: Trauma causing a piece of bone or cartilage to break free and enter the joint space.
Inspection	Swelling around the joint may be noted. The athlete tends to hold the joint in a pain-free position.	
Palpation	The affected joint feels warm secondary to inflammation. Pain may become specific on palpation along the joint line.	
Functional tests	Active, passive, and resisted range of motion may be reduced secondary to the loose body lodging between the joint surfaces, creating a mechanical block against movement. AROM: Also may be limited by pain and/or **contracture**. PROM: Also may be limited by pain and/or contracture. RROM: Also may be limited by pain and/or contracture.	

Contracture: A pathological shortening of muscular fibers inhibiting the lengthening of the muscle.

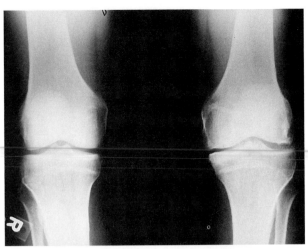

Figure 2–8. X ray of an arthritic joint. Note the loss of definition in the joint space of the athlete's left knee.

Bony Injuries

Although soft tissue injuries are more prevalent in athletes, bony injuries tend to be more traumatic because of the high forces producing them. The fracture of a bone usually creates a scene in which the athlete is in obvious distress. The clinician must perform a thorough, but quick, evaluation. In cases of fractures to the **long bones**, the ribs, and the spine, the utmost dedication to detail during the evaluation and management must be used to minimize the deleterious outcomes of such injuries.

Injuries to bones in the pediatric and adolescent athletic populations present with a set of entirely different challenges to the clinician. The presence of **growth plates** as a weak link in the skeleton presents problems in traumatic fractures as well as in overuse injuries. The clinician should always be cognizant of the potential for growth plate injury in this population.

Exostosis

Wolff's law states that a bone remodels itself in response to forces placed on it, a naturally occur-

even simple movement resulting in profound pain. The athlete may have a family history of rheumatoid arthritis, will have multiple joints affected, and may have associated medical complications from the disease.

Examination Segment	Clinical Findings of Arthritis		
History	Onset: Location of pain: Mechanism:	Insidious. Pain occurs throughout the involved joint. Osteoarthritis develops secondary to trauma and irregular biomechanical stresses being placed across the joint. Rheumatoid arthritis is caused by a systemic disorder that activates an inflammatory response in the body's joints.	
Inspection	In chronic cases, gross deformity of the joint is noticed. Individuals with cases of shorter duration present with mild swelling and redness. When arthritis affects the joints of the lower extremity, an **antalgic** gait is produced.		
Palpation	Warmth and swelling are identified in the affected joint. The articular surfaces, when and where palpable, are tender to the touch.		
Functional tests	AROM: PROM: RROM:	This is limited by pain, often becoming contracted as the condition progresses. These findings are equal to those of active range of motion testing. This is decreased secondary to pain.	
Ligamentous tests	Results may be positive if a deformity has developed, causing the stressed capsule and ligaments to elongate over time.		
Special tests	X-ray examination and other imaging techniques show degenerative changes within the joint.		

Long bone: A bone possessing a base, shaft, and head.
Growth plate: The area of bone growth in skeletally immature athletes; the epiphyseal plate.
Antalgic: Having a pain-relieving quality; analgesic.

ring phenomenon that allows bones to adapt and become stronger.[18] Growth of extraneous bone, exostosis, can occur owing to a stress reaction from injury or from irregular forces on the bone (Fig. 2–9). This irregular force on the bone creates an exostosis at the site of the stress that becomes painful and, in some cases, forms a mechanical block that can be a barrier against movement.

Apophysitis

Sometimes termed "growing pains," apophysitis is an inflammatory condition involving a bone's growth plate. In adolescent athletes, the growth plate represents the weak link along the bone. Some of these growth areas serve as, or are close to, the attachment sites for the larger, stronger muscle groups in the body. Tightness of these muscles, or repetitive forces applied to the bone by these muscles, can result in inflammation and the eventual separation of these areas away from the rest of the bone (Fig. 2–10).

Typical findings of apophysitis include a history of recent rapid growth in the athlete. As the skeleton rapidly matures, the muscular tissues do not fully adapt and apply increased stress to the growth plate. Once apophysitis has occurred, the athlete experiences decreased flexibility in the muscle group attaching to the site. Resistance exercises (e.g., weight lifting) result in pain as the forces generated are transmitted to the affected area.

Fractures

Classification schemes of bony fractures must consider the location of the fracture relative to the

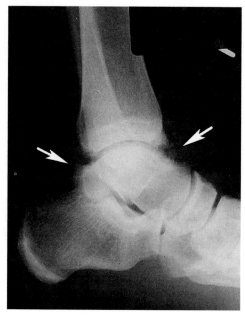

Figure 2–9. X ray of exostosis of the subtalar joint.

rest of the bone, the shape, direction, and magnitude of the fracture line(s), as well as the fracture's duration of onset. The use of relatively nondescriptive terms (e.g., boxer's fracture: a fracture of the fourth or fifth metacarpal) or the identification of a fracture type by an individual's name (e.g., Colles' fracture: fracture of the distal radius that is displaced posteriorly), although common practice, tends to become corrupted over time and may be less accurate.

Examination Segment	Clinical Findings of Exostosis		
History	Onset:		Insidious.
	Location of pain:		Exostosis involving the extremities most often results in the localization of pain and other symptoms.
			Spinal exostosis can result in pain being referred along the distribution of any affected nerve root(s).
	Mechanism:		Exostosis is the result of repeated strain placed on a bone or the bony insertion of a tendon.
Inspection	Deformity may be noted over the site of pain.		
Palpation	Point tenderness is present.		
	A defect, in the form of a bony outgrowth, may be palpable.		
Functional tests	AROM:	This is limited secondary to pain.	
	PROM:	This is equal to active range of motion.	
	RROM:	This is reduced secondary to pain.	

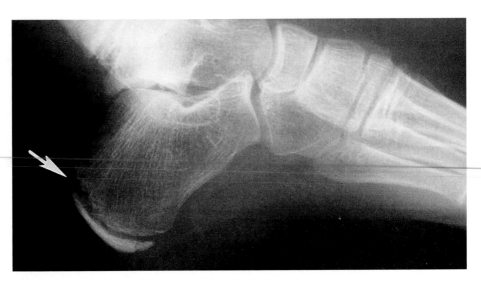

Figure 2–10. X ray of calcaneal apophysitis.

Fracture Location

	Diaphyseal fractures involve only the bone's *diaphysis* and are associated with a good *prognosis* for recovery, barring any extenuating circumstances.
	Epiphyseal fractures involve the fracture line crossing the bone's unsealed *epiphyseal line* and can have long-term consequences by disrupting the bone's normal growth. Epiphyseal fractures may mimic soft tissue injuries by resembling joint instability during stress testing.
	Articular fractures disrupt the joint's articular cartilage, which, if improperly healed, results in pain and decreased range of motion and can lead to arthritis of the joint.

Relative Severity of the Fracture Line

	Fracture lines not completely discommunicating the proximal end of the bone from its distal end are described as **incomplete fractures.**
	Fracture lines with complete disassociation between the two ends of the bone are termed **undisplaced fractures** if the two ends of the bone maintain their relative alignment to each other.
	Displaced fractures involve the loss of alignment between the two segments and may jeopardize the surrounding tissues.
	An **open fracture** (compound fracture) occurs when a displaced fracture exits the skin.

Diaphysis: The shaft of a long bone.
Prognosis: The course a disease or injury is expected to take.
Epiphyseal line: The area of growth found between the diaphysis and epiphysis in immature long bones.

Shape of the Fracture Line

	Depressed fractures occur from direct trauma to flat bones, causing the bone to fracture and depress.
	Transverse fractures are caused by a direct blow, *shear force*, or tensile force being applied to the shaft of a long bone and result in a fracture line that is perpendicular to the bone's long axis.
	Extremely high-velocity impact forces can result in the shattering of bone into multiple pieces, a **comminuted fracture**. This type of fracture often requires surgical correction.
	Compressive forces placed through the long axis of the bone can lead to a **compacted fracture**, in which one end of a fractured segment is driven into the opposite piece of the fracture, often leading to a shortening of the involved limb.
	A rotational force placed on the shaft of a long bone, such as twisting the tibia while the foot remains fixated, can result in a **spiral fracture**, in which the fracture line assumes an S-shape along the length of the bone.
	Longitudinal fractures, most commonly occurring as the result of a fall, have a fracture line that runs parallel to the bone's long axis.

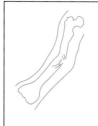 Generally specific to the pediatric and adolescent population, **greenstick fractures** involve a displaced fracture on one side of the bone and a compacted fracture on the opposite side. The name is derived from an analogy to an immature tree branch that has been snapped.

Avulsion Fractures

Avulsion fractures involve the tearing away of a ligament's or tendon's bony attachment (Fig. 2–11). Except for the case of large tendons (e.g., the patellar tendon), this injury is often missed because of the relatively small fracture site and the similarity to sprains or strains and their mechanisms. Tendon avulsions can also occur if a muscle is forcefully contracted and the attachment site is pulled away from the rest of the bone. When large tendons are involved, there is obvious deformity at the fracture site. In the case of smaller tendons or ligaments, the athlete describes pain at the fracture site and point tenderness is elicited. The stress testing of the joint may display the signs and symptoms of a third-degree sprain or strain.

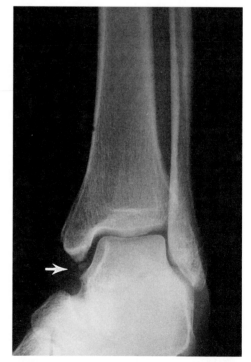

Figure 2–11. X ray of an avulsion fracture of the attachment of the deltoid ligament.

Shear forces: Forces from opposing directions that are applied perpendicular to a structure's long axis.
Compressive force: A force applied along the length of a structure, causing the tissues to approximate one another.

Stress Fractures

Although stress fractures most commonly occur in the lower extremity, this condition can be found in any bone that absorbs stress.[19,20] Stress fractures present as a complex injury because of their nondescript initial findings. The complaints reported by the athlete are nonspecific and tend to mimic those associated with soft tissue injuries. Stress fractures occur when the bone's *osteoclastic* activity outweighs osteoblastic activity, causing a weakened area along the line of stress. If the external stress is not reduced (e.g., running), the bone eventually fails.

The history reveals a chronic condition caused by repetitive stresses to the involved area. The athlete may have a recent change in his or her workout routine including changes in equipment, playing surfaces, frequency, duration, and/or intensity. With specific palpation, an area of exact tenderness can be discerned along any bony surface. Compression of long bones may result in increased pain.

Neurovascular Pathologies

Trauma to the neurovascular structures, that is, nerves, arteries, and veins, is often a consequence of joint dislocation, bony displacement, or concussive forces. Vascular disruption, if untreated, can lead to the loss of the affected body part; neurological inhibition can lead to the loss of the involved part.

Peripheral Nerve Injury

Entrapment injuries to the peripheral nerves are common at the ankle, elbow, wrist, and cervical spine. The closer to the CNS that this injury occurs, the greater the dispersion of the symptoms. Likewise, peripheral nerves distal to the spinal column have a greater probability of regeneration than a lesion that occurs more proximal to the CNS.

In some cases a nonneurological tissue or swelling entraps the nerve, causing dysfunction in the form of paresthesia and muscular weakness. In athletes, this is most commonly seen at the ulnar tunnel, pronator teres muscle, carpal tunnel, and tarsal tunnel. In each case the athlete complains of varying pain patterns and paresthesia. With careful manual muscle testing, muscle weakness may be elicited. Although these syndromes may be suspected on evaluation, they must be confirmed by a physician through electrodiagnostic testing.

Stretch injuries to peripheral nerves may be divided into three categories based on the pathology and the prognosis for recovery. **Neurapraxia** is the mildest form of peripheral nerve stretch injury. The nerve, *epineurium*, and *myelin sheath* are stretched but remain intact. Symptoms are usually transient and include burning pain, numbness, and temporary weakness on clinical evaluation.

Axonotmesis involves a disruption of the axon and the myelin sheath, but the epineurium remains intact. The signs and symptoms are the same as for neurapraxia, but axonotmesis has a longer duration.

Examination Segment	Clinical Findings of Stress Fractures	
History	Onset:	Insidious. The athlete cannot report a single traumatic event causing the pain.
	Location of pain:	Pain tends to radiate from the involved bone but may become diffuse.
	Mechanism:	Cumulative microtrauma causes stress fractures.
Inspection	Usually no bony abnormality is noted. Soft tissue swelling and redness may be present.	
Palpation	Point tenderness exists over the fracture site.	
Functional tests	AROM: This is usually within normal limits. PROM: This is usually within normal limits. RROM: This is usually within normal limits.	
Special tests	Long bone compression test. Percussion along the length of the bone. Bone scans or other imaging techniques.	

Osteoclasts: Cells that absorb and remove unwanted bone.
Epineurium: Connective tissue containing blood vessels surrounding the trunk of a nerve, binding it together.
Myelin sheath: A fatty-based lining of the axon of myelinated nerve fibers.

Because the axon undergoes **wallerian degeneration**, the return of function is unpredictable and sustained weakness may be experienced.

Neurotmesis, a complete disruption of the nerve, is the most severe form of peripheral nerve injury. The prognosis for the return of normal function is poor. This injury occurs under extremely high forces and usually entails **concurrent** injury to bones, ligaments, and tendons. Many times a nerve **graft** or tendon transfer is required to return function to the extremity. It should be noted that these procedures meet with limited success and are not conducive to the return to competitive athletics.

Reflex Sympathetic Dystrophy

Reflex sympathetic **dystrophy** (RSD) is an exaggerated, generalized pain response following injury, involving intense or unduly prolonged pain that is out of proportion to the severity of the injury, **vasomotor** disturbances, delayed functional recovery, and various associated **trophic** changes.[21] Although RSD must be definitively diagnosed by a physician, the clinician must be aware of the common early findings so that a timely referral can be made (Table 2–2). The prognosis for RSD is extremely variable, but early intervention appears to improve the probability of a favorable outcome, making early recognition and referral a priority.

IMAGING TECHNIQUES

Various forms of imaging techniques used to view the body's subcutaneous structures are referenced throughout this text. Although the physician orders and subsequently interprets these results, a knowledge of the application of these techniques is valuable to the clinician. The athlete, or the athlete's

Table 2–2. Clinical Findings of Reflex Sympathetic Dystrophy

- Pain that is disproportionately increased relative to the severity of the injury
- Superficial hypersensitive areas (e.g., pain when clothing touches the skin)
- Edema
- Decreased motor function, leading to dystrophy
- Muscle spasm
- Dermatologic alterations including the integrity of the skin, skin temperature changes, hair loss, and changes in the nailbed
- Vasomotor instability: **Raynaud's phenomenon, vasoconstriction, vasodilation, hyperhidrosis**
- Skeletal changes including **osteoporosis**

parents, may desire information regarding the procedures, their uses, and the eventual outcome. Table 2–3 presents these imaging techniques and their most advantageous uses.

Radiographs

The most common imaging technique used in the evaluation of athletic injuries is radiography, or x-ray examinations (Fig. 2–12). Discovered in 1895, the use of x rays marked the first time in the history of medicine that the internal structures could be viewed without invasive techniques.[22] Before this, the only method of viewing the internal structures was to actually cut the individual open.

X-ray examination uses **ionizing radiation** to penetrate the body. Depending on the density of the underlying tissues, the radiation is absorbed or dispersed in varying degrees. High-density tissues such as bone absorb more radiation and are therefore more difficult to penetrate than less-dense tissue. The exposure to radiation leaves an imprint on

---

Wallerian degeneration: Degeneration of a nerve's axon that has been severed from the body of the nerve.
Concurrent: Occurring at the same time.
Graft: An organ or tissue used for transplantation. In an allograft, tissue is received from the same species. In an autograft, tissue is transplanted from within the same individual.
Dystrophy: The progressive deterioration of muscle.
Vasomotor: Pertaining to nerves controlling the muscles within the walls of blood vessels.
Trophic: Pertaining to efferent nerves controlling the nourishment of the area they innervate.
Raynaud's phenomenon: A reaction to cold consisting of bouts of pallor and cyanosis, causing exaggerated vasomotor responses.
Vasoconstriction: A decrease in a vessel's diameter.
Vasodilation: An increase in a vessel's diameter.
Hyperhidrosis: Excessive or profuse sweating.
Osteoporosis: Decreased bone density common in postmenopausal women.
Ionizing radiation: Electromagnetic energy that causes the release of an atom's protons, electrons, or neutrons. Ionizing radiation is potentially hazardous to human tissue.

Table 2–3. Various Imaging Techniques and Their Use in Diagnosing Athletic Injuries

Technique	Best Use
Radiography (x ray)	Standard: Bone lesions, joint surfaces, and joint spaces Arthrogram: Capsular tissue tears and articular cartilage lesions Myelogram: Pathologies within the spinal canal
Computed tomography (CT)	Bony or articular cartilage lesions and some soft tissue lesions, especially when quantifying detailed lesions (e.g., size and location; useful in identifying tendinous and ligamentous injuries in varying joint positions)
Magnetic resonance imaging (MRI)	Soft tissue structures, especially ligamentous and meniscal injuries
Bone scan	Acute bony change determination but may produce false-positive findings, especially in endurance athletes
Ultrasonic imaging	Tendon and other soft tissue imaging

special x-ray film, producing the familiar x-ray image. Overexposure to ionizing radiation is hazardous, and care must be taken to protect the reproductive organs through the use of a lead apron.

The interpretation of x-ray images can be simplistically based on the ABCs method:[23]

A Alignment: The clinician observes for the normal continuity of the bones and joint surfaces and the alignment of one bone to another, relative to the uninvolved extremity.

B Bones: Bones should have normal density patterns, presenting with uniform color throughout the bone as compared bilaterally. Areas of decreased density appear as darkened areas within the bone. Fractures and abnormal bony outgrowths such as exostosis should be appreciated by the examiner.

C Cartilage: Although cartilage itself does not produce an x-ray image, the cartilage and ligamentous structures are appreciated for what does not appear. The spaces should be smooth, uniform, and of equal sizes when compared bilaterally.

s Soft tissue: Although soft tissue cannot be appreciated, swelling within the confines of the soft tissue or between the soft tissue and the bones can be determined. Additionally, the outline of soft tissues and even pockets of edema within soft tissue can be identified with adjusted exposure techniques.

Assessment of a joint's ligamentous integrity often requires the use of imaging techniques, during which stress is applied to a joint to measure the amount of laxity, a **stress x ray** (Fig. 2–13). This requires application of a force across a ligament by a physician during the x-ray exposure, allowing for the measurement of excessive motion, determining a third-degree ligament injury, or ascertaining the amount of overall joint laxity.

Various other forms of x-ray screening involve the use of radio-opaque dyes that are absorbed by the tissues, allowing for their visualization by x-ray examination. Collectively known as **contrast**

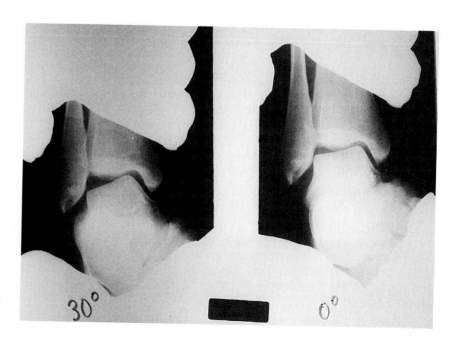

Figure 2–12. Stress x ray for inversion of the ankle.

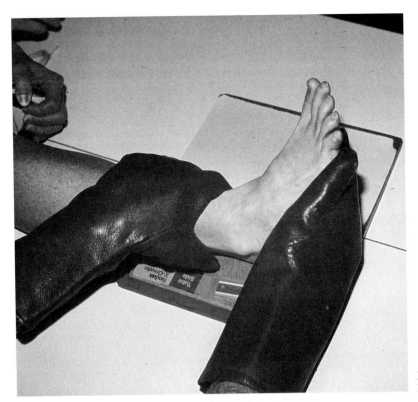

Figure 2-13. Setup of the stress x ray shown in Figure 2-12.

imaging, arthrograms, myelograms, and angiograms have various applications to specific body systems. With the availability of magnetic resonance imaging techniques, these types of studies are less frequently used in the diagnosis of athletic injuries.

Computed Tomography

Computed tomography (CT) uses much of the same principles and technology as radiography but is used to determine and quantify the presence of a specific pathology rather than as a general screening tool. In the case of CT scans, the x-ray source and x-ray detectors rotate around the body (Fig. 2-14). Instead of the image being produced on film, a computer determines the density of the underlying tissues based on the absorption of x rays by the body, allowing for more precision in viewing soft tissue. This information is then used to create a two-dimensional image, or slice, of the body.[22] These slices can be obtained at varying positions and thicknesses, allowing the physician to study the area and its surrounding anatomical relationships (Fig. 2-15).

Magnetic Resonance Imaging

Perhaps the greatest innovation in the noninvasive diagnosis of subcutaneous pathology, magnetic resonance imaging (MRI) acquires a detailed picture of the body's soft tissues (Fig. 2-16). Like CT, MRI is used to identify specific pathology or visualize a soft tissue structure (e.g., an anterior cruciate ligament sprain) rather than as a general screening tool. MRI offers superior visualization of the body's soft tissues, including swollen and inflamed tissues.

These images are obtained by placing the athlete in an MRI tube that produces a magnetic field, causing the body's hydrogen nuclei to align with the magnetic axis (Fig. 2-17). The tissues are then bombarded by radio waves, causing the nuclei to resonate as they absorb the energy. When the energy to the tissues ceases, the nuclei return to their state of equilibrium by releasing energy, which is then detected by the MRI unit and transformed by a computer into mages.[22]

Unlike the ionizing radiation associated with radiographs and CT scans, the energy used during the MRI process produces no known harmful effects. The only known limitations to the administration of this procedure lie with athletes suffering

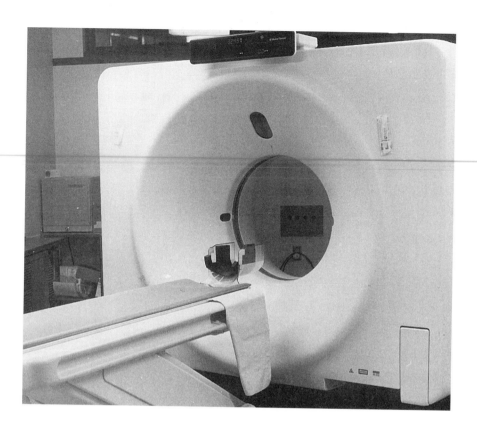

Figure 2–14. Setup of a CT scan.

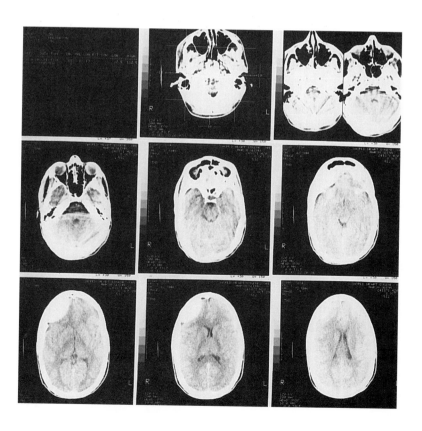

Figure 2–15. CT scan of the cranium.

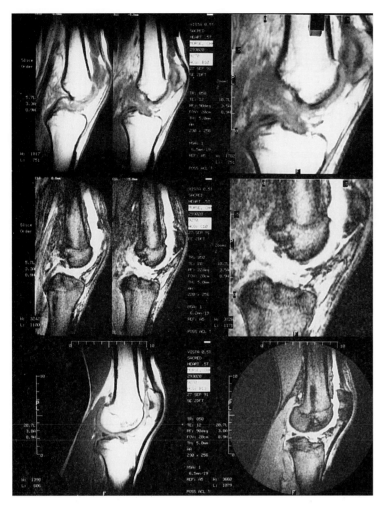

Figure 2–16. MRI image showing the knee in cross section.

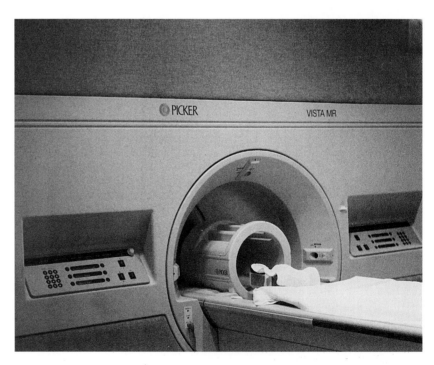

Figure 2–17. MRI generator.

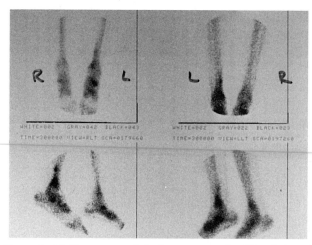

Figure 2–18. Bone scan of the lower extremity. The darkened areas indicate "hot spots" of high uptake of the tracer element.

quires that the athlete be injected with the ***radionu-clide*** Tc-99m, a ***tracer element*** that is absorbed by areas of bone undergoing remodeling. These areas appear as darkened spots on the image and must be correlated with clinical signs and symptoms (Fig. 2–18). Common pathologies that bone scans are used to identify include degenerative disease, bone tumors, and stress fractures of the long bones and the vertebrae.[24]

Ultrasonic Imaging

Many internal organs and certain soft tissue structures, such as tendons, may be visualized through the use of ultrasonic energy. The energy produced by ultrasonic imaging devices is quite similar to that used during therapeutic ultrasound treatments but has a frequency of less than 0.8 MHz. Through a technique similar to sonar on a submarine, a computer detects the amount of sound that is reflected away from the tissues and creates a two-dimensional image of the subcutaneous structures (Fig. 2–19).

from claustrophobia (who are fearful of entering the imaging tube) or the presence of implanted metal plates or screws. Further technological advances will soon eliminate these contraindications by minimizing the effects of the imaging tube and reducing the level of magnetism to the point that metal implants can be safely exposed.

Bone Scan

Bone scans are a form of nuclear medicine used to detect bony abnormalities that are not normally visible on a standard radiograph. This procedure re-

REFERENCES

1. Garrett, WE, Duncan, PW, and Malone, TR: Muscle Injury and Rehabilitation. Williams and Wilkins, Baltimore, 1988, p 9.
2. Rachun, A (ed): Standard Nomenclature of Athletic Injuries. American Medical Association, Monroe, WI, 1976.

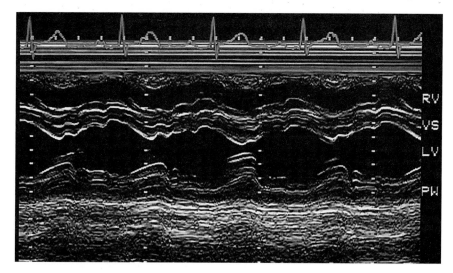

Figure 2–19. Ultrasonic image (mode echocardiogram) of the heart, showing normal left ventricular size and wall thickness. (RV = right ventricle; LV = left ventricle; VS = ventricular septum; PW = posterior wall.

Radionuclide: An atom that, when disintegrating, emits electromagnetic radiation.

Tracer element: A substance that is introduced into the tissues to follow or trace an otherwise unidentifiable substance or event.

3. Almekinders, LC, Garrett, WE, and Seaber, AV: Pathophysiologic response to muscle tears in stretching injuries. Transactions of the Orthopedic Research Society 9:307, 1984.

4. Almekinders, LC, Garrett, WE, and Seaber, AV: Histopathology of muscle tears in stretching injuries. Transactions of the Orthopedic Research Society 9:306, 1984.

5. Garrett, WE, et al: Biomechanics of muscle tears in stretching injuries. Transactions of the Orthopedic Research Society 9:384, 1984.

6. Garrett, WE, et al: The effect of muscle architecture on the biomechanical failure properties of skeletal muscle under passive extension. Am J Sports Med 16:7, 1988.

7. Davies, GL, Wallace, LA, and Malone, TR: Mechanisms of selected knee injuries. Phys Ther 60:1590, 1980.

8. Gross, MT: Chronic tendinitis: Pathomechanics of injury, factors affecting the healing response, and treatment. Journal of Orthopedic and Sports Physical Therapy 16:248, 1992.

9. Frey, CC, and Shereff, MJ: Tendon injuries about the ankle in athletes. Clin Sports Med 7:103–118, 1988.

10. Comb, JA: Myositis ossificans traumatica. Pathogenesis and management. Athletic Training: Journal of the National Athletic Training Association 22:193, 1987.

11. Estwanik, JJ: Contusions and the formation of myositis ossificans. Physician and Sportsmedicine 18:53, 1990.

12. It's bursitis, but which type? Emerg Med 21:71, 1989.

13. Distefano, VJ: Anatomy and biomechanics of the ankle and foot. Athletic Training: Journal of the National Athletic Trainers Association 16:43, 1981.

14. Garrick, JG, and Requa, RK: Role of external support in the prevention of ankle sprains. Med Sci Sports Exerc 5:200, 1973.

15. Gardiner, JB: Osteochondritis dessicans in three members of a family. J Bone Joint Surg Br 37:139, 1955.

16. Woodward, AH, and Bianco, AJ: Osteochondritis dessicans of the elbow. Clin Orthop 110:35, 1975.

17. Lindholm, TS, Osterman, K, and VanKkae, E: Osteochondritis dessicans of the elbow, ankle, and hip. Clin Orthop 148:245, 1980.

18. Starkey, C: The injury response process. In Starkey, C: Therapeutic Modalities for Athletic Trainers. FA Davis, Philadelphia, 1993, p 4.

19. Ward, WG, Bergfeld, JA, and Carson, WG: Stress fracture of the base of the acromial process. Am J Sports Med 22:146:1994.

20. Yasuda, T, et al: Stress fracture of the right distal femur following bilateral fractures of the proximal fibulas. A case report. Am J Sports Med 20:771, 1992.

21. Schutzer, SF, and Gossling, HR: The treatment of reflex sympathetic dystrophy syndrome. J Bone Joint Surg Am 66:625, 1984.

22. D'Orsi, CJ: Radiology and magnetic resonance imaging. In Greene, HL, Glassock, RJ, and Kelley, MA: Introduction to Clinical Medicine. BC Decker, Philadelphia, 1991, p 91.

23. Schuerger, SR: Introduction to critical review of roentgengrams. Phys Ther 68:1114, 1988.

24. Patton, DO, and Doherty, PN: Nuclear medicine studies. In Greene, HL, Glassock, RJ, and Kelley, MA: Introduction to Clinical Medicine. BC Decker, Philadelphia, 1991, p 81.

3

The Foot and Toes

The foot and toes, in combination with the ankle and lower leg, are called on to perform a diverse range of tasks. When a person is standing, the foot must provide a stable platform to balance and support the body. When a person is walking or running, the foot must serve as a rigid lever during the toe-off phase of gait and as a shock absorber during the heel-strike phase (Fig. 3–1). In conjunction with the ankle, the foot and toes must possess the flexibility required to adapt to uneven terrain.

As the function of the foot, toes, and ankle are highly interrelated, so too is the evaluation of these structures. This text describes the evaluation of the foot and toes in this chapter and the ankle and lower leg in the next. Despite this artificial delineation between the two areas, a thorough evaluation of the foot and toes should also encompass a thorough evaluation of the ankle complex and vice versa. Some conditions may also necessitate the examination of the entire lower extremity and the lumbar spine, and an analysis of gait.

CLINICAL ANATOMY

The foot relies on the intimate and precise relationships among various structures. True one-on-one articulation between its bones is rare and tends to be limited to the joints of the toes; the majority of the remaining bones have multiple articulations with their contiguous structures. Muscular action and support is provided from the foot's *intrinsic* muscles, as well as those muscles originating from the lower leg.

Anatomically as well as functionally, the foot can be divided into three zones: the **hindfoot**, the **midfoot**, and the **forefoot and toes** (Fig. 3–2). The foot is formed by 26 bones; the **tarsals** consist of the calcaneus, talus, navicular, cuboid, and three cuneiforms; each of the five **metatarsals** leads to the **phalanges**. Each toe is formed by three phalanges, with the exception of the great toe, which is formed by only two bones.

Formed by the calcaneus and the talus, the **hindfoot** provides stability during the heel-strike phase of gait and serves as a lever arm for the Achilles tendon during **plantarflexion** of the foot. Serving as the shock-absorbing segment, the **midfoot** is composed of the navicular, three cuneiforms, and cuboid. The **forefoot**, formed by the five metatarsals and 14 phalanges, acts as a lever during the toe-off phase of gait. As a unit, the foot is required to absorb and dissipate a force equal to seven times the athlete's body weight when running.[1] Each of these three sections must work in concert for the foot to function properly.

The Hindfoot

The calcaneus is the largest of the tarsal bones, and its most prominent feature is the posteriorly projecting **calcaneal tubercle**. The size of this tubercle is important in providing a mechanically powerful lever for increasing the muscular force produced by the gastrocnemius, soleus, and plantaris (triceps surae). The large calcaneal body serves as the origin and insertion for many of the ligaments and muscles acting on the foot and ankle.

Arising off the calcaneal body's anterior medial surface is the **sustentaculum tali** that assists in supporting the talus (Fig. 3–3). On this structure's inferior surface is a groove through which the tendon of the flexor hallucis longus passes. The lateral portion of the anterior calcaneus articulates with the cuboid. Projecting off the lateral side of the calcaneus, the **peroneal tubercle** assists in maintaining the alignment of the peroneal tendons. This is the point where the peroneal tendons *diverge*, with the peroneus brevis running superior to the tubercle and the peroneus brevis traveling inferior to it.

On the inferior surface are medial and lateral *facets*, which provide a base for weight bearing and serve as the site for muscular and ligamentous attachments. The superior surface is marked with

---

Intrinsic: Arising from within the body or within the body part being described.
Diverge: To split.
Facet: A small, smooth, articular surface on a bone.

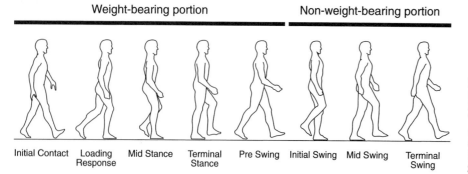

Figure 3–1. Phases of gait for the right foot as defined by the Los Ranchos Medical Center system of gait analysis. This system, described in Chapter 8, divides the gait into weight-bearing and non–weight-bearing portions. (Adapted from Norkin and Levangie.[3])

facets that, in combination with the sustentaculum tali, provide for articulation with the talus.

The saddle-shaped **talus** acts as the interface between foot and ankle function. Its unique shape is necessitated by its five functional articulations: (1) superiorly with the distal end of the tibia, (2) medially with the medial malleolus, (3) laterally with the lateral malleolus, (4) inferiorly with the calcaneus, and (5) anteriorly with the navicular. There are no muscular attachments on the talus.

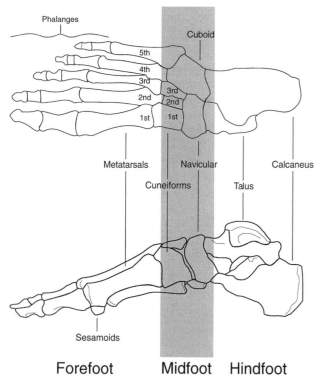

Figure 3–2. Anatomical zones of the foot. The talus and calcaneus form the hindfoot (rearfoot); the 3 cuneiform, the navicular, and the cuboid form the midfoot; and the 5 metatarsals, 14 phalanges, and 2 sesamoid bones form the forefoot.

The Midfoot

Playing a key function in supporting the medial longitudinal arch, the **navicular** articulates anteriorly with the three cuneiforms, the cuboid laterally, and the talus posteriorly. The medial aspect of the navicular gives rise to the navicular *tuberosity*, the insertion of the tibialis posterior muscle.

In addition to the navicular, the **cuboid** articulates with the third cuneiform medially, the fourth and fifth metatarsals anteriorly, and the calcaneus posteriorly. A palpable *sulcus* is formed anterior to the tuberosity of the cuboid and posterior to the base of the fifth metatarsal where the peroneus longus begins its course along the foot's plantar surface.

Adding to the flexibility of the midfoot and forefoot, the three **cuneiforms** are referenced numerically from medial to lateral. Each cuneiform articulates with the navicular posteriorly, the corresponding metatarsal anteriorly, and with the contiguous cuneiform medially and laterally. The third cuneiform also articulates with the cuboid laterally.

The Forefoot

The five **metatarsals** (MTs) may be conceptualized as miniature long bones, each having a base (proximal), body, and head (distal). The MTs are referenced numerically from medial (first) to lateral (fifth). The metatarsal heads each articulate with the proximal phalanx of the corresponding toe and loosely with the neighboring metatarsal heads. Proximally, the bases of the first three MTs articulate with the corresponding cuneiform, although the second MT has an articulation with the first and second cuneiform. The lateral two MTs articulate with the cuboid. Like the heads, the bases articulate with the contiguous MTs, but with a tighter fit.

Each **phalanx** also has a base, shaft, and head, al-

Tuberosity: A nodulelike projection off a bone, serving as an attachment site for muscles and ligaments; referred to as a tubercle in the upper extremity.
Sulcus: A groove or depression within a bone.

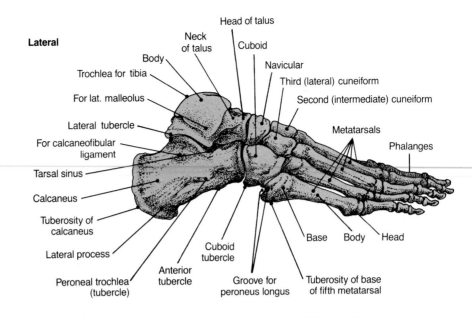

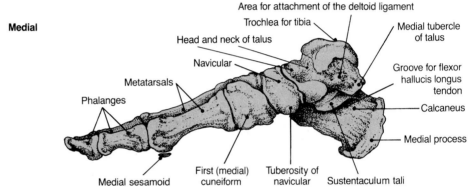

Figure 3–3. Anatomy of the foot showing prominent bony landmarks and sites of ligamentous and muscular attachments. (From Rothstein, JM, Roy, SH, and Wolf, SL,[1a] p 5, with permission.)

beit on a much smaller scale, and the toes are numbered from 1, the great toe (hallux), to 5, the little toe.

Articulations and Ligamentous Support

The ligaments joining the tarsal bones of the foot may be collectively grouped into three sets: (1) the thin *dorsal* tarsal ligaments, (2) the relatively thick plantar tarsal ligaments, and (3) the *interosseous* tarsal ligaments that stretch between contiguous bones and interrupt the synovial cavities. The specific names given to these ligaments tend to reflect the bones that they connect.[2] The myriad ligaments found in the foot prohibit a complete and detailed discussion in this section. The reader is encouraged to refer to anatomy resources for further explanation.

The Subtalar Joint

Located at the junction between the inferior surface of the talus and the superior surface of the calcaneus, the subtalar (talocalcaneal) joint provides articulation at three points. The **posterior articulation** is a concave facet on the talus, whereas the **anterior** and **middle articulations** are convex facets. Obliquely crossing the talus and calcaneus is the tarsal canal, a sulcus that allows for the attachment of an intra-articular ligament.

It is often incorrectly stated that the motions occurring at the subtalar joint are inversion and *eversion*. The subtalar joint is a uniaxial joint with 1 degree of *freedom of movement*: supination and pronation.[3] The triplanar motion of the talus occurs around a single joint axis, allowing the component elements of pronation and supination to occur

---

Dorsal: Referring to the superior portion of the foot and toes.
Interosseous: Between two bones.
Eversion: The movement of the plantar aspect of the calcaneus away from the midline of the body.
Freedom of movement: The number of cardinal planes in which a joint allows motion.

Table 3–2. Posterior and Plantar Musculature Acting on the Ankle, Foot, and Toes

Muscle	Action	Origin	Insertion	Nerve	Root
Abductor digiti minimi	Flexion of the 5th MTP joint Abduction of the 5th MTP joint	• Lateral portion of the tuber calcanei • Proximal lateral portion of calcaneus	• Lateral portion of the proximal 5th phalanx	Lateral plantar	S1, S2
Abductor hallucis	Abduction of the 1st MTP joint Assists in flexion of the 1st MTP joint	• Medial calcaneus tuberosity • Flexor retinaculum	• Plantar surface of the medial base of the 1st toe's proximal phalanx	Medial plantar	L4, L5, S1
Adductor hallucis	Assists forefoot adduction Adduction of the 1st MTP joint Assists flexion of the 1st MTP joint	• Plantar aponeurosis Oblique head • Bases of 2nd through 4th metatarsals • Tendon sheath of peroneus longus Transverse head • Plantar surface of 3rd, 4th, and 5th metatarsal heads	• Lateral surface of the base of the 1st toe's proximal phalanx	Lateral plantar	S1, S2
Flexor digiti minimi brevis	Flexion of the 5th MTP joint	• Plantar surface of the cuboid • Base of the 5th metatarsal	• Plantar aspect of the base of the 5th metatarsal	Lateral plantar	S1, S2
Flexor digitorum brevis	Flexion of the 2nd through 5th PIP joints Assists in flexion of the 2nd through 5th MTP joints	• Medial calcaneal tuberosity • Plantar fascia	• Via four tendons, each having two slips, into the medial and lateral sides of the proximal 2nd through 5th phalanges	Medial plantar	L4, L5, S1
Flexor digitorum longus	Flexion of 2nd through 5th PIP and DIP joints Flexion of 2nd through 5th MTP joints Assists in ankle plantarflexion	• Posterior medial portion of the distal two-thirds of the tibia • From fascia arising from the tibialis posterior	• Plantar base of distal phalanges of the 2nd through 5th toes	Tibial	L5, S1
Flexor hallucis brevis	Assists in foot inversion Flexion of 1st MTP joint	• Medial side of the cuboid bone's plantar surface • Slip from the tibialis posterior tendon	• Via two tendons into the medial and lateral sides of the proximal phalanx of the first toe	Medial plantar	L4, L5, S1

Muscle	Action	Attachment	Nerve	Root
Flexor hallucis longus	Flexion of 1st IP joint Assists in flexion of 1st MTP joint Assists in foot inversion Assists in plantarflexion of the ankle	• Plantar suface of the proximal phalanx of the 1st toe	Tibial	L4, L5, S1
		• Posterior distal two-thirds of the fibula • Associated interosseous membrane and muscular fascia		
Gastrocnemius	Ankle plantarflexion Assists in knee flexion	• To the calcaneus via the Achilles tendon	Tibial	S1, S2
		Medial head • Posterior surface of the medial femoral condyle • Adjacent portion of the femur and knee capsule Lateral head • Posterior surface of the lateral femoral condyle • Adjacent portion of the femur and knee capsule		
Interossei, dorsal	Abduction of the 3rd, 4th, and 5th digits Assists in flexion of the MTP joints Assists in extension of the 3rd, 4th, and 5th IP joints	• Via two heads to the contiguous sides of the metatarsal bones	Lateral plantar	S1, S2
		• Lateral portion of the bases of the 2nd, 3rd, 4th, and 5th proximal phalanges • The medial border of the second phalanx also receives the interossei arising between the 2nd and 3rd metatarsal		
Interossei, plantar	Adduction of the 3rd, 4th, and 5th digits Assists in flexion of the MTP joint Assists in extension of the 3rd, 4th, and 5th IP joints	• Base and medial aspect of the 3rd, 4th, and 5th metatarsals	Lateral plantar	S1, S2
		• Medial portion of the bases of the 3rd, 4th, and 5th proximal phalanges		
Lumbricals	Flexion of 2nd through 5th MTP joints Assists in extension of the 2nd through 5th IP joints	• Tendons of flexor digitorum longus	1st: Medial plantar 2nd–5th: Lateral plantar	1st: L4, L5, S1 2nd–5th: S1, S2
		• Posterior surfaces of 2nd through 5th toes via the tensor digitorum longus tendons		
Peroneus brevis	Eversion of foot Assists in ankle plantarflexion	• Distal two-thirds of the lateral fibula	Superficial peroneal	L4, L5, S1
		• Styloid process at the base of the 5th metatarsal		

continued

Table 3–2. Posterior and Plantar Musculature Acting on the Ankle, Foot, and Toes—*Continued*

Muscle	Action	Origin	Insertion	Nerve	Root
Peroneus longus	Eversion of the foot Assists in ankle plantarflexion	• Lateral tibial condyle • Fibular head • Upper two-thirds of the lateral fibula	• Lateral aspect of the base of the 1st metatarsal • Lateral and dorsal aspect of the 1st cuneiform	Superficial peroneal	L4, L5, S1
Plantaris	Ankle plantarflexion Assists in knee flexion	• Distal portion of the supracondylar line of the lateral femoral condyle • Adjacent portion of the femoral popliteal surface • Oblique popliteal ligament	• To the calcaneus via the Achilles tendon	Tibial	L4, L5, S1
Quadratus plantae	Modifies the flexor digitorum's angle of pull Assists in flexion of the 2nd through 5th MTP joints	Medial head • Medial calcaneus Lateral head • Lateral calcaneus	• Dorsal and plantar surfaces of the flexor digitorum longus	Lateral plantar	S1, S2
Soleus	Ankle plantarflexion	• Posterior fibular head • Upper one-third of the fibula's posterior surface • Soleal line located on the posterior tibial shaft • Middle one-third of the medial tibial border	• To the calcaneus via the Achilles tendon	Tibial	S1, S2
Tibialis posterior	Inversion of the foot Assists in ankle plantarflexion	• Length of the interosseous membrane • Posterior, lateral tibia • Upper two-thirds of the medial fibula	• Navicular tuberosity • Via fibrous slips to the sustentaculum tali; cuneiforms, cuboid, and bases of the 2nd, 3rd, and 4th metatarsals	Tibial	L4, S1

Muscle actions, origins, and insertions adapted from Kendall and McCreary[4a]; innervations adapted from Daniels and Worthingham.[4b]

Table 3-3. Anterior and Dorsal Musculature Acting on the Ankle, Foot, and Toes

Muscle	Action	Origin	Insertion	Nerve	Root
Extensor digitorum longus	Extension of the 2nd through 5th MTP joints Assists in extending 2nd through 5th PIP and DIP joints Assists in foot eversion Assists in ankle dorsiflexion	• Lateral tibial condyle • Proximal three-fourths of anterior fibula • Proximal portion of the interosseous membrane	• Via four tendons to the distal phalanges of the 2nd through 5th toes	Deep peroneal	L4, L5, S1
Extensor digitorum brevis	Extension of the 1st through 4th MTP joints Assists in extension of the 2nd, 3rd, and 4th PIP and DIP joints	• Distal portion of the superior and lateral portion of the calcaneus • Lateral talocalcaneal ligament • Lateral portion of the inferior extensor retinaculum	• To the dorsal surface of the base of the first phalanx (this tendon is also referred to as the extensor hallucis brevis) • Proximal phalanges of the 2nd, 3rd, and 4th toes and to the distal phalanges via an attachment to the extensor digitorum longus tendon	Deep peroneal	L5, S1
Peroneus tertius	Eversion of the foot Dorsiflexion of the ankle	• Distal one-third of the anterior surface of the fibula • Adjacent portion of the interosseous membrane	• Dorsal surface of the base of the 5th metatarsal	Deep peroneal	L4, L5, S1
Extensor hallucis longus	Extension of 1st MTP joint Extension of 1st IP joint	• Middle two-thirds of the anterior surface of the fibula • Adjacent portion of the interosseous membrane	• Base of the distal phalanx of the 1st toe	Deep peroneal	L4, L5, S1
Tibialis anterior	Dorsiflexion of the ankle Inversion of the foot	• Lateral tibial condyle • Upper one-half of the tibia's lateral surface • Adjacent portion of the interosseous membrane	• Medial and plantar surfaces of the 1st cuneiform • Medial and plantar surfaces of the 1st metatarsal	Deep peroneal	L4, L5, S1

Muscle actions, origins, and insertions adapted from Kendall and McCreary[4a]; innervations adapted from Daniels and Worthingham.[4b]

metatarsal heads, the arches become further extenuated, owing to a windlass effect (Fig. 3-7).

During static weight bearing, muscles provide little support to the medial arch. However, during walking a force couple is formed between the tibialis anterior, pulling the arch upward, and the tibialis posterior, drawing the arch proximally.

The Lateral Longitudinal Arch

Lower and more rigid than the medial longitudinal arch, the lateral arch is composed of the calcaneus, the cuboid, and the fifth metatarsal. Although the lateral longitudinal arch is often considered to be a unique structure, it is actually a contin-

Table 3–4. Layers of the Foot's Intrinsic Muscles

Layer	Muscles
Superficial layer	Abductor hallucis
	Flexor digitorum brevis
	Abductor digiti minimi
Middle layer	Tendon of flexor hallucis longus
	Tendons of flexor digitorum longus
	Quadratus plantae
	Lumbricals
Deep layer	Flexor hallucis brevis
	Adductor hallucis
	Flexor digiti minimi brevis
Interosseous layer	Plantar interossei
	Dorsal interossei

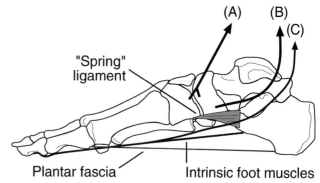

Figure 3–5. Soft tissue support of the medial longitudinal arch. Dynamic support is obtained through the (A) tibialis anterior, (B) tibialis posterior, (C) flexor hallucis longus muscles. The spring ligament is assisted by the plantar fascia and intrinsic foot muscle in bowing the arch.

uation of the medial arch. The arch itself is rarely the site of injury. Injuries to the lateral foot take the form of fractures to the fifth MT from compensatory weight bearing, owing to other foot and ankle pathology.

The Transverse Metatarsal Arch

The transverse metatarsal arch, formed by the lengths of the metatarsals and tarsals, originates at the metatarsal heads and remains present to the point where it fades on the calcaneus. The weight-bearing structures are the first and fifth metatarsal heads, whereas the second metatarsal forms the apex of the arch. Structural support of this arch is derived from the intermetatarsal ligaments and transverse head of the adductor hallucis muscle.

CLINICAL EVALUATION OF FOOT AND TOE INJURIES

As noted in this chapter's introductory section, the evaluation of foot injuries should also encompass a thorough evaluation of the ankle complex and may also necessitate the evaluation of the lower extremity, lumbar spine, and gait (Table 3–5). To

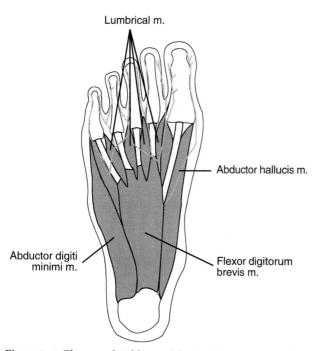

Figure 3–4. The superficial layer of the foot's intrinsic muscles is formed by the abductor digiti minimi, the abductor hallucis, and the flexor digitorum brevis muscles. The lumbrical muscles are a component of the middle muscle layer. The blood supply to the toes is also shown.

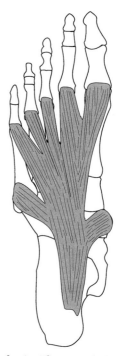

Figure 3–6. Plantar fascia. The central slip attaches to each of the five toes. Extending the toes tightens the fascia, increasing the curvature of the medial longitudinal arch.

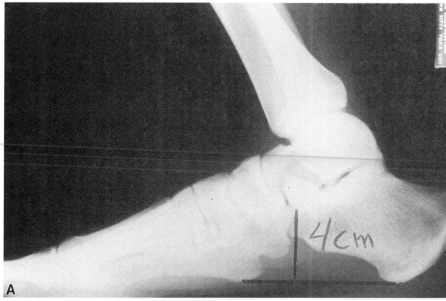

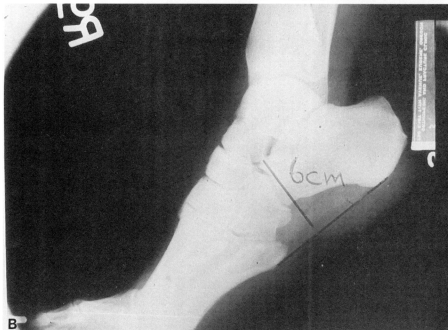

Figure 3–7. Windlass effect of the plantar fascia on the medial longitudinal arch. (*A*) The height of the medial arch when the foot is fully weightbearing (*B*) Extending the toes causes the plantar fascia to tighten, resulting in an increase in the height of the arch.

permit a thorough evaluation of these structures, the athlete should be dressed in shorts during the examination.

History

The importance of gaining a detailed and accurate history of recent and prior incidence of foot pain cannot be understated. An acute onset of symptoms should lead the examiner to suspect bony trauma until it is ruled out. Insidious pain may arise from inflammation of a ligamentous or muscular structure or from the development of a stress fracture.

- **Location of the pain:** Pain in the foot may arise from trauma to its intrinsic structures or from compensation for improper lower leg biomechanics, or it may be referred from trauma to the lumbar or sacral nerve roots, the sciatic nerve, the femoral nerve, or the common plantar nerve (Table 3–6).
  - ○ **Heel pain:** Pain in the athlete's heel may be the result of plantar fasciitis or a heel spur, especially if the pain is located on the medial plantar aspect. In the absence of a mechanism of injury to this area, pain may be referred from the lumbar nerve roots or their peripheral nerves.
  - ○ **Medial arch pain:** The medial arch can be

Table 3–5. Evaluation of the Foot and Toes

History	Inspection	Palpation	Functional Tests	Ligamentous Tests	Neurological Tests	Special Tests
Location of the pain	General inspection	Medial structures	Active range of motion	MTP and IP joints	Tarsal tunnel	Arch pathologies
Heel pain	Callus and blisters	First MTP joint	Flexion	Valgus stress testing	Peroneal nerve	Pes planus
Medial arch pain	Foot type	First metatarsal	Extension	Varus stress testing	Sciatic nerve	Test for supple pes planus
Metatarsal pain	Toes	First cuneiform	Passive range of motion	Proximal inter-metatarsal joints	Lumbar or sacral nerve root impingement	Feiss' line
Great toe pain	Morton's alignment	Navicular	Flexion	Intermetatarsal glide		Navicular drop test
Lateral arch pain	Claw toes	Talar head	Extension	Ligaments of the midfoot		Pes cavus
Onset of injury	Hammer toe	Sustentaculum tali	Resisted range of motion			Transverse meta-tarsal arch
Acute onset	Hallux valgus	Spring ligament	Flexion			Plantar fasciitis
Insidious onset	Bunion	Medial talar tubercle	Extension			Heel spur
Mechanism of injury	Corns	Calcaneal dome	Mobility of the first ray			Plantar fascia rupture
Playing surface	Ingrown toenail	Flexor hallucis longus	Related motions			Tarsal tunnel syndrome
Running distance	Subungual hematoma	Flexor digitorum longus	Subtalar joint			Tarsal coalition
Running duration	Medial structures	Tibialis posterior	Inversion			Metatarsal fractures
Shoes	Medial arch	Lateral structures	Eversion			Interdigital neuroma
	Lateral structures	Fifth MTP joint	Talocrural joint			Hallux rigidus
	Fifth metatarsal	Fifth metatarsal	Dorsiflexion			Sprains of the first MTP joint
	Dorsal structures	Styloid process	Plantarflexion			Phalanx fractures
	Plantar surface	Cuboid				
	Plantar warts	Lateral border of the calcaneus				
	Callus	Peroneal tendons				
	Posterior structures	Dorsal structures				
	Achilles tendon	Sinus tarsi				
	Foot alignment	Dome of the talus				
	Forefoot varus	Cuneiforms				
	Forefoot valgus	Rays				
	Hindfoot varus	Tibialis anterior				
	Hindfoot valgus	Extensor hallucis longus				
	Non–weight-bearing inspec-tion of foot alignment	Extensor digitorum longus				
	Assessment of talar position	Extensor digitorum brevis				
		Inferior extensor retinaculum				
		Dorsalis pedal artery				
		Plantar structures				
		Medial calcaneal tubercle				
		Plantar fascia				
		Sesamoid bones of the great toe				
		Metatarsal heads				
		Interdigital neuroma				

Table 3–6. Possible Trauma Based on the Location of Pain

Location of Pain

	Proximal (Calcaneus)	Distal (Toes)	Plantar	Dorsal	Medial	Lateral
Soft tissue	Calcaneal bursitis Retrocalcaneal bursitis	Corns Hallux rigidus IP sprain MTP sprain	Callus Plantar fascia rupture Plantar fasciitis Plantar warts Interdigital neuroma	Tarsal tunnel syndrome	Medial arch pathology Plantar fasciitis Tarsal tunnel syndrome	Peroneal tendinitis
Bony injury	Calcaneal fracture	Phalanx fracture Sesamoid fracture Arthritis/ inflammation	Sesamoiditis Heel spur	Metatarsal stress fracture Talus fracture Tarsal coalition	Navicular stress fracture Bunion	Cuboid fracture Fifth metatarsal fracture (esp. base)

the site of pain for tarsal tunnel syndrome. A compression of the medial plantar branch of the posterior tibial nerve, tarsal tunnel syndrome will radiate a sharp, burning pain and paresthesia to the medial arch.

○ **Metatarsal pain:** Pain that is specifically located on a metatarsal and has worsened over time can indicate a stress fracture. This pain should be differentiated from pain arising from between the metatarsals, which could be caused by impingement of the interdigital nerves. The pain caused by both conditions carries the common trait of worsening with activity.

○ **Great toe pain:** Pain and dysfunction in the great toe can be disabling to the athlete by altering the gait cycle. Pathology within the MTP joint is characterized by diffuse pain throughout the joint during hyperextension. Pain localized to the plantar surface of the joint may be caused by a *sesamoid* fracture or inflammation of the sesamoids (sesamoiditis).

○ **Lateral arch pain:** Compression of the lateral branch of the plantar nerve as it passes through the tarsal tunnel can cause pain radiating along the lateral arch. Acutely, pain may be isolated to the lateral arch following fractures of the fifth MT.

• **Onset and Mechanism of Injury:** As mentioned previously, the length of time the athlete's symptoms have been present, as well as pain that is worsened or diminished with activity, are significant findings.

Acute Onset

○ The acute onset of injuries to the foot may occur from a twisting along its longitudinal axis as the foot lands on an uneven surface. These irregular positions place an increased force across the bones and ligamentous structures as they are stressed beyond their end ranges. A direct blow to the phalanges or metatarsals may result in their fracture.

Insidious Onset

○ **Playing surface:** Has the athlete changed from training on a surface of one density to a surface with a different density? For example, a change from running on an indoor rubberized track to running outdoors on pavement alters the ground reaction forces that are distributed through the foot, ankle, and lower leg. Moving to a harder surface may result in an increased load being placed through these structures, whereas moving to a softer or rubberized surface increases eccentric loading of the muscles due to the surface's rebounding effect.

○ **Distance and duration:** Has the athlete significantly increased the distance, duration, or intensity of training? Athletes who alter these components of their training regimen may increase or alter the forces placed on the body and hinder the foot's ability to accommodate, resulting in overuse injuries. The increased stresses placed on the muscles providing dynamic support to the foot become fatigued, resulting in altered biomechanics.

○ **Shoes:** Has the athlete been wearing shoes that are excessively worn or of an inappropriate type, or does he or she have a new pair of shoes for competition or daily wear? Training shoes that no longer provide adequate support may allow injury-causing forces to reach the foot. Changing either competitive or casual footwear (such as high heels) may alter the biomechanics of the lower extremity and redistribute forces about the foot.

A broad scope of questions is appropriate for the history-taking process. Throughout the remainder of the examination more information detailing the onset of the injury and the factors that increase or decrease the athlete's pain should be obtained.

Inspection

The inspections process may begin before the formal evaluation process by observing the athlete entering the facility. At this time it should be noted whether the athlete was assisted into the facility, is currently using crutches or a cane, or has any gross dysfunction in gait. During the history-taking process the examiner should note any bilateral gross deformity, swelling, or redness in the foot, toes, and ankle (Fig. 3–8). In addition to the inspection of the body area involved, the evaluation of chronic conditions should also encompass the inspection of the athlete's daily casual and participation footwear.

The inspection should be performed while the feet are non–weight bearing and then compared with the findings while the feet are weight bearing. In the non–weight-bearing position the foot is allowed to assume its natural alignment. When weight bearing, the foot reveals the way it compensates for structural abnormalities of the foot, the lower extremity, and the body as a whole.

General Inspection of the Foot

• Calluses and blisters: The entire foot should be inspected for blisters and calluses, as they may indicate improperly fitting shoes, poor biomechanics, or underlying bony or soft tissue dysfunction. Blisters indicate areas of increased pressure caused by friction, rubbing, and/or irritation

---

Sesamoid bone: A bone that lies within a tendon.

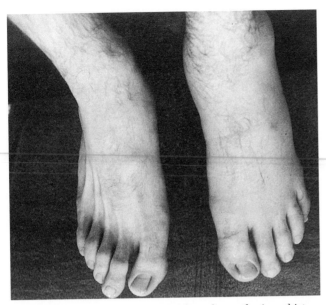

Figure 3–8. Swelling of the foot. Without first gathering a history of the injury, it cannot be determined whether this swelling is caused by trauma to the foot or ankle or by distal migration from a lower leg or knee injury.

of the foot against the shoe and tend to indicate a short-term problem. Calluses develop as the result of long-term pressures. Those located under the first and/or fifth metatarsal heads may indicate a biomechanical deficit such as supination, whereas those under the calcaneus are usually the result of an improper gait pattern.[5]

• **Foot type:** The foot should be observed from the anterior and posterior views to determine its general type: pronated, neutral, or supinated (Fig. 3–9). Feet that are deviated from the neutral classification represent either a structural abnormality within the foot or the foot's adaptation to a structural deficit in the leg, pelvis, or spine. A method of objectively classifying foot type has been proved to have a moderate to high interrater reliability.[6] To be classified as pronated or supinated, the observations must meet the extremes of each of the three categories presented in Table 3–7; otherwise, the foot should be classified as neutral.

Inspection of the Toes

• **Morton's alignment:** This condition, also referred to as **Morton's toe,** is identified by the second toe's being longer than the first toe (Fig. 3–10). This results in a greater amount of force transmitted along the second ray, causing *hypertrophy* of the second metatarsal. A callus may be present under the second metatarsal head.

• **Claw toes:** Characterized by hyperextension of the MTP joint and flexion of the PIP and DIP joints, claw toes are commonly associated with high arches (**pes cavus**) and tend to involve the lateral four toes simultaneously (Fig. 3–11). It is common to find a callus over the dorsal portion of the PIP joint and on the plantar surface of the MTP joint.

• **Hammer toe:** Hammer toe involves the hyperextension of the MTP and DIP joints and flexion of the PIP joint (Fig. 3–12). This position is the result of contractures of the associated toe extensors and flexors and is extenuated by the inability of the interosseous muscles' ability to hold the proximal phalanx in the neutral position. A callus may be found on the dorsal surface of the PIP joint resulting from friction against the shoe. In most cases this deformity affects only one ray and may be caused by improperly fitting shoes (especially during the growth years), hereditary factors, or hallux valgus.[1]

• **Hallux valgus:** The normal alignment of the first MTP joint is 8 to 20 degrees of valgus. When this range is exceeded, the great toe is forced to overlap the second toe, forming what is termed as hallux valgus (Fig. 3–13). Although the overlapping of the toes is the most noticeable trait of hallux valgus, it is generally a benign concern. Pain and dysfunction may result from a bunion over the first MTP joint that occurs secondary to the valgus. Hallux valgus may be congenital or may result from improperly fitting footwear such as pointed-toed shoes.

• **Bunion:** Caused by the development and subsequent inflammation of a bursa, bunions are characterized by redness, inflammation, and tenderness. Causes of bunions include hallux valgus and poorly fitting shoes (Fig. 3–13).

• **Corns:** Also referred to as clavus, corns are a thickening of the stratum corneum and tend to occur in non–weight-bearing areas. **Hard corns** are located in areas that receive excessive pressure and appear as hard, granular nodules on the skin. Hard corns tend to be formed on the proximal portion of the foot and, owing to the resulting biomechanical changes in foot function, progress distally.[7]

Soft corns form between the toes, with the web space between the fourth and fifth toes being the most common site. Dampness in the web space serves to moisten the corn, thus keeping it soft. Both types of corns may be sensitive to the touch and soft corns run the risk of developing an infection because of the moist, warm, dark environment.

• **Ingrown toenail:** These most often involve the

Hypertrophy: The increase in the cross-sectional size of a muscle, bone, or organ.

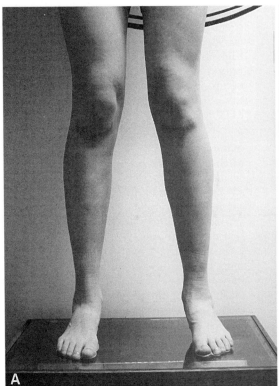

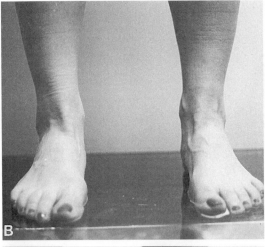

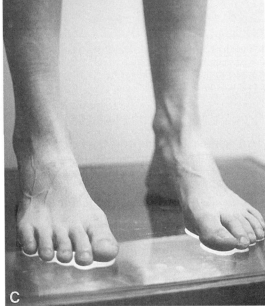

Figure 3–9. Three classifications of feet: (*A*) pronated, (*B*) normal, (*C*) supinated.

great toe. The corners of the nail should be inspected for intrusion into the skin (Fig. 3–14). The areas of ingrowth cause disruption and subsequent infection of the skin surrounding and beneath the nailbed, causing it to appear red and swollen.

• **Subungual hematoma**: A localized trauma to the toenail can result in the formation of a hematoma beneath the nail, a subungual hematoma (Fig. 3–15). Commonly found in the great toe, the resulting collection of blood turns the nail a dark purple and causes a great deal of pain from pressure being placed on the involved nerve endings. Subungual hematoma may form secondary to a fracture of the distal phalanx.

Inspection of the Medial Structures

• **Medial longitudinal arch**: Spanning from the calcaneus to the first MTP joint, the medial longi-

tudinal arch is more prominent when the foot is non–weight bearing. In the non–weight-bearing position, it should be noted whether the arch is abnormally flattened (**pes planus**) or heightened (**pes cavus**). A thorough evaluation of the arch is presented in the Pathologies and Related Special Tests Section of this chapter.

Inspection of the Lateral Structures

• **Fifth metatarsal**: The foot's lateral border normally is relatively straight, especially along the shaft of the fifth MT. The length of the bone should be inspected for deviation of its contour, which indicates a fracture.

Inspection of the Dorsal Structures

The dorsal surface of the foot is thinly covered by the long toe extensors and the small mass of the ex-

Table 3–7. Classification Scheme for Defining Foot Type (Weight Bearing)

Pronated Foot	Supinated Foot
• The calcaneus must be everted greater than 3° from perpendicular relative to the position of the ground.	• The calcaneus must be inverted greater than 3° from perpendicular relative to the position of the ground.
• A medial bulge must be present at the talonavicular joint, indicating excessive talar adduction.	• A medial bulge must *not* be present at the talonavicular joint, indicating excessive talar adduction.
• The medial arch must be low. This is determined by Feiss' line, formed by connecting the points formed by the head of the first MT, the navicular tubercle, and the medial malleolus (see the description of Feiss' line in the Arch Pathologies section of this chapter). If this angle is in the range of 30°–90°, the arch is considered low.	• Using Feiss' line, the arch must be high (150°–180°).

Each of the three criteria under each of the foregoing headings must be met for the foot to be classified as such. Otherwise the foot should be categorized as neutral.

Adapted from Dahle.[6]

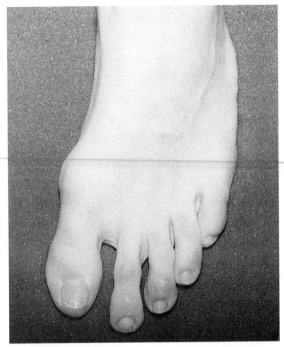

Figure 3–10. Morton's toe. The second toe extends past the great toe. Note also the presence of a bunion over the lateral aspect of the first metatarsophalangeal joint and callus development over the interphalangeal joints.

tensor digitorum brevis laterally. The dorsal aspect of the foot should be observed for swelling, discoloration, or abnormal bony alignment.

Inspection of the Plantar Surface

The length of the plantar surface of the foot should be inspected, paying particular attention to the condition of the skin and the presence of callus formation or blisters as noted previously.

• **Plantar warts**: A common dermatological abnormality afflicting the foot's plantar aspect are plantar warts (Fig. 3–16). These tend to be localized in areas of calloused skin in areas of excessive weight-bearing stresses. They are more focal than an ordinary callus and can be point-tender. Plantar warts mask the normal **whorls** and skin markings, thus differentiating them from callus build-up.

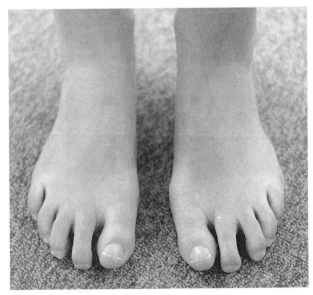

Figure 3–11. "Claw toe" deformity that is caused by hyperextension of the metatarsophalangeal joints and flexion of the proximal and distal interphalangeal joints. This condition is often associated with pes cavus.

___

Whorls: Swirl markings in the skin. Fingerprints are images formed by the whorls on the fingertips.

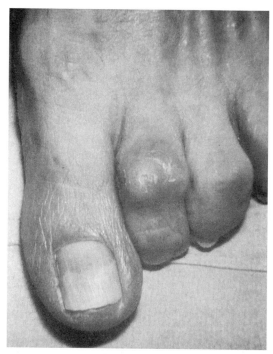

Figure 3–12. "Hammer toe" deformity resulting from hyperextension of the metatarsophalangeal and distal interphalangeal joints combined with flexion of the proximal interphalangeal joint.

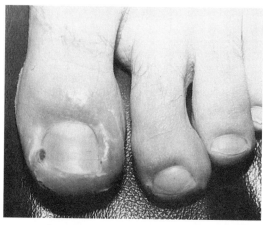

Figure 3–14. Ingrown toenail. This painful condition results from abnormal growth patterns of the nail, causing it to imbed with the skin.

Inspection of the Posterior Structures

• **Achilles tendon:** With the athlete in the weight-bearing position, the relationship of the Achilles tendon to the tibia should be observed. Normally these two structures should be in alignment. Bowing of the tendon may be an indication of pes planus (Fig. 3–17).

Inspection of Foot and Calcaneal Alignment

The following inspection of the relative alignment of the forefoot, midfoot, and hindfoot are performed with the athlete weight bearing (Fig. 3–18).

• **Forefoot varus:** This condition involves inversion of the forefoot on the hindfoot so the medial side of the forefoot is higher than the lateral side. The normal valgus tilt (35 to 45 degrees) of the talar head and neck is not present, resulting in a resemblance to pes planus.

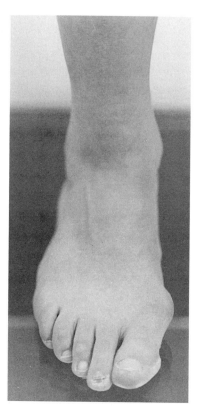

Figure 3–13. Increased angle between the long axis of the first metatarsal and the great toe, hallux valgus. Over time, this condition leads to the development of a bunion over the medial border of the metatarsophalangeal joint. In more severe cases, the great toe rests on top of the second toe.

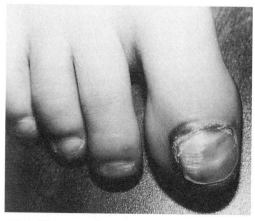

Figure 3–15. Trauma to the toe can result in bleeding under the nail, a subungual hematoma. Often, the blood must be drained from beneath the nail.

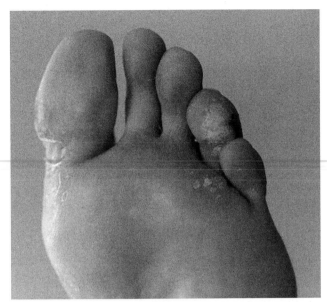

Figure 3–16. Plantar warts. This condition results in point tenderness and masks the normal skin markings, thus distinguishing it from callus.

- **Forefoot valgus:** Clinically resembling pes cavus, the midtarsal joint is supinated so that the lateral aspect of the foot contacts the ground. In this case the normal valgus tilt of the talar head has been exceeded.

- **Hindfoot varus:** During inspection of the weight-bearing foot and ankle, hindfoot varus is indicated by inversion of the calcaneus owing to the bony configuration of the foot and ankle complex, a varus alignment of the tibia, or a congenital defect in which the calcaneus does not completely derotate from its fetal position.[8] The hindfoot becomes rigid, increasing supination and decreasing the amount of pronation available to the foot. Chronic cases may result in retrocalcaneal exostosis "pump bumps" (Fig. 3–19).

- **Hindfoot valgus:** Taking an opposite alignment of hindfoot varus, the calcaneus is everted in athletes suffering from hindfoot valgus. The hindfoot becomes more mobile, resulting in increased pronation of the foot.

Non–Weight-Bearing Inspection of Foot and Calcaneal Alignment

A thorough assessment of foot alignment requires comparative measures taken when the foot is weight bearing and again when the foot is non–weight bearing. To assess the position of the foot while it is non–weight bearing, the athlete is positioned prone so that the feet and ankles are lying over the edge of the examination table.

- **Assessment of talar position:** With the right foot as an example, the examiner places the left thumb and index fingers over the sides of the talar dome. The examiner's right hand should dor-

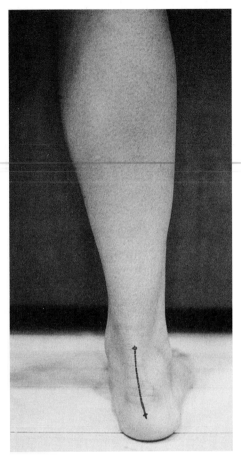

Figure 3–17. Achilles tendon alignment in an individual with pes planus.

siflex the ankle and begin to invert and evert the foot (Fig. 3–20). The neutral position of the talus is determined by the symmetry of the talus within the mortise. When the talus is in its neutral position, the alignment of the forefoot and hindfoot should be noted.

- **Mobility of the first ray:** The metatarsonavicular joint and the first MPT joint should be as-

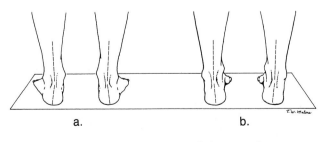

a.	b.
Calcaneovarus	Calcaneovalgus

Figure 3–18. (a) Rearfoot valgus (calcaneovalgus), pronation of the subtalar joint caused by eversion of the calcaneus. (b) Rearfoot varus (calcaneovarus), supination of the subtalar joint associated with calcaneal inversion. (From Norkin, CC, and Levangie, PK,[3] p 390, with permission.)

sessed for normal mobility. Pes cavus is often marked by hypermobility of the first ray; pes planus may result in a rigid ray.

Palpation

To increase the ease of palpation, the athlete should be positioned so that the foot and ankle extend off the end of the evaluation table. The related ankle structures should be included during the palpation phase of a foot evaluation.

Palpation of the Medial Bony and Ligamentous Structures

• **First metatarsophalangeal joint**: The clinician should locate the articulation between the proximal phalanx of the first toe and the first metatarsal. This area is palpated for any tenderness or increased skin temperature that may indicate acute injury to the ligamentous structures, chronic inflammatory conditions of the tendons or articular structures, or disease states such as *gout*.

• **First metatarsal**: The clinician should palpate the length of the first metatarsal, noting any crepitus, bony deformity, or pain elicited along the shaft. Because the dorsal and medial surfaces and part of the plantar surface of this bone are easily palpated, gross fractures can be identified with relative ease. If a fracture is suspected, the evaluation should be terminated, the foot immobilized, and the athlete referred to a physician.

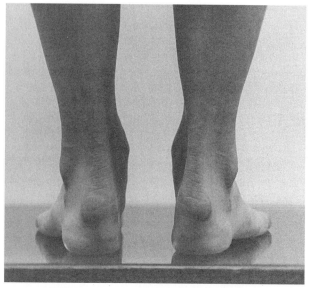

Figure 3–19. Retrocalcaneal exostosis, "pump bumps."

• **First cuneiform**: The base of the first metatarsal articulates with the first cuneiform and can be identified by the attachment of the tibialis anterior. During active plantarflexion, the peroneus longus causes the base of the first metatarsal to be depressed on the cuneiform, making this junction more palpable.

• **Navicular**: The clinician should continue to palpate proximally and identify where the first

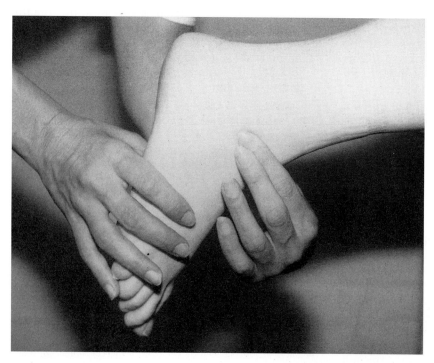

Figure 3–20. Finding the neutral position of the talus. Subtalar neutral is found when the talus fits symmetrically within the mortise.

Gout: A form of acute arthritis marked by inflammation and pain in the distal joints.

cuneiform articulates with the medial border of the navicular. The navicular serves as the keystone of the medial longitudinal arch. As such, any dysfunction of this bone results in dysfunction of the arch as a whole.

• **Talar head**: Immediately proximal to the navicular is the talar head. This structure is more easily located by inverting and everting the forefoot. When the forefoot is in eversion, the talar head is more prominent medially.

• **Sustentaculum tali**: Located distal to the medial malleolus is the sustentaculum tali, a protrusion off the calcaneus. Serving as an attachment site for the spring ligament and providing inferior support to the talus, this structure is not always easily identifiable.

• **Spring ligament**: The plantar calcaneonavicular ligament may be palpated from its origin off the sustentaculum tali to its insertion on the navicular. In cases of pes planus or forefoot sprains, this ligament may become very tender to the touch.

• **Medial talar tubercle**: The clinician should palpate proximally and superiorly to locate the small projection off the proximal-medial border of the talus, immediately adjacent to the posterior margin of the medial malleolus. The medial talar tubercle serves as a site of attachment for a portion of the ankle's deltoid ligament.

• **Calcaneal dome**: From the medial talar tubercle, the clinician should palpate inferiorly to locate the posterior flair of the calcaneus and continue to palpate to the site of the Achilles tendon attachment.

Palpation of the Medial Musculature

• **Flexor hallucis longus**: The bulk of this muscle is hidden beneath the gastrocnemius and soleus and is not palpable until its tendon begins its path behind and around the medial malleolus. It is difficult to distinguish this tendon from the other structures in the area. As the tendon begins its course along the plantar aspect of the foot it once again is no longer palpable until it inserts on the distal phalanx of the great toe.

• **Flexor digitorum longus**: Like the flexor hallucis longus, the mass of the flexor digitorum longus is not identifiable as it lies beneath the bulk of the gastrocnemius and soleus muscles. Its tendon is palpable, although not uniquely identifiable, as it passes behind and around the medial malleolus. As it passes along the plantar aspect of the foot it is no longer palpable until it inserts on the plantar aspect of the second through fifth toes.

• **Tibialis posterior**: Palpation of this muscle is described in Chapter 4. Its attachment site on the

medial aspect of the navicular may elicit tenderness in the presence of pathology.

Palpation of the Lateral Bony Structures

• **Fifth metatarsophalangeal joint**: The articulation between the fifth toe and fifth metatarsal must be located. The joint should be palpated for tenderness arising from ligaments or articular damage.

• **Fifth metatarsal**: The clinician should palpate the length of the fifth metatarsal and note any pain or discontinuity in the bone's shaft. This structure, especially at its proximal end, is the site of many acute and stress fractures.

• **Styloid process**: The base of the fifth metatarsal is marked by a laterally projecting styloid process where the peroneus brevis muscle attaches. Covered by a bursa, this is a common site for stress fractures as well as for an avulsion fracture of the peroneus brevis tendon from its attachment (Jones fracture).

• **Cuboid**: By palpating immediately proximal to the styloid process the cuboid may be identified. At the middle portion of the lateral cuboid is the groove through which the peroneus longus passes beneath the foot.

• **Lateral border of the calcaneus**: From the cuboid, one should continue to palpate toward the hindfoot. The junction between the cuboid and the calcaneus is often indistinct. The most prominent bony landmark on the calcaneus is the **peroneal tubercle**, located inferiorly and slightly distal to the most distal portion of the lateral malleolus. The peroneal tubercle marks the point at which the peroneus longus and brevis tendons diverge after jointly slinging behind the lateral malleolus.

Palpation of the Lateral Musculature

• **Peroneal tendons**: Palpation of the peroneus longus and brevis is described in Chapter 4. Injury to these structures may result in pain at the base of the fifth MT and cuboid.

Palpation of the Dorsal Bony Structures

• **Sinus tarsi**: Located anteriorly to the lateral malleolus is the sinus tarsi. Normally this landmark appears as a depression in the forefoot and marks the site of the extensor digitorum brevis muscle. Following acute trauma including ankle sprains, tarsal fractures, or dislocations or with chronic conditions such as arthritis, the sinus may fill with fluid and become sensitive to the touch.

• **Dome of the talus**: The clinician should palpate medially to find the dome of the talus. This structure is more easily located if the foot and ankle are placed in inversion and plantarflexion, allowing the dome's lateral border to become palpable from under the ankle mortise.

- **Cuneiforms:** The cuneiforms are virtually indistinguishable from each other to the touch, but their locations can be approximated relative to the first three metatarsals. The three cuneiforms each articulate with the first three metatarsals; by palpating the length of the metatarsals to their bases, the individual cuneiforms can be identified (see Fig. 3–2).

- **Rays:** Starting with the distal phalanx, the clinician should palpate the length of the toes through the length of its associated metatarsal, noting any deformity, crepitus, or pain elicited during this process.

Palpation of the Dorsal Musculature and Related Soft Tissue

- **Tibialis anterior:** The tendon of the tibialis anterior is more prominent when the foot is inverted and the ankle dorsiflexed, allowing its insertion on the first cuneiform to be located. As it crosses the talocrural joint, the tendon is quite palpable, but it quickly loses its identity as it flairs into its musculotendinous junction.

- **Extensor hallucis longus:** Locate the extensor hallucis longus (EHL) tendon by palpating laterally from the tibialis anterior tendon. When the athlete actively extends the great toe, the length of the tendon from its point of deviation from the tibialis anterior to its flair into the distal phalanx can be easily seen and palpated. One should continue to palpate the length of the EHL to the point of insertion along the middle half of the anterior fibula and adjacent interosseous membrane.

- **Extensor digitorum longus:** Lateral to the extensor hallucis longus is the tendon of the extensor digitorum longus. Although the central portion of the tendon is difficult to palpate, its individual slips to the lateral four toes are prominent on the dorsal aspect of the foot when the toes are extended.

- **Extensor digitorum brevis:** The origin and proximal body of the extensor digitorum brevis can be palpated in the sinus tarsi when the toes are actively extended. The tendinous slips to each of the toes become indistinguishable as they pass under the long toe tendons. The most medial portion of the extensor digitorum brevis muscle and its tendon attaching on the first toe is often referred to as a separate muscle, the **extensor hallucis brevis**.

- **Inferior extensor retinaculum:** As the tendons of tibialis anterior, extensor hallucis longus, and extensor digitorum longus pass over the talus and tarsals, their proximity to the bones during dorsiflexion is maintained by the inferior extensor **retinaculum**. The inferior extensor retinaculum traverses the entire upper portion of the foot and should be palpated along its entire length.

- **Dorsalis pedal artery:** Lying between the extensor hallucis longus tendon and the extensor digitorum longus tendon is the dorsalis pedal artery, whose pulse may be felt over the area of the talus. Although this pulse may not be felt in all individuals, the clinician should attempt to detect the presence of a pulse and compare it with the opposite extremity. A unilateral absence or decreased pulse may be indicative of a vascular obstruction such as **anterior compartment syndrome** (see Chapter 4).

Palpation of the Plantar Bony Structures

The plantar surfaces of the calcaneus and the metatarsal heads are padded by fatty deposits and overlying thick skin, making the identification of specific structures difficult. The examiner must rely on approximations and functional tests in identifying and determining many painful tissues.

- **Medial calcaneal tubercle:** The medial calcaneal tubercle can be located by identifying the point that the heel pad begins to thin and merge into the medial longitudinal arch. From this point, the clinician moves to the medial ridge and applies pressure upward and toward the calcaneus. The anterior ridge of the medial calcaneal tubercle is the attachment site of the plantar fascia and the flexor digitorum brevis muscle. The medial border of this structure is the site of origin of the abductor hallucis.

Pain elicited during palpation of this area may be indicative of **plantar fasciitis** or a **heel spur**. A form of exostosis, heel spurs are an abnormal bony outgrowth of the plantar fascia's attachment to the calcaneus (Fig. 3–21).

- **Plantar fascia:** From its origin on the calcaneus, the plantar fascia is palpated through its length and breadth to its attachment on each of the metatarsal heads. Athletes suffering from plantar fasciitis may demonstrate tenderness along the length of the fascia, and the examiner should note the presence of any painful areas within this structure.

- **Sesamoid bones of the great toe:** One palpates along the plantar surface of the first metatarsal to reach the first MTP joint. At this point two small

---

Retinaculum: A ligamentous tissue serving as a restraining band to hold other tissues in place.

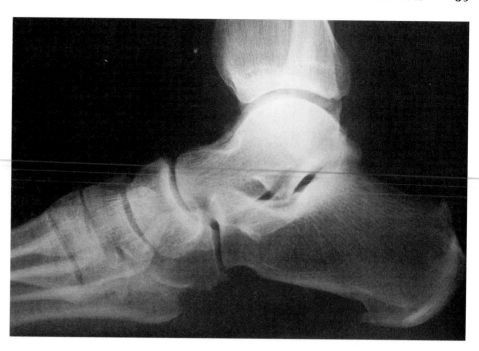

Figure 3–21. X ray of a heel spur. Note the hooklike projection arising from the anterior border of the calcaneal tuberosity.

sesamoid bones may be palpated in the flexor hallucis brevis tendon. Inflammatory conditions of these bones, **sesamoiditis**, or fractures elicit pain to the touch or while weight bearing, especially during the toe-off phase of gait, when pressure is applied to the ball of the foot and the joint is extended. The onset of sesamoiditis has been linked to rigidity of the first ray.[9]

• **Metatarsal heads:** From the first MTP joint, each of the metatarsal heads is palpated, with the examiner noting for the presence and integrity of the transverse arch located beneath the heads. The pads under the first and fifth metatarsal heads should be the thickest, as they are the primary weight-bearing areas of the forefoot.

• **Interdigital neuroma:** During the palpation of the metatarsal heads, a gentle pressure to the area between the metatarsals should be applied. Nerves located in this area can become inflamed and cause dysfunction of the foot and lower extremity.

Palpation of the Plantar Musculature

The intrinsic muscles of the plantar aspect of the foot cannot be palpated directly.

Functional Tests

This section describes the range of motion tests for the MTP joints only. A relatively small amount of motion is available at the IP joint and is difficult to accurately measure. The results of these tests should be compared bilaterally to determine any pathological conditions at these joints. Plantarflex-

ion, dorsiflexion, inversion, and eversion tests for the ankle are described in Chapter 4.

Active Range of Motion

• **Flexion and extension:** The greatest amount of range of motion occurs at the first MTP joint, allowing 75 to 85 degrees of extension and 35 to 45 degrees of flexion (Fig. 3–22). The first MTP joint must permit 60 to 65 degrees of extension; otherwise compensatory excessive pronation occurs during gait.[10] The range of motion available to the MTP joints decreases at each subsequent lateral joint. Active motion at the fifth MTP joint is negligible.

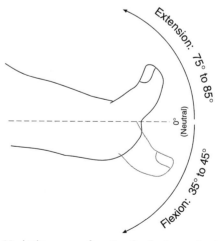

Figure 3–22. Active range of motion for flexion and extension of the great toe's metatarsophalangeal joint. The range of motion decreases with each subsequent joint.

Passive Range of Motion

Because the muscles acting on the lateral four toes are different from those acting on the hallux, passive motion should be determined for the first toe by itself and the motion at the lateral four toes as a unit.

- **Flexion**: The forefoot should be stabilized proximal to the MT heads. To prevent contribution from the IP joints, pressure should be applied on the dorsal portion of the proximal phalanx when testing both the hallux and the lateral four toes (Fig. 3–23). The normal end-feel for flexion is firm owing to tension of the dorsal fibers of the joint capsule and the collateral ligaments.

- **Extension**: Stabilization is maintained as described for measurement of passive flexion, but pressure is applied to the proximal phalanx's plantar aspect (Fig. 3–24). A firm end-feel arises from the capsule's plantar fibers and the short flexor muscles.

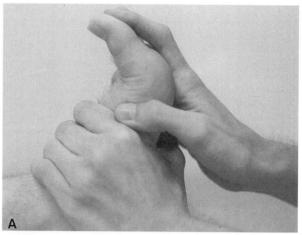

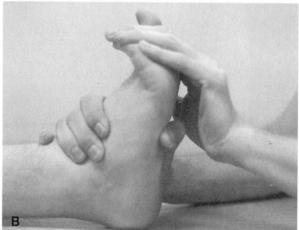

Figure 3–24. Passive extension of the (A) great toe and (B) lateral four toes.

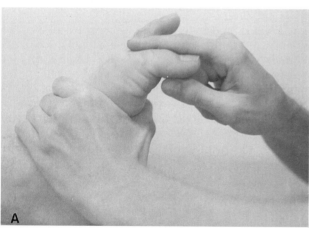

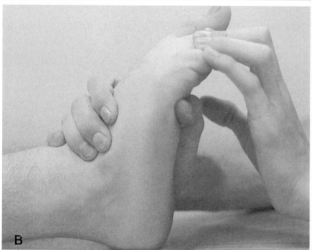

Figure 3–23. Passive flexion of the (A) great toe and (B) lateral four toes.

Resisted Range of Motion

- **Flexion**: The forefoot is stabilized by grasping the metatarsals proximal to their heads. Resistance is provided to the hallux along the entire length of the toe to discount any contribution that may be provided by flexion of the IP joint. Resistance is provided to the lateral four toes by using two or three fingers along the toe's plantar aspect (Fig. 3–25).

- **Extension**: While stabilizing the forefoot in the same manner described for resisted toe flexion, resistance is provided to extension along the dorsal aspect of the toes. The great toe should be tested individually from the lateral four toes.

Ligamentous and Capsular Testing

With the exception of the MTP and IP joints, it is difficult, if not impossible, to identify trauma to

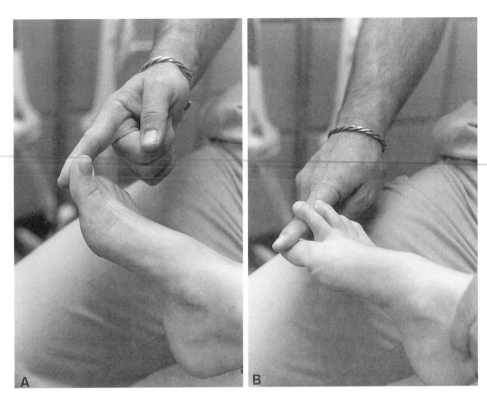

Figure 3–25. Resisted (*A*) flexion and (*B*) extension of the great toe.

specific ligaments of the foot because of its flexibility and their number. This section describes how to isolate stresses to the ligaments stabilizing the toes and less definitive ligamentous stresses to the foot itself.

Metatarsophalangeal and Interphalangeal Joints

Medially and laterally the MTP and IP joints are supported by the collateral ligaments, and the dorsal and plantar surfaces of these articulations are reinforced by the joint capsule. Passive overpressure in flexion, as described in the Passive Range of Motion section of this chapter, is used to determine the integrity of the dorsal joint capsule; passive overpressure in extension checks the integrity of the plantar capsule.

The application of a ***valgus force*** stresses the medial collateral ligaments of the joint. A ***varus force*** stresses the lateral collateral ligaments (Fig. 3–26). The results of this examination should be compared with those obtained when the test is repeated on the same joint on the opposite extremity.

Valgus Stress Testing of the MTP and IP Joints (Fig. 3–26A)

Position of athlete	Supine or sitting with the knees extended.
Position of examiner	Standing lateral to the involved foot. The proximal bone is stabilized close to the joint to be tested. The bone distal to the joint being tested is grasped near the middle of its shaft. Care must be taken to isolate the joint being tested.
Evaluative procedure	The distal bone is moved laterally, attempting to open up the joint on the medial side.
Positive tests	Increased laxity when compared to the same joint on the opposite extremity, or pain.
Implications	Medial collateral ligament sprain of the involved joint.

Valgus force: A force applied toward the body's midline (medially).
Varus force: A force applied from the body's midline outward (laterally).

Varus Stress Testing of the MTP and IP Joints (Fig. 3–26*B*)

Position of athlete	Supine or sitting with the knees extended.
Position of examiner	Standing lateral to the involved foot. The proximal bone is stabilized close to the joint to be tested. The bone distal to the joint being tested is grasped near the middle of its shaft. Care must be taken to isolate the joint being tested.
Evaluative procedure	The distal bone is moved medially, attempting to open up the joint on the lateral side.
Positive tests	Increased laxity when compared to the same joint on the opposite extremity, or pain.
Implications	Lateral collateral ligament sprain of the involved joint.

Proximal Intermetatarsal Joints

The deep transverse metatarsal ligaments and the interosseous ligaments secure the MT heads in a relatively immobile alignment. Forces that cause an abnormal amount of glide between any two MT heads can result in these ligaments being traumatized. Forcing a glide, thus duplicating the mechanism of injury, can be used to check the integrity of these structures (Fig. 3–27). The amount of glide should be compared bilaterally.

Intermetatarsal Glide (Fig. 3–27)

Position of athlete	Supine or sitting with the knees extended.
Position of examiner	Standing in front of the athlete's feet. One hand grasps the first MT head; the other grasps the second MT head.
Evaluative procedure	The two MT heads are moved in opposite directions. This procedure is repeated by moving to the lateral MT heads until all four intermetarsal joints have been evaluated.
Positive test results	Pain or increased glide compared with the opposite extremity.
Implications	Trauma to the deep transverse metatarsal ligament and/or interosseous ligament.

Ligaments of the Midfoot

The ligaments of the midfoot cannot be accurately isolated for ligamentous testing. An evaluation that leads the clinician to believe that a midfoot sprain exists is made from a history involving twisting, pain with gross movements of the ankle and foot, and pain during palpation following an x ray to rule out the presence of a fracture.

Neurological Examination

Neurological dysfunction can radiate into the foot secondary to lumbar nerve root impingement or trauma to the peripheral nerves. Pathologies such as **peroneal nerve palsy** and **anterior compartment syndrome** (both covered in Chapter 4) can result in symptoms radiating into the foot (see page 73 for Neurological Screen).

Pathologies and Related Special Tests

Many of the conditions affecting the normal function of the foot may be traced to improper biomechanics of the foot itself or are caused by the foot's compensating for biomechanical deficits elsewhere in the lower extremity.

Arch Pathologies

Abnormalities of the arch may be caused by acute trauma or disease states or, more commonly, may

Neurological Screen

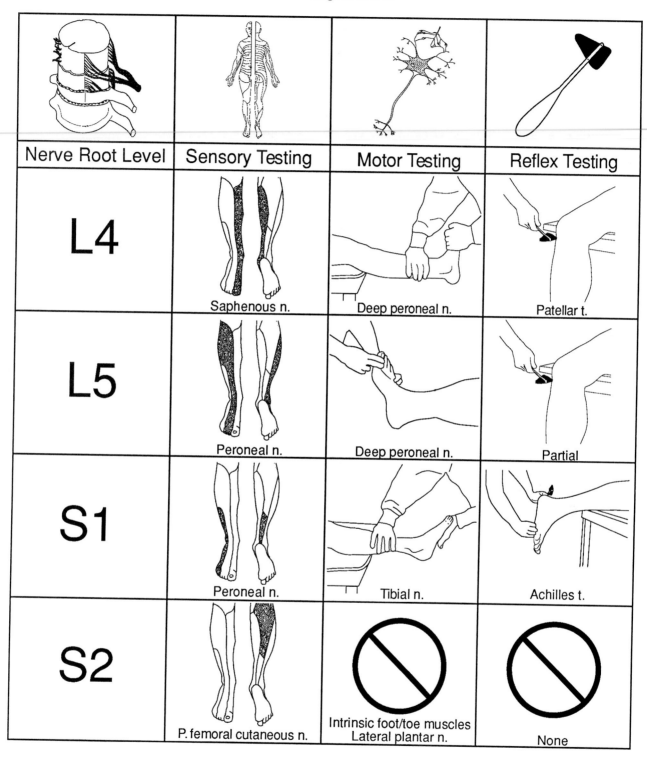

Nerve Root Level	Sensory Testing	Motor Testing	Reflex Testing
L4	Saphenous n.	Deep peroneal n.	Patellar t.
L5	Peroneal n.	Deep peroneal n.	Partial
S1	Peroneal n.	Tibial n.	Achilles t.
S2	P. femoral cutaneous n.	Intrinsic foot/toe muscles Lateral plantar n.	None

occur congenitally. Many athletes successfully compete throughout long careers with pes planus or pes cavus. It is only when these conditions become painful or cause pain or biomechanical dysfunction elsewhere that they become of concern. Possible ramifications of altered arch structure include plantar fasciitis, heel spurs, and patellofemoral pain for pes planus and claw toes, metatarsal stress fractures, or a plantar fascia rupture for pes cavus.

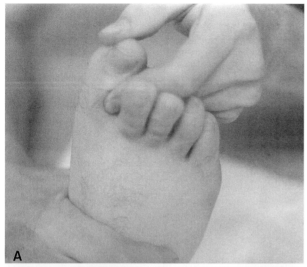

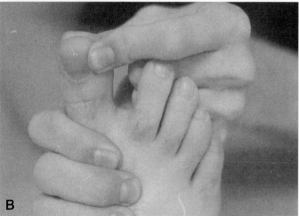

Figure 3–26. Stress testing of the toe's capsular ligaments: (*A*) valgus stress applied to the interphalangeal joint; (*B*) varus stress applied to the metatarsophalangeal joint.

Pes Planus

Pes planus is characterized by a flattening of the medial longitudinal arch, hence its colloquial name, "flat feet" (Fig. 3–28). Although pes planus may result from acute trauma, its onset is usually gradual or congenital. The depression of the arch is closely associated with pronation of the foot (the talus being tilted toward the midline of the body) and often subluxation of the navicular, resulting in the talar head's becoming more prominent.

Traumatic, symptomatic pes planus can be related to a fracture of an **accessory navicular**.[11] The accessory navicular is an abnormal osseous outgrowth on the navicular, which, when present, serves as a partial attachment site for the tibialis posterior. When the union between the accessory navicular and the navicular itself is "fractured," the effectiveness of the tibialis posterior in supporting the medial arch is decreased. Furthermore, the motion between the two bony segments results in pain.

Mechanical factors leading to pes planus include weakness of the tibialis posterior, tibialis anterior, and the short and long flexors of the toes. Stretching or weakness of the supporting ligaments, especially the spring ligament, results from the plantarmedial displacement of the talus and further extenuates the amount of weight-bearing pronation. These events may be triggered or exaggerated by postural abnormalities of the spine and lower extremity to which the foot must adapt during weight bearing.

Pes planus may be classified as being either rigid (structural) or flexible (supple). Rigid pes planus is marked by the absence of the medial longitudinal arch when the foot is both weight bearing and non–weight bearing. With supple pes planus,

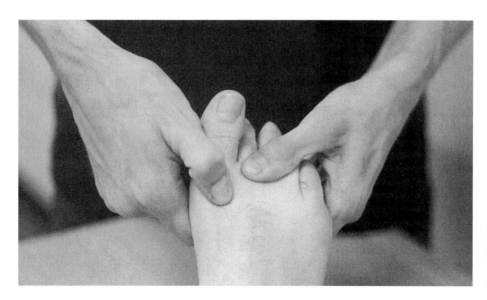

Figure 3–27. Testing the amount of intermetatarsal glide between the first and second metatarsal heads. This test should be performed for each of the four articulations formed between the five metatarsals.

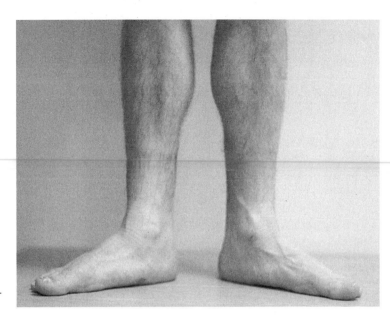

Figure 3–28. Pes planus. Note the absence of the medial longitudinal arch.

the arch appears normal when it is non–weight bearing, but the arch disappears when the foot is weight bearing. Supple pes planus may be corrected with the use of firm orthotics, but semirigid orthotics may be used with athletes with rigid pes planus to decrease certain biomechanical deficiencies.

Two tests may be used to determine the severity of downward displacement of the navicular while the foot is weight bearing. A rough estimation of the downward displacement may be made using **Feiss' line**, in which the amount of navicular drop is estimated relative to a line spanning the distance from the plantar aspect of the first MTP joint and the me-

dial malleolus. A more quantitative measure can be performed using the **navicular drop test**, in which the distance the navicular is displaced inferiorly is calculated.

Test for Supple Pes Planus. This test is meaningful only in those cases where a normal longitudinal arch is present during non–weight bearing. During this test, the examiner simply observes if a normal-appearing medial longitudinal arch disappears during weight bearing (Fig. 3–29). If this test result is positive, the presence of a supple flat foot may be confirmed by having the athlete perform a heel-raise. The arch should reappear because of the windlass effect of the plantar fascia.

Test for Supple Pes Planus (Fig. 3–29)

Position of athlete	Sitting on the edge of the examination table.
Position of examiner	Positioned on a stool facing the athlete.
Evaluative procedure	With the athlete in a non–weight-bearing position the examiner notes the presence of a medial longitudinal arch. The examiner asks the athlete to stand so that the body weight is evenly distributed.
Positive test results	Presence of a medial longitudinal arch.
Implications	If the medial longitudinal arch disappears when weight bearing, a supple pes planus is present.

Feiss' Line. This method of determining the amount of navicular drop during weight bearing relies on the examiner's estimating the proportion of the drop based on units of thirds (Fig. 3–30).

Feiss' Line (Fig. 3–30)

Position of athlete	Sitting with the feet off the end of the table.
Position of examiner	At the feet of the athlete. With the athlete non–weight bearing, the examiner identifies and marks the apex of the medial malleolus, the navicular tubercle, and the plantar aspect of the first MTP joint. A line is drawn connecting the marks over the first MTP joint and the medial malleolus.
Evaluative procedure	The athlete stands with the feet approximately 1 ft apart and the weight evenly distributed. The new position of the navicular tubercle is marked.
Positive test results	A navicular that drops two-thirds of the distance to the floor or greater.
Implications	Hyperpronation of the foot.

Navicular Drop Test. The degree of weight-bearing foot pronation may be determined by the navicular drop test.[12,13] Using a 3 × 5 index card, the level of the navicular is marked when the athlete is non–weight bearing and weight bearing (Fig. 3–31). The degree of navicular drop is then calculated by measuring the distance, in millimeters, between the two positions.

Navicular Drop Test (Fig. 3–31)

Position of athlete	Sitting with both feet on the floor. A noncarpeted surface is recommended. With the athlete non–weight bearing, a dot is placed over the navicular tuberosity.
Position of examiner	Kneeling in front of the athlete.
Evaluative procedure	The subtalar joint is placed in the neutral position with the athlete's foot flat against the ground, but non–weight bearing. A 3 × 5 index card is positioned next to the medial longitudinal arch. A mark is made on the card corresponding to the level of the navicular. The athlete stands with the body weight evenly distributed between the two feet, and the foot is allowed to relax. The new level of the navicular is marked on the index card. The relative displacement (drop) of the navicular is determined by measuring the distance between the two marks (in millimeters).
Positive test results	The navicular drops greater than 10 mm.
Implications	Hyperpronation of the foot.

Pes Cavus

Appearing as a high medial longitudinal arch, pes cavus is a congenital foot deformity, although certain disease states may result in its presence. Upon inspection, the examiner notes a spreading of the forefoot and the apparent drop of the forefoot relative to the hindfoot caused by the depression of the metatarsal heads (Fig. 3–32). The dorsal pads under the calcaneus and the metatarsal heads appear smaller than in a "normal" foot. The lateral four toes are normally clawed and calluses may be found over the PIP joints. This foot type is associated with a generalized stiffness and impaired ability to adapt to ground contact forces.

Transverse Metatarsal Arch

Pain may be present over the heads of the second through fifth MTs as the result of a deficit in the transverse metatarsal arch. This can be inspected and palpated from the plantar aspect of the involved foot and compared with the uninvolved side.

Plantar Fasciitis

The plantar fascia has been implicated as the most common site of heel pain in runners.[14] Trauma to the plantar fascia may lead to its inflammation, a pulling away of its origin from the calcaneus, a strain of its tissues, or its complete rupture. Inflam-

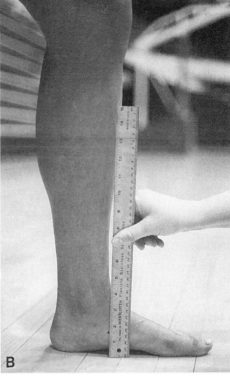

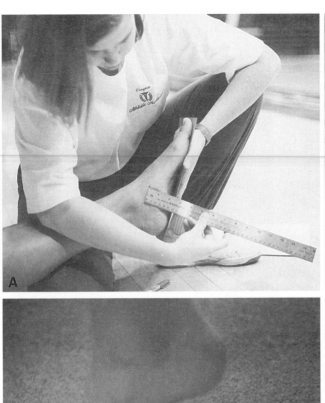

Figure 3–29. Supple pes planus. (*A*) The athlete displays a normal arch in the non–weight-bearing position. (*B*) In weight bearing, the arch disappears (ruler added for demonstrative purposes). (*C*) When the athlete performs a toe-raise, the arch returns by means of the windlass effect.

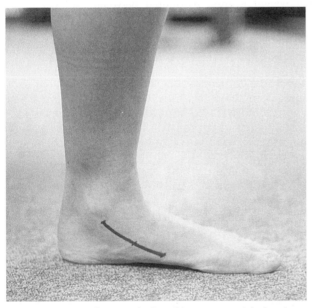

Figure 3–30. Feiss' line. With the athlete non–weight bearing, a line is drawn from the apex of the medial malleolus, navicular tubercle, and the plantar aspect of the first metatarsophalangeal joint. The displacement of the navicular tubercle is marked when the athlete bears weight.

mation of this structure may predispose it to tearing-type injuries secondary to the functional shortening of its tissues.

Inflammation of the plantar fascia may result from a single traumatic episode, or more commonly, secondary to repeated stress. Abnormal foot construction, pes planus or pes cavus, predisposes the athlete to the onset of this condition.

Pain tends to be centralized around the plantar fascia's origin on the medial calcaneal tubercle, but the length of the fascia may be tender as well. The classic symptom is pain when stepping out of bed in the morning. Initially the athlete complains of pain in the heel when resting after activity. As this injury progresses, pain is experienced with the onset of activity, subsiding secondary to stretching of the tissues and increased blood flow to the area. In the chronic stage, the athlete complains of almost constant pain (Table 3–8).

Tightness of the triceps surae muscle group is another common clinical finding associated with plantar fasciitis. These muscles pull upward on the calcaneus, moving it into plantarflexion, increasing and prolonging the tension on the plantar fascia as it attaches at the calcaneal tubercle.

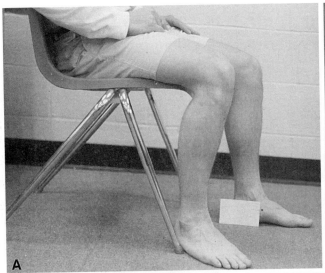

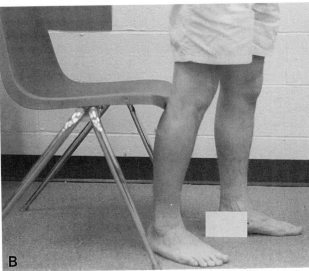

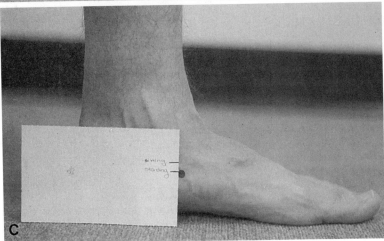

Figure 3–31. Navicular drop test. (*A*) The level of the navicular tuberosity is identified with the athlete seated and the foot non–weight bearing. (*B*) With the athlete standing and the weight evenly distributed between the two feet, the level of the navicular tuberosity is marked. (*C*) The functional measure of this test is the distance in millimeters that the navicular displaces inferiorly.

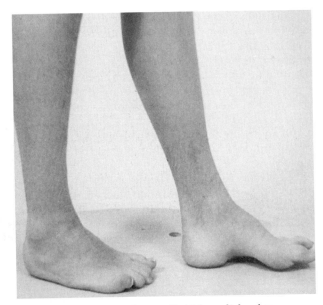

Figure 3–32. Pes cavus, abnormally high medial arches.

When accompanied by pes planus or pes cavus, plantar fasciitis may be considered a symptom of changes in the foot's biomechanics.[15] In this event, the problem with the arch must be corrected to alleviate the plantar fasciitis. Chronic cases of plantar fasciitis may lead to the development of a heel spur and/or hallux rigidus, leading to a significant decrease in the amount of strength and range of motion available to the foot and its plantarflexors and dorsiflexors.[16]

Heel Spur

Prolonged inflammatory conditions of the plantar fascia or pes planus can lead to exostosis at the site where the plantar fascia attaches to the calcaneus. The shortening of the plantar fascia increases the amount of tension placed on the attachment site of the fascia. This results in a bony outgrowth (exostosis) of the attachment site, which generally assumes a hooked shape (see Fig. 3–21).

Table 3–8. Evaluative Findings of Plantar Fasciitis

Examination Segment	Clinical Findings	
History	Onset:	Either acute or insidious.
	Location of pain:	Pain is centralized near the medical calcaneal tubercle and can be spread throughout the fascia. The athlete may describe pain when stepping, especially after being in a non–weight-bearing position and especially upon weight bearing when awakening in the morning.
	Mechanism:	Acute: Forced dorsiflexion of the ankle combined with toe extension.
		Insidious: Increased activity, additional distance when running, changing surface, or new or different shoes.
Inspection	In some cases swelling may be noted on the plantar aspect near the calcaneus. Pes planus may be noted.	
Palpation	Pain is at or near the origin of the plantar fascia and, on occasion, runs the length of the plantar fascia.	
Functional tests	Pain may be experienced during both active and passive ankle dorsiflexion and toe extension because of the stretch placed on the plantar fascia.	
Ligamentous tests	Not applicable.	
Neurological tests	Not applicable.	
Special tests	None.	
Comments	Plantar fasciitis may result secondary to pes planus and may lead to the development of heel spurs.	

The signs and symptoms of a heel spur are similar to those of plantar fasciitis (see Table 3–8). However, heel spurs tend to have a gradual onset and the athlete complains of pain during the heel-strike phase of gait. However, 15 percent of *asymptomatic* adults have been found to have spurs.[17] Once again, a thorough assessment of the triceps surae group for tightness is necessary with this condition.

Plantar Fascia Rupture

A single tensile force applied to the plantar fascia involving dorsiflexion of the foot combined with extension of the toes may cause avulsion from its calcaneal bony attachment or rupture of its central slip. The athlete has immediate difficulty bearing weight secondary to pain at the plantar fascia. Push-off during the gait cycle is extremely difficult because of pain. The area may be swollen and discolored secondary to soft tissue swelling and bleeding.

Tarsal Tunnel Syndrome

Involving pressure caused by entrapment of the posterior tibial nerve or one of its branches as it passes through the tarsal tunnel, this syndrome produces a wide range of symptoms that may easily be confused with other foot and ankle maladies. The tarsal tunnel's bony floor is formed by the talus and calcaneus and is lined by the tendons of tibialis posterior, flexor digitorum longus, and flexor hallucis longus. Its roof is formed by the extensor retinaculum. The posterior tibial nerve and/or its branches pass through this nonyielding space, where it becomes vulnerable to increased pressure.

A complete biomechanical evaluation of the biomechanics of the lower extremity is required of athletes suffering from tarsal tunnel syndrome. Common findings include supple flat feet, in which hyperpronation increases the stress placed on the nerve, prolonging its recovery. The use of an orthotic to control the amount of pronation is recommended when treating athletes with this condition.[18]

The onset of tarsal tunnel syndrome (TTS) may be caused by acute trauma such as fracture, dislocation, hyperplantarflexion, or eversion; overuse responses; or ganglion formation, fibrosis, arthritis, or other disease states.[19–23] The primary complaint is that of pain, burning, numbness, or paresthesia at the medial malleolus radiating to the sole of the foot, heel, and up the calf with the symptoms worsening when standing or running. Muscular function is often normal (Table 3–9). A positive Tinel's sign is often elicited along the path of the nerve (Fig. 3–33).

Tarsal tunnel syndrome may easily be confused with the symptoms produced by plantar fasciitis. However, a close examination of the symptoms assists in differentiating between the two.[19] Pain pro-

---

Asymptomatic: Without symptoms.

Table 3–9. Evaluative Findings of Tarsal Tunnel Syndrome

Examination Segment	Clinical Findings
History	Onset: Acute or insidious. Location of pain: Pain, numbness, and paresthesia occur along the plantar, lateral and/or medial aspects of the foot. Mechanism: Compression of the posterior tibial nerve (or its branches) within the tarsal tunnel. This pressure may also involve the vascular structures within the tunnel. A history of a plantarflexion-plantareversion mechanism injury to the ankle may be described.
Inspection	Inspection of the foot is normally unremarkable. However, in chronic cases trophic changes of the foot and nails may be noted. Inspect the medial longitudinal arch for signs of pes planus, a condition often associated with TTS.
Palpation	Palpation over the tibial nerve and its branches results in tenderness, especially in the area of the tarsal tunnel and with nerve passage beneath the flexor retinaculum.
Functional tests	AROM: Motor function of the intrinsic and extrinsic muscles is often normal. PROM: Forced plantarflexion may increase symptoms secondary to pressure from the extensor retinaculum. RROM: This is normal.
Ligamentous tests	Not applicable.
Neurological tests	There is a positive Tinel's sign inferior and distal to the medial malleolus. Sharp/dull and two-point discrimination may be decreased along the medial and plantar aspects of the foot.
Special tests	Not applicable.
Comments	Symptoms of TTS may closely resemble those of other foot maladies, especially plantar fasciitis. Presence of TTS is confirmed through electrical diagnostic studies.

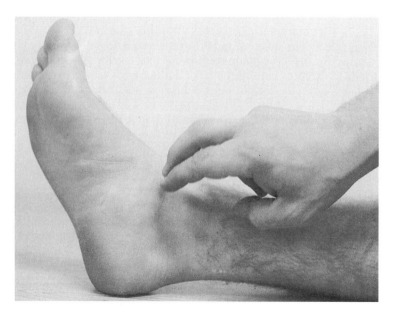

Figure 3–33. Location of Tinel's sign for tarsal tunnel syndrome. Tapping over this area refers pain into the foot and toes.

duced by TTS tends to be along the medial portion of the heel and arch; plantar fasciitis is localized near the fascia's insertion on the calcaneus. Stretching and exercise often decrease the pain produced by plantar fasciitis; activity increases the pain caused by TTS. A definitive diagnosis of TTS is made through electrodiagnostic studies.

Tarsal Coalition

A bony, fibrous, or cartilaginous union between two or more tarsal bones, tarsal coalition is thought to be a hereditary condition that most often affects the calcaneonavicular joint.[24,25] The athlete displays limitation in the subtalar motions leading to further stress at the midtarsal area and the eventual collapse of the longitudinal arches. Any *rigidity* in the hindfoot may be indicative of tarsal coalition and warrants the referral of the athlete to a physician for further evaluation. Tarsal coalition is differentiated from other foot problems because of the limitations in subtalar motion and can be identified by a physician through the use of an x-ray examination.

Metatarsal Fractures

Any of the metatarsals may be fractured secondary to direct trauma. The fracture site may be visibly deformed and locally swollen. Crepitus and deformity may be felt during palpation. Range of motion above and below the fracture site may be limited because of pain. Any suspected fracture to the metatarsals requires immediate immobilization and non–weight bearing as the athlete is referred for evaluation by a physician (Table 3–10). The presence of acute fractures may be further substantiated by the use of the long bone compression test (Fig. 3–34).

Stress fractures, common in the metatarsals, may be related to excessive foot mobility. As the athlete bears weight, the excessive mobility increases stress on the second, third, and fourth MTs. Over time the athlete begins to experience local pain that is asso-

Table 3–10. Evaluative Findings of Metatarsal Fractures

Examination Segment	Clinical Findings	
History	Onset:	Acute, or in the case of stress fractures, insidious.
	Location of pain:	Pain occurs along the shaft of the metatarsal, radiating into the intermetatarsal space and proximally up the foot.
	Mechanism:	Acute: Direct trauma to the metatarsal (e.g., being stepped on), dynamic overload (e.g., avulsion of the peroneus brevis tendon), or rotational (e.g. inversion of the foot).
		Insidious: Repetitive stresses placed along the shaft of the metatarsal or compression arising from the contiguous metatarsals (e.g., "march fracture"). The athlete's symptoms typically increase with activity and decrease with rest.
Inspection	In acute injuries, gross deformity and/or swelling may be visible along the shaft of the bone. Stress fractures may reveal no significant signs, but inflammation around the painful area may be present.	
Palpation	Tenderness and crepitus may be present over the site of acute fractures or maturing stress fractures. A *false joint* may be present with acutely fractured metatarsals.	
Functional tests	AROM and PROM:	Movements that compress the bone, mainly dorsiflexion of the ankle or rotation of the foot, typically result in pain.
	RROM:	In all planes resisted range of motion normally results in pain. These symptoms are replicated when weight bearing.
Ligamentous tests	Not applicable.	
Neurological tests	Not applicable.	
Special tests	Long bone compression test.	
Comments	The presence of acute fractures must be confirmed through x-ray examination. Bone scans are required to definitively diagnose stress fractures in their early stages.	

Rigidity: A pathological loss of a joint's motion or a soft tissue's elasticity.
False joint: Abnormal movement along the length of a bone caused by a fracture or incomplete fusion.

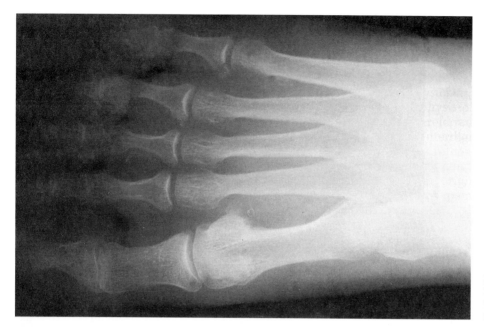

Figure 3–38. Fracture of the proximal phalanx of the fifth toe. Note the fracture line crossing the proximal medial process.

the metatarsal or phalanx are negative. This condition is often referred to as "turf toe" because of the reportedly high instance of this injury during competition on artificial turf. However, the working definition of turf toe has expanded to the point that its label is placed on any condition afflicting the first MTP joint.

Athletes, especially those who compete barefooted, are also susceptible to varus and valgus sprains of the MTP joints. A varus force is applied to the joint capsule and collateral ligaments when the toes are bent toward the body's midline. An outward bending results in a varus force being placed on the capsule.

Phalanx Fractures

Fractures of the toes' phalanges occur when a longitudinal force is applied to the bone, as when an immovable object is kicked, or secondary to a crushing force, as when a weight is dropped on the toes or the toes are stepped on (Fig. 3–38). Signs and symptoms of a fracture phalanx include deformity, pain, and crepitus. While running or walking, pain is experienced during toe-off. Although this condition results in great pain and is disabling to the gait, few treatment options exist. Once the presence of a fracture has been confirmed through x-ray examination, the treatment consists of rest, the use of a hard-soled shoe to prevent flexion of the toes, and perhaps the use of crutches.

ON-FIELD EVALUATION AND MANAGEMENT OF FOOT INJURIES

The on-field evaluation and management of foot and toe injuries are discussed as a single unit.

Acutely, significant trauma to the foot and toes manifests itself through the athlete's inability to bear weight, although it is possible for an athlete to walk off the playing area with a fracture, especially if it involves the toes.

The most important finding during the on-field evaluation of foot injuries is the history relating to the mechanism of injury, any sounds associated with its onset, and the athlete's ability to bear weight on the injured limb. Range of motion testing during this phase of the evaluation is most likely limited to inversion and eversion of the foot and plantarflexion and dorsiflexion of the ankle. If these can be performed pain-free, the athlete can attempt to bear weight as described in Chapter 1. Only the most severe cases, based on the degree of pain, reports of a "crack" or "pop," or obvious trauma such as bleeding through the shoe, warrant removal of the shoe or sock while on the playing surface.

The remaining evaluation proceeds as described earlier in this chapter. During the inspection phase, any gross deformity of the metatarsal shafts or malalignment of the bony structure of the foot and toes should be noted. With the exceptions of the plantar and superior aspects of the calcaneus and the talus, the bones of the foot are relatively subcutaneous, assisting in the identification of crepitus or other deformities through palpation.

On any sign or symptom indicating a bony fracture or joint dislocation, the evaluation should be terminated, the foot and ankle splinted, and the athlete referred to a physician.

REFERENCES

1. Hossler, P, and Lipp, RM: Podiatry and the athletic trainer. Athletic Training: Journal of the National Athletic Trainers Association 17:93, 1982.

1a. Rothstein, JM, Roy, SH, and Wolf, SL: The Rehabilitation Specialist's Handbook. FA Davis, Philadelphia, 1991.

2. Hollinshead, WH, and Jenkins, DB: The foot. In Hollinshead, WH, and Jenkins, DB: Functional Anatomy of the Limbs and Back, ed 5. WB Saunders, Philadelphia, 1981, pp 316–338.

3. Norkin, CC, and Levangie, PK: The foot-ankle complex. In Norkin, CC, and Levangie, PK: Joint Structure and Function: A Comprehensive Analysis, ed 2. FA Davis, Philadelphia, 1992, pp 388–393.

4. DiStefano, VJ: Anatomy and biomechanics of the ankle and foot. Athletic Training: Journal of the National Athletic Trainers Association 16:43, 1981.

4a. Kendall, FP, and McCreary, EK: Muscles: Testing and Function, ed 3. Williams & Wilkins, Baltimore, 1983.

4b. Daniels, L, and Worthingham, C: Muscle Testing: Techniques of Manual Examination, ed 5. WB Saunders, Philadelphia, 1986.

5. Hossler, P, and Maffei, P: Podiatric examination techniques for in-the-field assessments. Athletic Training: Journal of the National Athletic Trainers Association 25:311, 1990.

6. Dahle, LK, et al: Visual assessment of foot type and relationship of foot type to lower extremity injury. Journal of Orthopedic and Sports Physical Therapy 14:70, 1991.

7. Brainard, BJ: Managing corns and plantar calluses. Physician and Sportsmedicine 19:61, 1991.

8. Tiberio, D: Pathomechanics of structural foot deformities. Phys Ther 68:1840, 1988.

9. Wilcox, S, and Draper, DO: Reusable slip-on padding for painful foot conditions. Athletic Training: Journal of the National Athletic Trainers Association 26:265, 1991.

10. Root, ML, Orien, WP, and Weed, JH: Clinical Biomechanics, Vol II. Normal and Abnormal Function of the Foot. Clinical Biomechanics, Los Angeles, 1977.

11. Richardson, EG: Symptomatic pes planus. Operative Techniques in Sports Medicine 2:33, 1994.

12. Brody, D: Techniques in the evaluation and treatment of the injured runner. Orthop Clin North Am 13:542, 1982.

13. Beckett, ME, et al: Incidence of hyperpronation in the ACL injured knee: A clinical perspective. Journal of Athletic Training 27:58, 1992.

14. Bujsen-Muller, F, and Flagsted, KE: Plantar aponeurosis and integral architecture of the ball of the foot. Anatomy 121:599, 1976.

15. Middleton, JA, and Kolodin, EL: Plantar fasciitis—Heel pain in athletes. Journal of Athletic Training 27:70, 1992.

16. Kibler, WB, Goldberg, C, and Chandler, TJ: Functional biomechanical deficits in running athletes with plantar fasciitis. Am J Sports Med 19:66, 1991.

17. Leach, RE, Seavey, MS, and Salter, DK: Results of surgery in athletes with plantar fasciitis. Foot and Ankle 7:156, 1986.

18. Mann, RA, and Baxter, DE: Diseases of the nerves. In Mann, RA, and Coughlin, MJ (eds): Surgery of the Foot and Ankle, ed 6. CV Mosby, St Louis, 1992, p 543.

19. Jackson, DL, and Haglund, B: Tarsal tunnel syndrome in athletes. Case reports and literature review. Am J Sports Med 19:61, 1991.

20. Kaplan, PE, and Kernahan, WT: Tarsal tunnel syndrome: An electrodiagnostic and surgical correlation. J Bone Joint Surg Am 63:96, 1981.

21. Frey, C: Magnetic resonance imaging and the evaluation of tarsal tunnel syndrome. Foot and Ankle 14:159, 1993.

22. Stefko, RM, Lauerman, WC, and Heckman, JD: Tarsal tunnel syndrome caused by an unrecognized fracture of the posterior process of the talus (Cedell fracture). J Bone Joint Surg Am 76:116, 1994.

23. Sammarco, GJ, Chalk, DE, and Feibel, JH: Tarsal tunnel syndrome and additional nerve lesions in the same limb. Foot and Ankle 14:71, 1993.

24. Jayakumar, S, and Cowell, HR: Rigid flatfoot. Clin Orthop 122:77, 1977.

25. Stormont, DM, and Peterson, HA: The relative incidence of tarsal coalition. Clin Orthop 181:24, 1983.

26. Thompson, FM, and Deland, JT: Occurrence of two interdigital neuromas in one foot. Foot and Ankle, 14:15, 1993.

27. Mann, RA, and Thompson, FM: Rupture of the posterior tibial tendon causing flat foot. J Bone Joint Surg Am 67:556, 1985.

4

The Ankle and Lower Leg

Injury to the ankle is the most common joint trauma in athletics, accounting for 20 to 25 percent of all athletic time-lost injuries.[1-5] During athletic competition, the ankle is often placed in a position in which abnormal forces must be absorbed and dissipated by its ligamentous and capsular structures. Ankle sprains have a relatively high reinjury rate because of the residual instability and loss of the joint's sense of position caused by subsequent injuries to its ligaments.

The lower leg offers a significant challenge to the clinician's evaluation and management skills. Trauma or dysfunction of the muscles originating from or attaching to the tibia or fibula can lead to biomechanical changes and potentially can cause injurious gait problems. Seemingly minor injuries, such as contusions, can result in severe consequences from compression of the neurovascular structures leading to and from the ankle, foot, and toes.

CLINICAL ANATOMY

The lower leg is formed by the tibia and fibula (Fig. 4-1). The junction of the distal tibia, fibula, and talus is referred to as the **ankle mortise** (Fig. 4-2). However, any discussion of the ankle must also include the calcaneus, navicular, cuboid, and fifth metatarsal because of the important ligamentous and muscular attachments to these structures.

Maintenance of the normal relationship between the tibia and fibula is required for function and stability of the knee proximally and the ankle and foot distally. The primary function of these bones is to distribute the weight-bearing forces along the limb while still providing the ankle mortise the ability to produce the range of motion needed for walking and running.

The **tibia** is the primary weight-bearing bone of the lower leg. Its distal articular surface forms the roof of the ankle mortise; the medial malleolus forms the shallow medial border of the mortise and provides a broad site for the attachment of the ligaments. This strong ligamentous arrangement, coupled with the lateral bony block formed by the fibula, limits eversion of the ankle.

The anterolateral and posterior borders of the tibial shaft serve as the origin for many of the muscles acting on the ankle, foot, and toes. The **periosteum** of the tibial shaft may become inflamed secondary to overuse syndromes of these muscles at their attachment sites. The relatively flat anteromedial border is thinly covered by soft tissue, predisposing the periosteum to contusions in this area.

Lateral to the tibia is the **fibula**. A long, thin bone, the fibula (1) serves as a site of muscular origin and attachment, (2) serves as a site of ligamentous attachment, (3) provides lateral stability to the ankle mortise, and (4) serves as a pulley for increasing the efficiency of muscle action.

The role of the fibula as a weight-bearing bone is not fully understood. The amount of force transmitted through the fibula has been reported to range from 0 to 12 percent of the athlete's total body weight.[1,2,6] To the practicing clinician the percentage of body weight carried along this bone is inconsequential. Of significance is that trauma to the fibula decreases its ability to function properly.

With the exception of the fibular head, the upper two-thirds of the fibular shaft sits in relative security covered by muscle. A close relationship is found between the proximal portion of the fibula and the peroneal nerve, which innervates the lower leg's lateral compartment (Fig. 4-3). The nerve courses subcutaneously just posterior to the fibular head, making it vulnerable to injury. The distal one-third of the fibula becomes more superficial and begins to thin prior to flaring out to form the lateral malleolus. Because of its slender shape at this point, the distal one-third of the fibular shaft is a common site for fractures.

The lateral malleolus provides a site of attachment for the lateral ankle ligaments. The lateral malleolus extends farther distally than does the medial malleolus, forming a wall of the ankle mortise that is mechanically superior at limiting eversion than the medial malleolus is at limiting inversion. The lateral ankle is a common site for sprains that may result in ligaments being avulsed from the lat-

---

Periosteum: A fibrous membrane containing blood vessels covering the shafts of long bones.

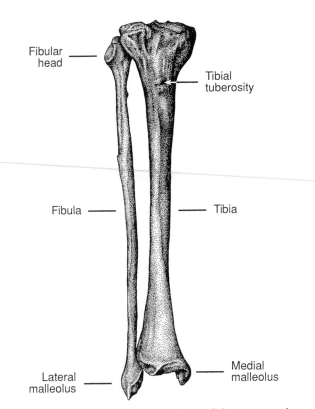

Figure 4–1. Long bones of the lower leg and their primary bony landmarks.

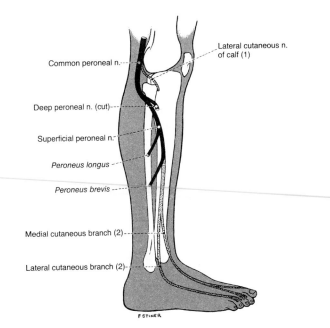

Figure 4–3. Path of the peroneal nerve. The common peroneal nerve courses over the lateral portion of the fibular head, exposing it to potential injury. Trauma at this site causes a weakness in plantarflexion, eversion, and dorsiflexion. (From Rothstein, JM, Roy, SH, and Wolf, S,[6a] p 322, with permission.)

eral malleolus, especially when the ankle is inverted.

The superior articulating portion of the **talus**, the **trochlea**, is quadrilateral, with the anterior surface broader than the posterior surface (Fig. 4–4). Its body is almost entirely covered with articular cartilage. The medial border of the talus articulates with the tibia's medial malleolus, its lateral border with the lateral malleolus, and its superior surface with the tibia. Its inferior surface articulates with the calcaneus, forming the subtalar joint.

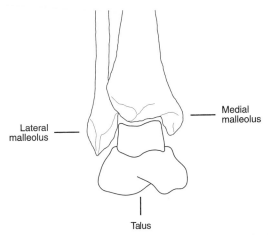

Figure 4–2. Ankle mortise—the articulation formed by the distal end of the tibia and its medial malleolus, the fibula's lateral malleolus, and the talus.

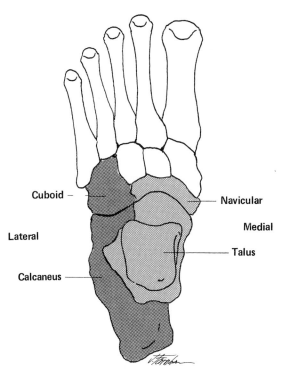

Figure 4–4. View of the superior articular surface of the talus. Its wide anterior edge fits tightly in the mortise when the ankle is dorsiflexed. (From Norkin, CC, and Levangie, PK,[9] p 394, with permission.)

Related Bony Structures

The **calcaneus** plays an important role in foot and ankle function. The Achilles tendon insertion on the calcaneal tubercle provides the foot with a mechanical advantage, forming a long lever arm that adds increased power during gait (see Fig. 3–3). The large body of the calcaneus also provides a site of attachment for some of the ankle's ligaments.

The **navicular** is located anterior to the talus along the foot's medial arch. This bone serves as the site of insertion for the tibialis posterior and tibialis anterior muscles and offers support of the medial longitudinal arch via the plantar calcaneonavicular "spring" ligament.

Positioned laterally along the lateral longitudinal arch, the **cuboid** is anterior to the calcaneus while the base of the **fifth metatarsal** articulates distally with the anterolateral portion of the cuboid. These bones serve primarily as the site of attachment for the peroneus brevis and provide a passageway for the route of the peroneus longus along the foot's plantar aspect.

Articulations and Ligamentous Support

Isolated movements of a single joint in a single plane do not occur during functional movements of the ankle complex. Pure **uniplanar** injuries are almost nonexistent because of the ankle's intimate physiological relationship with the structures of the foot. The majority of injuries to the ankle involve the lateral structures and are the result of an inversion stress accompanied by plantarflexion and/or internal rotation of the foot.

The Talocrural Joint

Formed by the articulation between the talus, the tibia, and the fibula, the talocrural joint is a congruent articulation, especially as it nears its **closed-packed position** of dorsiflexion. A modified **synovial hinge joint**, the talocrural articulation has one degree of freedom of movement: dorsiflexion and plantarflexion. The axis of rotation runs in an oblique direction, connecting the points just distal to the inferior tips of the lateral and medial malleolus (Fig. 4–5).[7]

The joint is surrounded by a joint capsule and most of the supportive ligaments are areas of increased density in the capsule. Tearing of the ankle ligaments almost always results in damage to the joint capsule and irritation of the synovial lining.

Three ligaments provide lateral support to the talocrural joint in a manner such that at least one is taut regardless of the relative position of the ankle mortise (Fig. 4–6). The **anterior talofibular (ATF) ligament** originates off the anterolateral surface of the lateral malleolus and follows an anterior path to insert on the talus near the sinus tarsi. This ligament is tight during plantarflexion, resists the motion of inversion of the talocalcaneal unit in the plantarflexed position, and limits anterior translation of the talus on the tibia. The **calcaneofibular (CF) ligament** is an extracapsular structure that has an attachment on the outermost portion of the lateral malleolus and courses 133 degrees inferiorly and posteriorly to its insertion on the calcaneus.[8] The CF ligament is taut in the extreme range of dorsiflexion and is the primary restraint of talar inversion within the midrange of motion. Arising from the posterior portion of the lateral malleolus, the

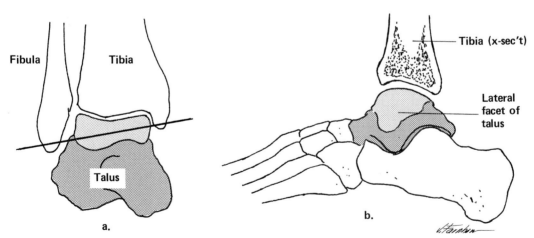

Figure 4–5. Axis of movement of the talocrural joint in the (a) transverse and (b) frontal planes. (From Norkin, CC, and Levangie, PK,[9] pp 382, 384, with permission.)

Uniplanar: Occurring in only one of the cardinal planes.
Closed-packed position: The point in a joint's range of motion at which its bones are maximally congruent; the most stable position of a joint.
Synovial hinge joint: A joint separated by a space filled with synovial fluid.

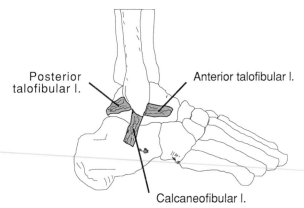

Figure 4-6. Lateral ankle ligaments. The calcaneofibular ligament is an extracapsular structure; the anterior and posterior talofibular ligaments are thickenings in the joint capsule.

posterior talofibular (PTF) ligament takes an inferior and posterior course to attach on both the talus and calcaneus. This is the strongest of the three lateral ligaments and is responsible for limiting posterior displacement of the talus on the tibia.

Medial ligamentous support is provided by four ligaments that, as a group, are termed the **deltoid ligament** (Fig. 4-7). The **anterior tibiotalar (ATT) ligament** originates off the anteromedial portion of the tibia's malleolus and inserts on the superior portion of the medial talus. Arising from the apex of the medial malleolus and having attachment on the calcaneus below the medial malleolus is the **tibiocalcaneal (TC) ligament**. The **posterior tibiotalar (PTT) ligament** spans the posterior aspect of the medial malleolus to attach on the posterior portion of the talus. As a group these three ligaments prevent eversion of the talus. The **tibionavicular (TN) ligament** runs beneath and slightly posterior to the ATT to insert on the medial surface of the navicular to check lateral translation and lateral rotation of the tibia on the foot. The ATT and TN ligaments are taut when the subtalar joint is plantarflexed, whereas the TC and PTT ligaments become tight during dorsiflexion.

The Interosseous Membrane

Spanning the entire length between the tibia and fibula is the interosseous membrane, a strong fibrous tissue that fixates the fibula to the tibia and serves as the site of origin for many of the muscles acting on the foot and toes. A small proximal opening allows for the passage of the tibia's anterior neurovascular structures. Distally, the membrane blends into the anterior and posterior tibiofibular ligaments to form the tibiofibular **syndesmosis joint**.

The Distal Tibiofibular Syndesmosis

The integrity of the ankle mortise is dependent on the functional relationship between the tibia and fibula. This union is a syndesmosis joint in which a convex facet on the fibula is buffered from a concave tibial facet by dense, fatty tissue. The syndesmosis is maintained by the **anterior and posterior tibiofibular (tib-fib) ligaments** and an extension of the interosseous membrane, the **crural interosseous (CI) ligament** (Fig. 4-8). This structural arrangement allows for rotation and slight abduction (spreading) while still maintaining **joint stability**. The CI ligament functions as a fulcrum to motion at the lateral malleolus, so a small amount of malleolar movement results in a large degree of movement at the tibiofibular joint.[9] Excessive eversion and/or dorsiflexion can result in a widening of the ankle mortise, with possible injury to the ligaments supporting the syndesmosis (Fig. 4-9).

The Subtalar Joint

The subtalar joint, along with the other tarsal joints, contributes to the movements of pronation and supination. In conjunction with the other tarsal joints, the subtalar joint contributes to the isolated movement of inversion and eversion.

Muscles of the Lower Leg and Ankle

The lower leg may be divided into four distinct compartments, each containing muscles and neurovascular structures (Fig. 4-10). Tightly bound by fascial linings, any intracompartmental injury can result in the accumulation of fluids that subsequently increase the pressure within the compart-

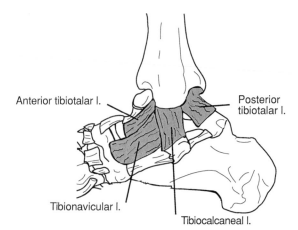

Figure 4-7. Medial "deltoid" ankle ligament showing the four individual ligaments.

Syndesmosis joint: A relatively immobile joint in which two bones are bound together by ligaments.
Joint stability: The integrity of a joint when it is placed under a functional load.

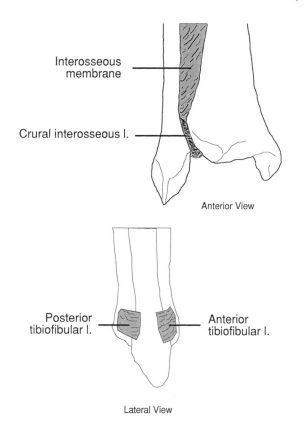

Figure 4-8. Distal tibiofibular syndesmosis with the talus removed for clarity. The anterior view shows the role of the interosseous membrane and the crural interosseous ligament in maintaining lateral restraint of the fibula. The lateral view shows the role of the tibiofibular ligaments in preventing anterior and posterior displacement of the fibula on the tibia.

ment, obstructing the flow of blood to and from the area and placing pressure on the nerves. The action, origin, insertion, and innervation of each muscle are described in Table 4–1.

Structures of the Anterior Compartment

The muscles of the anterior compartment, the tibialis anterior, the extensor hallucis longus (EHL), the extensor digitorum longus (EDL), and the peroneus tertius all act to dorsiflex the ankle (Fig. 4–11). The most superficial of these muscles, the **tibialis anterior**, is the prime mover for ankle dorsiflexion and subtalar joint inversion. The **extensor hallucis longus** assists as a foot invertor, whereas the **extensor digitorum longus** contributes to eversion. The **peroneus tertius** runs parallel with the fifth tendon of the EDL, but its attachment on the dorsal surface of the fifth MT causes this muscle to make a stronger contribution to eversion than dorsiflexion.[10]

Crossing the anterior portion of the ankle mortise is the **extensor retinaculum**, whose superior and inferior bands give it a Z shape (Fig. 4–12). Serving to bind down the distal portion of the muscles of the anterior compartment, the retinaculum prevents a bowstring effect during dorsiflexion and/or toe extension. The medial portion of the inferior band holds the tibialis anterior and extensor hallucis longus close to the dorsum of the foot. A loop on the lateral border wraps around the four tendinous slips of the extensor digitorum longus, holding them laterally and against the dorsum of the foot.

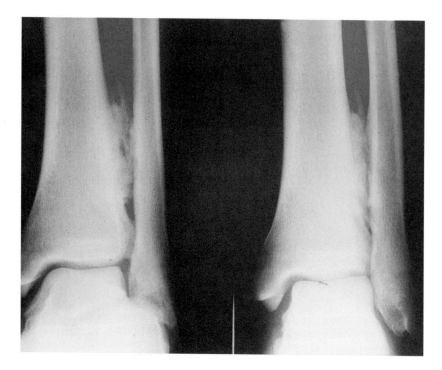

Figure 4-9. X-ray view of a syndesmosis sprain. Note the wide gap between the tibia and fibula on the left image versus the image on the right. This injury results from the wide anterior border of the talus being forced into the mortise during hyperdorsiflexion, from external rotation of the foot, or both.

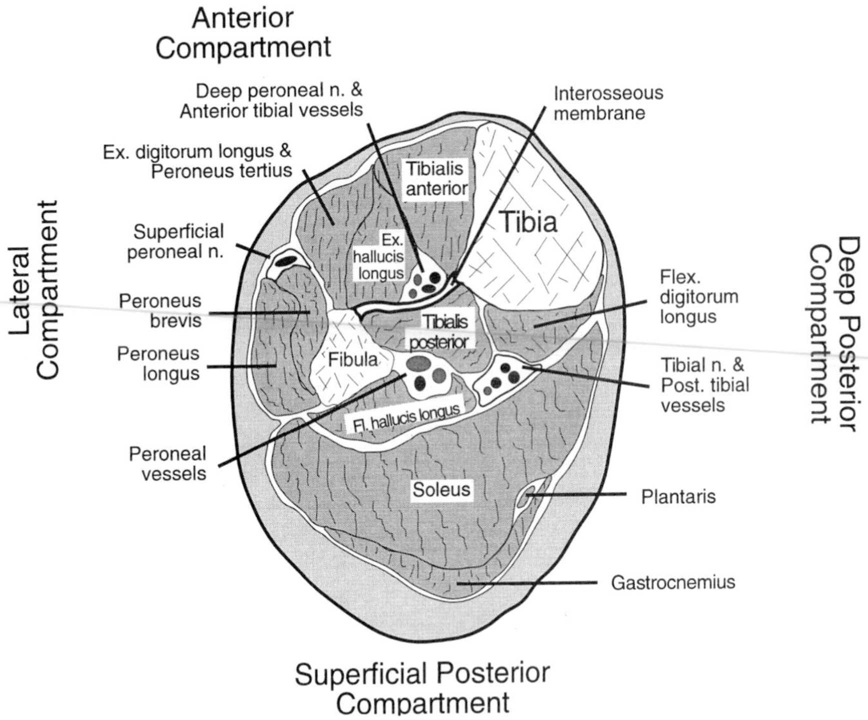

Anterior
Compartment

Figure 4-10. Cross section of the lower leg, indicating the muscles and neurovascular structures located in each of the four compartments. "Vessels" refer to the associated artery, vein, and lymphatic vessel.

Branching off the common peroneal nerve near the fibular head, the **deep peroneal nerve** runs a course from the upper portion of the fibula along the interosseous membrane behind the tibialis anterior. This nerve and its subsequent branches innervate most of the muscles located within the anterior compartment and on the dorsum of the foot. Supplying the anterior compartment with its blood, the **anterior tibial artery** passes through the superior portion of the interosseous membrane to follow the path taken by the deep peroneal nerve. A branch of the anterior tibial artery, the **dorsalis pedis artery**, supplies blood to the dorsum of the foot. Following trauma such as fracture, dislocation, and hemorrhage within the anterior compartment, it is important to establish the presence of this pulse.

Structures of the Lateral Compartment

The **peroneus longus** and **peroneus brevis** form the bulk of the lateral compartment. The peroneus longus is the most superficial of these muscles, with its bulk covering all but the most inferior portion of the peroneus brevis and its tendon. The two tendons share a common synovial sheath as they pass behind and around the lateral malleolus, where their positions are maintained by the **superior and inferior peroneal retinacula**. Their paths diverge as they clear the retinaculum and approach the peroneal tubercle. The peroneus brevis tendon courses to the dorsal aspect of the base of the fifth MT, while the peroneus longus tendon runs a path along the plantar aspect of the foot to attach to the base of the first MT and first cuneiform. As a group, these

muscles are strong evertors of the foot and contribute to plantarflexion (Fig. 4-13).

The lateral compartment contains the **superficial peroneal nerve**, which innervates the peroneus brevis, peroneus tertius, and, in conjunction with the common peroneal nerve, the peroneus longus. Arising off the posterior tibial artery, the **peroneal artery** runs a course next to the interosseous membrane, supplying blood to the lateral compartment and lateral ankle.

Structures of the Superficial Posterior Compartment

The gastrocnemius, soleus, and plantaris collectively form the triceps surae muscle group (Fig. 4-14). The **gastrocnemius** and **plantaris** are two-joint muscles, each having origins on the femoral condyles. The **soleus** is the only member of the triceps surae group to cross only one joint line. The gastrocnemius and soleus have a common insertion on the calcaneus via the Achilles tendon. Some anatomy texts also include the plantaris as a part of the Achilles tendon complex. Whether a formal attachment is present or not, the plantaris tendon represents the anteromedial portion of the Achilles tendon complex and insertion. The gastrocnemius and soleus are prime movers during plantarflexion, with the gastrocnemius most involved when the knee is extended.

Traveling between the two heads of the gastrocnemius and running deep to lie between the soleus and the tibialis posterior (located in the deep posterior compartment) is the longest branch of the sci-

Table 4–1. Muscles Acting on the Foot and Ankle

Muscle	Action	Origin	Insertion	Nerve	Root
Extensor digitorum longus	Extension of the 2nd through 5th MTP joints Assists in extending 2nd through 5th PIP and DIP joints Assists in foot eversion Assists in ankle dorsiflexion	Lateral tibial condyle Proximal three-fourths of anterior fibula Proximal portion of the interosseous membrane	Via four tendons to the distal phalanges of the 2nd through 5th toes	Deep peroneal	L4, L5, S1
Extensor hallucis longus	Extension of the 1st MTP joint Extension of the 1st IP joint	Middle two-thirds of the anterior surface of the fibula Adjacent portion of the interosseous membrane	Base of the distal phalanx of the 1st toe	Deep peroneal	L4, L5, S1
Flexor digitorum longus	Flexion of 2nd through 5th PIP and DIP joints Flexion of 2nd through 5th MTP joints Assists in ankle plantarflexion Assists in foot inversion	Posterior-medial portion of the distal two-thirds of the tibia From fascial arising from the tibialis posterior	Plantar base of distal phalanges of the 2nd through 5th toes	Tibial	L5, S1
Flexor hallucis longus	Flexion of 1st IP joint Assists in flexion of 1st MTP joint Assists in foot inversion Assists in plantarflexion of the ankle	Posterior distal two-thirds of the fibula Associated interosseous membrane and muscular fascia	Plantar surface of the proximal phalanx of the 1st toe	Tibial	L4, L5, S1
Gastrocnemius	Ankle plantarflexion Assists in knee flexion	Medial Head Posterior surface of the medial femoral condyle Adjacent portion of the femur and knee capsule Lateral Head Posterior surface of the lateral femoral condyle Adjacent portion of the femur and knee capsule	To the calcaneus via the Achilles tendon	Tibial	S1, S2
Peroneus brevis	Eversion of foot Assists in ankle plantarflexion	Distal two-thirds of the lateral fibula	Styloid process at the base of the 5th metatarsal	Superficial peroneal	L4, L5, S1
Peroneus longus	Eversion of the foot Assists in ankle plantarflexion	Lateral tibial condyle Fibular head Upper two-thirds of the lateral fibula	Lateral aspect of the base of the 1st metatarsal Lateral and dorsal aspect of the 1st cuneiform	Superficial peroneal	L4, L5, S1

Table 4–1. Muscles Acting on the Foot and Ankle (*Continued*)

Muscle	Action	Origin	Insertion	Nerve	Root
Peroneus tertius	Eversion of the foot Dorsiflexion of the ankle	Distal one-third of the anterior surface of the fibula Adjacent portion of the interosseous membrane	Dorsal surface of the base of the 5th metatarsal	Deep peroneal	L4, L5, S1
Plantaris	Ankle plantarflexion Assists in knee flexion	Distal portion of the supracondylar line of the lateral femoral condyle Adjacent portion of the femoral popliteal surface Oblique popliteal ligament	To the calcaneus via the Achilles tendon	Tibial	L4, L5, S1
Soleus	Ankle plantarflexion	Posterior fibular head Upper one-third of the fibula's posterior surface Soleal line located in the posterior tibial shaft Middle one-third of the medial tibial border	To the calcaneus via the Achilles tendon	Tibial	S1, S2
Tibialis anterior	Dorsiflexion of the ankle Inversion of the foot	Lateral tibial condyle Upper one-half of the tibia's lateral surface Adjacent portion of the interosseous membrane	Medial and plantar surfaces of the 1st cuneiform Medial and plantar surfaces of the 1st metatarsal	Deep peroneal	L4, L5, S1
Tibialis posterior	Inversion of the foot Assists in ankle plantarflexion	Length of the interosseous membrane Posterior, lateral tibia Upper two-thirds of the medial fibula	Navicular tuberosity Via fibrous slips to the sustentaculum tali, the cuneiforms, cuboid, and the bases of the 2nd, 3rd, and 4th metatarsals	Tibial	L4, S1

Muscle actions, origins, and insertions adapted from Kendall and McCreary[12]; innervations adapted from Daniels and Worthingham.[10a]

atic nerve, the **tibial nerve.** Supplying the innervation for all of the muscles in the superficial and deep posterior compartment, branches of the tibial nerve continue to the plantar aspect of the foot after slinging around the medial malleolus. Following the same course as the tibial nerve is the **posterior tibial artery**.

Structures of the Deep Posterior Compartment

The **tibialis posterior** is the only muscle of the deep posterior compartment acting exclusively on the ankle complex (Fig. 4–15). Its angle of pull makes it a primary adductor of the forefoot while assisting in plantarflexion and inversion. The remaining two muscles of the deep posterior compartment, the **flexor digitorum longus** and the **flexor hallucis longus,** serve as secondary plantarflexors and invertors of the ankle and foot.

A common mnemonic, "**T**om, **D**ick, **A**nd **N**ervous **H**arry," is used to describe the structures that sling behind the medial malleolus: **t**ibialis posterior, flexor **d**igitorum longus, tibial **a**rtery, tibial **n**erve, and the flexor **h**allucis longus.

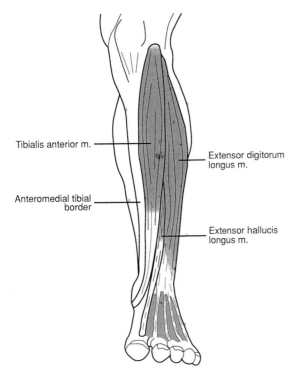

Figure 4–11. Muscles of the anterior compartment: the tibialis anterior, extensor hallucis longus, and extensor digitorum longus.

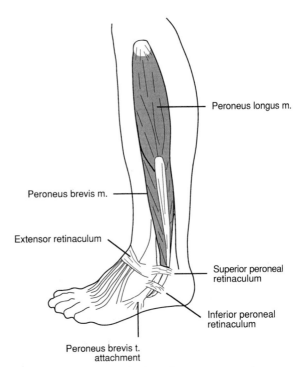

Figure 4–13. Muscles of the lateral compartment: the peroneus longus and brevis. The superior and inferior retinacula maintain the alignment of the peroneal tendons so that their angle of pull plantarflexes and everts the foot.

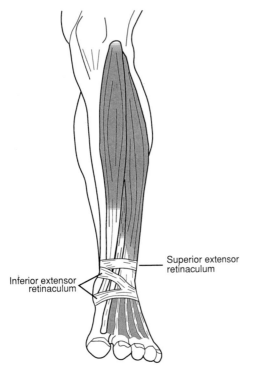

Figure 4–12. Extensor retinaculum formed by the inferior and superior bands. These structures prevent the muscles of the anterior compartment from bowing during dorsiflexion.

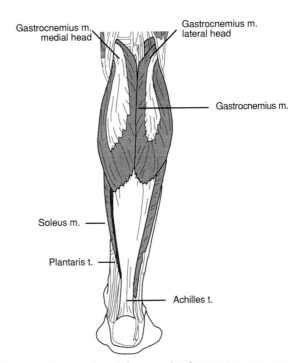

Figure 4–14. Muscles of the superficial posterior compartment: the gastrocnemius, soleus, and plantaris. This group of muscles is collectively referred to as the "triceps surae."

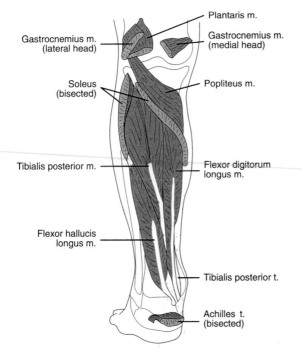

Gastrocnemius m.
(lateral head)

Plantaris m.

Gastrocnemius m.
(medial head)

Soleus
(bisected)

Popliteus m.

Tibialis posterior m.

Flexor digitorum
longus m.

Flexor hallucis
longus m.

Tibialis posterior t.

Achilles t.
(bisected)

Figure 4–15. Muscles of the deep posterior compartment: the tibialis posterior, flexor hallucis longus, and flexor digitorum longus. The superficial muscles have been removed to show the deep compartment.

Bursae

Two major bursae are associated with the lower leg and ankle. The **calcaneal bursa** is found between the Achilles tendon and the calcaneus, functioning to decrease friction between these two structures. Lying between the posterior aspect of the Achilles tendon and the skin is the **retrocalcaneal bursa**, which protects the Achilles tendon from direct trauma and decreases friction from the skin and footwear.

CLINICAL EVALUATION OF THE ANKLE AND LOWER LEG

The following describes a model evaluation of the ankle and lower leg, and its components are presented in Table 4–2. Depending on the circumstances surrounding the injury, this model may be condensed or expanded. During the initial evaluation of an acute injury the clinician should be aware of those conditions warranting the termination of the evaluation and the immediate referral to a physician. Both ankles should be exposed during this examination to facilitate inspection and palpation of the foot and ankle. A complete examination of an ankle injury may require a concurrent evaluation of the foot and knee.

History

During the history-taking process for an ankle or lower leg injury, the onset and mechanism of injury, the duration of the symptoms, and any previous history of injury to the involved or uninvolved limb must be established. The athlete's responses to the following list guide the remainder of the history-taking process and form the framework on which the rest of the examination is based.

- **Location of the pain:** The area of pain must be identified as specifically as possible so that the subsequent portions of the evaluation emphasize the suspected structures involved (Table 4–3). The lower leg and ankle may also be areas of referred pain arising from anterior compartment syndrome, tarsal tunnel syndrome, and sciatic nerve or lumbar nerve root impingement.

- **Nature or type of pain:** Specific questions must be posed to determine how the athlete's symptoms are aggravated by certain activities and how these symptoms are affecting the athlete's activity or normal daily activities.

- **Onset:** The onset of symptoms assists in determining if there has been an acute traumatic incident such as a sprain, strain, or fracture, or if there has been a gradual onset of symptoms as with overuse syndromes.

- **Injury mechanism:** In the case of macrotrauma the mechanism of injury can assist in identifying the general area of the structures and the type of injury involved (Table 4–4). Chronic or insidious disorders require more in-depth questioning to determine the factors surrounding the cause of pain.

- **Level of activity and conditioning regimen:** Developing a "picture" of the athlete's recent training habits is necessary when evaluating chronic or insidious conditions. For overuse injuries it should be established whether the athlete has:
  ○ Significantly increased the duration, intensity, or type (i.e., added hills) of exercise (When available, the athlete's personal training log is useful in determining excessive increases in exercise intensity.)
  ○ Changed shoe brands or styles or is competing in old, worn-out shoes
  ○ Switched from participating on a surface of one texture and density to one of a different type
  ○ Recently begun wearing orthotics or changed the type of orthotic worn

- **Prior history of injury:** The athlete should be thoroughly questioned and, if available, the athlete's medical file reviewed regarding the history of injury to both the involved and the uninvolved limb. Athletes with a history of previous ankle sprains may present with excess laxity and de-

Table 4–2. Evaluation of the Ankle

History	Inspection	Palpation	Functional Tests	Ligamentous Tests	Neurological Tests	Special Tests
Location of the pain	General inspection	Lateral structures	Active range of motion	Anterior talofibular ligament instability	Anterior compartment syndrome	Ankle sprains
Nature or type of pain	Weight-bearing status	Fibular shaft	Plantarflexion and dorsiflexion	Anterior drawer test	Peroneal nerve involvement	Inversion ankle sprains
Onset	General bilateral comparison	Interosseous membrane	Inversion and eversion	Calcaneofibular ligament instability	Sciatic nerve involvement	Syndesmosis sprains
Injury mechanism	Lateral structures	Anterior and posterior tibiofibular ligaments	Passive range of motion	Inversion stress test (talar tilt)	Lumbar nerve involvement	Eversion ankle sprains
Level of activity and conditioning regimen	Peroneal muscle group	Calcaneofibular ligament	Plantarflexion and dorsiflexion	Deltoid ligament instability		Ankle dislocations
Prior history of injury	Distal one-third of the fibula	Anterior talofibular ligament	Inversion and eversion	Eversion stress test (talar tilt)		Lower leg fractures
	Lateral malleolus	Posterior talofibular ligament	Resistive range of motion	Kleiger's test		Stress fractures
	Anterior structures	Peroneal tubercle	Dorsiflexion	Ankle syndesmosis instability		Squeeze test
	Appearance of the anterior lower leg	Cuboid	Tibialis anterior	Kleiger's test		Bump test
	Contour of the malleoli	Base of the 5th metatarsal	Peroneus tertius			Achilles tendon Pathology
	Talus	Peroneus longus and brevis	Plantarflexion			Achilles tendinitis
	Sinus tarsi	Peroneal retinaculum	Gastrocnemius			Achilles tendon rupture
	Medial structures	Anterior structures	Soleus			Thompson test
	Medial malleolus	Anterior tibial shaft	Inversion			Subluxating peroneal tendons
	Medial longitudinal arch	Dome of the talus	Tibialis posterior			Neurovascular deficit
	Posterior structures	Extensor retinacula	Other muscles			Anterior compartment syndrome
	Gastrocnemius-soleus complex	Sinus tarsi	Eversion			Deep vein thrombophlebitis
	Achilles tendon	Tibialis anterior				
	Bursae	Long toe extensors				
	Calcaneus	Peroneus tertius				
		Medial structures				
		Medial malleolus				
		Deltoid ligament				
		Sustentaculum tali				
		Spring ligament				
		Navicular and navicular tubercle				
		Talar head				
		Tibialis posterior				
		Long toe flexors				
		Posterior structures				
		Gastrocnemius-soleus complex				
		Achilles tendon				
		Calcaneal bursa				
		Retrocalcaneal bursa				
		Dome of the calcaneus				
		Palpation of pulses				
		Posterior tibial artery				
		Dorsalis pedis artery				

96

Table 4–3. Possible Trauma Based on the Location of Pain (Excluding Gross Injury)

| | *Location of Pain* | | | |
	Lateral	Anterior	Medial	Posterior

Soft tissue	Inversion ankle sprain
	Syndesmosis sprain
	Capsular impingement
	Subluxating peroneal
	   tendons
	Peroneal muscle strain
	Peroneal tendinitis
	Interosseous mem-
	   brane trauma
	Peroneal nerve trauma
		Extensor retinaculum
		   sprain
		Tibialis anterior or
		   long toe extensor
		   strain
		Tibialis anterior or
		   long toe extensor
		   tendinitis
		Anterior compartment
		   syndrome
			Eversion ankle sprain
			Capsular impingement
			Tibialis posterior strain
			Tibialis posterior ten-
			   dinitis
				Triceps surae strain
				Achilles tendinitis
				Achilles tendon rupture
				Calcaneal bursitis
				Retrocalcaneal bursitis
				Deep vein thrombophlebitis

Bony	Lateral ligament avul-
	   sion
	Lateral malleolus frac-
	   ture
	Fibular stress fracture
	Peroneal tendon avul-
	   sion (Jones frac-
	   ture)
		Tibial stress fracture
		Talar fracture
		Talar osteochondritis
		Arthritis
		Periosteitis
			Medial ligament avul-
			   sion
			Medial malleolus avul-
			   sion
				Calcaneal fracture

creased proprioception, while athletes with other injuries to the lower extremity or lumbar spine may present with biomechanical changes in gait.

Inspection

As with any paired body part, the involved lower leg or ankle should always be compared with the uninvolved side. Much of the observation phase should be performed while the athlete is non–weight bearing and then compared with the weight-bearing findings.

General Inspection

• **Weight-bearing status:** The inspection process begins as the athlete enters the facility or walks off the field. At this point the weight-bearing ca-

pacity of the involved limb should be noted, including:
   ○ Did the athlete enter the facility with ease or was an antalgic gait present, signifying pain?
   ○ Was the limb externally rotated, suggesting a lack of ankle dorsiflexion secondary to pain or restriction?

• **General bilateral comparison:** Both lower extremities should be observed, while noting any gross swelling, redness, pallor, or other obvious deformity.

Inspection of the Lateral Structures

• **Peroneal muscle group:** The peroneal muscle group should be observed in its entirety. The tendons may be seen as they course posteriorly and inferiorly around the lateral malleolus, being held tightly in position by the superior and inferior peroneal retinacula (see Fig. 4–13).

Table 4–4. Mechanism of Ankle Injury and the Resultant Tissue Damage

Uniplanar Motion	Tensile Forces	Compressive Forces

Inversion	Lateral structures: ATF, CF, PTF, lateral capsule,
	   and peroneal tendons
		Medial structures: medial malleolus, deltoid
		   ligament, and medial neurovascular bundle

Eversion	Medial structures: deltoid ligament, tibialis
	   posterior, and long toe flexors
		Lateral structures: lateral malleolus and lateral
		   capsule

Plantarflexion	Anterior structures: anterior capsule, long toe
	   extensors, extensor retinaculum
		Posterior structures: posterior capsule,
		   retrocalcaneal bursa

Dorsiflexion	Posterior structures: Achilles tendon
	Lateral structures: tibiofibular syndesmosis,
	   posterior talofibular ligament
		Anterior structures: anterior capsule,
		   syndesmosis, extensor retinaculum

• **Distal one-third of the fibula:** The examiner should observe the contour and symmetry of the distal one-third of the fibula as it becomes superficial prior to forming the lateral malleolus. Any discontinuity in the bone's shaft or the formation of edema over this portion of the shaft should be noted, as this may indicate a possible syndesmosis sprain or fibular fracture.

• **Lateral malleolus:** Normally very little soft tissue covers the lateral malleolus, making its shape easily identifiable. Even the mildest of ankle sprains may result in swelling, masking the malleolus and peroneal tendons (Fig. 4–16). Any formation of ecchymosis around and distal to the lateral malleolus, signifying acute trauma such as a sprain or fracture, must be noted.

Inspection of the Anterior Structures

• **Appearance of the anterior lower leg:** The anterior lower leg should be inspected for skin color and edema. Athletes with **anterior compartment syndrome** may present with reddened or shiny skin and/or pitting edema. If these signs coincide with paresthesia in the web space between the first and second toes, decreased dorsiflexion strength, and/or absence of the dorsalis pedis pulse, the athlete should be immediately referred to a physician.

• **Contour of the malleoli:** The malleoli should be prominent as they project from the tibia and

fibula. Swelling can obscure these prominences. Swelling between the tibia and fibula above the distal tibiofibular joint and the distal one-third of the interosseous membrane may indicate a syndesmotic sprain.

• **Talus:** If the athlete is capable of bearing weight, the examiner should observe the bilateral symmetry of the tali. In athletes with leg-length discrepancies, one foot has a prominent medial talus caused by pronation of the longer leg, whereas the shorter leg maintains a somewhat neutral or supinated position.

With the athlete still standing, the examiner should note the presence of the medial longitudinal arch. If this arch is not adequately supported, the medial aspect of the talus rotates inward and the navicular drops inferiorly. This excessive protrusion of the talus can be appreciated from the anterior as well as the posterior view. Athletes suffering from lower leg pain such as periosteitis or tendinitis of the tibialis anterior or tibialis posterior muscles often display this deformity. The medial movement of the talus and subsequent flattening of the medial longitudinal arch fatigue the musculature and place strain on their periosteal attachments on the tibia.

• **Sinus tarsi:** The sinus tarsi is not a specific anatomical structure but rather an indentation formed over the talus next to the extensor digitorum brevis. This area should be observed, noting its normally concave shape. After injury to the

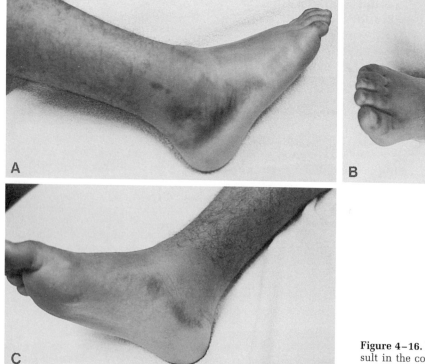

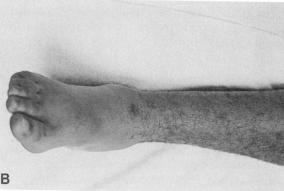

Figure 4–16. Damage to the lateral ankle capsule can result in the collection of edema around and distal to the malleolus. Note the medial formation of ecchymosis.

anterior talofibular ligament or talar fractures, the area fills with fluid, resulting in loss of its normal indentation in the proximal foot.

Inspection of the Medial Structures

- **Medial malleolus:** Like the lateral malleolus, the medial malleolus is relatively superficial, with little soft tissue covering it. Its appearance should be distinct without disruption or the presence of edema.

- **Medial longitudinal arch:** The normal concave appearance of the medial longitudinal arch should be maintained with the athlete both weight bearing and non–weight bearing. Pes planus (flatfoot) results in the talus shifting medially, causing increased stress on its supportive ligamentous and muscular structures as well as altering gait biomechanics. Pes cavus, a high medial arch, results in a supinated foot, predisposing the athlete to inversion ankle sprains.

Inspection of the Posterior Structures

- **Gastrocnemius-soleus complex:** Bilateral comparison should indicate calf musculature of approximately equal size, shape, and mass. *Atrophy* may be present owing to impairment of the S1 or S2 nerve root or to the tibial or sciatic nerve. Tearing of the musculature may result in depressions in the skin, especially at the musculotendinous junction with the Achilles tendon. Redness and swelling of the posterior calf could indicate deep vein *thrombophlebitis*.

- **Achilles tendon:** The prominent Achilles tendon may be seen as it tapers from the musculotendinous junction to its insertion on the calcaneus. Achilles tendon ruptures may present with a visible defect if the tear occurs in its middle or distal portion, whereas proximal tears may present with no visible defects. Achilles tendon ruptures should be confirmed through the Thompson test.

- **Bursae:** The calcaneal and retrocalcaneal bursae should be inspected for swelling, redness, or other signs of inflammation.

- **Calcaneus:** The calcaneus is normally very distinct, with little soft tissue covering its medial and lateral borders. The presence of a thickened area at the insertion of the Achilles tendon is sometimes found in athletes with retrocalcaneal pain. This thickening, an exostosis, may be caused by the athlete's footwear rubbing on this area and may be associated with retrocalcaneal bursitis.

Palpation

Most examiners palpate the lateral bony structures first because most injuries to the lower leg and ankle occur to either the lateral ligamentous structures or the fibula. The sequence of the palpation should be altered according to the location of pain and crepitus and the type of injury, but it should always start away from the site of pain and work toward it.

Palpation of the Lateral Bony and Ligamentous Structures

- **Fibular shaft:** The examiner begins by locating the fibular head superiorly and palpating along the length of the shaft over the bulk of the peroneals until it re-emerges. One continues to palpate the mass and circumference of the lateral malleolus, noting any crepitus or point tenderness.

The examiner applies gentle pressure over the distal one-third of the fibular shaft, noting any pain and discontinuity in the bone, which may indicate the presence of a fracture. The lateral ligamentous structures may be avulsed from their origin on the malleolus or their insertion on the talus or calcaneus through the tensile forces associated with inversion. This pathology causes point tenderness, swelling, and crepitus. The distal portion of the lateral malleolus may be "knocked off" by the calcaneus during excessive inversion of the calcaneus. Long bone fractures may be ruled out using the **squeeze** or **bump test**. If a fracture is suspected, one must terminate the evaluation, splint the ankle so that it is non–weight bearing, and refer the athlete to a physician so that a definitive diagnosis may be made via x-ray examination.

- **Interosseous membrane:** An area of the interosseous membrane may be palpated in the ankle syndesmosis between the distal fibula and tibia.

- **Anterior and posterior tibiofibular ligaments:** The attachment of the anterior and posterior tibiofibular ligaments on the fibula may be located just superior to the lateral malleolus (Fig. 4–17). Palpate anteriorly along the length of the anterior tib-fib ligament to its attachment on the anterolateral portion of the tibia. Direct palpation of the posterior tib-fib ligament is difficult because of the mass of the peroneal group. Tenderness along these structures and/or the interosseous membrane may indicate a syndesmotic ankle sprain.

Atrophy: A wasting or decrease in the size of a muscle or organ.
Thrombophlebitis: Inflammation of a vein and the subsequent formation of blood clots.

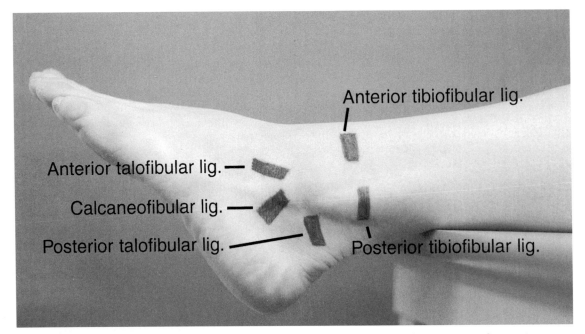

Figure 4–17. Surface anatomy of the anterior and posterior tibiofibular, the anterior and posterior talofibular, and the calcaneofibular ligaments. The calcaneofibular ligament, when intact, is palpable when the ankle is slightly inverted.

• **Calcaneofibular ligament:** From the tib-fib ligaments the examiner palpates down the lateral malleolus to the origin of the CF ligament on the distal tip of the malleolus (Fig. 4–17). As the ligament leaves the malleolus and crosses the joint space it becomes palpable. This ligament is usually the secondary structure damaged during inversion ankle sprains and absorbs the greatest amount of stress when the talocrural joint is in the neutral position.

• **Anterior talofibular ligament:** One should locate the origin of the calcaneofibular ligament and move anteriorly on the malleolus to find the origin of the ATF ligament on the inferior portion of the anterior malleolus. Running a course somewhat parallel to the plantar surface of the foot when the foot is in neutral position, the ATF ligament attaches on the anterolateral aspect of the talus near the sinus tarsi. This structure is not distinctly identifiable.

• **Posterior talofibular ligament:** From the origin of the calcaneofibular ligament, the examiner moves upward and posteriorly around the malleolus to locate the PTF ligament. This ligament is not directly palpable, but pressure should be applied over the point of its insertion on the posterior portion of the talus. In most cases the PTF ligament is damaged only in severe ankle sprains or dislocations.

• **Peroneal tubercle:** Felt as a small nodule located just anterior to the attachment of the CF ligament and inferior to the distal tip of the lateral malleolus, the peroneal tubercle marks the point on the calcaneus at which the peroneus longus

and brevis tendons diverge. In cases of peroneal tendinitis or rupture of the distal peroneal retinaculum, this area is tender to the touch.

• **Cuboid:** Palpate anteriorly from the peroneal tubercle to locate the cuboid as it lies proximal to the base of the fifth MT. This bone is rarely injured but may become tender secondary to ligamentous injury or inflammation of the peroneal tendons.

• **Base of the fifth metatarsal:** Flaring from the base of the fifth MT is the styloid process. This structure may be avulsed from the shaft following the forceful contraction of the peroneus brevis muscle as occurs when the muscle attempts to counteract inversion of the ankle.

Palpation of the Lateral Musculature and Related Soft Tissue

• **Peroneus longus and brevis:** The examiner locates the peroneus longus muscle from its origin on the fibular head and palpates the muscle belly along the upper two-thirds of the lateral fibula. The tendon becomes palpable along the distal one-third of the fibula and may be palpated along with the peroneus brevis tendon as they course posterior to the lateral malleolus and sling beneath it. As these tendons approach the peroneal tubercle, they diverge so that the peroneus longus tendon passes through the groove in the cuboid to follow a course along the plantar aspect of the foot, at which point it is no longer palpable, while the peroneus brevis tendon attaches to the base of the fifth MT.

• **Peroneal retinaculum:** The space between the posterior portion of the lateral malleolus and the calcaneus is palpated for pain elicited over the superior peroneal retinaculum where the peroneal tendons pass beneath it. The clinician continues to follow the length of the tendons to locate the inferior peroneal retinaculum immediately below the lateral malleolus. Tears in these structures, especially the superior retinaculum, result in **dislocating** or **subluxating peroneal tendons**.

Palpation of the Anterior Bony and Ligamentous Structures

• **Anterior tibial shaft:** Palpation of the tibia should begin by locating the site at which the patellar tendon attaches to the tibial tuberosity. The anteromedial portion of this bone is subcutaneous and therefore is palpable along its length to its distal termination as the medial malleolus. Special attention should be given to the anterior ridge of the tibia where the tibialis anterior and long toe flexors attach, as well as to the periosteum and posterior border of the shaft near the area of the tibialis posterior. These areas may become inflamed secondary to overuse, such as with shin splints (Box 4–1).

Box 4–1. Shin splints

The term "shin splints" has been applied to myriad conditions affecting the lower leg. Among the many causes of this pain are (1) tibialis anterior tendinitis, (2) tibialis posterior tendinitis, (3) periosteitis, (4) tibial stress fractures, (5) fibular stress fractures, (6) recurrent chronic anterior compartment syndrome, and (7) inflammation of the interosseous membrane. Rather than using an obscure term that may refer to a wide number of injuries, the clinician should fully ascertain the cause of the lower leg pain. This is important not only to clarify the exact nature of the athlete's pain but also to properly plan the athlete's treatment and rehabilitation regimen.

• **Dome of the talus:** Plantarflexing the foot allows the anterior dome of the talus to be exposed from under the ankle mortise. Pain along this area is common with ankle synovitis and impact injuries to the ankle joint.

• **Extensor retinacula:** The reader should refer to Figure 4–12 to determine the approximate location of the superior and inferior extensor retinacula. These structures are palpated for signs of tenderness as the tendons pass under them. The retinacula may become traumatically injured during forceful, sudden dorsiflexion, or the tendons

passing under it may become inflamed owing to friction.

• **Sinus tarsi:** Located between the lateral malleolus and the neck of the talus, the area of the sinus tarsi may become swollen and painful to the touch following ATF ligament injury, arthritic changes in the ankle, or fracture of the talus (Fig. 4–18).

Palpation of the Anterior Musculature and Related Soft Tissue

• **Tibialis anterior:** The clinician begins palpating the tibialis anterior from its origin on the anterolateral portion of the proximal tibia and continues to palpate distally along the length of the muscle belly. Near the distal portion of the medial tibia the belly begins to merge into a thick, round tendon. The examiner proceeds to palpate the tendon to the point at which it inserts on the cuneiform and first metatarsal.

• **Long toe extensors:** The extensor hallucis longus and extensor digitorum longus may be injured secondary to ankle plantarflexion or from dynamic overload during eccentric dorsiflexion. In Chapter 3 one finds the description of the palpation technique for these two muscles.

• **Peroneus tertius:** The examiner locates the peroneus tertius as it arises from the distal one-half of the anterior surface of the fibula. It is then

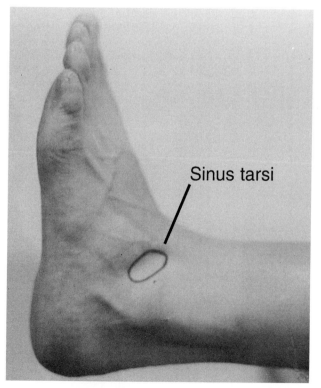

Figure 4–18. Location of the sinus tarsi. This depression may become swollen and painful secondary to anterior talofibular ligament sprains, arthritis, or talar fractures.

palpated distally along the length of the muscle belly and tendon to its insertion point on the dorsal aspect of the base of the fifth MT. The tendon is most palpable as it crosses the joint anterior to the lateral malleolus and is identifiable by being the most lateral of the muscles. The peroneus tertius is not present in the entire population.

Palpation of the Medial Bony and Ligamentous Structures

• **Medial malleolus:** The entire border of the medial malleolus is palpated, noting any pain that may be elicited at the attachment sites of the medial ligaments on this structure, or crepitus, indicative of a fracture. One continues to palpate up the posteromedial tibial border, noting any pain that arises along the periosteal lining.

• **Deltoid ligament:** The mass of the deltoid ligament may be palpated as it encircles the lower portion of the medial malleolus, but for all practical purposes the individual ligaments forming this complex cannot be distinguished from each other (Fig. 4–19).

• **Sustentaculum tali:** One should palpate approximately one finger's width inferior from the medial malleolus to locate the area of the calcaneal sustentaculum tali. This small and often impalpable structure serves two important functions: (1) supporting the talus and (2) serving as the site of attachment for the spring ligament.

• **Spring ligament:** This ligament's origin may be located from the sustentaculum tali and it may be palpated along its route distally to its insertion on the navicular. Serving to maintain the medial longitudinal arch, this ligament becomes stretched in cases of chronic pes planus or torn in acute pronation or rotation of the forefoot.

• **Navicular and navicular tubercle:** The navicular tubercle is easily identified by the attachment of the tibialis posterior. The clinician palpates the navicular itself for signs of tenderness that may be indicative of tibialis posterior tendinitis, a sprain of the spring ligament, or a stress fracture. Pain elicited during palpation of this structure can also indicate an inflamed accessory navicular.

• **Talar head:** The examiner palpates posteriorly from the navicular to locate its articulation with the head of the talus, detectable anterior to and distal to the malleoli. The talus can be located by palpating the area between the malleoli as the athlete inverts and everts the plantarflexed foot.

Palpation of the Medial Musculature and Related Soft Tissue

• **Tibialis posterior:** The belly of the tibialis posterior is not distinctly palpable, as it lies under the gastrocnemius and soleus muscles. Its tendon passes behind and around the medial malleolus and becomes most palpable at its insertion on the navicular tubercle.

• **Long toe flexors:** Palpation of the flexor hallucis longus and flexor digitorum longus muscles and their tendons is described in Chapter 3. These tendons may be pinched between the medial malleolus and the calcaneus during inversion of the ankle.

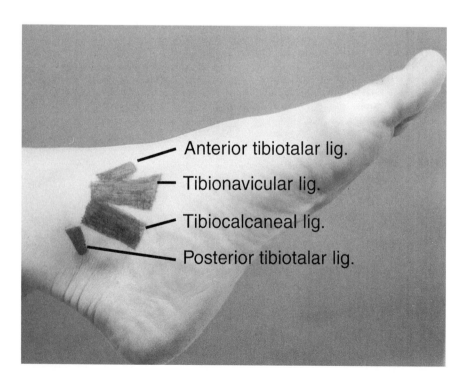

Anterior tibiotalar lig.

Tibionavicular lig.

Tibiocalcaneal lig.

Posterior tibiotalar lig.

Figure 4–19. Surface anatomy of the deltoid ligaments. During palpation these ligaments are not distinguishable from one another.

Palpation of the Posterior Bony and Ligamentous Structures

The posterior tibial shaft is covered by the bulk of the calf musculature, the Achilles tendon, and bursae and thus is not palpable.

Palpation of the Posterior Musculature and Related Soft Tissue

• **Gastrocnemius-soleus complex:** The gastrocnemius is palpable from its dual origin on the lateral and medial femoral condyles. Giving rise to a large muscle mass, the belly of the gastrocnemius should be palpated in its entirety as it forms the bulk of the posterior calf musculature.

• **Achilles tendon:** From its insertion on the calcaneus, the attachment of the Achilles tendon is located and its length palpated. This tendon should feel firm and ropelike, with a gradual, symmetrical increase in its width. The Achilles tendon and its musculotendinous junction should be palpated for symptoms of tendinitis or an **Achilles tendon rupture**, in which a gross discontinuity may be noted.

• **Calcaneal bursa:** Found between the posterior aspect of the calcaneus and the anterior portion of the Achilles tendon, this structure may be isolated by squeezing the soft tissue anteriorly on either side of the Achilles tendon.

• **Retrocalcaneal bursa:** Located between the posterior aspect of the Achilles tendon and the skin, the calcaneal bursa may be isolated by pinching the skin that overlies the tendon. In chronic inflammatory conditions, this bursa may be enlarged and thickened, forming "pump bumps" (see Fig. 3–9).

• **Dome of the calcaneus:** Just anterior to the calcaneal bursa, the calcaneal dome is located. Pain elicited from adolescent athletes during palpation of this area may indicate calcaneal apophysitis near the Achilles tendon's insertion on the calcaneus, as described in Chapter 3.

Palpation of Pulses

• **Posterior tibial artery:** The posterior tibial artery is located between the flexor digitorum longus and flexor hallucis longus tendons, as they sling behind the medial malleolus. Supplying a significant amount of blood to the foot, the presence of this pulse should be established following any significant lower extremity bone fracture or joint dislocation. It should be noted that swelling along the medial joint line may mask the presence of this pulse and make its detection difficult.

• **Dorsalis pedis artery:** A branch of the anterior tibial artery, the dorsalis pedis pulse may be palpated between the extensor digitorum longus and extensor hallucis longus tendons as they pass over the cuneiforms. It is important to establish the presence of this pulse following lower extremity fracture or dislocation and in those individuals suspected of having an **anterior compartment syndrome**. This pulse is not readily detectable in all people. In the absence of a pulse on the involved side, make sure that the pulse is identifiable on the uninvolved extremity.

Functional Tests

The amount of active and passive range of motion available to the talocrural joint can be affected by muscular tightness. To allow for proper gait, the talocrural joint must provide 10 degrees of dorsiflexion during walking and 15 degrees during running. Athletes displaying tightness in the gastrocnemius-soleus complex pronate the foot during weight bearing to compensate for the lack of dorsiflexion, leading to biomechanical changes in the lower extremity and predisposing the athlete to overuse injuries.

Subtalar joint motion is relatively difficult to measure accurately. The range of motion available to this joint is influenced by the bony structure of the ankle mortise, the position of the talocrural joint, and past injury to the ligaments supporting this joint.

For the purposes of this section, plantarflexion and dorsiflexion are defined as the movement taking place at the talocrural joint, while inversion and eversion describe the motion occurring at the subtalar joint (Table 4–5; see Table 4–1 for nerve innervations).

Range of motion is influenced by the athlete's age and gender. In the high school and college–aged population, women have a greater range of motion in all planes than do men. Range of motion decreases after age 20 for both genders, but to a greater extent in women.[11, 12]

Table 4–5. Muscles Contributing to Foot and Ankle Movements

Dorsiflexion	Inversion
Extensor digitorum longus	Extensor hallucis longus
Extensor hallucis longus	Flexor digitorum longus
Peroneus tertius	Flexor hallucis longus
Tibialis anterior	Tibialis anterior
	Tibialis posterior

Plantarflexion	Eversion
Flexor digitorum longus	Extensor digitorum longus
Flexor hallucis longus	Peroneus brevis
Gastrocnemius	Peroneus longus
Peroneus brevis	Peroneus tertius
Peroneus longus	
Plantaris	
Soleus	
Tibialis posterior	

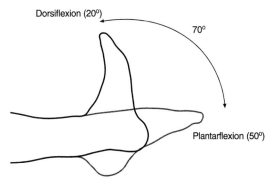

Figure 4-20. Range of motion for plantarflexion and dorsiflexion. Tightness of the Achilles tendon limits dorsiflexion.

Active Range of Motion

• **Plantarflexion and dorsiflexion:** Spanning a range of 70 degrees, normal active range of motion occurs as 20 degrees of dorsiflexion and 50 degrees of plantarflexion from the neutral position (Fig. 4-20). When using a goniometer for this measurement, one must ensure that the movement arm is aligned with the talus parallel to the metatarsals to isolate true talocrural motion from accessory foot motion.

• **Inversion and eversion:** Accounting for a total of 25 degrees, the predominant movement occurs as 20 degrees of inversion from the neutral position and 5 degrees of eversion from neutral (Fig. 4-21).

Passive Range of Motion

• **Plantarflexion and dorsiflexion:** Dorsiflexion should be measured once with the knee flexed and then again with the knee extended to determine tightness of the gastrocnemius. The normal end-feel for both plantarflexion and dorsiflexion is firm owing to soft tissue stretch of the anterior joint capsule, deltoid ligament, and ATF ligament during plantarflexion and of the Achilles

tendon during dorsiflexion. Following injury, the lost range of motion is greater in plantarflexion than in dorsiflexion, although loss of dorsiflexion is more debilitating in the long term because of the resultant changes in gait mechanics.

• **Inversion and eversion:** The athlete should be lying prone during the measurement of subtalar inversion and eversion, although less reliable measurements may be made with the athlete sitting. The tibia and fibula should be stabilized to prevent hip or lower leg rotation. The normal end-feel during neutral inversion is firm secondary to soft tissue stretch from the lateral ankle ligaments (especially the CF ligament) and the peroneus longus and brevis muscles. A hard end-feel may be presented during eversion as the result of the fibula's striking the calcaneus or it may be firm because of stretching of the medial joint capsule and musculature. After injury the capsular pattern lost is greater for inversion than for eversion.

Resistive Range of Motion

• **Dorsiflexion:** The athlete should be placed in either the sitting or the supine position so that the foot hangs over the edge of the table. To measure resistive dorsiflexion of the foot as a whole, stabilization is provided to the lower leg just above the ankle joint, while resistance is provided to the distal aspect of the dorsal foot (Fig. 4-22).

Isolated resistive dorsiflexion may be performed for the following muscles:

○ **Tibialis anterior:** By providing resistance against dorsiflexion and inversion, the tibialis anterior may be isolated if the athlete does not compensate with the extensor hallucis longus.

○ **Peroneus tertius:** Moving the resistance to the lateral portion of the dorsal foot and applying pressure against dorsiflexion and eversion isolates the peroneus tertius if the athlete does not compensate with the extensor digitorum longus as indicated by extension of the lateral four toes during testing.

• **Plantarflexion:** The athlete sits or lies prone with the foot reaching past the edge of the table. The lower leg is stabilized just above the ankle joint while resistance is provided to the distal portion of the foot's plantar surface (Fig. 4-23). Because the plantarflexor group is so powerful, it is often necessary to test these muscles through the use of a unilateral heel-raise. Using a tabletop for balance, the athlete is asked to perform a set of 10 toe-raises (Fig. 4-24). Weakness in the plantarflexor group is evidenced by being unable to complete the test, by inclining forward, or by bending the knee when the gastrocnemius is being isolated.[12]

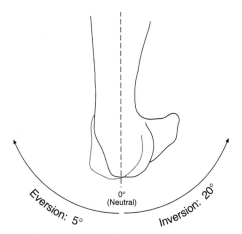

Figure 4-21. Range of motion for inversion and eversion.

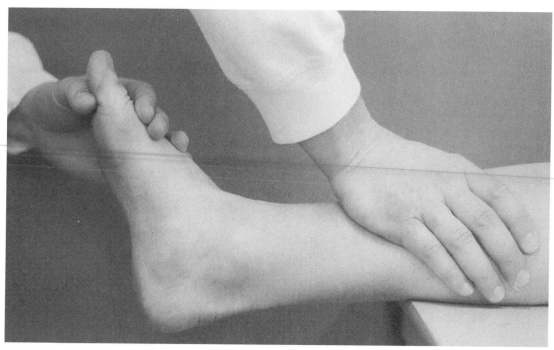

Figure 4–22. Hand placement for testing resisted dorsiflexion.

Individual plantarflexors may be isolated through the following techniques:

○ **Gastrocnemius:** The contribution of the gastrocnemius to ankle plantarflexion is greatest when the knee is extended. This position also allows for contribution from the plantaris muscle.

○ **Soleus:** To isolate the soleus muscle, flex the knee off the end of the table so that it is bent to 90 degrees (a minimum of 30 degrees' flexion is required to remove the influence of the gastrocnemius). The examiner stabilizes the lower leg with one hand just above the posterior ankle joint and provides resistance with the other hand at the distal portion of the foot's plantar surface.

○ **Other muscles contributing to plantarflexion**: The flexor digitorum longus and the flexor hallucis longus contribute slightly to plantarflexion.

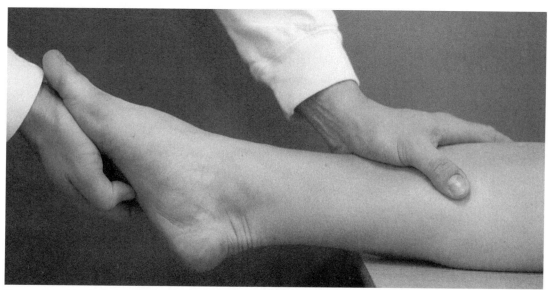

Figure 4–23. Hand placement for testing resisted plantarflexion.

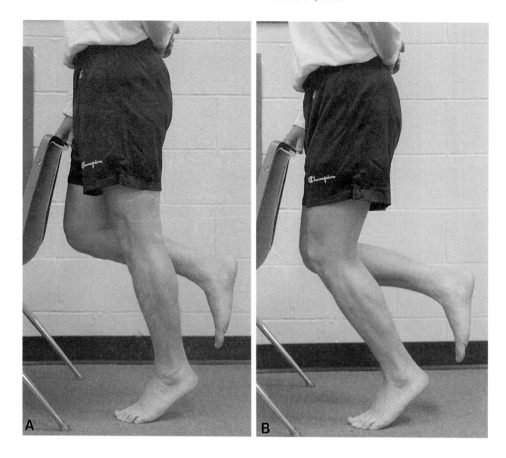

Figure 4–24. Toe-raise test for plantarflexion. (*A*) With the knee extended to involve the triceps surae group. (*B*) With the knee flexed to isolate the soleus muscle.

• **Inversion:** The athlete sits or lies supine with the lower leg externally rotated or side-lies on the side that is being tested. The lower leg is stabilized with one hand while resistance is provided along the medial aspect of the foot as the athlete attempts to invert the plantarflexed foot (Fig. 4–25).

Specific muscles contributing to inversion may be isolated using the following techniques:

○ **Tibialis posterior:** The lower leg is stabilized while resistance is provided along the medial aspect of the foot while the athlete attempts to plantarflex and invert. During this test any flexion of the toes should be noted, indi-

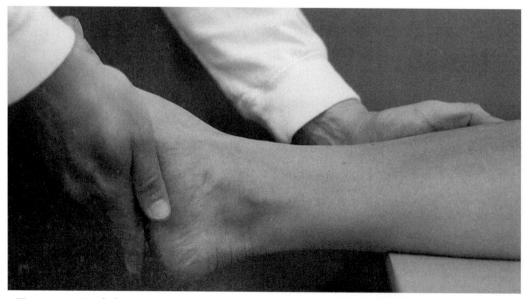

Figure 4–25. Hand placement for testing resisted inversion.

cating possible substitution of the flexor hallucis longus or flexor digitorum longus muscles.

○ **Other muscles contributing to inversion:** The combined force of the flexor digitorum longus, flexor hallucis longus, and extensor hallucis longus provides significant contribution to subtalar inversion, as described in Chapter 3. Another powerful invertor, the tibialis anterior, is described in the Resistive Dorsiflexion Testing section of this chapter.

• **Eversion:** The athlete is seated or positioned supine with the leg internally rotated, or side-lying on the opposite side as that being tested. The lower leg is stabilized above the ankle and resistance is provided along the lateral aspect of the foot while the athlete attempts to evert the plantarflexed foot (Fig. 4–26).

It is difficult, if not impossible, to differentiate between the contribution to eversion of the peroneus longus and the peroneus brevis. The peroneus tertius contributes to eversion and is described in the Resistive Dorsiflexion section of this chapter. The role and description of the extensor digitorum longus is discussed in Chapter 3.

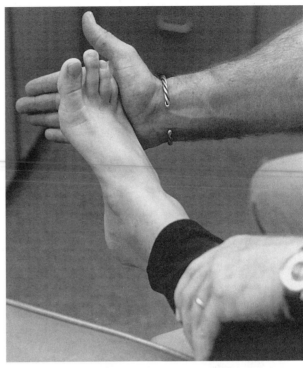

Figure 4–26. Hand placement for testing resisted eversion.

Tests for Ligamentous Stability

The range of motion tests also serve to stress the ligaments of the ankle complex, especially during the passive range of motion testing (see Table 4–4). Tests for ligamentous stability should still be performed as a unique section of the clinical examination with emphasis placed on joint play and ligament-specific tenderness and pain.

Test for Anterior Talofibular Ligament Instability

The motions of ankle plantarflexion and subtalar inversion (supination) place a great deal of strain on the ATF. Indeed, this is the most common position of the foot and ankle during injury of this structure. The ATF serves to prevent anterior translation of the talus relative to the ankle mortise. Using the anterior drawer test, the presence of tears to the ATF may be determined (Fig. 4–27).

Anterior Drawer Test (Fig. 4–27)

Position of athlete	Sitting over the edge of the table with the knee bent to prevent gastrocnemius tightness influencing the outcome of the test.
Position of examiner	Sitting in front of the athlete. One hand stabilizes the lower leg, taking care not to occlude the mortise. The other hand cups the calcaneus while the forearm supports the foot in a position of slight plantarflexion.
Evaluative procedure	The examiner draws the calcaneus and talus forward while providing a stabilizing force to the tibia.
Positive test results	The talus slides anteriorly from under the ankle mortise as compared with the opposite side (assuming it is normal). There may be an appreciable "clunk" as the talus subluxes and relocates, or the athlete describes pain.
Implications	Tear of the anterior talofibular ligament and the associated capsule.
Modification	The test may be performed with the athlete supine, but the knee must be kept in a minimum of 15° flexion to eliminate the influence of the gastrocnemius muscle.

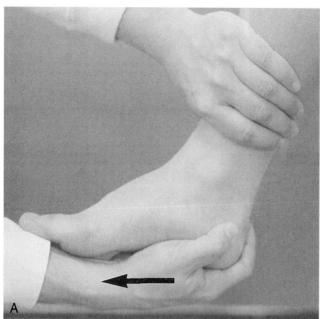

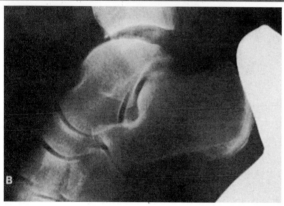

Figure 4–27. (*A*) Anterior drawer test to check the integrity of the anterior talofibular ligament. (*B*) X-ray view of a positive anterior drawer test. Note the anterior displacement of the talus relative to the tibia. (*B* from Donatelli, R,[12a] FA Davis, Philadelphia, 1990, p 13, with permission.)

Test for Calcaneofibular Ligament Instability

The inversion stress test (talar tilt test) is used to determine whether the calcaneofibular ligament has been compromised (Fig. 4–28). This test also stresses the anterior and posterior talofibular ligaments.

Inversion Stress Test (Talar Tilt) (Fig. 4–28)

Position of athlete	Sitting with legs over the edge of a table.
Position of examiner	In front of the athlete. One hand grasps the calcaneus and maintains the foot in neutral. The opposite hand stabilizes the lower leg. The thumb or forefinger may be placed along the calcaneofibular ligament so that any gapping of the talus away from the mortise can be felt.
Evaluative procedure	The hand holding the calcaneus provides an inversion stress by rolling the calcaneus inward, causing the talus to tilt.
Positive test results	The talus tilts or gaps excessively, as compared with the uninjured side; or pain is produced.
Implications	Involvement of the calcaneofibular ligament, possibly along with the anterior talofibular and posterior talofibular ligament.

Tests for Deltoid Ligament Instability

The distal expanse of the lateral malleolus makes it difficult to evert the ankle; thus many of the injuries to the deltoid ligament are caused by rotational stresses about the ankle joint. The eversion stress test (Fig. 4–29) is used to evaluate injury resulting from a pure eversion mechanism. Kleiger's test (Fig. 4–30) is used to determine injury to the deltoid ligament caused by a rotatory stress or injury to the syndesmosis, with the results differentiated by the location of pain.

Eversion Stress Test (Talar Tilt) (Fig. 4–29)

Position of athlete	Sitting with legs over the edge of a table.
Position of examiner	In front of the athlete. One hand grasps the calcaneus and maintains the foot in neutral. The opposite hand stabilizes the lower leg. The thumb or forefinger may be placed along the deltoid ligament so that any gapping of the talus away from the mortise can be felt.
Evaluative procedure	The hand holding the calcaneus rolls it outward, attempting to tilt the talus, causing a gap on the medial side of the ankle mortise.
Positive test results	The talus tilts or gaps excessively as compared with the uninjured side, or pain is described during this motion.
Implications	The deltoid ligament has been compromised.

Kleiger's Test (Fig. 4–30)

Position of athlete	Sitting with legs over the edge of the table.
Position of examiner	In front of the athlete. One hand stabilizes the lower leg in a manner that does not compress the distal tibiofibular syndesmosis. The other hand grasps the medial aspect of the foot while supporting the ankle in neutral.
Evaluative procedure	The foot is rotated laterally.
Positive test results	Deltoid ligament involvement: The athlete complains of medial and/or lateral joint pain. The examiner may feel displacement of the talus away from the medial malleolus. Syndesmosis involvement: Pain is described above the lateral malleolus.
Implications	Medial pain is indicative of trauma to the deltoid ligament, whereas pain in the area of the lateral malleolus reflects syndesmosis pathology.

Test for Ankle Syndesmosis Instability

Injury to the supporting structures of the ankle syndesmosis, the anterior tibiofibular ligament, the interosseous membrane, and the posterior tibiofibular ligament may be determined through pressure at the end of dorsiflexion range of motion or through an external rotation placed on the talus. Kleiger's test is used to determine damage to this structure.

Neurological Testing

Neurological dysfunction can occur secondary to compartmental syndromes or direct trauma in the case of the tibial or peroneal nerves. The nerve most prone to trauma may be the common peroneal nerve. The possible mechanisms for trauma to this nerve are presented in Table 4–6 (see Neurological Screen on page 110).

Pathologies and Related Special Tests

Although sprains are the predominant type of injury suffered by the lower leg and ankle, the evaluation process must not discount other potential injuries. Other acute injuries to this body area include fractures, dislocations, and tendon ruptures. Additionally, many overuse conditions plague the lower leg.

Neurological Screen

Nerve Root Level	Sensory Testing	Motor Testing	Reflex Testing
L4	Saphenous n.	Deep peroneal n.	Patellar t.
L5	Peroneal n.	Deep peroneal n.	Partial
S1	Peroneal n.	Tibial n.	Achilles t.
S2	P. femoral cutaneous n.	Intrinsic foot/toe muscles Lateral plantar n.	None

Ankle Sprains

Ankle sprains are common in competitive athletics. Most of these injuries are inversion ankle sprains, resulting in trauma to the lateral ligament complex. A lesser, yet significant percentage of sprains also involve the medial ankle ligaments and the ankle syndesmosis. Because of the close association of many of the ankle ligaments with the joint capsule, ligament injury often results in trauma to the capsule. Ankle sprains may also be complicated by fractures of the ankle mortise, avulsion of the lig-

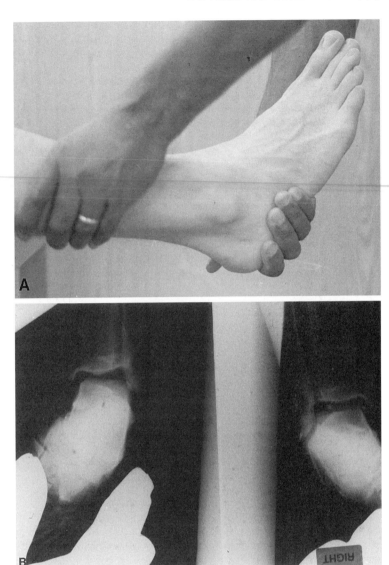

Figure 4–28. (*A*) Inversion stress test (talar tilt test) to check the integrity of the calcaneofibular ligament. (*B*) X-ray view of an inversion stress.

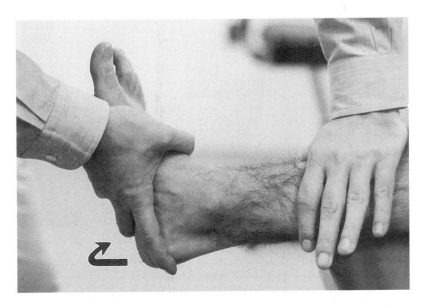

Figure 4–29. Eversion stress test to determine the integrity of the deltoid ligament, especially the tibiocalcaneal ligament.

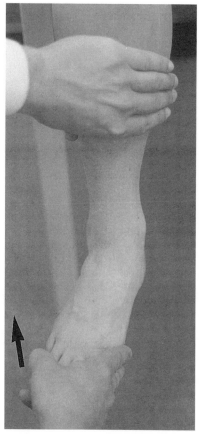

Figure 4–30. Kleiger's test for determination of rotatory damage to the deltoid ligament or the distal tibiofibular syndesmosis. The implication is based on the area of pain that is elicited.

aments from their site of origin or attachment, or dislocation of the talus.

Inversion Ankle Sprains. Damage to the lateral ligament complex tends to occur when the foot is in the **open-packed position** of plantarflexion, thus predisposing the ATF ligament to damage. Most athletic movements place the foot in plantarflexion, such as

Table 4–6. Mechanisms of Injury of the Common Peroneal Nerve

Mechanism	Causal Factor
Lesion	Fracture of the fibular head
Concussive	Contusion to the superior portion of the fibula
Compression	Knee braces or elastic wraps
Internal pressure	Prolonged squatting (e.g., baseball or softball catcher)
Entrapment	Exertional compartment syndromes
Traction	Varus stress to the knee, plantarflexion and inversion of the ankle, hyperextension of the knee

Adapted from Coombs.[13]

when landing from a jump, during the push-off phase of gait, or when cutting to change direction.

Calcaneofibular ligament damage occurs secondary to ATF ligament trauma when the foot is plantarflexed and inverted. When the ankle is inverted in the neutral position, the CF ligament is the primary restraint against inversion, and injury may be isolated to this structure.

Athletes with this injury describe a mechanism of inversion and/or plantarflexion or rotation (see Table 4–4) and may report a "pop" at the time of injury. With the exception of an isolated CF ligament sprain, swelling may rapidly develop around the lateral malleolus secondary to an associated tear in the joint capsule. Palpation elicits tenderness along the involved ligament(s) and capsule (Table 4–7). Special attention must be paid to pain and crepitus elicited over the origin and insertion of the ligament, indicating a possible avulsion fracture. Pain is demonstrated during the movements of inversion and/or plantarflexion, as described in the Ligamentous and Capsular Testing portion of this chapter.

The presence of an inversion mechanism should not limit suspicion of injury to only the lateral ligaments. This mechanism can also result in impingement of the medial capsule and the structures passing behind and beneath the medial malleolus, especially the tibialis posterior. Excessive inversion of the talus and calcaneus can result in the fracture of the distal medial malleolus or base of the fifth MT in addition to avulsing the lateral ligaments from their site of origin or insertion (Fig. 4–31). Additionally, this mechanism may result in traction injuries to the peroneal nerve.[13] Extra caution should be exercised when evaluating apparent ankle sprains in adolescent athletes. Those athletes displaying excessive laxity should be referred to a physician to rule out the presence of epiphyseal fractures through radiography.[14]

Athletes who have suffered an inversion ankle sprain are predisposed to subsequent injury, with residual symptoms appearing in 11 to 33 percent of the individuals suffering "severe" ankle sprains.[15] Two theories have been suggested to account for the high recurrence of ankle sprains[16]: (1) Ligaments lose their ability to passively support and protect the joint and the peroneal reflex arc is too slow to evoke a contraction in these muscles in time to contract, limiting the force and speed of inversion[17]; and (2) there is a decrease in the proprioceptive ability of the capsule, ligaments, and peroneal muscles, occurring secondary to the initial trauma of injury.[18,19] Although much reliance has been placed on the use of tape and braces to prevent recurrence of ankle sprains, all ankle sprains should be followed by a complete rehabilitation program.

Chronic or severe inversion ankle sprains often result in a number of secondary conditions. Following a tear of the anterior talofibular and calcane-

---

Open-packed position: The joint position at which its bones are maximally incongruent.

Table 4–7. Evaluative Findings of Inversion Ankle Sprains

Examination Segment	Clinical Findings
History	Onset: Acute. Location of pain: Lateral border of the ankle around the area of the malleolus and sinus tarsi. Mechanism: Inversion, plantarflexion, or talar rotation in any combination.
Inspection	Findings include swelling and redness around the lateral joint capsule, which may seep to the dorsum of the foot. Ecchymosis may be present around the lateral malleolus.
Palpation	Pain is elicited along the involved ligaments. Crepitus at the site of ligamentous origin or insertion may indicate an avulsion fracture.
Functional tests	AROM: Pain on the lateral side of the ankle during plantarflexion and inversion indicates stretching of the lateral ligaments. Pain medially indicates a pinching of the medial structures. Lateral pain during dorsiflexion and eversion indicates a pinching of the lateral capsule. PROM: Motion produces pain along the ligaments as described in the Ligamentous and Capsular Testing section of this chapter (also see Table 4–2). RROM: Decreased strength or pain during most motions is found secondary to stretching of the ligaments or of the peroneal muscles. Isometric contractions may not elicit pain.
Ligamentous testing	Positive inversion stress test and/or anterior drawer test results.
Neurological testing	This is not required in normal ankle sprain evaluation. Hyperplantarflexion and inversion may result in stretching of the peroneal nerve.
Special tests	None.
Comments	The clinician must be aware of avulsion fracture of the lateral ligaments, impingement of the medial joint capsule, impingement of the structures beneath the medial malleolus, and possible fracture of the medial malleolus or base of the 5th MT. Adolescent athletes displaying ankle instability should be referred for x-ray examination to rule out the possibility of an epiphyseal injury.

ofibular ligaments, the anterolateral capsule may develop a dense area of thickened connective tissue that becomes impinged between the lateral malleolus and calcaneus when the foot and ankle are dorsiflexed and everted.[20]

Repeated episodes of inversion sprains, as well as those involving a single incident, may have an associated talar chondral lesion. These lesions are not easily identifiable by standard x-ray examination and have a common trait of pain of unidentified origin and tenderness along the superior anteromedial (tibial) portion of the ankle mortise. Innovations in diagnostic imaging techniques such as magnetic resonance imaging (MRI) and bone scans have greatly increased the frequency of diagnosis of this injury.[21,22] If this condition goes unchecked, osteochondritis dissecans of the talocrural joint is likely to develop.[23]

Syndesmosis Sprains. Injury to the tibiofibular syndesmosis has been estimated to account for as much as 10 percent of all ankle sprains[24] and as high as 18 percent in professional football players, which may be attributed to their increased participation on artificial surfaces.[25] Other factors contributing to the occurrence of syndesmotic ankle sprains include *collision sports* in which the mechanism of injury involves planting the foot and "cut-

ting" so that the talus is externally rotated and the foot dorsiflexed. Another common mechanism is an athlete's being fallen on while lying on the ground, causing external rotation of the foot.

The athlete describes lateral ankle pain, especially above the lateral malleolus, that is intensified during forced dorsiflexion or Kleiger's test or that is reduced when the syndesmosis is compressed. The widening of the ankle mortise (see Fig. 4–9) results in instability of the ankle as the talus is allowed a greater amount of glide within the joint. Although less common, syndesmotic sprains require a longer recovery period than do inversion sprains.[25]

Eversion Ankle Sprains. As previously described, the strength of the deltoid ligament combined with the mechanical superiority of the lateral malleolus limits eversion, so that injury to the deltoid ligament accounts for only 15 percent of all ankle sprains.[26] Because of the small amount of eversion normally associated with the subtalar joint (5 degrees), the primary mechanism for damage to this ligament group is external rotation of the talus on the ankle mortise. Pain is present along the medial joint line and swelling tends to be more localized than lateral ankle sprains (Table 4–8). If an eversion mechanism is described, the lateral malle-

---

Collision sports: Individual or team sports relying on the physical dominance of one athlete over another. By their nature, these sports mandate violent physical contact.

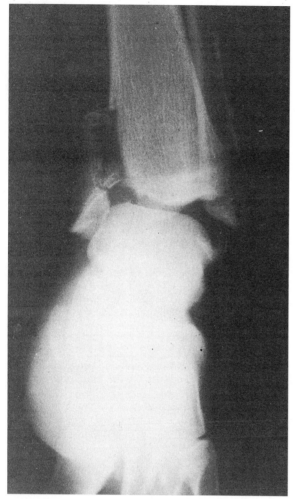

Figure 4–31. Fracture of the medial malleolus caused by excessive inversion of the ankle.

olus should be carefully evaluated for the presence of a "knock-off" fracture (Fig. 4–32).

Ankle Dislocations. Resulting from excessive rotation combined with inversion or eversion, dislocations of the talocrural joint result in major disruption of the joint capsule and associated ligaments and often have an associated fracture of the malleoli, long bones, and/or talus. Normally resulting in immediate pain and loss of function, the athlete may report an audible snap or crack and report pain in the ankle and lower leg. The foot may be grossly malaligned and, if the defect is not visible, the superior portion of the talus may be palpated as it protrudes anteriorly from the ankle mortise (Fig. 4–33).[27] The evaluation should also confirm the presence of the distal pulses and include a secondary survey of the ankle mortise and long bones for possible fracture. The ankle is then immobilized and the athlete transported for medical intervention.

Lower Leg Fractures

Many acute fractures of the lower leg, especially those involving the tibial shaft, exhibit obvious gross deformity (Fig. 4–34). In many instances the athlete and others in the vicinity of the injury report an audible snap (or crack) at the time of injury. Pain is reported along the fracture site and may radiate up the lower leg and extremity. Palpation may reveal crepitus or discontinuity along the bone shaft; if a bony defect is visible, palpation should not be performed. Although long bone fractures normally result in immediate dysfunction and an inability to bear weight, athletes suffering from fibular fractures may still be

Table 4–8. Evaluative Findings of Eversion Ankle Sprains

Examination Segment	Clinical Findings
History	Onset: Acute. Location of pain: Medial border of the ankle and foot, radiating from the medial malleolus. Mechanism: Eversion and/or rotation.
Inspection	Swelling and redness around the medial joint capsule.
Palpation	Pain is located near the deltoid ligaments. Crepitus at the site of ligamentous origin or insertion may indicate an avulsion fracture.
Functional tests	AROM: Pain on the medial side of the ankle during plantarflexion indicates stretching of the anterior tibiotalar and/or the tibionavicular ligaments. Pain during dorsiflexion indicates trauma to the posterior tibiotalar ligament. PROM: Motion produces pain along the ligaments, as described in the Ligamentous and Capsular Testing section of this chapter (also see Table 4–2). RROM: Decreased strength or medial pain during most motions secondary to stretching of the medial ligaments.
Ligamentous testing	Positive eversion stress test and/or Kleiger's test results.
Neurological testing	Not applicable.
Special tests	None.
Comments	Excessive calcaneal eversion can result in a fracture of the lateral malleolus, talar dome, or disruption of the syndesmosis.

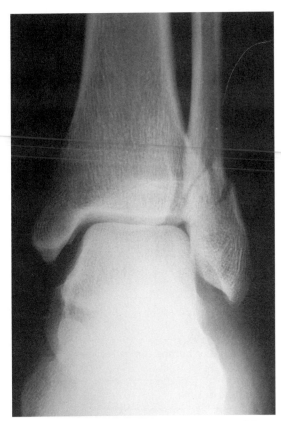

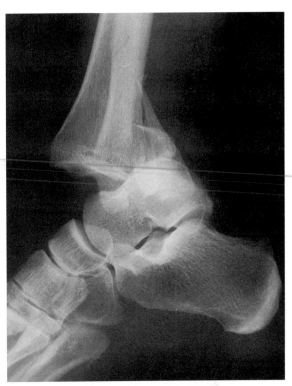

Figure 4–33. Posterior ankle dislocation. Often the talus displaces anteriorly relative to the tibia. This x ray shows the talus being displaced posteriorly relative to the tibia. Note the fracture of the malleolus caused by the wide anterior talar border's being forced into the mortise.

Figure 4–32. Fracture of the lateral malleolus caused by excessive eversion of the ankle. This type of fracture to the lateral malleolus is more common as it extends farther inferiorly than does the medial malleolus.

capable of walking. In cases when deformity or other signs of a gross fracture are absent, the squeeze test may be used to confirm fracture of the fibula (Fig. 4–35). The bump test may be used for calcaneal or talar fractures or hairline fractures of the tibia (see Stress Fractures later in this chapter).

Nondisplaced fibular or tibial fractures may be treated by simple casting. However, comminuted or displaced fractures often require the use of internal or external fixation devices to realign and stabilize the fracture sites. A fracture of the distal fibula involving the syndesmosis may require an internal fixation device or a screw to maintain the alignment of the fibula with the tibia during the healing process and to prevent subsequent rotational instabilities of the talus (Fig. 4–36).[28]

Squeeze Test (Fig. 4–35)

Position of athlete	Sitting or lying with the knee extended.
Position of examiner	Standing next to, or in front of, the injured leg. The evaluator's hands are cupped behind the tibia and fibula *away* from the site of pain.
Evaluative procedure	The evaluator gently squeezes (compresses) the fibula and tibia, gradually adding more pressure if no pain or other symptoms are elicited. The pressure is progressed toward the injured or painful site until pain is elicited.
Positive test results	Pain is elicited, especially when it is away from the compressed area.
Implications	Gross fracture or stress fracture of the fibula.
Comments	One should avoid applying too much pressure too soon into the test. Pressure should be applied gradually and progressively.

Stress Fractures. The tibia, fibula, and talus may be the site of stress fractures that are the result of the accumulation of microtraumatic forces. Having symptoms of gradual onset, the athlete complains of a burning pain along the shaft of the bone or, as is often the case with fibular stress fractures, proximal to the lateral malleolus. The athlete often describes pain along the bone that worsens with activity and subsides with rest. During activity, decreased muscular strength and cramping may be reported. Palpation may reveal crepitus and point tenderness isolated to a single spot along the shaft of the bone and, in many cases, the painful area is visually unremarkable (Table 4–9). Individuals having a narrow tibial shaft or a high degree of hip external rotation are predisposed to the onset of stress fractures.[29]

Acute stress fractures are not visible on standard x-ray examination and require the use of diagnostic techniques such as bone scans. Advanced stress fractures may be manifest through the squeeze test, as described in the previous section, or through the bump test (Fig. 4–37). Pain guides the management of stress fractures. Many athletes respond to rest and anti-inflammatory medication, whereas advanced cases may require casting or a walker boot.

Bump Test (Fig. 4–37)

Position of athlete	Sitting with the involved leg off the end of the table and the knee straight, or lying supine. The ankle is in the neutral position.
Position of examiner	Standing in front of the heel of the involved leg. The posterior portion of the lower leg is stabilized with the nondominant hand.
Evaluative procedure	Using the palm of the dominant hand, the examiner bumps the calcaneus with progressively more force until pain is elicited.
Positive test results	Pain emanating from the calcaneus, talus, fibula, or tibia.
Implications	Possible advanced stress fracture.

Achilles Tendon Pathology

Because of its dual association with the two prime plantarflexors, the gastrocnemius and the soleus, any injury to the Achilles tendon results in decreased plantarflexion strength. The disrupted plantarflexion may cause significant changes in the athlete's gait, impairing the ability to walk, run, and jump normally.

Achilles Tendinitis. Factors such as running mechanics, duration and intensity of running, the type of shoe and running surface, as well as the biomechanics of the foot and ankle may all result in inflammation of the Achilles tendon and its related structures. It has been suggested that this inflammatory condition does not actually afflict the Achilles tendon but, rather, the peritendinous tissues surrounding it.[30,31]

Most cases of Achilles tendinitis are traced to overuse syndromes and repeated eccentric loading of the tendon. Athletes with foot rigidity are predisposed to this condition, as the gait must be modified to compensate for a valgus or varus hindfoot. Improperly fitting footwear may cause friction between the heel counter and the tendon, while shoes with a very rigid heel may not permit adequate range of motion in the midfoot and forefoot, altering the foot's biomechanics. Achilles tendinitis may also have an acute onset resulting from a direct blow to the tendon.

Athletes suffering from Achilles tendinitis describe pain (sometimes as "burning") radiating along the length of the tendon. The area is tender to the touch and crepitus may be elicited, particularly with active range of motion. This condition may be the result of, or may result in, tightness of the gastrocnemius-soleus muscle group (Table 4–10).

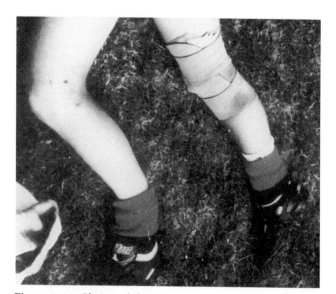

Figure 4–34. Obvious deformity caused by a lower leg fracture and possible ankle dislocation.

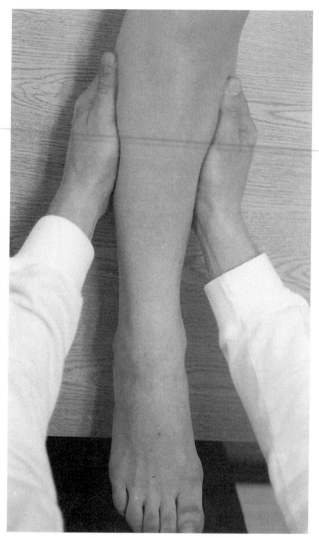

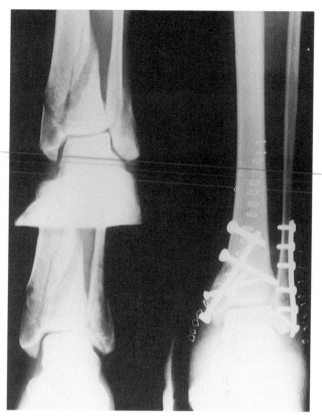

Figure 4-36. X ray showing screws and plates used to set a fracture and dislocation of the ankle mortise.

Figure 4-35. Squeeze test to identify fibular fractures. Pressure is applied to the fibula away from the athlete's site of pain. A positive test result, as shown in this photograph, is pain along the distal fibula.

Achilles Tendon Rupture. Forceful, sudden contraction, such as that which occurs when a defensive back or basketball player changes direction, when a gymnast dismounts from a piece of apparatus, or when a softball player plants and pivots to make a throw, results in a large amount of tension developing in the Achilles tendon. If this tension becomes too great the tendon fails, resulting in an Achilles tendon rupture. Although this injury is liable to occur in any athlete in any age group, it tends to be predominant in men over the age of 30.

The athlete reports the immediate inability to push off with the injured leg during ambulation and often describes the sensation of being "kicked." If the lesion occurs in the tendon's midsubstance, the defect may be observable and/or palpable (Fig. 4-38). Even in cases when the tendon is completely ruptured, the athlete is able to actively plantarflex the ankle through contraction of the per-

oneus longus and brevis, long toe flexors, plantaris, and the tibialis posterior muscles, although the strength of the contraction is markedly decreased (Table 4-11). The presence of an Achilles tendon rupture is confirmed through the Thompson test.

Thompson Test

The ability to actively plantarflex the foot should not be construed as absolute evidence that the Achilles tendon is intact and functioning. The Thompson test provides information about the integrity of the Achilles tendon and should be performed any time injury to this complex is suspected (Fig. 4-39) (see top of page 118).

Subluxating Peroneal Tendons

Forceful, sudden dorsiflexion and inversion or plantarflexion and eversion may stretch or rupture the superior peroneal retinaculum that functions to hold the peroneal tendons behind the lateral malleolus. Extreme cases may involve the inferior peroneal retinaculum as well (see Fig. 4-12). When these tendons lose their alignment from behind the lateral malleolus and are allowed to cross laterally to it, the peroneals, which are normally plantarflexors, become dorsiflexors (Fig. 4-40). The peroneal tendons may dislocate from the groove behind the lateral malleolus and may be observed as they "snap" into

Thompson Test (Fig. 4–39)

Position of athlete	Prone, with the foot off the edge of the table.
Position of examiner	At the side of the athlete, with one hand over the muscle belly of the calf musculature.
Evaluative procedure	The examiner squeezes the calf musculature while observing for plantarflexion of the foot.
Positive test results	When the calf is squeezed, the foot does not plantarflex.
Implications	The Achilles tendon has been ruptured.

and out of position during plantarflexion and dorsiflexion or active eversion. This biomechanical change alters the biomechanics of the foot and ankle, resulting in pain and dysfunction (Table 4–12).

In cases in which the retinaculum is stretched, the degree of subluxation may be controlled by rehabilitation exercises and taping. However, once the retinaculum has been stretched, it does not return to its original state.[32] When the retinacula have been completely disrupted or pain and dysfunction become great, surgical intervention is required.

Neurovascular Deficit

Disruption of the blood or nerve supply to or from the lower leg may be the result of acute trauma, overuse conditions, congenital defects, or surgery. A complete examination of the dermatomes, reflexes, and pulses of the lower leg and foot should be conducted to rule out the possibility of neurovascular involvement.

Anterior Compartment Syndrome

Resulting from increased pressure within the anterior compartment, anterior compartment syndrome threatens the integrity of the lower leg, foot, and toes through the obstruction of the neurovascular network (the deep peroneal nerve and anterior tibial artery) contained within this compartment. The bony posterolateral border and dense fibrous fascial lining of the compartment possess poor elas-

Table 4–9. Evaluative Findings of Lower Leg Stress Fractures

Examination Segment	Clinical Findings	
History	Onset:	Insidious, secondary to repetitive running and/or jumping.
	Location of pain:	Along the shaft of the tibia or fibula; initially, localized occurring only after exercise.
	Mechanism:	No known origin of pain. Interviewing the athlete may indicate a sudden increase in the duration or intensity of exercise or a change in playing surface or shoe worn.
	Predisposing factors:	Individuals having a narrow tibial shaft and/or an externally rotated hip have a higher rate of injury.
Inspection	This is normally unremarkable; however, localized swelling may be present in advanced stages.	
Palpation	Pain along the fracture site.	
Functional tests	All functional test results may be normal in the acute stages of stress fractures. In advanced cases or immediately following exercise, decreased strength may be evident owing to inflammation of the muscles near the site of the stress fracture.	
Ligamentous testing	Not applicable.	
Neurological testing	Not applicable.	
Special tests	The squeeze test is performed for advanced fibular stress fractures. The bump test is performed for advanced fibular, tibial, calcaneal, or talar stress fractures.	
Comments	Early stages of stress fractures may clinically resemble those of periosteitis. Early signs of stress fractures appear on bone scans. Healing bone does not appear on standard x-ray examination for 4 to 6 wk after the onset of symptoms.	

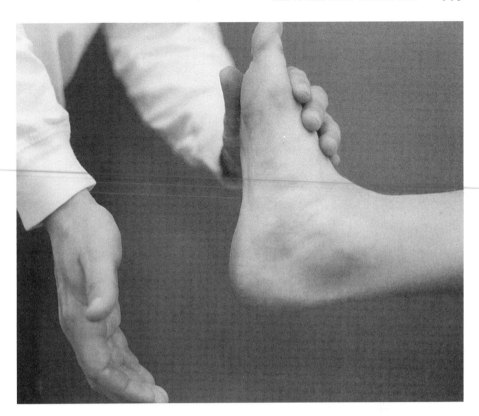

Figure 4–37. Bump test to identify stress fractures of the lower leg or talus. The examiner's hand is bumped against the athlete's foot. The subsequent shock waves elicit pain in areas of stress fractures. Note that this test is not definitive.

tic properties required to accommodate for expansion of the intracompartmental tissues.

Acutely, anterior compartment syndrome occurs from intracompartmental hemorrhage secondary to a blow to the anterolateral portion of the tibia. The subsequent bleeding and edema formation result in an increased pressure within the compartment, obstructing the neurovasculature network to and from the dorsum of the foot and causing ischemic destruction of the involved tissues.

Table 4–10. Evaluative Findings of Achilles Tendinitis

Examination Segment	Clinical Findings	
History	Onset:	Insidious, or the result of trauma to the Achilles tendon.
	Location of pain:	Along the length of the Achilles tendon.
	Mechanism:	Overuse or secondary to acute trauma, such as a blow to the Achilles tendon. It may also occur secondary to an improperly fitting shoe rubbing against the tendon.
Inspection	Discoloration and/or edema may be visible along the length of the tendon. The tendon may seem thicker on the affected side than on the opposite side.	
Palpation	Pain is elicited during palpation of this structure. Crepitus may be evident.	
Functional tests	AROM:	Pain and crepitus occur during plantarflexion and dorsiflexion.
	PROM:	Pain is present during dorsiflexion, resulting from stretching the tendon. Dorsiflexion range of motion may be diminished secondary to Achilles tendon tightness.
	RROM:	Pain and decreased strength are present during plantarflexion.
Ligamentous testing	Not applicable.	
Neurological testing	Not applicable.	
Special tests	None.	
Comments	Achilles tendinitis is often associated with foot rigidity. It may also be associated with calcaneal or retrocalcaneal bursitis.	

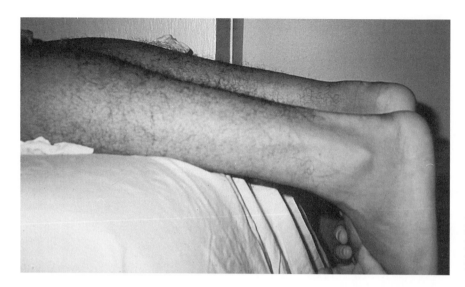

Figure 4–38. Ruptured Achilles tendon. The athlete's right (far) Achilles tendon has been ruptured. Note the depression proximal to the calcaneus and the involved swelling.

Compartmental syndromes may also have an insidious or chronic onset, with symptoms occurring during and after exercise. Chronic compartment syndrome (CCS), also referred to as recurrent compartment syndrome and intermittent claudication, is an exertional malady occurring secondary to anatomical abnormalities obstructing the blood flow in exercising muscles. Factors predisposing athletes to CCS include[33,34]:

• Herniation of muscle, occluding the neurovascular network as it transverses the interosseous membrane

• Fascia that fails to accommodate the increase in muscle volume during exercise

• Excessive hypertrophy of the muscles within an otherwise normal fascial network

Table 4–11. Evaluative Findings of Achilles Tendon Rupture

Examination Segment	Clinical Findings	
History	Onset:	Acute
	Location of pain:	Achilles tendon and/or lower portion of the gastrocnemius. The athlete often reports the sensation of being "kicked."
	Mechanism:	Forceful plantarflexion, usually the result of eccentric loading or plyometric contraction of the calf musculature.
	Predisposing factor:	A relationship may exist between a history of Achilles tendinitis and a rupture of the tendon.
Inspection	A defect *may* be visible in the Achilles tendon or at the musculotendinous junction, but rapid swelling may obscure this. Discoloration may be present around the tendon.	
Palpation	A palpable defect exists in the Achilles tendon, although it may quickly become obscured by swelling. Pain elicited along the tendon and lower gastrocnemius-soleus muscle group.	
Functional tests	AROM: The athlete is unable to bear weight on the involved extremity. Plantarflexion may still be present owing to the tibialis posterior, plantaris peroneals, and long toe flexors, although the athlete may describe pain during this motion and during dorsiflexion (because of the stretching of the Achilles tendon). PROM: Pain is elicited during dorsiflexion. RROM: There is a weak or nonexistent ability to plantarflex.	
Ligamentous testing	Not applicable.	
Neurological testing	Not applicable.	
Special tests	Positive Thompson test result.	
Comments	This injury tends to occur more frequently in male athletes over age 30, although any age group is susceptible. In acute conditions, the status of the dorsalis pedis pulse should be monitored.	

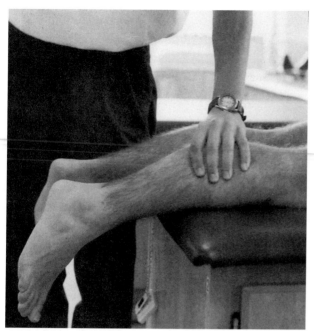

Figure 4–39. Thompson test for an Achilles tendon rupture. When the Achilles tendon is intact, squeezing the calf muscle results in slight plantarflexion. A positive Thompson test occurs when the calf is squeezed but no motion is produced in the foot, indicating a tear of the Achilles tendon.

- Increased capillary permeability

- Postexercise fluid retention

- Decreased venous return

Signs and symptoms of anterior compartment syndrome include pain within the compartment, numbness at the web space between the first and second toes, decreased strength during dorsiflexion,

and drop foot. A dramatic increase in pain or pain that seems disproportionate with the other examination findings is another factor identifying anterior compartment syndrome[35,36] (Table 4–13).

The presence of the dorsalis pedis pulse must be established in the involved limb (Fig. 4–41). Because this pulse is not detectable in all individuals, both limbs must be examined. If the pulse is present in the uninvolved extremity but not in the involved extremity, then one may assume that the blood flow to the foot has been compromised. Even though the blood pressure within the tibial artery may be sufficient to produce a palpable dorsalis pedis pulse, the pressure increase may be great enough to inhibit flow within the smaller vessels and capillaries.[33]

Acute anterior compartment syndrome should be considered a medical emergency and the athlete immediately referred for medical treatment. Chronic compartment syndromes tend to present symptoms during exercise that subsequently subside with rest. Confirmation of CCS requires the measurement of the intracompartmental pressure directly during and after exercise, an invasive technique that is performed in a medical facility.[37]

Deep Vein Thrombophlebitis

Thrombophlebitis, the inflammation of veins with associated blood clots, is most commonly found in postsurgical athletes, but it may also occur secondary to any trauma to the lower extremity. Athletes with this condition complain of pain and tightness in the calf during walking. Inspection of the calf may reveal swelling, and palpation tends to indicate tightness of the calf musculature and to elicit pain.

Homans' Sign. A test for the Homans' sign is indicated whenever deep vein thrombophlebitis (DVT) is suspected in the lower leg (Fig. 4–42). A positive

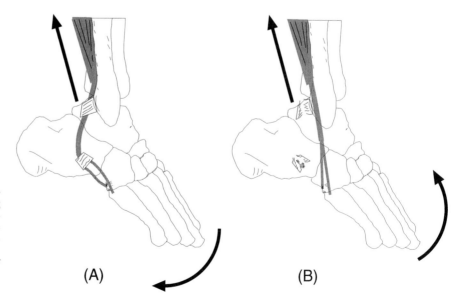

Figure 4–40. Illustration showing biomechanical changes with subluxating peroneal tendon. (*A*) When the peroneal retinacula is intact, the peroneals serve as plantarflexors of the foot. (*B*) Subluxating peroneal tendons, caused by the rupture or stretching of the retinacula, change the angle of pull to that of a dorsiflexor.

(A)   (B)

Homans' Test for Deep Vein Thrombosis (Fig. 4–42)

Position of athlete	Sitting or supine, with the knee extended.
Position of examiner	At the end of the athlete's leg, with one hand supporting the calcaneus and the other hand on the plantar surface of the foot.
Evaluative procedure	The foot is passively dorsiflexed while the knee is kept extended.
Positive test results	Pain in the calf.
Implications	Possible deep vein thrombophlebitis. This should be in agreement with other clinical findings of pain with deep palpation, swelling, heat, and dysfunction.
Note	A strain of the gastrocnemius or soleus may produce a false-positive result with this examination.

Homans' sign is not absolute proof of DVT; a definitive diagnosis must be made through a physician via the use of ultrasonic images.

ON-FIELD EVALUATION OF LOWER LEG AND ANKLE INJURIES

Injuries to the lower leg and ankle are prevalent in athletics and the majority of the athletic trainer's on-field evaluation is dedicated to this body region. The goals of the on-field evaluation of these injuries are to rule out fractures and dislocations, determine the athlete's weight-bearing status, and identify the best method for removing the athlete from the field.

Equipment Considerations

The very nature of competitive athletics mandates ever more specialized footwear, braces, and tape. Although designed to protect the athlete from injury while also improving performance, these devices may hinder the evaluation and management of acute injuries.

Footwear Removal

Once a gross fracture or dislocation has been ruled out, it is often necessary to remove the athlete's shoe so that a thorough examination of the injury can be conducted once the athlete has reached the sideline.

Table 4–12. Evaluative Findings of Subluxating/Dislocating Peroneal Tendons

Examination Segment	Clinical Findings	
History	Onset:	Acute or insidious.
	Location of pain:	Behind the lateral malleolus in the area of the superior peroneal retinaculum, across the lateral malleolus, length of the peroneal tendons, and, in some cases, at the site of the inferior peroneal retinaculum.
	Mechanism:	Forceful dorsiflexion and eversion or plantarflexion and inversion.
Inspection	Swelling and ecchymosis may be isolated behind the lateral and inferior lateral malleolus (see under functional tests).	
Palpation	Tenderness behind the lateral malleolus and perhaps over the site of the inferior patellar retinaculum (see under functional tests).	
Functional tests	AROM:	The peroneal tendon may be seen, felt, or heard as it subluxates while the foot and ankle move from plantarflexion and inversion to dorsiflexion and eversion and back.
	PROM:	There are no significant clinical findings.
	RROM:	Findings are the same as for AROM. The clinician should palpate the area behind the lateral malleolus to identify any abnormal movement of the peroneal tendons.
Ligamentous testing	No significant findings.	
Neurological testing	Not applicable.	
Special tests	None.	

Table 4–13. Evaluative Findings of Acute and Chronic Anterior Compartment Syndrome

Examination Segment	Clinical Findings	
History	Onset:	Acute or chronic.
	Location of pain:	Anterolateral portion of the lower leg, being described as "achy," "sharp," or "dull."
		Other complaints such as muscle tightness, cramping, swelling, weakness, or the inability to exercise owing to pain may also be described.
	Mechanism:	Acute: direct blow to the anterolateral tibia.
		Chronic: symptoms reported during or after running or other prolonged activity.
Inspection	The anterior compartment may appear red, shiny, and swollen. In advanced cases, the dorsum of the foot may also be discolored.	
Palpation	The anterior compartment feels hard and edematous. After an acute onset the area is painful to to the touch.	
	The presence of a normal dorsalis pedis pulse should be determined.	
Functional tests	AROM: Decreased (or absent) ability to dorsiflex the ankle or extend the toes. Drop foot syndrome may be observed in the athlete's gait.	
	PROM: Pain may be elicited during plantarflexion secondary to stretching of the tendons of tibialis anterior and the long toe extensors caused by stretching of tissues within the compartment.	
	RROM: Weakness is exhibited during dorsiflexion and toe extension.	
Ligamentous testing	Not applicable.	
Neurological testing	Numbness may be present in the web space between the 1st and 2nd toes and possibly on the dorsum of the foot.	
Special tests	There are no clinician tests for these conditions. Chronic anterior compartment syndrome is confirmed by measuring the intracompartmental pressure during exercise.	
Comments	The clinician should not apply a compression wrap during the treatment of anterior compartment syndrome, as this technique increases the intracompartmental pressure and may exacerbate the condition.	
	Bilateral involvement in chronic anterior compartment syndromes is common.	

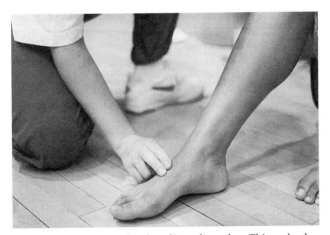

Figure 4–41. Locating the dorsalis pedis pulse. This pulse becomes diminished in the presence of anterior compartment syndrome or proximal joint dislocations. It is not always palpable and the findings of the involved limb should be compared to the uninvolved extremity.

Most shoes may be easily removed by completely unlacing them, spreading the sides and pulling the tongue down to the toes (Fig. 4–43). The athlete is asked to plantarflex the foot, if possible. The shoe is then removed by sliding the heel counter away from the foot and then lifting the shoe up and off the foot. Apprehensive athletes may be allowed to remove the shoe themselves. If a fracture or dislocation is suspected, the examiner should loosen the shoe enough to allow for palpation of the dorsalis pedis and posterior tibial pulses and transport the athlete with the shoe in place and the leg splinted.

Removal of Tape and Braces

Prophylactic devices such as tape or ankle braces must be removed to allow for the complete examination of the foot and ankle. Braces are tightened by

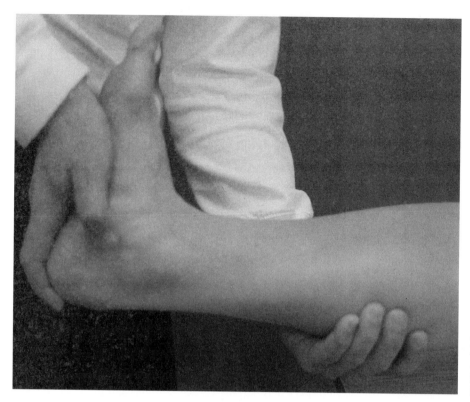

Figure 4–42. Homans' test for deep vein thrombosis. The calf is squeezed while the ankle is passively dorsiflexed. Indication of a positive result is a burning pain within the calf.

laces or Velcro straps and may be removed in a manner such as described for shoe removal. Ankle tape can be removed by cutting along a line parallel to the posterior portion of the malleolus on the side opposite the site of pain. The cut is then continued along the plantar aspect of the foot.

On-Field Inspection

During the on-field inspection of ankle and lower leg injuries, any gross bony or joint injury must be ruled out before progressing to the other elements of the evaluation.

The contour and alignment of the lower leg, foot, and ankle should be examined, noting any discontinuity or malalignment of the structures that may indicate a fracture or dislocation.

On-Field Palpation

Assuming normal alignment of the lower leg, the evaluation proceeds to palpation of the bony structures and related soft tissue.

• **Bony palpation:** The examiner begins by palpating the length of the tibia and fibula and continuing on to the talus, the remaining tarsals, and metatarsals. Any incongruencies, crepitus, or areas of point tenderness, especially in the area in which the athlete describes pain, should be noted. If a disruption of a long bone or joint is

felt, the joint should be splinted and the athlete transported to a hospital.

• **Soft tissue palpation:** A quick, yet thorough evaluation of the major soft tissues is performed, emphasizing the ligamentous structures for point tenderness and the tendons for signs of rupture.

On-Field Functional Tests

Once the possibility of a gross fracture or dislocation has been ruled out, the athlete's ability to move the limb and subsequently bear weight must be established.

• **Willingness to move the involved limb:** If the athlete displays normal alignment of the limb, the athletic trainer should observe the athlete's willingness to move the injured body part through the full range of motion. This task should be performed with a minimal amount of discomfort. If the athlete has no ability or is unwilling to move the involved limb, the athlete should be removed from the field with assistance.

• **Willingness to bear weight:** If the athlete describes no pain and there are no signs of restriction in the range of motion, the athlete is assisted to the standing position, bearing weight on the uninvolved leg. The athletic trainer then assumes a position under the athlete's arm on the involved side, providing some support. The athlete walks off the

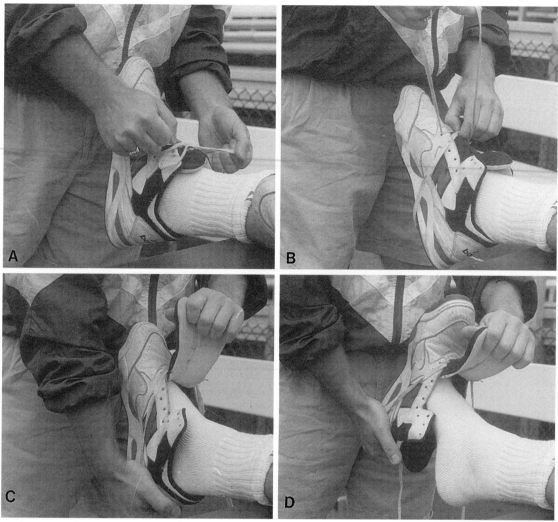

Figure 4–43. (*A*) Removing the shoe following a foot or ankle injury. (*B*) Completely remove the laces, (*C*) withdraw the tongue, and (*D*) slide the shoe from the foot.

field, attempting to place as little weight as possible on the involved limb.

INITIAL MANAGEMENT OF ON-FIELD INJURIES

This section describes the emergency management procedures for major trauma occurring to the ankle and lower extremity. Although fractures, dislocations, and acute anterior compartment syndrome are discussed, any suspicions of major trauma or of injury that is outside of the scope of the clinician's knowledge should be referred for further evaluation.

Fractures and Dislocations

Any obvious fracture or joint dislocation should immediately be immobilized using a moldable or vacuum splint (see Fig. 1–11). In most instances it is recommended that the shoe be left in place while the athlete is being transported to the hospital because it may be more safely removed in the emergency room after further diagnostic tests, such as x-ray examination, to determine the full extent of the injury (Fig. 4–44). The laces and tongue of the shoe should be loosened and the sock cut to permit palpation of the dorsalis pedis and the posterior tibial pulses, which are then compared bilaterally.

Anterior Compartment Syndrome

Unlike other acute soft tissue injuries, suspected anterior compartment syndromes should *not* be treated with compression. The use of external compression devices such as wraps or compression boots functions to increase the pressure within the anterior compartment and thus exacerbates the condition. If acute gross hemorrhage is present and/or

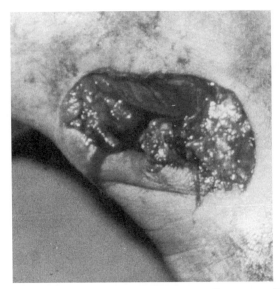

Figure 4–44. This apparent laceration is actually an open dislocation of the talus.

the dorsalis pedis pulse is absent, the athlete must be immediately referred for medical intervention. If, at the time of the injury, the athlete does not display signs of intracompartmental hemorrhage but there is reason to suspect such a response, the athlete should be presented with a list of the signs and symptoms to be aware of (see Table 4–13) and instructed whom to contact if the symptoms worsen.

REFERENCES

1. Campbell, DG, et al: Dynamic ankle ultrasonography. A new imaging technique for acute ankle ligament injuries. Am J Sports Med 22:855, 1994.
2. Garrick, JM: The frequency of injury, mechanism of injury, and epidemiology of ankle sprains. Am J Sports Med 5:241, 1971.
3. Lassiter, TE, Malone, TR, and Garrett, WE: Injury to the lateral ligaments of the ankle. Orthop Clin North Am 20:629, 1989.
4. Glick, JM, Gordon, RB, and Nishimoto, D: The prevention and treatment of ankle injuries. Am J Sports Med 4:136, 1976.
5. Garrick, JG, and Requa, RK: The epidemiology of foot and ankle injuries in sports. Clinics in Sports Medicine 7:29, 1988.
6. Takebe, K, et al: Role of the fibula in weight-bearing. Clin Orthop 184:2899, 1984.
6a. Rothstein, JM, Roy, SH, and Wolf, S: The Rehabilitation Specialist's Handbook, FA Davis, Philadelphia, 1991.
7. Inman, VT: The Joints of the Ankle. Williams & Wilkins, Baltimore, 1976.
8. Burks, RT, and Morgan, J: Anatomy of the lateral ankle ligaments. Am J Sports Med 22:72, 1994.
9. Norkin, CC, and Levangie, PK: The ankle-foot complex. In Norkin, CC, and Levangie, PK: Joint Structure and Function: A Comprehensive Analysis, ed 2. FA Davis, Philadelphia, 1992, p 383.
10. Hollinshead, WH, and Jenkins, DB: The leg. In Hollinshead, WH, and Jenkins, DB: Functional Anatomy of the Limbs and Back, ed 5. WB Saunders, Philadelphia, 1981, p 305.
10a. Daniels, L, and Worthingham, C: Muscle Testing: Techniques of Manual Examination, ed 5. WB Saunders, Philadelphia, 1986.
11. Grimston, SK, et al: Differences in ankle joint complex range of motion as a function of age. Foot and Ankle 14:215, 1993.
12. Kendall, FP, and McCreary, EK: The lower extremity. In Kendall, FP, and McCreary, EK: Muscles: Testing and Function, ed 3. Williams & Wilkins, Baltimore, 1983, p 145.
12a. Donatelli, R: Biomechanics of the Foot and Ankle. FA Davis, Philadelphia, 1990.
13. Coombs, JA: Peroneal nerve palsy complicating an ankle sprain. Athletic Training: Journal of the National Athletic Trainers Association 25:247, 1990.
14. Collins, WJ, and Hofner, RG: A lower leg epiphyseal plate injury in a young athlete: Is it just an ankle sprain? Athletic Training: Journal of the National Athletic Trainers Association 19:61, 1984.
15. Löfvenberg, R, and Kärrholm, J: The influence of an ankle orthosis on the talar and calcaneal motions in chronic lateral instability of the ankle: A stereophotogrammetric analysis. Am J Sports Med 21:224, 1993.
16. Johnson, MB, and Johnson, CL: Electromyographic response of peroneal muscles in surgical and nonsurgical injured ankles during sudden inversion. Journal of Orthopedic and Sports Physical Therapy 18:497, 1993.
17. Isalov, E: Response of peroneal muscles to sudden inversion of the ankle during standing. International Journal of Sports Biomechanics 2:100, 1986.
18. Freeman, MAR: Treatment of ruptures of the lateral ligament of the ankle. J Bone Joint Surg Br 47:661, 1965.
19. Freeman, MAR, et al: The etiology and prevention of functional instability of the foot. J Bone Joint Surg Br 47:678, 1965.
20. Meislin, RJ, et al: Arthroscopic treatment of synovial impingement of the ankle. Am J Sports Med 21:186, 1993.
21. Taga, I: Articular cartilage lesions in ankles with lateral ligament injury: An arthroscopic study. Am J Sports Med 21:120, 1993.
22. Loomer, R, et al: Osteochondral lesions of the talus. Am J Sports Med 21:13, 1993.
23. Bassett, FH: A simple surgical approach to the posteromedial ankle. Am J Sports Med 21:144, 1993.
24. Cedal, CA: Ankle lesions. Acta Orthop Scand 46:425, 1975.
25. Boytim, MJ, Fischer, DA, and Neumann, L: Syndesmotic ankle sprains. Am J Sports Med 19:294, 1991.
26. Garrick, JG, and Requa, RK: Role of external support in the prevention of ankle sprains. Med Sci Sports Exerc 5:200, 1973.
27. Savoie, FH, et al: Maisonneuve fracture dislocation of the ankle. Journal of Athletic Training 27:268, 1992.
28. Michelson, J: Controversies in ankle fractures. Foot and Ankle 14:170, 1993.
29. Giladi, M, et al: Stress fractures. Identifiable risk factors. Am J Sports Med 19:647, 1991.
30. O'Connor, P, and Kersey, RD: Achilles peritendinitis. Athletic Training: Journal of the National Athletic Trainers Association 15:159, 1980.
31. Puddu, G, et al: A classification of Achilles tendon disease. Am J Sports Med 4:145, 1976.
32. Wilkins, DR: Taping the subluxating peroneal tendon. Athletic Training: Journal of the National Athletic Trainers Association 26:370, 1991.
33. Pedowitz, RA, and Gershuni, DH: Diagnosis and treatment of chronic compartment syndrome. Critical Reviews in Physical and Rehabilitation Medicine 5:301, 1993.
34. Genuario, SE: Differential diagnosis: Exertional compartment syndromes, stress fractures, and shin splints. Athletic Training: Journal of the National Athletic Trainers Association 24:31, 1989.
35. Blick, SS, et al: Compartment syndrome in open tibial fractures. J Bone Joint Surg Am 68:1348, 1986.
36. Detmer, DE, et al: Chronic compartment syndrome: Diagnosis, management, and outcomes. Am J Sports Med 13:162, 1985.
37. Whitesides, TE, et al: Tissue pressure measurements as a determinant for the need of fasciotomy. Clin Orthop Rel Res 113:43, 1975.

5

The Knee

Ligamentous injury to the knee can be the most devastating orthopedic injury suffered by athletes. Having little architectural bony support, the knee complex is a tenuously constructed joint; yet it is required to transmit forces to and from the lower leg and at the same time receive blows and dissipate potentially injurious forces. Paradoxically, the most massive muscles of the body serve to flex and extend the joint, but they provide relatively little protection to the joint itself. Conceptually, the tendons and ligaments crossing the joint are roughly equivalent to tying two logs end-to-end.

This chapter discusses injury to the knee and related muscles. The patella, as it relates to the knee joint proper, is described in this chapter. Those conditions particular to the patellofemoral articulation are described in Chapter 6 and injury to the quadriceps and hamstring muscle groups, in Chapter 7.

CLINICAL ANATOMY

The term "tibiofemoral joint" seems to imply that the knee involves articulation between the tibia and femur only, when, in fact, it involves articulation among the femur, menisci, and tibia, all of which must act in concert. The patellofemoral mechanism must be functioning properly as well, to ensure adequate tibiofemoral mechanics. The superior tibiofibular syndesmosis, although not a part of the knee articulation, must also be intact. The tibiofemoral articulation is the articulation between the femur and tibia, the two longest bones of the body, as they lie end-to-end. This type of bony arrangement requires unique ligamentous and muscular support.

The length of the **femur**, the longest and strongest bone in the body, is approximately one-quarter of the body's total height.[1] The femur's posterior aspect is demarcated by the **linea aspera**, a bony ridge spanning the length of the shaft (Fig. 5–1). As it reaches its distal end, the shaft broadens to form the medial and lateral epicondyles.

The **lateral epicondyle** is wider and exits the femoral shaft at a lesser angle than the **medial epicondyle**. Arising off the superior crest of the medial epicondyle is the **adductor tubercle**. Inferior to each epicondyle are the **medial and lateral condyles**. Covered with hyaline cartilage, these convex structures form the articular surfaces of the knee's articulation with the tibia and have a discrete anteroposterior curvature that is convex in the *frontal plane*. The articular surface of the medial condyle is longer than that of the lateral condyle and flares outward posteriorly. Sharing a common anterior surface, the condyles diverge posteriorly and are separated by the deep **intercondylar notch**. An anterior depression forms the **femoral trochlea** through which the patella glides as the knee moves in flexion and extension.

Corresponding to the femoral condyles are the **tibia's** proximal articular plateaus. The medial tibial plateau is concave in both the frontal and sagittal planes, whereas the lateral articular plateau is concave in the frontal plane and convex in the *sagittal plane*. The medial tibial condyle (plateau) is 50 percent larger than the lateral condyle to accommodate for the flare of the medial femoral condyle. Separating the two condyles are the intercondylar eminences, raised areas that match the femur's intercondylar notch (Fig. 5–2). On the anterior portion of the tibia is the **tibial tuberosity**, representing the site of the patellar tendon's distal attachment.

Two bones outside the tibiofemoral articulation have a direct impact on the knee's function and stability. The **patella** is a sesamoid bone located in the patellar tendon (ligament) that improves the mechanical function of the quadriceps when extending the knee, dissipates the forces received from the *extensor mechanism*, and protects the anterior portion of the knee. Several of the soft tissues about the knee attach to the **fibular head**. Instability of this structure owing to fracture or syndesmotic injury decreases the stability and function of the knee.

Frontal plane: A vertical plane passing through the body, dividing it into anterior and posterior portions.
Sagittal plane: A vertical plane passing through the body, dividing it into left and right sides.
Extensor mechanism: The mechanism formed by the quadriceps and patellofemoral joint that is responsible for causing extension of the lower leg at the knee joint.

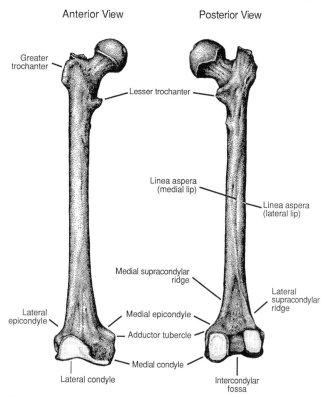

Figure 5–1. Anterior and posterior view of the femur. Note that the single anterior articular surface on the femur's condyles diverges posteriorly.

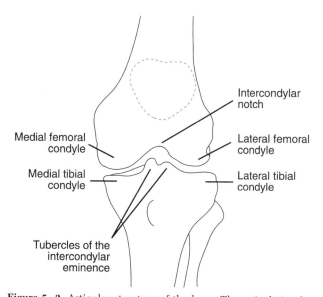

Figure 5–2. Articular structure of the knee. The articulation between the femoral and tibial condyles is aided by the menisci. The tubercles of the intercondylar eminence align with the intercondylar notch.

Articulations and Ligamentous Support

The presence of the medial and lateral articular condyles classifies the tibiofemoral joint as a **double condyloid articulation**, capable of freedom of motion in two planes: (1) flexion and extension and (2) internal and external rotation of the tibia on the femur. The other movements that occur between the tibia and femur, such as valgus and varus bending and anterior and posterior glide, are **accessory motions** attributed to the joint's construction. These motions can be increased following damage to one or more of the knee's ligaments.

Joint Capsule

Surrounding the circumference of the knee joint is a fibrous joint capsule. Along the medial, anterior, and lateral aspects of the joint, the capsule arises superior to the femoral condyles and fixates distal to the tibial condyles. Posteriorly the capsule attaches to the posterior margins of the femoral condyles above the joint line, and inferiorly, to the posterior tibial condyle. The strength of the capsule is reinforced by the collateral ligaments medially and laterally, the retinaculum medially and laterally, the oblique popliteal ligament and arcuate ligaments posteriorly, and the patellar tendon anteriorly. Further reinforcement is gained from the muscles that cross the knee joint.

Lining the articular portions of the fibrous joint capsule is a **synovial capsule**. The synovium surrounds the articular condyles of the femur and tibia medially, anteriorly, and laterally. On the posterior portion of the articulation, the synovial capsule invaginates anteriorly along the femur's intercondylar notch and the tibia's intercondylar tubercles, excluding the cruciate ligaments from the synovial membrane (Fig. 5–3).

The Collateral Ligaments

Supporting the medial joint line is the **medial collateral ligament (MCL)**. Formed by two layers, the **deep layer** is a thickening of the joint capsule having an attachment to the medial meniscus. Separated from the deep layer by a bursa, the **superficial layer** arises from a broad band just below the adductor tubercle to insert on a relatively narrow site 7 to 10 cm below the joint line (Fig. 5–4). As a unit, the two layers of the MCL are tight in complete extension. As the knee is flexed to the midrange, its anterior fibers are taut; in complete flexion the posterior fibers are tight. The MCL serves primarily to protect the knee against valgus forces while also providing a secondary restraint against external rotation of the tibia and anterior translation of the

---

Accessory motion: Motion that accompanies active movement and is necessary for normal motion but can not be voluntarily isolated.

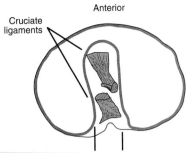

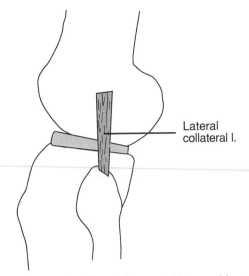

Figure 5–3. The knee's joint capsules. The fibrous capsular membrane completely envelops the bony surface of the knee. The synovial capsular membrane surrounds the medial and lateral articular surfaces but invaginates to exclude the cruciate ligaments.

Figure 5–5. Lateral collateral ligament. This ropelike structure originates from the lateral femoral condyle and attaches to the apex of the fibular head. The lateral collateral ligament is an extracapsular structure.

tibia on the femur, especially in the absence of an intact anterior cruciate ligament.

Unlike the MCL, the **lateral collateral ligament (LCL)** has no attachment to the joint capsule or meniscus. This prominent, cordlike structure arises from the lateral femoral condyle, sharing a common site of origin with the lateral joint capsule, and inserts off the proximal aspect of the fibular head (Fig. 5–5). The LCL is the primary restraint against varus forces when the knee is between full extension and 30 degrees of flexion. This structure also provides secondary restraint against external rotation of the tibia on the femur.

The Cruciate Ligaments

The cruciate ligaments are considered to be intra-articular, yet are located outside of the synovial capsule (see Fig. 5–3). Named according to their relative attachments on the tibia, the **anterior cruciate**

ligament **(ACL)** arises from the anteromedial intercondylar tubercle of the tibia and travels posteriorly and laterally to insert on the medial wall of the lateral femoral condyle (Fig. 5–6). The ACL serves as a static stabilizer against:

1. Anterior translation of the tibia on the femur
2. Internal rotation of the tibia on the femur
3. External rotation of the tibia on the femur
4. Hyperextension of the tibia

The ACL has two discrete segments: an **anteromedial bundle** and a **posterolateral bundle.**[2] A third band, an **intermediate bundle**, located between the anteromedial and posterolateral bundles, has been described in the early literature but is no longer considered true by anatomists.[3]

As the knee moves from extension into flexion there is a juxtaposition of the ACL's attachment sites. When the knee is fully extended, the femoral attachment of the anteromedial bundle is anterior to the attachment of the posterolateral bundle. When the knee is flexed, the relative positions are reversed, causing the ACL to wind upon itself (Fig. 5–7). This leads to varying portions of the ACL being taut as the knee progresses through its range of motion. When the knee is fully extended, the posterolateral bundle is tight; when the knee is fully flexed, the anteromedial bundle is taut.

Throughout the midrange of motion, the amount of stress placed on the ACL is minimized when the tibia remains in the neutral positions.[3] In the terminal 15 degrees of extension, internally rotating the tibia greatly increases the strain placed on the ACL, whereas externally rotating the tibia markedly reduces this strain. Both valgus and varus stresses increase the strain placed on the ACL throughout the entire range of motion (Fig. 5–8).

Shorter and stronger than the ACL, the **posterior**

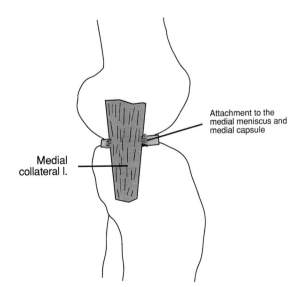

Figure 5–4. Medial collateral ligament. Arising from a broad band on the medial femoral epicondyle just below the adductor tubercle, it tapers inward to attach on the medial tibial plateau. Consisting of two layers separated by a bursa, the deep layer is continuous with the medial joint capsule and has an attachment on the medial meniscus.

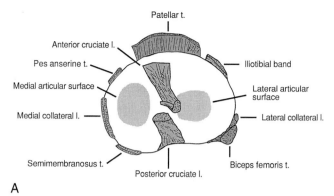

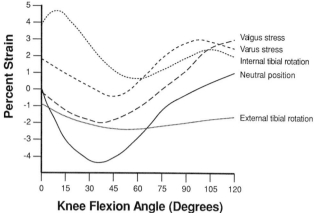

Figure 5–8. Strain placed on the anterior cruciate ligament through the range of motion. Altering the relative alignment of the tibia to the femur increases the strain on the ligament throughout the range of motion. (Adapted from Arms.[3])

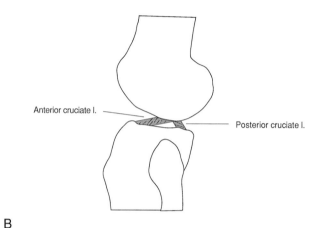

Figure 5–6. Cruciate ligaments. (*A*) Superior view referencing the cruciate ligaments to each other and to other supportive structures about the knee. (*B*) Lateral view of the cruciate ligaments.

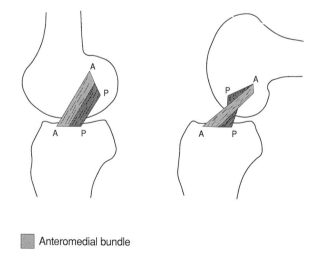

Anteromedial bundle

Posterolateral bundle

Figure 5–7. Biomechanics of the anterior cruciate ligament. When the knee is fully extended, the femoral attachment site of the anteromedial bundle (A) is proximal to the attachment site of the posterolateral bundle (P). When the knee is flexed, these attachment sites juxtapose their positions, causing the anterior cruciate to wind upon itself. (Adapted from Fu.[2])

cruciate ligament (PCL) arises from the posterior aspect of the tibia approximately 1 cm distal to the joint surface and takes a superior and anterior course passing medially to the ACL to attach to the lateral portion of the femur's medial condyle. Although not receiving as much attention as the ACL, the PCL has been described as the primary stabilizer of the knee.[4] The primary restraint against posterior displacement of the tibia on the femur, the PCL's posterior fibers are taut when the knee is fully extended and the anterior fibers when it is fully flexed. During the screw home mechanism the PCL and ACL wind upon each other in flexion and unwind in extension. With this concept in mind, it is easy to see how damage to the PCL can result in an inherently unstable knee, not only in the frontal plane but also in the transverse plane by removing the axis of tibial rotation.

The Arcuate Ligament Complex

Formed by the oblique popliteal ligament and the arcuate popliteal ligament, the **arcuate ligament complex** provides support to the posterior joint capsule. The oblique popliteal ligament, an expansion of the semimembranosus tendon, arises off the tibia's medial condyle and travels superiorly and laterally to attach on the middle portion of the posterior joint capsule (Fig. 5–9). Arising from the fibular head, the arcuate ligament passes over the popliteus muscle, where it diverges to insert on the intercondylar area of the tibia and the posterior aspect of the femur's lateral epicondyle. The ACL limits anterior displacement of the tibia relative to the femur, hyperextension and hyperflexion of the knee, and becomes tight during internal and external tibial rotation as well as during valgus and varus loading of the knee.

Superior Tibiofibular Syndesmosis

Similar to the inferior tibiofibular syndesmosis, the superior junction between the tibia and fibula is an immovable joint. The superior syndesmosis is

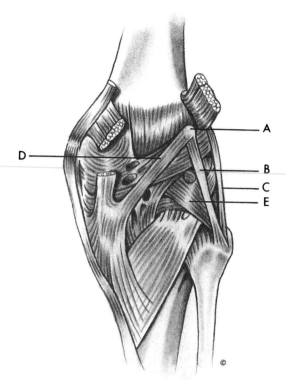

Figure 5–9. Ligaments of the posterolateral knee. (A) Fabella, (B) fabellofibular ligament, (C) lateral collateral ligament, (D) oblique popliteal ligament, and (E) arcuate ligament. (From Greenfield, BH,[4a] p 27, with permission.)

more stable than its distal counterpart because of the alignment between the fibular head and the indentation on the proximal tibia. This joint is stabilized by the superior anterior and posterior tibiofibular ligaments and, to a lesser degree, by the interosseous membrane. Anterior displacement of the fibula is partially blocked by a bony outcrop from the tibia. Therefore, most fibular instabilities tend to occur posteriorly and may affect the peroneal nerve.

The Menisci

An examination of a skeletal model of the knee joint reveals incongruencies between the articular surfaces of the tibia and fibula. This problem is at least partially remedied by the presence of the fibrocartilaginous medial and lateral menisci. These structures serve to:

1 Deepen the articulation and fill the gaps that normally occur during the knee's articulation

2 Provide lubrication for the articulating surfaces

3 Provide shock absorption

4 Increase the stability of the joint

When viewed in cross section, the menisci are wedge-shaped, with their outer borders thicker than their inner rims. When viewed from above, this wedge creates a concave area on the tibia to accept

the femur's articulating surfaces. The **medial meniscus** resembles a half-crescent, or C, that is wider posteriorly than anteriorly. The **lateral meniscus** is more circular in shape (Fig. 5–10). Both menisci are attached at their periphery to the tibia via the **coronary ligament**. The anterior horns of each meniscus are joined together by the **transverse ligament** and are connected to the patellar tendon via **patellomeniscal ligaments**.

The lateral meniscus is smaller and more mobile than the medial meniscus. In addition to the aforementioned attachments to the medial meniscus and the patellar tendon, the lateral meniscus also attaches to the ACL, to the femur via the **ligament of Wrisberg**, and to the popliteus muscle via the joint capsule and coronary ligament.

During knee extension the lateral femoral condyle pushes the lateral meniscus anteriorly, distorting its shape in the anteroposterior plane. In the early degrees of flexion the popliteus pulls the lateral meniscus posteriorly, and in the later range of motion the posterior horn is pulled medially and anteriorly by the meniscofemoral ligament.

Each meniscus may be divided into a **vascular zone**, which runs contiguously with its peripheral attachment to the coronary ligament and joint capsule, and an **avascular zone**, formed by the inner portion of the meniscus. Because of the presence of an active blood supply, meniscal tears occurring within the vascular zone have an improved chance of healing compared with tears within the avascular zone, which rely on nutrients being delivered via the synovial fluid.

Muscles of the Knee

The muscles acting on the knee serve primarily to flex or extend it. The flexor musculature have the secondary responsibility of rotating the tibia. Those flexors attaching on the tibia's medial side internally rotate it, while those attaching on the lateral side externally rotate it. The muscles acting on the knee, their origins, insertions, and innervation are presented in Table 5–1.

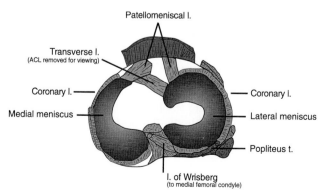

Figure 5–10. Superior view of the medial and lateral meniscus and their associated ligamentous structures. The peripheral border of the menisci is fixated to the tibia by the coronary ligament.

Table 5–1. Muscles Acting on the Knee

Muscle	Action	Origin	Insertion	Nerve	Root
Biceps femoris	Knee flexion External rotation of the tibia Long head Hip flexion Hip external rotation	Long head Ischial tuberosity Sacrotuberous ligament Short head Lateral lip of the linea aspera Upper two-thirds of the supracondylar line	Lateral fibular head Lateral tibial condyle	Long head Tibial Short head Common peroneal	Long head S1, S2, S3 Short head L5, S1, S2
Gastrocnemius	Assists in knee flexion Ankle plantarflexion	Medial head Posterior surface of the medial femoral condyle Adjacent portion of the femur and knee capsule Lateral head Posterior surface of the lateral femoral condyle Adjacent portion of the femur and knee capsule	To the calcaneus via the Achilles tendon	Tibial	S1, S2
Gracilis	Knee flexion Internal rotation of the tibia Hip adduction	Symphysis pubis Inferior ramus of the pubic bone	Proximal portion of the anteromedial tibial flair	Obturator (posterior)	L3, L4
Popliteus	Open chain Internal rotation of the *tibia* Knee flexion Closed chain External rotation of the *femur* Knee flexion	Lateral femoral condyle Oblique popliteal ligament	Posterior tibia superior to the soleal line Fascia covering the soleus	Tibial	L4, L5, S1
Rectus femoris	Knee extension Hip flexion	Anterior inferior iliac spine Groove located superior to the acetabulum	To the tibial tubercule via the patella and patellar ligament	Femoral	L2, L3, L4
Sartorius	Knee flexion Internal rotation of the tibia Hip flexion Hip abduction Hip external rotation	Anterior superior iliac spine	Proximal portion of the anteromedial tibial flair	Femoral	L2, L3
Semimembranosus	Knee flexion Internal rotation of the tibia Hip extension Hip internal rotation	Ischial tuberosity	Posteromedial portion of the tibia's medial condyle	Tibial	L5, S1
Semitendinosus	Knee flexion Internal rotation of the tibia Hip extension Hip internal rotation	Ischial tuberosity	Medial portion of the tibial flair	Tibial	L5, S1, S2
Vastus intermedius	Knee extension	Anterolateral portion of the upper two-thirds of the femur Lower one-half of the linea aspera	To the tibial tubercle via the patella and patellar ligament	Femoral	L2, L3, L4

Table 5-1. Muscles Acting on the Knee *(Continued)*

Muscle	Action	Origin	Insertion	Nerve	Root
Vastus lateralis	Knee extension	Proximal interochanteric line Greater trochanter Gluteal tuberosity Upper one-half of the linea aspera	To the tibial tubercle via the patella and patellar ligament	Femoral	L2, L3, L4
Vastus medialis	Knee extension	Distal one-half of the intertrochanteric line Medial portion of the linea aspera Oblique portion Tendons from adductor longus and adductor magnus	To the tibial tubercle via the patella and patellar ligament	Femoral	L2, L3, L4

Muscle actions, origins, and insertions adapted from Kendall and McCreary,[4b] with permission; innervations adapted from Daniels and Worthingham,[4c] with permission.

Anterior Muscles

Although its name implies the presence of four muscles, the **quadriceps femoris** muscle group is best described as consisting of five muscles, the **vastus lateralis, vastus intermedius, vastus medialis, vastus medialis oblique**, and **rectus femoris**, each having a common attachment to the tibial tuberosity via the patella and patellar tendon (Fig. 5-11). The vastus medialis has a discrete group of fibers arising from the medial femoral condyle and the fascia of the adductor magnus, referred to as the vastus medialis oblique (VMO). As a group, the quadriceps femoris extends the knee, while the rectus femoris also serves as a hip flexor, especially when the knee is flexed; and the VMO guides the patella medially. In addition to extending the tibia, the vastus lateralis (VL) also causes the patella to glide laterally.

Posterior Muscles

The posterior muscles, the **semitendinosus, semimembranosus**, and **biceps femoris**, are collectively known as the **hamstring muscle group** and act as a unit to flex the knee and extend the hip (Fig. 5-12). The biceps femoris serves to externally rotate the tibia while the semimembranosus and semitendinosus act to internally rotate the tibia.

The posterior knee capsule is reinforced by the **popliteus** muscle (see Fig. 5-9). In an **open kinetic chain** the popliteus causes internal rotation of the tibia on the femur; in a **closed kinetic chain**, the popliteus externally rotates the femur on the tibia.

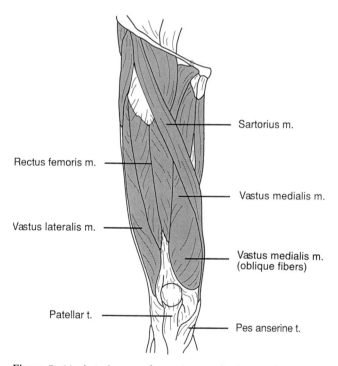

Figure 5-11. Anterior muscles acting on the knee. The vastus lateralis, rectus femoris, vastus intermedius (hidden beneath the rectus femoris), and vastus medialis share a common insertion via the patellar tendon.

Responsible for unscrewing the knee from its locked position in extension, its remaining influence on knee flexion is slight. However, when the athlete is weight bearing with the knee partially

---

Open kinetic chain: Motion that occurs when the distal portion of the extremity is non-weight bearing.
Closed kinetic chain: Motion that occurs when the distal portion of the extremity is weight bearing or otherwise fixed.

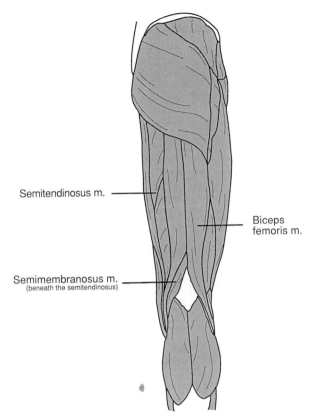

Semitendinosus m.

Biceps femoris m.

Semimembranosus m.
(beneath the semitendinosus)

Figure 5–12. Posterior muscles acting on the knee. In addition to flexing the joint, the biceps femoris externally rotates the tibia while the semimembranosus and semitendinosus internally rotate it.

flexed, the popliteus assists the posterior cruciate ligament in preventing posterior displacement of the tibia on the femur.

A diamond-shaped **popliteal fossa** is formed by the leg's posterior musculature (Fig. 5–13). Although its inner boundaries are largely devoid of muscles (with the exception of the popliteus) the popliteal fossa contains the popliteal artery and vein; the tibial, common peroneal, posterior femoral cutaneous, and obturator nerves; and the small saphenous vein.

The Pes Anserine Muscle Group

The **gracilis** and **sartorius**, along with the **semitendinosus**, form the **pes anserine** muscle group (Latin for "goose's foot," the shape of the tendons as they insert on the tibia). The **sartorius** is an unusual muscle in that, although it arises from the anterior superior iliac spine, crosses over the quadriceps femoris muscles, and inserts on the tibia inferior to the tuberosity, it is a flexor of the knee joint (see Fig. 5–11). This occurs because the sartorius crosses the knee posterior to its axis. In addition to flexing the knee, the pes anserine group internally rotates the tibia and externally rotates the femur. The sartorius also flexes the hip.

The Iliotibial Band

Originating from the anterior superior iliac crest is the **tensor fasciae latae**. This small muscle inserts into the **iliotibial band (ITB)**, travels down the lateral aspect of the femur to insert on the anterolateral tibia (Gerdy's tubercle), and attaches to the lateral patellar retinaculum and the biceps femoris tendon through divergent slips. Although the tensor fasciae latae and ITB make a relatively insignificant contribution to knee motion, the deep fibers of the ITB attaching to the lateral joint capsule function as an anterolateral knee ligament.[5]

The angle at which the ITB addresses the tibia varies according to the relative position of the lower leg, which, in turn, alters the knee's biomechanics. When the knee is fully extended, the ITB is anterior to or located over the lateral femoral condyle. When the knee is flexed beyond 30 degrees, the ITB shifts behind the lateral femoral condyle, giving it an angle of pull as if it were a knee flexor (Fig. 5–14). This posterior shift is greatly influenced by the biceps femoris, which has a fibrous expanse attaching to the ITB. During contraction of the biceps femoris, the ITB is drawn posteriorly.

The Screw Home Mechanism

The unequal sizes of the femoral condyles and the tightening of the cruciate ligaments as they wind upon themselves necessitate a locking mechanism (screw home mechanism) as the knee nears its final degrees of extension.[6] As the knee is extended to its terminal end ranges, the medial articulation serves as a pivot point as the lateral tibial plateau glides posteriorly on the lateral femoral condyle. This effect results in external rotation on the femur at terminal extension, the screw home mechanism.

During extension of the non–weight-bearing knee this mechanism occurs as 5 to 7 degrees of external rotation of the tibia on the femur. However, when weight bearing, the tibia is fixated so the terminal range of motion is accomplished by a combination of the tibial external rotation and femoral internal rotation. To initiate flexion the knee must be unlocked. When non–weight bearing, this is accomplished by the popliteus muscle; when weight bearing it is by contraction of the popliteus, semimembranosus, and semitendinosus muscles.

CLINICAL EVALUATION OF KNEE AND LEG INJURIES

During the clinical evaluation of the knee and leg the athlete should be wearing shorts to permit inspection of the muscles originating off the femur and pelvis. The approach described in this chapter may be modified, based on the clinical findings (Table 5–2). With the detection of any signs or

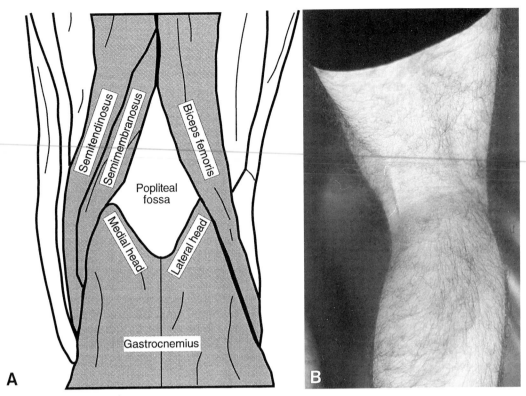

Figure 5–13. Popliteal fossa. (*A*) Anatomical reference and (*B*) surface anatomy.

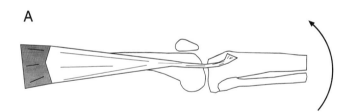

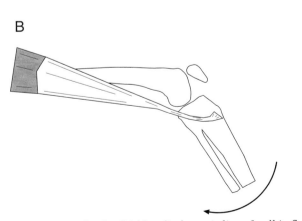

Figure 5–14. The iliotibial band's dynamic line of pull in flexion and extension. (*A*) When the knee is fully extended, the iliotibial band's angle of pull is that of a knee extensor. (*B*) When it is flexed past 30°, it assumes an angle of flexor.

symptoms of fracture or gross instability of the knee the evaluation should be terminated, the limb properly splinted, and the athlete referred to a physician for medical evaluation. The patella is described in this section only as it relates to tibiofemoral function. Chapter 6 presents the detailed evaluation of patellofemoral conditions.

History

A detailed history of the athlete's injury will greatly assist in determining the nature of the trauma. Blows to the knee place a compressive force on the joint structures at the point of the blow, tensile forces on the side opposite, and shear forces across the joint. Rotatory forces about the knee, such as those experienced when an athlete cuts to change direction, place tensile forces about the joint capsule and cruciate ligaments. The menisci may also be torn by this mechanism secondary to impingement and shearing between the articular condyles. A tearing of muscle fibers or tendon may result from a concentric dynamic overload of the muscles, such as occurs with the quadriceps group when jumping, or an eccentric overload, such as occurs when the hamstrings contract to slow the lower limb during sprinting.

- **Screw home mechanism test:** This test is used to approximate the amount of internal and exter-nal tibial rotation occurring during active knee flexion and extension (Fig. 5–23).[9]

Screw Home Mechanism Test (Fig. 5–23)

Position of athlete	Sitting on the edge of the table.
Position of examiner	Standing or sitting in front of the athlete.
Evaluative procedure	With the knee flexed, a dot is placed on the center of the patella. A dot is placed on the tibial tubercle so that it is aligned immediately below the dot on the patella. The athlete then completely extends the knee, at which point the tibial dot should rotate laterally relative to the dot on the patella.
Positive test results	The tibial dot fails to move laterally relative to the patella.
Implications	Inhibition of the screw home mechanism (external rotation of the tibia) caused by a mechanical block or muscular insufficiency.

Passive Range of Motion

- **Flexion and extension:** Passive range of motion measurements should be taken in the supine position, with the femur slightly elevated by placing a folded towel under it. The normal end-feel for flexion is soft because of the approximation of the gastrocnemius group with the hamstrings or the heel striking the buttock. Extension produces a firm end-feel because of stretching of the posterior capsule and the cruciate ligaments. Tightness of the hamstring group may limit extension.

Resisted Range of Motion

- **Extension:** The athlete is positioned in the seated position with the knee flexed over the side. Resistance is provided over the anterior tibia just proximal to the ankle. While stabilizing the distal

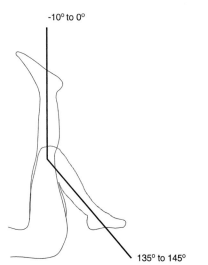

-10° to 0°

135° to 145°

Figure 5–22. Range of motion for flexion and extension of the knee.

quadriceps group, resistance is provided as the athlete moves through extension (Fig. 5–24). Isometric break pressure may be applied when the knee is flexed to 10, 45, and 90 degrees unless this protocol is contraindicated by the athlete's postoperative notes.

- **Flexion:** The athlete is positioned prone on the examination table. To measure resisted flexion, resistance is applied over the Achilles tendon while the thigh is stabilized. Resistance may be provided through the full range of motion, or break pressure may be applied with the knee flexed to 15, 45, 90, and 120 degrees (see Fig. 5–24).

Obvious internal or external rotation of the tibia during resisted flexion can specify weakness in the medial or lateral hamstrings, especially if this rotation is greater than that observed during testing of the uninvolved side. Excessive internal rotation is indicative of biceps femoris weakness, whereas external rotation is indicative of semimembranosus and/or semitendinosus pathology.

- **Isolating the sartorius:** Sometimes referred to as the "tailor's muscle," the sartorius has the ability to flex the hip and knee while concurrently abducting and externally rotating the hip (tailors sometimes develop pathology after sitting with their legs crossed for long periods of time). The sartorius can be isolated during manual muscle testing by resisting knee and hip flexion, external rotation, and abduction of the hip (Fig. 5–25). This motion is easily performed by asking the athlete to run the heel up the length of the opposite anterior tibia.

Criteria for Return to Competition

An athlete's return to competition following a knee injury has traditionally been based on measures such as isokinetic bilateral quadriceps and hamstring strength, isokinetic quadriceps/

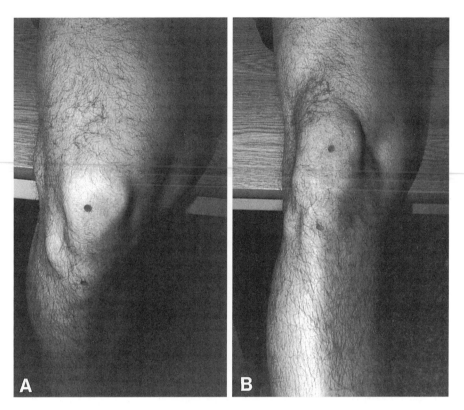

Figure 5–23. Screw home mechanism test. (*A*) When the knee is flexed to 90°, the tibial tuberosity is positioned lateral to the center of the patella. (*B*) When the knee is extended, the centers of the tibial tuberosity and the patella align.

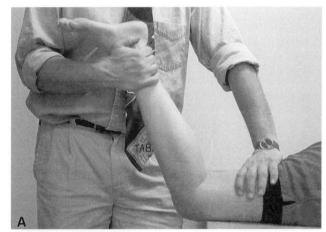

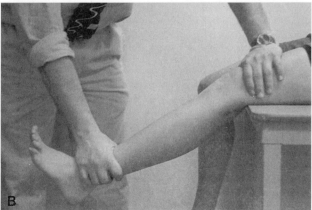

Figure 5–24. Resistive range of motion testing for the knee: (*A*) flexion and (*B*) extension.

hamstring ratios, thigh girth measurements, active range of motion, and pain. The following sport-specific functional activities have been described as valid criteria for return to full athletic participation.[10] The athlete should be able to perform these tests pain- free with no residual swelling or sense of instability before being allowed to return to activity:

Co-contraction test: A semicircle with an 8-ft diameter is marked on the floor. The athlete stands 48 inches within the semicircle's diameter, and surgical tubing, 48 inches long and 1 inch in diameter, is securely fastened 5 ft above the floor. A belt harness is used to secure the other end of the tubing to the athlete with no tension as to cause a recoil. The athlete then steps behind the semicircle at one of its terminal ends. Using a sidestep (not crossing one leg over the other), the athlete is to complete five lengths following the semicircle in as little time as possible (Fig. 5–26).

Carioca test: Using a crossover step so that the athlete's body stays perpendicular to the direction of travel, the athlete completes two lengths of a 40-ft circuit as quickly as possible.

Shuttle run test: Cones or lines are marked at 20-ft distances from each other. The athlete starts at one point, runs to the other, reaches down to the ground, and reverses direction. This test should be performed so that the athlete covers a total of 80 ft.

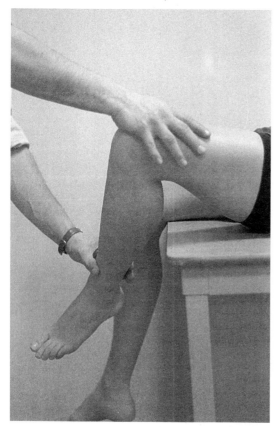

Figure 5-25. Isolating the sartorius during resisted range of motion testing. The examiner provides resistance while the athlete moves the heel up the anterior tibial border of the opposite leg.

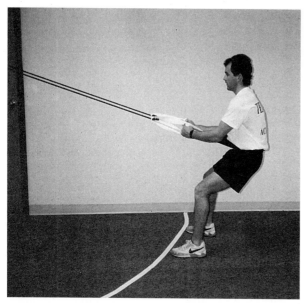

Figure 5-26. Co-contraction test to determine the functional capacity of the athlete with anterior cruciate ligament injury.

Tests for Ligamentous Stability

Ligamentous stability of the knee may occur in one plane, either as anteroposterior instability in the frontal plane or as valgus/varus instability in the sagittal plane, or it may occur as a multidirectional rotatory instability. This section presents tests for uniplanar instabilities. Tests for rotatory instabilities are discussed in the Pathologies and Related Special Tests section of this chapter.

Tests for Anterior Cruciate Ligament Instability

Two basic tests are used to determine the relative stability of the ACL by attempting to displace the tibia anteriorly on the femur. The ACL provides 86 percent of the restraint against this motion.[11] In the case of a complete ACL disruption this force is checked by the posterior capsule, the deep layer of the MCL, and the arcuate ligament complex.

The **anterior drawer test** involves placing the knee in 90 degrees of flexion and attempting to displace the tibia anteriorly (Fig. 5–27). In this position the anterior drawer test yields a positive result only if the ACL's anteromedial bundle has been damaged.[12–15] The clinician must be aware of contraction of the hamstrings during this test. In this position, the line of pull from the hamstrings complements the function of the ACL, possibly masking an otherwise positive test result (Fig. 5–28). Common pitfalls of the anterior drawer test are:

1 The effects of gravity

2 Guarding by the hamstring group masking anterior displacement of the tibia on the femur

3 Effusion within the capsule providing resistance to movement

4 The geometry of the articular condyles causing the triangular shape of the menisci to form a block against anterior movement of the tibia

5 Flexing the knee to 90 degrees causing anterior displacement of the tibia, masking the amount of further displacement during the drawer test.[16]

6 Because the knee is placed in 90 degrees of flexion, the anterior drawer test may be more sensitive to lesions localized within the anteromedial bundle.

A modification of the anterior drawer test, **Lachman's test** tends to isolate the posterolateral bundle of the ACL because the knee is flexed to 20 degrees (Fig. 5–29 and see Fig. 5–8). This test is generally considered to be more reliable than the anterior drawer test for determining ACL damage.

Performing Lachman's test requires the clinician to firmly grasp and manipulate the athlete's tibia and femur. In many cases athletes have heavy, muscular legs, inhibiting the ability to properly perform

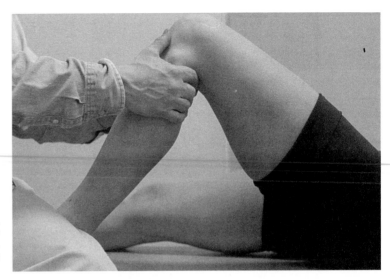

Figure 5–27. Anterior drawer test. The knee is flexed to 90°, the evaluator sits on the athlete's foot to provide stabilization, and the tibia is drawn forward. The hamstrings must be relaxed to produce accurate results.

the test. In these cases, the femur may be rested on a tightly rolled towel or stabilized by an assistant.[17] The tibia is drawn forward in a way similar to the drawer test procedure.

The art of manual ACL testing is being augmented and validated through the use of instrumented arthrometers (Fig. 5–30). These devices more accurately measure the amount of anterior tibial translation in a quantitative, reproducible manner and are less prone to the physical limitation faced by the clinician when performing the anterior drawer or Lachman's test.[18–21]

Any athlete with an apparently positive anterior drawer or Lachman's test result should also be screened for PCL insufficiency. If the PCL is deficient, tests for ACL insufficiency may appear positive as the tibia is moved anteriorly from its posteriorly subluxed position on the femur.[22]

As described by Draper, the **"alternate Lachman's test"** can be used to differentiate abnormal tibiofemoral glide caused by tears of the ACL from that caused by PCL deficiencies.[22] This test places the athlete in the prone, rather than the supine, position, thus preventing the posterior tibial sag resulting from the supine position (Fig. 5–31).

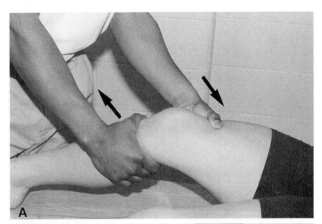

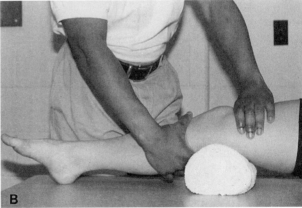

Figure 5–29. Lachman's test. (*A*) The knee is flexed to 15° and the tibia is drawn forward. (*B*) Lachman's test may be modified by placing a rolled towel beneath the athlete's knee to assist in stabilization of the femur.

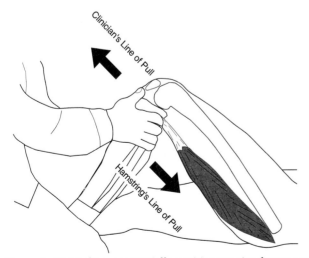

Figure 5–28. Masking a potentially positive anterior drawer test. Contraction of the hamstring group pulls the tibia posteriorly, the direction opposite the line of pull.

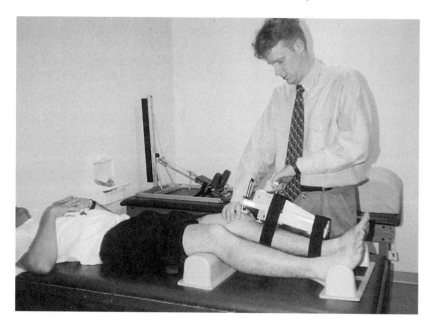

Figure 5–30. Instrumented testing of the anterior cruciate ligament using the KT-1000™ arthrometer.

The Anterior Drawer Test (Fig. 5–27)

Position of athlete	Lying supine. The hip is flexed to 45° and the knee to 90°.
Position of examiner	Sitting on the examination table in front of the involved knee. The athlete's foot is placed under the examiner's buttocks to fixate the tibia in the neutral position. The examiner grasps the tibia just below the joint line of the knee. The thumbs are placed along the joint line on either side of the patellar tendon. The index fingers are used to palpate the hamstring tendons to ensure that they are relaxed.
Evaluative procedure	The tibia is drawn forward toward the examiner.
Positive tests	An increased amount of anterior tibial translation compared with the opposite (uninvolved) limb or the lack of a firm end-point.
Implications	A tear of the anteromedial bundle of the anterior cruciate ligament.
Comments	Because the anterior drawer test primarily stresses the anteromedial bundle, damage to the posterolateral bundle may not be determined through the use of this test.

Lachman's Test (Fig. 5–29)

Position of athlete	Lying supine. The knee is passively flexed to 20°.
Position of examiner	The dominant hand grasps the tibia around the level of the tibial tuberosity. The non-dominant hand grasps the femur just above the level of the condyles.
Evaluative procedure	While the examiner supports the weight of the leg and the knee is flexed to 20°, the tibia is drawn anteriorly while a posterior pressure is applied to the femur. The process is then repeated so that the femur is pulled forward and the tibia driven backward.
Positive test results	An increased amount of anterior tibial translation compared with the opposite (uninvolved) limb or the lack of a firm end-point.
Implications	Damage to the anterior cruciate ligament.
Modifications	See Figures 5–29B and 5–31 for a modification of this procedure.

Alternate Lachman's Test (Fig. 5–31)

Position of athlete	Prone. The knee is passively flexed to 30°.
Position of examiner	Positioned at the legs of the athlete so that the athlete's ankle is supported by the examiner. The examiner's hand palpates the anterior joint line on either side of the patellar tendon.
Evaluative procedure	A downward pressure is placed on the proximal portion of the posterior tibia as the examiner notes any anterior tibial displacement.
Positive test results	Excessive anterior translation relative to the uninvolved knee (greater than 6 mm) indicates a tear of the anterior cruciate ligament.
Implications	Positive results found in the anterior drawer and/or Lachman's test and in the alternate Lachman's test indicate a tear of the ACL. A positive anterior drawer test and/or Lachman test result and a negative alternate Lachman's test result implicate a tear in the posterior cruciate ligament.

Tests for Posterior Cruciate Instability

Tests for damage of the PCL attempt to determine the amount of posterior displacement of the tibia on the femur relative to the uninvolved side. This motion places stress primarily on the PCL, followed by the arcuate ligament complex and the anterior joint capsule.

As noted during the inspection process, a posterior sag of the tibia may be evidenced when the flexed knee is viewed from the lateral side (see Fig. 5–19). Using the same positioning as the anterior drawer, the **posterior drawer test** attempts to displace the tibia posteriorly (Fig. 5–32). **Godfrey's test** uses gravity to extenuate the posterior sag as noted during the inspection process (Fig. 5–33).

Posterior Drawer Test (Fig. 5–32)

Position of athlete	Lying supine. The hip is flexed to 45° and the knee to 90°.
Position of examiner	Sitting on the examination table in front of the involved knee. The athlete's foot is placed under the examiner's buttocks to fixate the tibia in the neutral position. The examiner grasps the tibia just below the joint line of the knee. The thumbs are placed along the joint line on either side of the patellar tendon.
Evaluative procedure	The tibia is pushed posteriorly away from the examiner.
Positive test results	An increased amount of posterior tibial translation compared with the opposite (uninvolved) limb or the lack of a firm end-point.
Implications	A tear of the posterior cruciate ligament.

Godfrey's Test (Fig. 5–33)

Position of athlete	Lying supine, knees extended and legs together.
Position of examiner	Standing next to the athlete.
Evaluative procedure	The clinician lifts the athlete's lower legs and holds them parallel to the table so that the knees are flexed to 90°. The clinician then observes the level of the tibial tuberosities.
Positive test results	A unilateral posterior (downward) displacement of the tibial tuberosity.
Implications	A tear of the posterior cruciate ligament.
Comments	The lower leg must be stabilized as distally as possible; supporting the tibia proximally prevents it from sagging posteriorly.

Tests for Medial Collateral Ligament Instability

When the knee is fully extended the MCL is assisted in limiting valgus stress by the posterior oblique ligament, posteromedial capsule, and cruciate ligaments, as well as the muscles crossing the medial joint line. When the knee is flexed to 25 degrees, the MCL is the primary structure for checking valgus forces.[23]

The **valgus stress test** is performed once with the knee fully extended and again when the knee is flexed to 25 degrees (Fig. 5–34). Valgus laxity demonstrated on a fully extended knee indicates a major disruption of the medial supportive structures. Placing the knee in approximately 25 degrees of flexion isolates the stress to the MCL.

Valgus Stress Test (Fig. 5–34)

Position of athlete	Lying supine with the involved leg close to the edge of the table.
Position of examiner	Standing lateral to the athlete's involved limb. One hand supports the medial portion of the distal tibia while the other hand grasps the knee along the lateral joint line. To test the entire medial joint capsule the knee is kept in complete extension. To isolate the MCL the knee is flexed to 25°.
Evaluative procedure	A medial (valgus) force is applied to the knee while the distal tibia is moved laterally.
Positive test results	Increased laxity compared with the uninvolved limb.
Implications	In complete extension: A tear of the medial collateral ligament, medial joint capsule, and possibly the cruciate ligaments. In 25° of flexion: A tear of the medial collateral ligament.
Comments	When testing the knee in full extension it is recommended that the leg be left on the table, preventing shortening of the hamstring muscle group.
Modification	To promote greater relaxation of the athlete's musculature, the thigh may be left on the table with the knee flexed over the side.

Tests for Lateral Collateral Ligament Instability

The **varus stress test** is used to determine the integrity of the LCL, the lateral joint capsule, ITB, arcuate ligament complex, and lateral musculature when it is performed in complete extension (Fig. 5–35). When the knee is flexed to 25 degrees and the varus stress reapplied, the LCL is better isolated. As was described for the valgus stress test, a positive varus stress test result while the knee is fully extended may indicate trauma to the other lateral and/or internal structures.

Varus Stress Test (Fig. 5–35)

Position of athlete	Lying supine, with the involved leg close to the edge of the table.
Position of examiner	Sitting on the table with the athlete's involved leg supported under the clinician's arm. One hand supports the lateral portion of the distal tibia, while the other hand grasps the knee along the medial joint line. To test the entire lateral joint capsule, the knee is kept in complete extension. To isolate the LCL, the knee is flexed to 25°.
Evaluative procedure	A lateral (varus) force is applied to the knee, while the distal tibia is moved inward.
Positive test results	Increased laxity compared with the uninvolved limb.
Implications	In complete extension: A tear of the lateral collateral ligament, lateral joint capsule, and related structures, indicating possible rotatory instability of the joint. In 25° of flexion: A tear of the lateral collateral ligament.

Stability of the Proximal Tibiofibular Syndesmosis

The tibiofibular syndesmosis is of concern because of the attachment of the LCL and biceps femoris to the fibular head. Instability of the syndesmosis results in altered biomechanics and decreased lateral stability secondary to abnormal movement between the fibula and tibia, most commonly caused by a "glancing" blow to the superior fibula.[24] This movement occurs as an anterior and/or posterior displacement of the fibula on the tibia or a lateral movement of the fibula away from the tibia (Fig. 5–36).

Tibiofibular Translation Test (Fig. 5–36)

Position of athlete	Lying supine with the knee passively flexed to approximately 90°.
Position of examiner	Standing lateral to the athlete's involved side. One hand stabilizes the tibia while the other hand grasps the fibular head.
Evaluative procedure	While stabilizing the tibia, the examiner attempts to displace the fibular head anteriorly and then posteriorly.
Positive test results	Any perceived movement of the fibula on the tibia.
Implications	An anterior fibular shift indicates damage to the superior posterior tibiofibular ligament; posterior displacement reflects instability of the anterior tibiofibular ligament of the proximal tibiofibular syndesmosis.

Neurological Testing

A neurological examination is required when referred pain to the knee is suspected, the proximal tibiofibular joint displays laxity, or the athlete has suffered a dislocation of the tibiofemoral joint. Neurological involvement may also be associated with swelling within the popliteal fossa or lateral joint line. Additionally, athletes may display local or distal neurological involvement following surgery. Neurological testing is not required with most other acute or chronic injuries (see Neurological Screen on page 155).

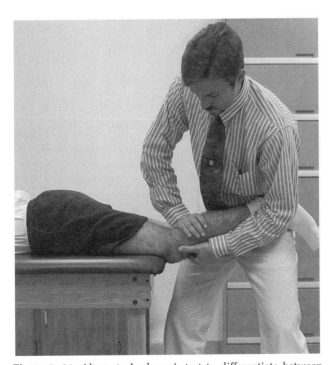

Figure 5–31. Alternate Lachman's test to differentiate between anterior tibial glide caused by anterior cruciate versus posterior cruciate ligament laxity.

Pathologies and Related Special Tests

Trauma to the knee may result from a contact-related mechanism, through rotational forces placed on the knee while weight bearing, or secondary to overuse. Knee injuries suffered by interscholastic or intercollegiate-aged athletes are most likely to be the result of a single traumatic episode. A small portion of this population and a larger percentage of older athletes are likely to suffer from degenerative changes within the knee.

Uniplanar Knee Sprains

Athletes with uniplanar knee sprains present with instability in only one of the body's cardinal planes: Damage to the MCL or LCL leads to valgus or varus instability in the frontal plane, whereas damage to the ACL or PCL results in instability in the sagittal plane in the form of anterior or posterior shifting of the tibia on the femur. This type of injury involves damage that is isolated to a single structure. When multiple structures are involved (e.g., the ACL and lateral joint capsule), a multiplanar or rotatory instability results.

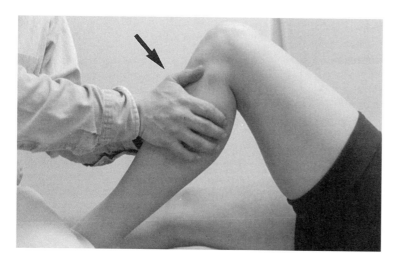

Figure 5–32. Posterior drawer test for posterior cruciate ligament laxity. The tibia is pushed posteriorly relative to the femur.

Medial Collateral Ligament Sprains

The MCL is damaged from tensile forces placed on this structure secondary to a valgus or rotatory stress on the knee. When the knee is fully extended, the valgus force is dissipated by the superficial and deep layers of the MCL, the anteromedial and posteromedial joint capsule, and the tendons of the pes anserine group. When the knee is flexed past 20 degrees, the superficial layer of the MCL becomes more responsible for resisting valgus forces (Table 5–5).

Medial collateral ligament sprains may occur in isolation, but, because of the deep layer's communication with the medial joint capsule and medial meniscus, damage to these structures should always be suspected. Rotational forces placed on the knee at the time of injury may also lead to the involve-

ment of the ACL. Damage to these two structures is the most common combination of ligamentous injury in the knee.[25] As described in Chapter 6, patellar dislocations can occur secondary to a valgus force placed on the knee. Therefore, all MCL sprains should include an evaluation of the patella for lateral dislocation.[26]

Lateral Collateral Ligament Sprains

Caused by a blow to the medial knee placing tensile forces on the lateral structures or by internal rotation of the tibia on the femur, LCL sprains result in varus laxity of the knee. The extracapsular nature of the LCL gives it a normally "springy" end-feel. A varus stress test result that feels empty when compared with the contralateral side should be considered positive for an LCL sprain (Table 5–6).

Because a varus force with concurrent internal tibial rotation can cause damage to the lateral capsular structures and the ACL, athletes suffering from LCL trauma should be suspected of suffering from anterolateral rotatory instability.

Anterior Cruciate Ligament Sprains

Injury to the ACL results from a force causing an anterior displacement of the tibia relative to the femur (the femur being driven posteriorly on the tibia), from non–contact-related rotational injuries, or from hyperextension of the knee. Unlike injury to the body's other ligaments, the majority of ACL sprains arise from non–contact-related torsional stress, such as when the athlete cuts or pivots.[12,13] Several anatomical factors that may predispose athletes to ACL injury have been suggested, including hyperpronation of the feet[27] and a small intercondylar notch.[28]

Associated with the injury mechanism, the

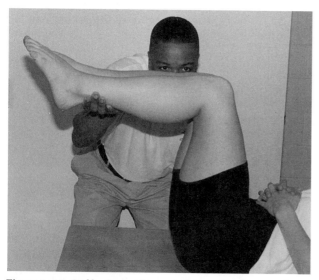

Figure 5–33. Godfrey's sign for posterior cruciate ligament laxity. Note the downward displacement of the left (facing) tibia.

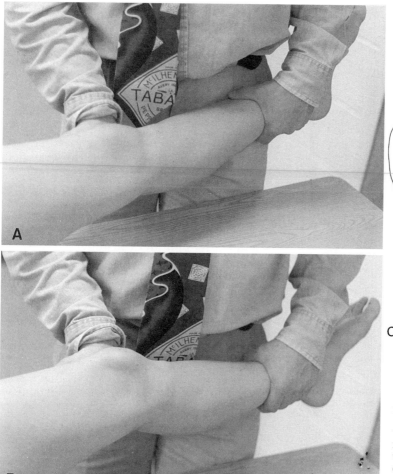

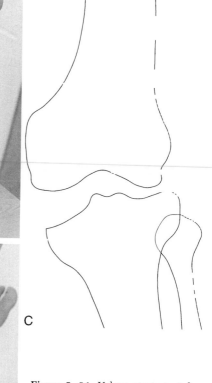

Figure 5-34. Valgus stress test for medial collateral ligament trauma. (*A*) In full extension to determine the integrity of the medial capsular restraints. (*B*) With the knee flexed to 15° to isolate the medial collateral ligament. (*C*) Schematic representation of the opening of the medial joint line.

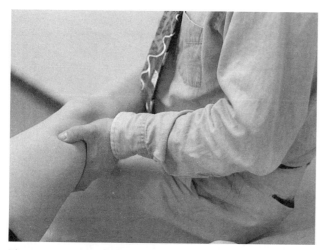

Figure 5-35. Varus stress test for lateral collateral ligament trauma. To isolate the lateral collateral ligament, flex the knee to between 20° and 30°.

athlete may describe the sensation of a "pop" emanating from within the knee joint and an immediate loss of knee function. Swelling occurs rapidly secondary to trauma of the medial geniculate artery, the ACL's primary blood supply. Normally this **hemarthrosis** remains within the fibrous capsule, but trauma to this structure results in diffuse swelling that may **extravasate** distally over time. Intracapsular swelling combined with the tension placed on the ACL limits the range of motion (see Fig. 5-8). Laxity of the ACL may be confirmed through Lachman's test and the anterior drawer test (Table 5-7). Because PCL deficiency can replicate positive test results for ACL involvement as the tibia is returned to its normal position, tests for PCL tears should be performed to rule out such false-positive results.

The term "partially torn ACL" is a functional mis-

Hemarthrosis: Blood within a joint cavity.
Extravasate: Fluid escaping from vessels into the surrounding tissue.

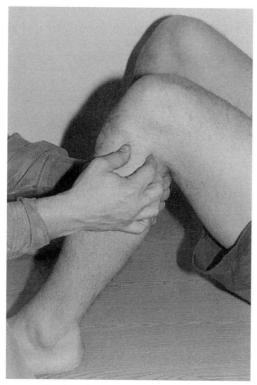

Figure 5–36. Testing the stability of the proximal tibiofibular syndesmosis. The examiner attempts to displace the proximal fibula anteriorly and posteriorly.

displacement of the tibia is extenuated and an anterior subluxation of the tibial condyles results when the anteromedial or anterolateral joint capsules, pes anserine, biceps femoris, or ITB are also traumatized.

Posterior Cruciate Ligament Sprains

Uniplanar PCL injury results from the tibia's being driven posteriorly on the femur or from hyperflexion or hyperextension of the knee when the joint is distracted (e.g., when the heel steps in a hole). Falling on a flexed knee can drive the tibia posteriorly, stressing the posterior cruciate ligament (Fig. 5–37). Immediately following the onset of injury the athlete may be relatively asymptomatic or may display the signs and symptoms of strain of the medial head of the gastrocnemius and/or a sprain of the posterior capsule.[29] Over time, symptoms such as pain in the posterior knee, weakness of the hamstring group, and reduced range of motion during flexion become evident (Table 5–8). The strength of the quadriceps group soon returns following a PCL sprain, but nonsurgically treated conditions rapidly lead to degeneration and instability of the joint.[30]

nomer. Because the bands of the ACL wind upon each other, even partial trauma to an individual band results in biomechanical dysfunction, instability, and increased stress on the remaining fibers, predisposing them to future injury.

The rotatory forces placed on the knee make "isolated" trauma to the ACL unlikely. Instability of the knee is greatly increased when trauma also damages one or more of the soft tissue constraints or the menisci.[20] As is described in the Rotatory Instabilities section of this chapter, the degree of anterior

Rotatory Knee Instabilities

Unlike uniplanar knee instabilities, rotatory (multiplanar) instabilities involve abnormal internal or external rotation of the tibia on the femur. The types of instabilities are named based on the relative direction in which the tibia subluxates on the femur. When this type of instability occurs, the axis of tibial rotation is shifted in the direction opposite that of the subluxation (Fig. 5–38). The four categories of rotatory instability are shown in the following table:

Instability	Tibial Displacement	Pathological Axis	Structural Instability
Anteromedial	Medial tibial plateau subluxates anteriorly	Posterolateral—resulting in abnormal external tibial rotation	ACL, anteromedial capsule, MCL, pes anserine, medial meniscus
Anterolateral	Lateral tibial plateau subluxates anteriorly	Posteromedial—resulting in abnormal internal tibial rotation	ACL, anterolateral capsule, LCL, ITB, biceps femoris, lateral meniscus
Posteromedial	Medial tibial plateau subluxates posteriorly	Anterolateral—resulting in abnormal internal tibial rotation	PCL, posterior oblique ligament, MCL, semimembranosus
Posterolateral	Lateral tibial plateau subluxates posteriorly	Anteromedial—resulting in abnormal external tibial rotation	PCL, arcuate ligament complex, LCL, biceps femoris

Neurological Screen

Nerve Root Level	Sensory Testing	Motor Testing	Reflex Testing
L2	Femoral n.	Femoral n.	Partial
L3	Femoral n.	Femoral n.	Partial
L4	Saphenous n.	Femoral n.	Patellar t.
L5	Peroneal n.	Semitendinosus Semimembranosus-Tibial n.	Partial
S1	Peroneal n.	Biceps femoris - Tibial n.	Achilles t.
S2	P. femoral cutaneous n.	Intrinsic foot/toe muscles Lateral plantar n.	None

Table 5–5. Evaluative Findings of a Medial Collateral Ligament Sprain

Examination Segment	Clinical Findings
History	Onset: Acute. Location of pain: Medial aspect of the knee, especially along the joint line. Mechanism: A valgus force to the knee or, less commonly, external rotation of the tibia.
Inspection	Immediate inspection of an MCL injury may produce unremarkable findings. Over time, swelling may be present along the medial aspect of the knee.
Palpation	Tenderness along the length of the MCL from its origin below the adductor tubercle to the insertion on the medial tibial flare.
Functional tests	AROM: Pain occurs during the terminal ranges of flexion and extension. Greater loss of range of motion occurs when the MCL is torn proximal to the joint line because of greater involvement of the capsule.[25] PROM: Pain occurs during the terminal ranges of flexion and extension. RROM: Decreased strength and/or pain occurs during resisted flexion and extension.
Ligamentous tests	Valgus laxity in complete extension indicates involvement of the medial capsular structures. Valgus laxity in flexion indicates involvement of the superficial layer of the MCL.
Neurological tests	Not applicable.
Special tests	Slocum drawer test for laxity of the anteromedial capsule.
Comments	If valgus laxity is present in full extension, tearing of the medial meniscus and other medial soft tissue damage should be suspected. Adolescent athletes displaying the valgus laxity should be referred to a physician to rule out the possibility of trauma to the epiphyseal plate. If a rotational force is suspected, laxity is displayed in complete extension, or the Slocum drawer test result is positive, pathology to the ACL and PCL should be ruled out. The patella should be checked for lateral stability.

Table 5–6. Evaluative Findings of a Lateral Collateral Ligament Sprain

Examination Segment	Clinical Findings
History	Onset: Acute. Location of pain: Lateral joint line of the knee and fibular head. Mechanism: Varus force placed on the knee or excess internal tibial rotation.
Inspection	If swelling is present it is likely to be diffuse, especially when trauma is isolated to the LCL, as it is an extracapsular structure.
Palpation	Palpation elicits tenderness along the length of the LCL and possibly the lateral joint line.
Functional tests	AROM: Pain may be experienced during flexion and at the terminal range of extension. PROM: Pain may be experienced during the terminal ranges of motion, although lack of such pain does not conclusively rule out LCL trauma. RROM: This is the same as for passive range of motion.
Ligamentous tests	Varus laxity in complete extension indicates involvement of the lateral capsular structures. Varus laxity in 20° to 30° of flexion isolates the LCL.
Neurological tests	Not applicable.
Special tests	Slocum drawer test for laxity of the anterolateral capsule.
Comments	The LCL has a normal "spring" when a varus force is applied. Adolescent athletes displaying varus laxity should be referred to a physician to rule out possible epiphyseal plate trauma. Athletes who have reported a rotatory mechanism of injury or who display LCL laxity through either a varus stress or a positive Slocum drawer test result should be suspected of having anterolateral rotatory instability.

Table 5–7. Evaluative Findings of an Anterior Cruciate Sprain

Examination Segment	Clinical Findings
History	Onset: Acute. Location of pain: Within the knee joint, sometimes described as "pain under the kneecap." Mechanism: A blow that drives the tibia anterior relative to the femur or the femur posterior relative to the tibia (shear force), hyperextension or rotation of the knee (tensile forces).
Inspection	Rapid effusion is present, usually forming within hours after the onset of injury.
Palpation	For isolated ACL injuries, pain is not normally reported during palpation (other than that resulting from a contusion caused by the traumatic force). The sweep and ballotable patella test results are positive if intracapsular swelling is present.
Functional tests	AROM: Pain or intracapsular swelling may prohibit any meaningful range of motion tests. Pain would be expected to be greatest at the extremes of the range of motion. PROM: Pain is likely throughout the range of motion (especially at the extremes) and may be intensified when the tibia is internally or externally rotated. RROM: Pain and limitation in the range of motion may preclude this portion of the examination being conducted in the acute stage of injury.
Ligamentous tests	Lachman's test and anterior drawer test.
Neurological tests	Not applicable.
Special tests	None for isolated ACL sprains (see anteromedial and anterolateral instability).
Comments	The anterior drawer and Lachman's tests may not produce positive results in the hours after the onset of the injury because of muscle guarding. Trauma to the posterior cruciate ligament may produce false-positive results for ACL insufficiency.

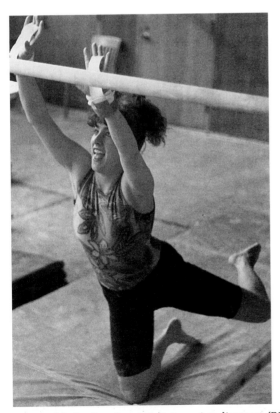

Figure 5–37. Mechanism for posterior cruciate ligament (PCL) trauma. Landing on a bent knee forces the tibia posteriorly relative to the femur.

Rotatory instabilities result when multiple structures are traumatized, often as the result of rotational forces placed on the knee. In each case, tests for laxity of the individual structures may produce only mildly positive results, but, when the combined laxity of each structure is summed, the degree of instability is marked.

Any injury to the knee's ligaments is suspect for causing rotatory instability. Therefore, any injury to the cruciate or collateral ligaments, the ITB, or the joint capsule should be presumed as potentially resulting in rotational instability. Clinically, athletes suffering from rotatory instability will report the knee "going out," decreased muscle strength, diminished performance, and a lack of confidence in the stability of the joint.

This text focuses only on tests for anteromedial and anterolateral rotatory instabilities. Tests for rotatory instability should not be performed as part of an on-field examination.

Anterolateral Rotatory Instability

Involving trauma to the ACL and the anterolateral capsular restraints, anterolateral rotatory instability (ALRI) results in a greater displacement of the tibia because of the keen role of the lateral extra-articular restraints.[31] Disruption of the LCL, ITB, biceps femoris, and lateral meniscus extenuates the amount of anterior tibial displacement and internal tibial rota-

Table 5–8. Evaluative Findings of a Posterior Cruciate Ligament Sprain

Examination Segment	Clinical Findings

History	Onset: Acute.
	Location of pain: Within the knee joint radiating posteriorly.
	Mechanism: Posterior displacement of the tibia on the femur (effect magnified when foot is plantarflexed).
	   Hyperflexion of the knee.
	   Hyperextension of the knee.

Inspection	The involved knee displays a posterior sag of the tibia. Swelling and effusion have a delayed onset.
Palpation	Tenderness may be elicited in the popliteal fossa.
Functional tests	AROM: Acutely, normal range of motion is present; pain may be produced as the knee nears full flexion. PROM: Pain is produced as the knee nears terminal flexion and with over-pressure during flexion. RROM: Normal strength during extension; pain as the knee nears terminal flexion.
Ligamentous tests	Posterior drawer test; Godfrey's sign.
Neurological tests	Not applicable.
Special tests	None.
Comments	Acutely, PCL sprains may resemble strains of the medial head of the gastrocnemius or a sprain of the posterior capsule.

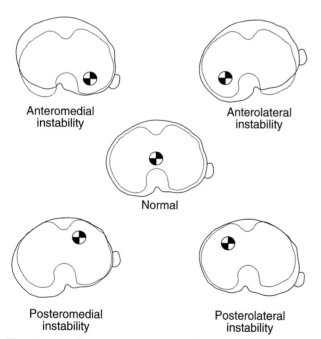

Figure 5–38. Classification of rotatory instabilities. The tibial articulating surface is shown in solid lines, the femoral articular surfaces in shaded lines. The type of instability is described based on the displacement of the tibia relative to the femur. Note that the axes of rotation are approximated.

tion, especially when combined with a tear of the ACL. Many special tests exist for determining the presence of ALRI, each with their own merits and limitations. The large number of tests is probably reflective of their relatively low reliability.

This test discusses three tests specific to this pathology: the lateral pivot shift, the Slocum ALRI test, and the flexion-rotation drawer. In addition, two tests, the Slocum drawer test and the crossover test, may be used to determine the presence of either ALRI or anteromedial rotatory instability (AMRI). Clinicians should remember that despite the myriad special tests at their disposal, a positive result for any one of the following techniques is sufficient to warrant further examination by an orthopedic physician.

Slocum Drawer Test for Rotatory Instability

A derivation of the anterior drawer test, the Slocum drawer test attempts to isolate either the anteromedial or the anterolateral joint capsule, depending on the position of the tibia. Internally rotating the tibia checks for the presence of anterolateral rotatory instability; externally rotating it checks for anteromedial rotatory instability (Fig. 5–39).

Slocum Drawer Test (Fig. 5–39)

Position of athlete	Lying supine with the knee flexed to 90°.
Position of examiner	Sitting on the athlete's foot. The tibia is internally rotated to 25° to test for anterolateral capsular instability. The tibia is externally rotated to 15° to test for anteromedial capsular instability.
Evaluative procedure	The tibia is drawn anteriorly.
Positive test results	An increased amount of anterior tibial translation compared with the opposite (uninvolved) limb or the lack of a firm end-point.
Implications	Test for anterolateral instability: Damage to the ACL, posterolateral capsule, LCL, ITB, and/or popliteus tendon. Test for anteromedial instability: Damage to the MCL, anteromedial capsule, and/or ACL.

Crossover Test

In this semifunctional test to determine the rotational stability of the knee, the athlete is asked to bear weight on the involved limb and step across with the uninvolved leg, similar to when the athlete "cuts" (Fig. 5–40). Because the foot of the weight-bearing leg remains fixed, the lateral femoral condyle is allowed to displace posteriorly relative to the tibia in the presence of laxity in the lateral capsular restraints. The clinician should be prepared to assist the athlete if the knee begins to give way.

This test is not as exacting as other tests for ligamentous instability but has the advantage of the athlete's somewhat replicating a sport-specific skill. Although primarily used to determine the presence of ALRI, the crossover test may be modified to test for AMRI by stepping behind with the uninvolved leg.

Crossover Test (Fig. 5–40)

Position of athlete	Standing with the weight on the involved limb.
Position of examiner	Standing in front of the athlete.
Evaluative procedure	ALRI: The athlete steps across and in front with the uninvolved leg, rotating the torso in the direction of movement. The weight-bearing foot remains fixated. AMRI: The athlete steps across and behind with the uninvolved leg, rotating the torso in the direction of movement. The weight-bearing foot remains fixated.
Positive test results	Pain, instability, or apprehension reported by the athlete.
Implications	ALRI: Instability of the lateral capsular restraints. AMRI: Instability of the medial capsular restraints.

Pivot Shift Test

Used to evaluate ALRI, the pivot shift test (also known as the lateral pivot shift) duplicates the anterior subluxation/reduction phenomenon that occurs during functional activities in ACL-deficient knees.[32] The tibia is internally rotated and a valgus force applied to the joint while the knee is moved from extension into flexion (Fig. 5–41). In the presence of a torn ACL, the femur is displaced posteriorly when the knee is placed in 10 to 20 degrees of flexion. As the knee continues into flexion, the ITB changes its angle of pull from that of an extensor to that of a flexor. When the knee reaches the range of 30 to 40 degrees of flexion,

the ITB causes the tibia to relocate, resulting in an appreciable "clunk." The pivot shift has been documented as being the most sensitive test for acute and chronic ACL injuries.[33] The presence of a negative pivot shift does not rule out the possibility of a partial ACL tear[34] (see top of page 160).

Slocum ALRI Test

The athlete's body weight is used to fixate the femur while the knee is flexed and a simultaneous valgus force is applied (Fig. 5–42). As the knee reaches 30 to 50 degrees, a subluxation of the tibia is reduced. This test is not as sensitive as the lateral

Pivot Shift Test (Fig. 5–41)

Position of athlete	Lying supine; the hip passively flexed to 30°.
Position of examiner	Standing lateral to the athlete, grasping the distal lower leg and/or ankle, maintaining 20° of internal tibial rotation. The knee is allowed to sag into complete extension. The opposite hand grasps the lateral portion of the knee at the level of the superior tibiofemoral joint, increasing the force of internal rotation.
Evaluative procedure	While maintaining internal rotation, a valgus force is applied to the knee while it is slowly flexed. To avoid masking any positive results, the athlete must remain relaxed throughout this test.
Positive test results	The tibia's position on the femur reduces as the leg is flexed in the range of 30° to 40°. During extension the anterior subluxation is felt.
Implications	Tear of the ACL, posterolateral capsule, arcuate ligament complex, and/or the ITB.
Modifications	This test may be performed with the tibia in the neutral position or externally rotated.
Comments	Meniscal involvement may limit range of motion to produce a false-negative test result. This test is most reliable when performed by a physician while the athlete is under anesthesia.

pivot shift but is useful when dealing with large or heavy athletes (see bottom of this page).

Flexion-Rotation Drawer Test for Anterolateral Rotatory Instability

This method of determining the presence of ALRI differs from the others presented in this text in that the flexion-rotation drawer (FRD) involves the stabilization of the tibia, resulting in the relative subluxation of the femur. In the presence of ALRI, the clinician's lifting and supporting the distal lower leg causes the femur to displace posteriorly and externally rotate (Fig. 5–43). The test then identifies the subsequent reduction of the femur relative to the tibia (see top of page 161).

Anteromedial Rotatory Instability

O'Donohue described a triad injury involving the ACL, MCL, and medial meniscus, resulting in AMRI. Recently this definition has been revised, with the lateral meniscus involved in this type of injury more frequently than in the medial one.[35] As described in the anterolateral rotatory instability section, the variants of the Slocum drawer test and the crossover test may be used to determine the presence of anteromedial rotatory instability. Additionally, isolated tests for ACL and MCL insufficiency yield positive results.

Meniscal Tears

It was once believed that the majority of meniscal tears involved the medial meniscus, but con-

Slocum ALRI Test (Fig. 5–42)

Position of athlete	Lying on the uninvolved side. The uninvolved leg is flexed at the hip and knee, moving it anterior to the involved extremity. The hip is rotated posteriorly. The involved leg is extended with the medial aspect of the foot resting against the table to provide stability.
Position of examiner	Standing behind the athlete, grasping the knee on the distal aspect of the femur and the proximal femur.
Evaluative procedure	A valgus force is placed on the knee, causing it to move into 30° to 50° of flexion.
Positive test results	An appreciable "clunk" or instability as the lateral tibial plateau subluxates or the athlete describes pain or instability.
Implications	Tear of the ACL, posterolateral capsule, arcuate ligament complex, and/or ITB.

Flexion-Reduction Drawer Test (Fig. 5–43)

Position of athlete	Lying supine.
Position of examiner	Standing lateral and distal to the involved knee. The clinician lifts the calf and ankle so that the knee is flexed to approximately 25°. Heavier athletes may require that the tibia be supported between the examiner's arm and torso.
Evaluative procedure	The tibia is depressed posteriorly to the femur. A valgus stress and axial compression along the tibial shaft are applied as the knee is slowly flexed.
Positive test results	The femur relocates itself on the tibia by moving anteriorly and internally rotating on the tibia.
Implications	Tear of the ACL, posterolateral capsule, arcuate ligament complex, and/or ITB.

temporary research has reversed this thought.[36,37] Many lateral meniscal tears are often asymptomatic and associated with ACL sprains. Improved diagnostic tests such as MRIs are now detecting lateral meniscal tears that once may have gone undetected.

Acute meniscal tears result from rotation and flexion of the knee, impinging the menisci between the articular condyles of the tibia and femur. Because of its greater mobility, the lateral meniscus may develop tears secondary to repeated stress, presenting with an insidious onset.

Two evaluative tests, McMurray's test and Apley's compression and distraction test, may be used to determine the presence of meniscal tears. However, the functional status of the athlete combined with the associated signs and symptoms may be the best model for determining trauma to these structures. Classic symptoms of meniscal tears involve "locking" of or "clicking" in the knee joint, especially when the athlete climbs stairs; pain and/or crepitus along the medial or lateral joint line, often with associated joint line swelling; and the knee's "giving way" during gait. The athlete may describe a rotational mechanism combined with flexion and a valgus or varus stress (Table 5–9). It should be noted that pain may not be described if the tear occurs in the avascular zone of the meniscus. Meniscal lesions may mimic the symptoms of patellofemoral dysfunction. Chapter 6 discusses the differential evaluation between these two conditions.

McMurray's Test for Meniscal Tears

McMurray's test attempts to replicate the impingement of the torn portion of the meniscus between the tibia and femur and to replicate the pain and locking of the knee described by the athlete. The method in this text describes a three-step process in which each pass attempts to isolate a distinct portion of each of the menisci (Fig. 5–44). Damage to the MCL or joint capsule may result in pain during this test secondary to the tensile forces placed on them during knee flexion and tibial rotation (see top of page 162).

Apley's Compression and Distraction Test for Meniscal Tears

Apley's compression and distraction test is used to differentiate pain caused by pressure on the

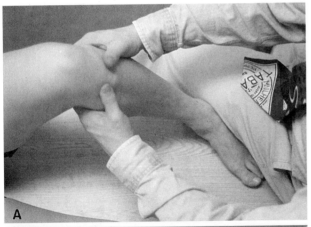

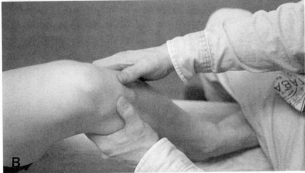

Figure 5–39. Slocum drawer test for rotatory instabilities. (*A*) With the tibia internally rotated to isolate the lateral capsular structures. (*B*) With the tibia externally rotated to isolate the medial capsule.

McMurray's Test for Meniscal Tears (Fig. 5–44)

Position of athlete	Lying supine.
Position of examiner	Standing lateral and distal to the involved knee. One hand supports the lower leg while the thumb and index finger of the opposite hand are positioned in the anteromedial and anterolateral joint line on either side of the patellar tendon.
Evaluative procedure	Pass one: With the tibia maintained in its neutral position, a valgus stress is applied while the knee is flexed through its available range of motion. A varus stress is then applied as the knee is returned to full extension. Pass two: The examiner internally rotates the tibia and applies a valgus stress while the knee is flexed through its available range of motion. A varus stress is then applied as the knee is returned to full extension. Pass three: With the tibia externally rotated, the examiner applies a valgus stress while the knee is flexed through its available range of motion. A varus stress is then applied as the knee is returned to full extension.
Positive test results	A popping, clicking, or locking of the knee, pain emanating from the menisci, or a sensation similar to that experienced during ambulation.
Implications	A meniscal tear on the side of the reported symptoms.
Comments	In acute injuries the available range of motion may not be sufficient to perform this test. Full flexion is required to isolate the posterior horns of the meniscus. Chondromalacia patellae or improper tracking of the patella may produce a click resembling that of a meniscal tear.

menisci versus pain arising from other soft tissue. This two-part test involves first a compression of the meniscus between the tibia and femur, then a distraction of the tibia, reducing the amount of pressure on the menisci (Fig. 5–45). Pain experienced during compression that disappears or is reduced during distraction is indicative of meniscal involvement (see top of page 163).

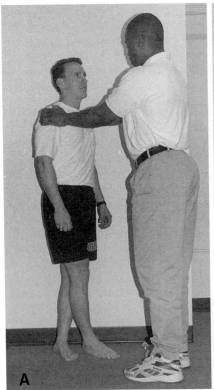
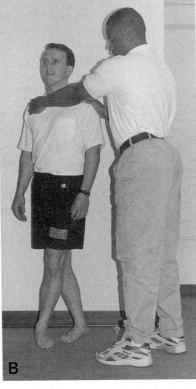

Figure 5–40. Crossover test for rotatory instabilities. (*A*) Stepping in front of the injured leg determines the presence of anterolateral rotatory instability. (*B*) Stepping behind the injured leg determines anteromedial rotatory instability.

Apley's Compression and Distraction Tests (Fig. 5–45)

Position of athlete	Lying prone. The knee is flexed to 90°.
Position of examiner	Standing lateral to the involved side.
Evaluative procedure	Compression test: The clinician applies pressure to the plantar aspect of the heel, applying an axial load to the tibia while simultaneously internally and externally rotating the tibia. Distraction test: The clinician grasps the lower leg and stabilizes the knee proximal to the femoral condyles. The tibia is distracted away from the femur while internally and externally rotating the tibia.
Positive test results	Pain experienced during compression that is reduced or eliminated during distraction.
Implications	Meniscal tear.
Comments	Pain that is experienced only during distraction or during both compression and distraction may indicate trauma to the collateral ligaments, joint capsule, or cruciate ligaments.

Osteochondral Defects

Osteochondral defects (OCDs) are localized areas of trauma to the tibial or femoral articular surfaces. OCDs are caused by tensile forces being placed on, or near, the attachment of the cruciate ligaments when the ACL or PCL is involved (see Fig. 2–7). Compressive and shear forces placed on the articular surfaces following abnormal joint stresses are other common mechanisms of OCDs in the knee.

The signs and symptoms of OCDs are often masked by those of the concurrent injury. Pain is increased during weight-bearing activities and an increase in pain and a decrease in strength are noted in closed kinetic chain activities relative to open chain motions. **Wilson's sign** can be used as a clinical evaluation tool for the presence of OCDs on the knee's articular surface. A definitive diagnosis must be made through the use of an x-ray examination or MRI.

Wilson's Sign

Wilson's sign is considered a pathological finding for osteochondritis dissecans in the knee and is positive if the lesion is found along the intercondylar area of the medial femoral condyle. The test is conducted by having the athlete extend the knee while the tibia is internally rotated (Fig. 5–46). The athlete is instructed to stop when pain is experienced and hold the knee in the position. If an OCD is present, usually at 30° of flexion, the pain is relieved by the athlete's externally rotating the tibia.

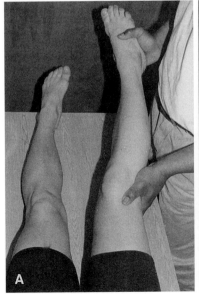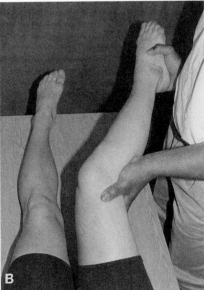

Figure 5–41. Lateral pivot shift test for anterolateral rotatory instability. (A) The knee is extended with the tibia internally rotated 20°. (B) Valgus force is applied to the knee while it is slowly flexed. The subluxation of the tibia and femur is felt in the presence of instability.

Wilson's Sign for Osteochondral Defects (Fig. 5–46)

Position of athlete	Sitting with the knee flexed to 90°.
Position of examiner	In front of the athlete to observe any reactions secondary to pain.
Evaluative procedure	The athlete actively extends the knee while the tibia is internally rotated. The athlete is told to stop the motion and hold the knee in the position in which pain is experienced. If pain is experienced, the athlete is allowed to externally rotate the tibia while the knee is held at its present point of flexion.
Positive test results	Pain experienced at about 30° of flexion that is relieved by externally rotating the tibia.
Implications	Osteochondral defect or osteochondritis dissecans on the intercondylar area of the medial femoral condyle.

Iliotibial Band Friction Syndrome

Resulting from friction between the ITB and the lateral femoral condyle, ITB friction syndrome tends to occur in sports requiring repeated knee flexion and extension, such as running, rowing, and cycling. Secondary to overuse, the bursa located between the distal ITB and the lateral femoral condyle becomes inflamed. This condition may progress to involve periosteitis of the condyle.

Several factors may predispose an athlete to ITB friction syndrome.[38–40] Genu varum may project the lateral femoral condyle laterally, increasing the friction as the ITB passes over it. Pronated feet, leg length differences, and other conditions resulting in internal tibial rotation alter the angle at which the ITB approaches its attachment on Gerdy's tubercle, increasing pressure at the lateral femoral condyle. Finally, a large lateral femoral condyle may result in increased irritation of the ITB as it passes over it.

The athlete typically describes a "burning" pain over the lateral femoral condyle that may radiate distally. Point tenderness is displayed at the point where the ITB passes over the condyle and may be described during resisted range of motion testing as the knee approaches 30° of flexion; however, no pain may be described during active and/or passive range of motion testing (Table 5–10). The athlete may describe increased pain while running down hills secondary to an increased stride length causing more pressure over the condyle. The presence of ITB friction syndrome may be confirmed through Noble's compression test, and ITB tightness, through Ober's test.

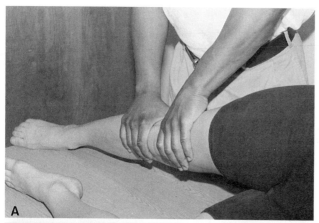

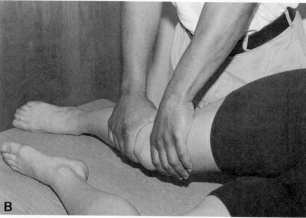

Figure 5–42. Slocum anterolateral rotatory instability test. (*A*) Athlete is side-lying with the involved foot stabilizing the tibia and with the superior pelvis rotated posteriorly. (*B*) Valgus force is applied to the knee. A positive test results in a noticeable clunk.

Noble's Compression Test for Iliotibial Band Friction Syndrome

In the Noble's compression test the examiner's thumb is used to increase the pressure on the ITB as it passes back and forth over the lateral femoral condyle (Fig. 5–47). The athlete describes pain similar to that experienced while exercising.

Noble's Compression Test (Fig. 5–47)

Position of athlete	Lying supine with the knee flexed.
Position of examiner	Standing lateral to the athlete on the involved side. The knee is supported above the joint line with the thumb over or just superior to the lateral femoral condyle. The opposite hand controls the lower leg.
Evaluative procedure	While applying pressure over the lateral femoral condyle, the knee is passively extended and flexed.
Positive test results	Pain under the thumb, most commonly as the knee approaches 30°.
Implications	Inflammation of the ITB, its associated bursa, or inflammation of the lateral femoral condyle.

Ober's Test for Iliotibial Band Tightness

Tightness of the ITB predisposes the athlete to ITB friction syndrome and, as is discussed in the next chapter, can result in lateral tracking of the patella. Ober's test is used to determine abnormal tightness of the ITB (Fig. 5–48). This test has many variations, but in each case it is necessary that the athlete's hip be positioned so that the tensor fasciae latae clears the greater trochanter. Failure to do this results in a false-positive test result (see top of page 166).

Popliteus Tendinitis

Popliteus tendinitis manifests itself in a manner similar to that of ITB friction syndrome, with the exception of the location of the pain. Athletes suffering from popliteus tendinitis describe pain in the proximal portion of the tendon, immediately anterior to the LCL. Like ITB friction syndrome, athletes with hyperpronation of the feet are predisposed to this condition, which worsens when the athlete is running downhill (Table 5–11). The popliteus acts to prevent a posterior shift of the tibia on the femur during midstance, and running downhill places excessive strain on the tendon. Palpation of the popliteus tendon is most easily conducted when the foot of the involved leg is placed on the uninvolved knee in the figure-4 position, a position that may produce pain in and of itself (Fig. 5–49).

ON-FIELD EVALUATION AND MANAGEMENT OF KNEE INJURIES

The process used during the on-field evaluation of knee injuries is similar to that described for the ankle. The athletic trainer must first rule out the presence of a gross fracture or dislocation of either

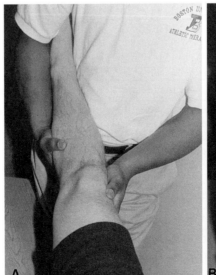
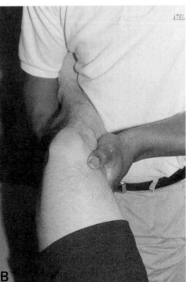

Figure 5–43. Flexion-reduction drawer test for anterolateral rotatory instability. (*A*) Knee is flexed to 25°. (*B*) Tibia is depressed posteriorly relative to the femur while a valgus stress and axial compression are applied.

Ober's Test for Iliotibial Tightness (Fig. 5–48)

Position of athlete	Lying on the side opposite that being tested.
Position of examiner	Standing behind the athlete. One hand stabilizes the pelvis, the other hand grasps the femur above the knee.
Evaluative procedure	The examiner abducts and extends the hip to allow the tensor fascia lata to clear the greater trochanter. The hip is then allowed to passively adduct to the table with the knee kept straight.
Positive test results	The leg does not adduct past parallel.
Implications	Tightness of the ITB, predisposing the athlete to ITB friction syndrome and/or lateral patellar malalignment.

the tibiofemoral joint or the patellofemoral joint (see Chapter 6) before conducting a more finite examination. It is vital that as much as possible regarding the injury history be gained while it is fresh in the athlete's mind. At this time the athlete should be questioned regarding the mechanism of injury, the fixation of the foot, and any associated sounds and sensations.

Equipment Considerations

Protective devices around the knee include both stabilizing and prophylactic braces, neoprene sleeves, and padding, each of which must be re-moved before evaluating the knee and patella. Most athletic uniforms include short pants, assisting in the ease of evaluation. However, football pants extend below the knee and have pockets in which a protective knee pad may be housed.

Football Pants

The pants worn for practice and competition in football are tight-fitting but fortunately are elastic. The knee may be exposed by reaching under the anterior portion of the pant and locating the attached pouch housing the knee pad. The knee pad is held down while the pant leg is pulled up and over the knee. The pad may then be removed and the pouch

Table 5–9. Evaluative Findings of Meniscal Tears

Examination Segment	Clinical Findings	
History	Onset:	Acute. Cases involving accumulated microtrauma still tend to present themselves as having an acute onset.
	Location of pain:	Along the medial or lateral joint line; however, tears to the avascular zone may not result in pain.
	Mechanism:	Tibial rotation combined with flexion and a varus or valgus stress.
Inspection	Inspection of an acutely torn meniscus normally does not present any conclusive findings. 　Over time, or in the case of a peripheral tear of the meniscus, swelling may be seen along the joint or in the popliteal fossa. Joint effusion may develop over 24 to 48 hours.	
Palpation	Peripheral tears may result in pain and crepitus along the joint line.	
Functional tests	The range of motion available may be limited owing to a mechanical block formed by a defect in the meniscus. AROM:　Range of motion may be decreased. PROM:　Pain is present near the extremes of flexion or extension. RROM:　Pain or locking is revealed as the torn portion of the meniscus passes beneath the femur's articular surface.	
Ligamentous tests	The integrity of the ACL and MCL should be established.	
Neurological testing	Not applicable.	
Special tests	Positive McMurray's test and/or Apley's compression/distraction test result.	
Comments	All suspected ACL or MCL injuries should be suspected of involving a meniscal tear until proven otherwise.	

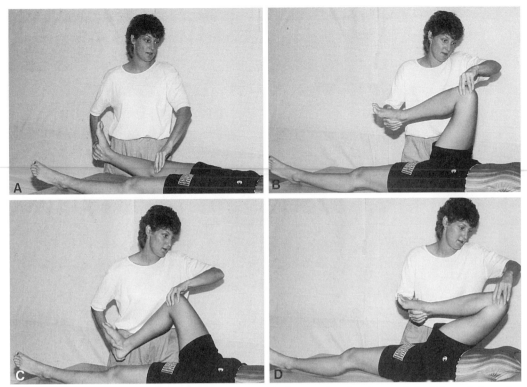

Figure 5–44. McMurray's test for meniscal lesions. The knee is flexed and extended while applying valgus and varus forces. A positive test is marked by a catching in the knee or palpable crepitus along the joint line. Patellofemoral conditions often mimic meniscal pathology.

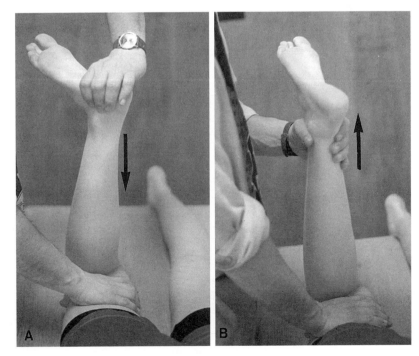

Figure 5–45. Apley's compression and distraction test for meniscal lesions. (*A*) Compression is applied while the tibia is internally and externally rotated. (*B*) The tibia is distracted and internally and externally rotated. Pain during compression that disappears during distraction implicates meniscal or articular cartilage involvement. Other results implicate ligamentous involvement.

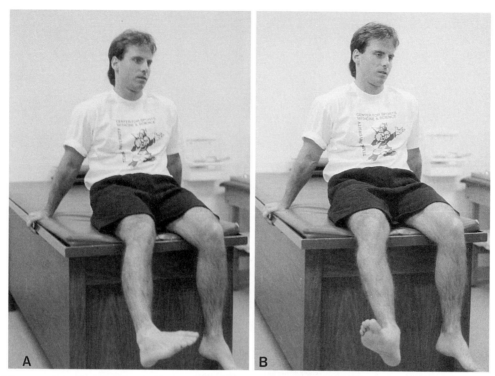

Figure 5–46. Wilson's sign for osteochondral defects. (*A*) The athlete extends the knee while the tibia is held in internal rotation. (*B*) When pain is experienced, the athlete holds the angle of flexion and externally rotates the tibia. In the presence of some osteochondral defects, the pain is relieved with external rotation.

Table 5–10. Evaluative Findings of Iliotibial Band Friction Syndrome

Examination Segment	Clinical Findings	
History	Onset:	Insidious.
	Location of pain:	Pain over the lateral femoral condyle proximal to the joint line that may radiate distally. Pain is increased when the athlete runs downhill.
	Mechanism:	Activities involving repeated knee flexion and extension.
Inspection	The athlete may present with one or more of the following bony alignments: Genu varum Pronated feet Leg length discrepancy	
Palpation	In advanced cases, pain may be elicited over the lateral femoral condyle, about 2 cm above the joint line.	
Functional tests	AROM: Range of motion is essentially normal. PROM: Range of motion is essentially normal. RROM: Pain may be described as the knee passes 30° during flexion and extension (representing the point where the ITB shifts over the lateral femoral condyle).	
Ligamentous tests	None.	
Neurological tests	Not applicable.	
Special tests	Positive Noble's compression test result.	
Comments	Iliotibial band tightness should be confirmed through Ober's test.	

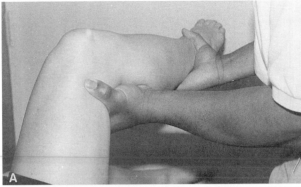

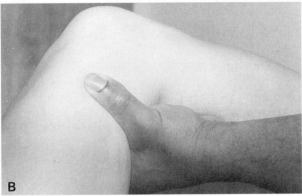

Figure 5–47. Noble's compression test for iliotibial band friction syndrome. (*A*) With the athlete's knee flexed to 45°, the examiner places pressure on the iliotibial band where it crosses the femoral condyle. The knee is then passively flexed and extended. In the presence of iliotibial band friction syndrome, pain is experienced when the knee approaches 30° of flexion, the point where the band crosses over the condyle. (*B*) Close-up of the pressure applied to the iliotibial band.

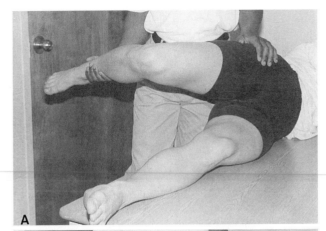

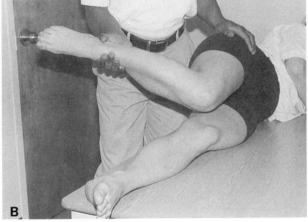

Figure 5–48. Ober's test for iliotibial band tightness. (*A*) To eliminate false-positive results, the greater trochanter must first be cleared from the tensor fasciae latae. (*B*) A positive result occurs when the knee does not adduct past parallel.

Table 5–11. Evaluative Findings of Popliteus Tendinitis

Examination Segment	Clinical Findings
History	Onset: Insidious. Location of pain: Pain in the popliteal fossa, radiating along the length of the popliteus tendon anterior to the LCL; increased when the athlete runs downhill. Mechanism: Overuse.
Inspection	In acute conditions, inspection is unremarkable; in chronic conditions, swelling or inflammation may be noted along the lateral joint line. The feet must be inspected for hyperpronation, a predisposing factor for popliteus tendinitis.
Palpation	Palpation is best performed in the figure-4 position (see Fig. 5–49). Pain and crepitus are elicited along the tendon anterior to the LCL.
Functional tests	AROM: Range of motion is full and normal. PROM: Range of motion is full and normal. RROM: Pain may be produced during resisted flexion from full extension as the popliteus "unscrews" the tibia.
Ligamentous tests	None.
Neurological tests	Not applicable.
Special tests	None.
Comments	The findings for popliteus tendinitis are similar to those of ITB friction syndrome, except for the location of the pain.

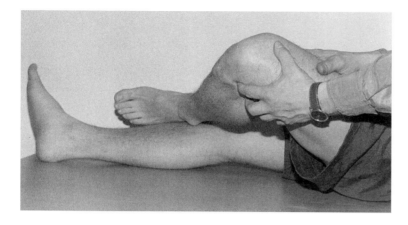

Figure 5–49. "Figure 4" position for palpating the popliteus tendon, located just anterior to the lateral collateral ligament.

flipped up and out of the way (Fig. 5–50). In cases when the pants are extraordinarily tight-fitting or inelastic, or when a brace is worn beneath the pants, making the preceding procedure difficult, the pant leg should be cut along one of the seams.

Removal of Knee Braces

Both prophylactic and stabilizing knee braces greatly hinder the on-field evaluation of knee in-juries. Once the pant leg has been pulled over the brace, prophylactic knee braces can be removed by loosening the lower Velcro strap, holding it in place, or cutting the tape. To remove the upper support, the examiner slides a hand under the strap or tape while pulling downwardly on the brace (see Fig. 5–50).

Because of the complexity of many of the stabilizing knee braces, it is easiest to first remove or detach all of the tibial straps, then the femoral ones. If

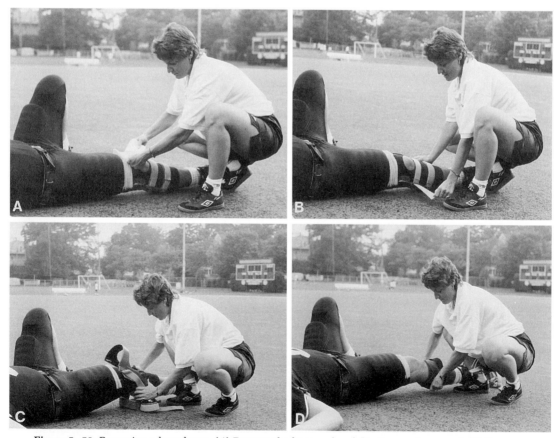

Figure 5–50. Removing a knee brace. (*A*) Remove the knee pad and flip its pouch upward. (*B*) Remove the Velcro straps. (*C*) Displace the distal (tibial) portion of the brace and slide the proximal portion from beneath the pant. (*D*) Remove any underlying padding.

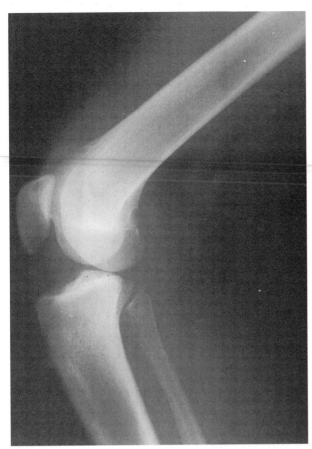

Figure 5–51. X-ray view of a tibiofemoral dislocation. Note the anterior displacement of the tibia relative to the femur.

Collateral and Cruciate Ligament Sprains

While the athlete is still on the playing field or court, only uniplanar ligamentous stress tests should be performed. This sequence should consist of valgus and varus stress testing for the collateral ligaments, Lachman's test for ACL deficiency, and the posterior drawer test for PCL laxity. For the basis of comparison and if the situation permits, the uninvolved knee should also be checked at this time. Laxity in the involved knee warrants the athlete being removed from the field in a non–weight-bearing manner, such as a two-person assist.

If significant laxity is demonstrated during the on-field examination, the athlete should be treated with ice, compression, and elevation and immediately referred to an orthopedic physician.

Meniscal Tears

The on-field determination of the possibility of a meniscal tear is based on the athlete's description of the injury mechanism. Athletes describing a "locking" or "giving way" at the time of the injury or who are hesitant to move the knee should be suspected of having a meniscal tear until otherwise ruled out. Likewise, any rotational mechanism or possible ACL or MCL sprain should also be assumed as involving the meniscus. The use of McMurray's test is not recommended during the on-field evaluation of possible meniscal injuries.

the athlete does not experience pain during knee flexion, the examiner should slightly flex the knee to allow the lower portion (tibial) of the brace, then lift the upper portion up and downward, away from the knee.

Tibiofemoral Joint Dislocations

Athletes with true dislocations of the tibiofemoral joint present with severe pain, muscle spasm, and obvious deformity of the joint. Because of the high probability of trauma to the neurovascular structures crossing the knee joint, this condition is considered a medical emergency. Most tibiofemoral dislocations occur with the tibia sliding anteriorly over the femur, resulting in a shortening of the involved leg, although the joint can dislocate perpendicular to the long axis of the femur (Fig. 5–51).

Management of this condition consists of establishing the presence of a distal pulse (e.g., dorsalis pedis), treating the athlete for shock, and activating the emergency medical squad for immediate physician intervention.

REFERENCES

1. Moore, KL: The lower limb. In Moore, KL: Clinically Oriented Anatomy, ed 2. Williams & Wilkins, Baltimore, 1985, p 403.
2. Fu, F, et al: Biomechanics of knee ligaments. Basic concepts and clinical application. J Bone Joint Surg Am 75:1716, 1993.
3. Arms, SW, et al: The biomechanics of anterior cruciate ligament rehabilitation and reconstruction. Am J Sports Med 12:8, 1984.
4. Van Dommelen, BA, and Fowler, PJ: Anatomy of the posterior cruciate ligament. A review. Am J Sports Med 17:24, 1989.
4a. Greenfield, BH: Rehabilitation of the Injured Knee: A Problem-Solving Approach. FA Davis, Philadelphia, 1993.
4b. Kendall, FP, and McCreary, EK: Muscles: Testing and Function, ed 3. Williams & Wilkins, Baltimore, 1983.
4c. Daniels, L, and Worthingham, C: Muscle Testing: Techniques of Manual Examination, ed 5. WB Saunders, Philadelphia, 1986.
5. Terry, GC, et al: How iliotibial tract injuries of the knee combine with acute anterior cruciate ligament tears to influence abnormal anterior tibial displacement. Am J Sports Med 21:55, 1993.
6. Soderberg, GL: Kinesiology: Application to pathological motion. Baltimore, Williams & Wilkins, 1986, p 207.
7. Reid, DC: Knee ligament injuries: Anatomy, classification, and examination. In Reid, DC: Sports Injury. Assessment and Rehabilitation. Churchill Livingstone, New York, 1992, p 449.
8. Voight, M, and Weider, D: Comparative reflex response times of vastus medialis oblique and subjects with extensor mechanism dysfunction. Am J Sports Med 19:131, 1991.

9. Hoppenfeld, S: Physical examination of the knee. In Hoppenfeld, S: Physical Examination of the Spine and Extremities. Appleton-Century-Crofts, New York, 1976, p 188.

10. Lephart, SM, et al: Functional performance tests for the anterior cruciate ligament insufficient athlete. Athletic Training: Journal of the National Athletic Trainers Association 26:44, 1991.

11. Blair, DF, and Willis, RP: Rapid rehabilitation following anterior cruciate ligament reconstruction. Athletic Training: Journal of the National Athletic Trainers Association 26:32, 1991.

12. Johnson, BC, and Cullen, MJ: The anterior cruciate ligament—Injuries and functions in anterolateral rotatory instability. Athletic Training: Journal of the National Athletic Trainers Association 17:79, 1982.

13. DiStefano, VJ: The enigmatic anterior cruciate ligament. Athletic Training: Journal of the National Athletic Trainers Association 16:244, 1981.

14. Girgis, FG, Marshall, JL, and Al Monajem, ARS: The cruciate ligaments of the knee joint. Anatomical, functional, and experimental analysis. Clin Orthop 106:216, 1975.

15. Furman, W, Marshall, JL, and Girgis, FG: The anterior cruciate ligament. A functional analysis based on post mortem studies. J Bone Joint Surg Am 58:178, 1976.

16. More, RC, et al: Hamstrings—an anterior cruciate ligament protagonist. Am J Sports Med 21:231, 1993.

17. Whitehill, WR, Wright, KE, and Nelson, K: Modified Lachman test for anterior cruciate ligament instability. Journal of Athletic Training 29:256, 1994.

18. Harter, RA, et al: A comparison of instrumented and manual Lachman test results in anterior cruciate ligament-reconstructed knees. Athletic Training: Journal of the National Athletic Trainers Association 25:330, 1990.

19. Barber-Westin, SD, and Noyes, FR: The effect of rehabilitation and return to activity on anterior-posterior knee displacements after anterior cruciate ligament reconstruction. Am J Sports Med 21:264, 1993.

20. Sgaglione, NA, et al: Arthroscopically assisted anterior cruciate ligament reconstruction with the pes anserine tendons. Am J Sports Med 21:249, 1993.

21. Cross, MJ, et al: Acute repair of injury to the anterior cruciate ligament. A long-term followup. Am J Sports Med 21:128, 1993.

22. Draper, DO, and Schulthies, S: A test for eliminating false positive anterior cruciate ligament injury diagnoses. Journal of Athletic Training 28:355, 1993.

23. Norkin, CC, and Levangie: PK: The knee complex. In Norkin, CC, and Levangie, PK: Joint Structure and Function: A Comprehensive Analysis, ed 2. FA Davis, Philadelphia, 1992, p 348.

24. Kladnik, KF: Subluxation and dislocation of the proximal tibiofibular joint. Athletic Training: Journal of the National Athletic Trainers Association 17:104, 1982.

25. Robbins, AJ, Newman, AP, and Burks, RT: Postoperative return of motion in anterior cruciate ligament and medial collateral ligament injuries. The effects of medial collateral ligament rupture location. Am J Sports Med 21:20, 1993.

26. Clancy, WG, and Bosanny, JJ: Functional treatment and rehabilitation of quadriceps contusions, patella dislocations and "isolated" medial collateral ligament injuries. Athletic Training: Journal of the National Athletic Trainers Association 17:249, 1982.

27. Beckett, ME, et al: Incidence of hyperpronation in the ACL injured knee: A clinical perspective. Journal of Athletic Training 27:58, 1992.

28. Schickendantz, MS, and Weiker, GG: The predictive value of radiographs in the evaluation of unilateral and bilateral anterior cruciate injuries. Am J Sports Med 21:110, 1993.

29. Sauers, RJ: Isolated posterior cruciate tear in a college football player. Athletic Training: Journal of the National Athletic Trainers Association 21:248, 1986.

30. Keller, PM, et al: Nonoperatively treated isolated posterior cruciate ligament injuries. Am J Sports Med 21:132, 1993.

31. Wroble, RR, et al: The role of the lateral extraarticular restraints in the anterior cruciate ligament-deficient knee. Am J Sports Med 21:257, 1993.

32. Magee, DJ: Knee. In Magee, DJ: Orthopedic Physical Assessment, ed 2. WB Saunders, Philadelphia, 1992, p 404.

33. Katz, JW, and Fingeroth, RJ: The diagnostic accuracy of ruptures of the anterior cruciate ligament comparing the Lachman test, the anterior drawer sign, and the pivot shift test in acute and chronic knee injuries. Am J Sports Med 14:88, 1986.

34. Lucie, RS, Wiedel, JD, and Messner, DG: The acute pivot shift: Clinical correlation. Am J Sports Med 12:189, 1984.

35. Shelbourne, KD, and Nitz, PA: The O'Donoghue triad revisited. Combined knee injuries involving anterior cruciate and medial collateral ligament tears. Am J Sports Med 19:474, 1991.

36. Krinskey, MB, et al: Incidence of lateral meniscus injury in professional basketball players. Am J Sports Med 20:17, 1992.

37. Scriber, K, and Mathney, M: Knee injuries in college football: An 18 year report. Athletic Training: Journal of the National Athletic Trainers Association 25:233, 1990.

38. Lebsack, D, Gieck, J, and Saliba, E: Iliotibial band friction syndrome. Athl Train JNATA 25:356, 1990.

39. Lucas, CA: Iliotibial band friction syndrome exhibited in athletes. Journal of Athletic Training 27:250, 1992.

40. Olsen, DW: Iliotibial band friction syndrome. Athletic Training: Journal of the National Athletic Trainers Association 21:32, 1986.

6

The Patellofemoral Articulation

Although the patellofemoral articulation is an integral part of the knee, it is separated in this text because of the differences in the mechanisms and onset of injury. With only a few exceptions, injury to the patellofemoral articulation is the result of overuse, congenital malalignment, or structural insufficiency.

CLINICAL ANATOMY

The patella is the largest sesamoid bone in the body, lying within the patellar tendon. Its design allows for increased efficiency of the quadriceps muscle group, protection of the anterior portion of the knee joint, and absorption and transmission of the patellofemoral *joint reaction forces*. In both the frontal and sagittal planes the patella is triangular. In the frontal plane the superior portion is wider than its distal apex; in the saggital plane it is marked with an anterior, nonarticulating surface and a narrower posterior articulating surface (Fig. 6–1).

The articular surface of the patella is composed of three distinct facets, each covered with up to a 5-mm thickness of hyaline cartilage. The medial and lateral facets each have superior, middle, and inferior articular surfaces. The odd facet, lying medial to the medial facet, has no articular subdivisions (Fig. 6–2).

During the movements of flexion and extension, the patella tracks within the femoral trochlear groove, an area between the two femoral condyles lined with articular cartilage. When the knee is fully extended, the patella rests on the distal portion of the femoral shaft, just proximal to the femoral groove. During flexion, the patella makes initial contact with the groove at 10 to 20 degrees of flexion and becomes seated within the groove as the knee approaches 20 to 30 degrees.[1] At this point the lateral border of the trochlea becomes prominent,

forming a strong barrier against lateral movement of the patella.

Distinct portions of the patella become involved in the articulation as the knee progresses through the range of motion (Table 6–1). The average patellofemoral contact area varies throughout the range of motion, with the greatest amount of surface area reported between 60 and 90 degrees of flexion.[2–4] Compressive forces are placed on the patella as it moves through the femoral trochlea, ranging from 0.5 times the body weight when walking to 3.3 times the body weight when walking up and down stairs or running on hills.[5] The maximum compressive force placed on the patella occurs at 30 degrees of flexion.[2,6]

The patella's position is maintained and restrained throughout the arc of motion by the patellar retinaculum (Fig. 6–3). The **lateral retinaculum** originates off the vastus lateralis and the iliotibial band and inserts on the patella's lateral border. Originating from the distal portion of the vastus medialis and adductor magnus and inserting on the medial border of the patella is the **medial retinaculum**. The superior portion of the knee's fibrous capsule thickens and inserts on the patella's superior border forming the **medial and lateral patellofemoral ligaments**.

Muscular Anatomy and Related Soft Tissues

This section discusses the specific effects that the quadriceps femoris muscles have on the patella's function. During flexion the patella is pulled inferiorly by the patellar tendon's attachment to the tibial tuberosity. During extension, the quadriceps femoris and its tendon pull the patella superiorly, forming the extensor mechanism.

Normally the length of the patellar tendon should be approximately the same length as the long axis of the patella (± 10 percent) (Fig. 6–4).[7] Abnormally

---

Joint reaction forces: Forces that are transmitted through a joint's articular surfaces.

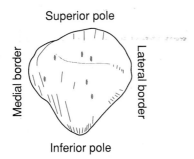

Figure 6-1. Anterior view of the left patella.

Table 6-1. Articulation of the Patellofemoral Joint

Position (Flexion)	Patellar Facet(s) in Contact With Femoral Trochlear Groove
0°	Patella rests on the distal femoral shaft
20°	Inferior portion of facets
45°	Medial and lateral facets
90°	Large area across the medial and lateral facets
135°	Odd facet

long or short tendons alter the mechanics of the extensor mechanism.

The **vastus lateralis** is the primary muscle pulling the patella laterally. Medially, the **oblique fibers of the vastus medialis (VMO)** approach the patella at a 55-degree angle, guiding the patella medially and controlling lateral patellar subluxation.[8] The adductor magnus, serving as part of the origin of the VMO, may have a secondary function in limiting the amount of lateral patellar tracking.[9,10] Tightness of the ITB can extenuate the lateral tracking of the patella, resulting in subluxations or patellar malalignment.

In healthy individuals, the VMO should contract simultaneously or before the vastus lateralis, whereas patellofemoral pain syndromes tend to cause latent VMO contraction timing.[11] This phenomenon may be due to pain or swelling. A buildup of 20 to 30 mL of excess fluid within the capsule neurologically inhibits the VMO, compared with 50 to 60 mL of fluid for the rest of the extensor mechanism.[12]

The alignment of the foot and normal flexibility of the triceps surae and hamstring muscle groups are needed to provide adequate knee range of motion. Tightness of the gastrocnemius and/or soleus may prohibit the 10 degrees of dorsiflexion required while walking and the 15 degrees required when running. The most common compensation for a lack of dorsiflexion is pronation of the foot. Likewise, increased foot pronation increases the amount of internal tibial rotation, affecting the relationship of the extensor mechanism by rotating the tibial tuberosity toward the midline.

Bursa of the Extensor Mechanism

Individual differences result in varying numbers of bursae being directly involved with the extensor mechanism. However, four bursae are considered to be consistent throughout the population (Fig. 6-5). Lying deep at the distal end of the quadriceps femoris muscle group and allowing free movement over the distal femur, the **suprapatellar bursa** is an extension of the knee's joint capsule. This bursa is held in place by the articularis genus muscle. The **prepatellar bursa** overlies the anterior portion of the patella and allows it to move freely beneath the skin. The distal portion of the patellar tendon receives protection against friction and blows by the **subcutaneous infrapatellar bursa**, overlying the tibial tuberosity, and the **deep infrapatellar bursa**, located between the tendon and the tibia. The **infrapatellar fat pad** separates the patellar tendon and the deep infrapatellar bursa from the joint capsule of the knee.

CLINICAL EVALUATION OF THE PATELLOFEMORAL JOINT

Dysfunction of joints superior to or inferior to the knee may manifest themselves as patellofemoral

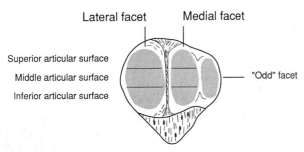

Figure 6-2. Posterior view of the left patella. The lateral and medial facets may be conceptualized as having superior, middle, and inferior articular surfaces. The odd facet has no such subdivisions.

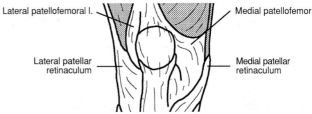

Figure 6-3. Patellar retinaculum and medial and lateral patellofemoral ligaments (partially hidden by the quadriceps muscle).

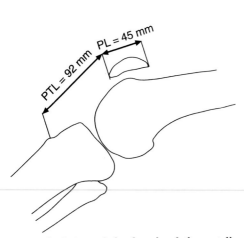

Figure 6–4. Calculation of the length of the patellar tendon (drawn from an x-ray view). PTL = patellar tendon length; PL = patellar length.

pain. Findings of the patellofemoral joint evaluation may necessitate adjunct evaluation of the hip, lower leg, ankle, foot, and related body areas. To meet this need the athlete should be dressed in shorts and bring his or her casual and competitive footwear to the evaluation.

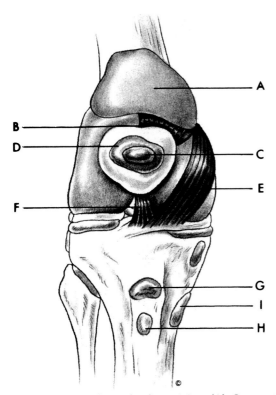

Figure 6–5. Bursae about the knee joint: (A) Suprapatellar pouch, (B) suprapatellar plica, (C) superficial prepatellar bursa, (D) deep prepatellar bursa, (E) medial plica, (F) infrapatellar bursa, (G) deep infrapatellar bursa, (H) superficial infrapatellar bursa, and (I) pes anserine bursa. (Adapted from Ficat, P, and Hungerford, DS,[12a] p 118, with permission.)

History

Many patellofemoral joint injuries are the result of overuse stresses, structural abnormalities, or biomechanical deficiencies of the lower leg. However, several acute, traumatic conditions can affect the patella and the extensor mechanism. During the history-taking process, the clinician must ascertain the onset and mechanism of injury, as well as pertinent past history of injury to the patellofemoral complex, the hip, knee, lower leg, and foot.

• **Mechanism and onset of injury:** The examiner should determine whether the athlete's chief complaint is the result of a single traumatic episode or stems from an insidious onset. Acute conditions affecting the patella include contusions and fractures resulting from direct blows and strains or ruptures of the patellar tendon caused by dynamic overload of the musculotendinous unit. A dislocated patella has an acute onset, but repeated subluxations are most likely the result of chronic conditions. Other chronic patellar conditions include chondromalacia patella, malalignment, tendinitis, bursitis, fat pad syndrome, or subtle subluxations (Box 6–1).

• **When pain occurs:** For chronic conditions the athlete should be questioned regarding when the pain occurs, what activities cause its onset, and how these symptoms affect the level of activity. Activities such as ascending or descending stairs or open chain knee extension exercises increase compressive forces of the patella on the knee.

Box 6–1. Chondromalacia Patella

Although it is often referred to and treated as a discernible ailment, chondromalacia patella (CP) is best thought of as a symptom. Chondromalacia patella is the softening and subsequent roughening of the patella's hyaline cartilage. This malady presents itself as grinding beneath the patella and may cause related swelling and pain. It is confirmed only through visual inspection during arthroscopy. CP is nebulous in nature because it is often found incidentally in otherwise normal knees.[33] Likewise, many individuals describing these symptoms before surgery have no signs of CP at the time of arthroscopy.[34–36]

Chondromalacia patella is most often, if not always, the result of biomechanical changes affecting the lower extremity. As such, chondromalacia may be treated symptomatically, but the key to its remedy is determining and correcting the underlying pathology.

Pain following prolonged periods of sitting, the **movie** or **theater sign**, may describe pain arising from prolonged pressure being placed on one or more facet. Athletes describing the knee as "locking" or "giving way" should be questioned more thoroughly. A distinction must be made between true locking of the knee and "clicking" beneath the patella. True locking of the knee is not indicative of patellofemoral pathology but, rather, of meniscal tears. Reports of the knee giving way may be the result of patellar subluxation or of internal derangement of the knee itself.

- **Location of the pain:** Pain radiating medially or laterally from the patella may indicate a pathological glide within the trochlea or an abnormal tilt of the patella. Posterior knee pain is a common complaint of athletes suffering from synovitis, although the pain may radiate to any area of the knee. Palpation is used to determine the source of the athlete's complaints.

- **Level of activity:** The athlete is questioned as to whether there has been an increase in the level of activity, a change in the surface on which the activity occurs, or a change of footwear or equipment (e.g., as occurs in changing from first base to catcher or bicycling to running). Each of these may place excessive or unaccustomed forces on the patellofemoral joint.

- **Prior surgery:** Knee surgery can result in inflammation, adhesion, or entrapment of the patella's restraints, resulting in painful movement and reduced range of motion.[13]

- **Relevant past history:** It is common for prior injuries to the lower leg to alter the biomechanics of the extensor mechanism. The athlete should be thoroughly questioned and the medical file examined for conditions such as foot pathologies, recurrent ankle sprains, Achilles tendon pathology, knee sprains, injury to the hip, or conditions involving the lumbar spine. Injury to the opposite limb may result in compensation by the currently involved knee.

Inspection

The entire knee complex should be observed for signs of gross deformity including patellar malalignment, dislocation, and the integrity of the patellar tendon. Any signs of inflammation, previous injury (e.g., scars), discoloration, or swelling around the knee and patellofemoral complex should be noted.

- **Patellar alignment:** With the knee fully extended and the athlete weight bearing, the patella

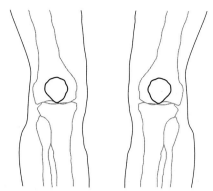

Figure 6-6. Normal patellar alignment with the knee extended. The patella's inferior pole should rest at the upper margins of the femoral trochlea.

should align at approximately the center of the femur, with the inferior pole located at the upper margin of the femoral trochlea (Fig. 6-6).

- **Patellar malalignment:** Several types of patellar malalignments may be displayed when the athlete is weight bearing.
  - ○ **Patella baja and patella alta:** Abnormal superior or inferior positioning may be demonstrated through gross inspection but often requires x-ray examination for definitive diagnosis. An abnormally long patellar tendon leads to a high-riding patella, patella alta. A shortened patellar tendon leads to a low-riding patella, patella baja (Fig. 6-7). Clinically, patella alta may be most easily identified through the **camel sign** (Fig. 6-8).
  - ○ **Squinting patellae:** This malalignment is identifiable by the patellae's being rotated medially on the femur, as if they were "looking" at one another while the feet are pointed straight ahead (Fig. 6-9). This alignment is caused by hip *anteversion*, internal rotation of the femur, or internal tibial rotation.
  - ○ **"Frog-eyed" patallae:** This patellar alignment is easily visualized from its comical name. The patellae take on a lateral and superior position so that they are "looking" up and away from each other (see Fig. 6-9B). This alignment is caused by a retroverted hip, external femoral rotation, or external rotation of the tibia.

- **Posture of the knee:** The knee should be inspected for the presence of genu valgum or genu varum, as described in Chapter 5. Genu varum places an increased compressive force on the lateral patellar facets, and genu valgum causes excessive lateral forces, increasing the pressure on the medial and odd facets. Genu recurvatum places additional pressure on the superior articular surfaces.

Anteversion: A forward bending or angulation of a bone or organ.

(A)

(A)

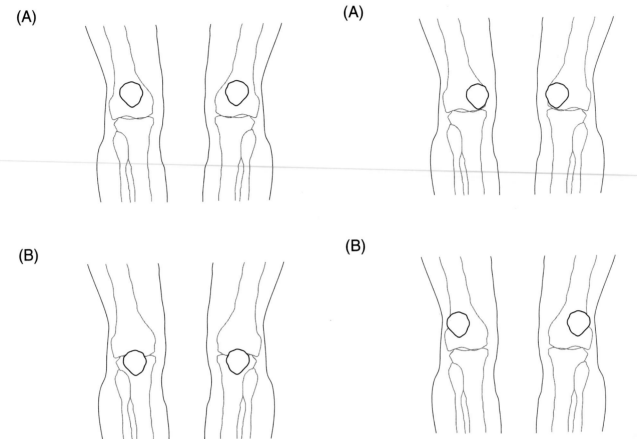

(B)

(B)

Figure 6–7. (*A*) Patella alta, a high-riding patella indicating a long patellar tendon. (*B*) Patella baja, a low-riding patella caused by shortness of the patellar tendon.

Figure 6–9. (*A*) Squinting patellae secondary to internal rotation of the lower extremity. (*B*) "Frog-eyed" patellae caused by external rotation of the lower extremity.

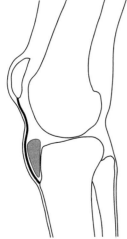

Figure 6–8. "Camel sign," a clinical indication of patella alta. The high-riding patella exposes the fat pad, forming a "double hump" when viewed from the lateral side.

• **Q angle:** The approximate tracking of the patella can be determined through the measurement of the Q angle. This angle describes the relationship between the line of pull of the quadriceps and the line of the tendon from the midpoint on the patella to its insertion on the tibial tuberosity. This measurement should be performed once with the knee extended and then again with the knee flexed to 90 degrees to account for increased lateral movement of the patella during flexion (Fig. 6–10). With the knee extended the normal Q angle is 13 degrees for men and 18 degrees for women. When the knee is flexed to 90 degrees, the Q angle should be 8 degrees for both genders.[14] Increased Q angles increase the forces placed on the lateral patellar facet, medial patellar retinaculum, and lateral border of the femoral trochlea secondary to an increased lateral glide of the patella.

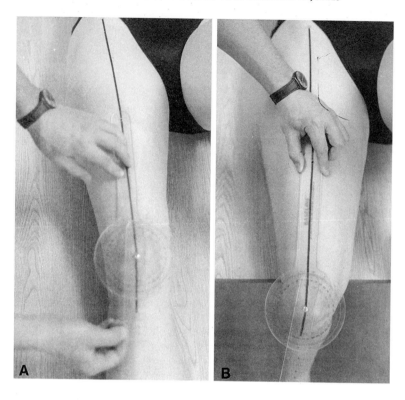

Figure 6–10. Measurement of the Q angle. (*A*) With the knee extended in a non–weight-bearing position. (*B*) With the knee flexed to 90°. The anatomical landmarks of the anterior superior iliac spine, center of the patella, and the tibial tuberosity are used to align the goniometer.

Measurement of the Q Angle
With the Knee Extended (Fig. 6–10A)

Position of athlete	Lying supine with the knee fully extended.
Position of examiner	Standing on the side of the limb to be measured.
Evaluative procedure	The examiner identifies and marks the anterior superior iliac spine (ASIS), the midpoint of the patella, and the tibial tuberosity. A goniometer is placed so that its axis is located over the patellar midpoint, the center of its stationary arm is over the line from the ASIS to the patella, and the moving arm is placed over the line from the patella to the tibial tuberosity.
Positive test results	A Q angle greater than 13° in men or 18° in women.
Implications	Increased lateral forces leading to a laterally tracking patella.

Measurement of the Q Angle With the Knee Flexed (Fig. 6–10B)

Position of athlete	Sitting with legs over the edge of the table with the knees flexed to 90°.
Position of e-p10.5aminer	Standing on the side of the limb to be measured.
Evaluative procedure	The examiner identifies and marks the ASIS, the midpoint of the patella, and the tibial tuberosity. A goniometer is placed so that its axis is located over the patellar midpoint, the center of its stationary arm parallels the line from the ASIS to the patella, and the moving arm is placed over the line from the patella to the tibial tuberosity.
Positive test results	A Q angle greater than 8°.
Implications	Increased lateral tracking in a functional position, predisposing the athlete to lateral patellar subluxations and/or dislocations.

- **Standing leg length difference:** A gross determination of leg length equality is made by placing the thumbs over the anterior superior iliac spine (ASIS). If the leg lengths are equal, the heights of the ASISs should be level; an unequal level may be indicative of a leg length discrepancy and should be measured more exactly (Fig. 6–11).

- **Foot positioning:** While weight bearing, the foot should maintain a neutral position. Excessive pronation results in the tibia's being internally rotated while excessive supination results in external tibial rotation. Pronation of one foot and supination of the other is indicative of a leg length discrepancy, with the supinated foot representing the shorter leg. If the athlete presents with a standing leg length difference, supinating the pronated foot should bring the ASISs to an equal level.

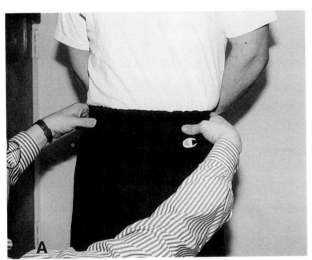

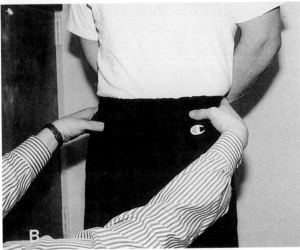

Figure 6–11. Gross determination of leg length difference. With the athlete standing with the feet shoulder-width apart and the knees extended, the examiner's thumbs are placed over the anterior superior iliac spine. With equal leg lengths the thumbs are level; unequal levels indicate shortness of the leg represented by the lower thumb.

Palpation

The complete palpation of the patellofemoral articulation must include the bony and soft tissue structures of the tibiofemoral articulation to rule out pathology of these structures. This section describes palpation of the knee and patella only as it relates to patellar dysfunction.

- Palpation of the bony and ligamentous structures
  - **Tibial tuberosity:** Identified by the insertion of the patellar tendon, the tibial tuberosity can become tender secondary to patellar tendinitis or a contusion. Tenderness and enlargement of the tuberosity in an adolescent athlete indicates the possibility of **Osgood-Schlatter disease.**
  - **Patella:** During palpation of the patella, pain arising from the bone itself must be distinguished from pain arising from the soft tissue. The patellar body is palpated to rule out the presence of fracture, indicated by pain, roughening, discontinuity, ridges, or crepitus. The examiner continues along the periphery of the four borders, attempting to elicit tenderness secondary to inflammatory conditions. Pain along the inferior pole is associated with **patellar tendinitis** and in the case of quadriceps tendinitis, pain is present along the superior pole.

In some instances the patella may be in two pieces, either from previous trauma or congenital defect (Fig. 6–12). This condition, a **bipartite patella**, reduces the efficiency of the extensor mechanism.

  - **Patellar articulating surface:** With the knee extended, the examiner moves the patella laterally to expose the outer portion of the lateral articular facet and medially to expose the odd facet. The exposed facets are palpated for signs of tenderness.
  - **Femoral trochlea:** In the patella's resting position on an extended knee, the medial and lateral femoral trochlear borders may be palpated for tenderness, with the lateral border more exposed than the medial. Moving the patella medially and laterally exposes more of the femoral articular surface.
  - **Presence of crepitus:** Grinding beneath the patella while it is compressed and moved against the femur suggests the presence of chondromalacia. Although this condition occurs in a significant portion of the population, its presence may reflect biomechanical changes in the extensor mechanism or elsewhere in the lower extremity. The presence of chondromalacia may further be substantiated through Clarke's sign (Fig. 6–13).

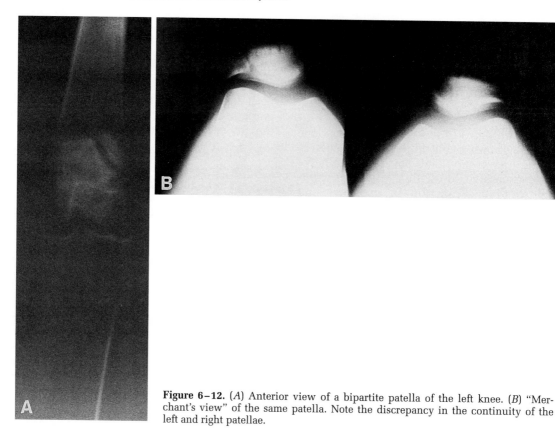

Figure 6–12. (*A*) Anterior view of a bipartite patella of the left knee. (*B*) "Merchant's view" of the same patella. Note the discrepancy in the continuity of the left and right patellae.

Clarke's Sign (Fig. 6–13)

Position of athlete	Lying supine with the knee extended.
Position of examiner	Standing lateral to the limb being evaluated. One hand is placed proximal to the superior patellar pole, applying a gentle downward pressure.
Evaluative procedure	The athlete is asked to contract the quadriceps muscle while a downward pressure is maintained on the patella.
Positive test results	The athlete experiences patellofemoral pain and cannot hold the contraction.
Implications	Possibly chondromalacia patella (examiner should be aware of false-positive results.)
Modification	The test may be performed with the knee flexed to various angles to assess different areas of patellofemoral contact.

○ **Retinacular and capsular structures:** The clinician palpates the medial and lateral retinacula and the medial and lateral patellofemoral ligaments for pain. The retinaculum and the associated structures may become painful with excessive movement of the patella.

○ **Synovial plica:** The anteromedial and anterolateral joint capsule is palpated for bands of thickened or folded tissue, denoting a synovial plica. These areas may become irritated and inflamed from being rubbed across bony structures or other tissues.

• Palpation of musculature and related soft tissue
  ○ **Quadriceps and superior patellar pole:** The site where the quadriceps muscle group inserts on the patella's superior pole should be located and the area palpated for tenderness or crepitus. If pain is present at the superior border, the examiner palpates up the length of the quadriceps group, noting the point at which the pain disappears.
  ○ **Suprapatellar bursa:** Located under the quadriceps group approximately 3 inches (four fingers' breadth) above the patella is the suprapatellar bursa. With the exception of puncture

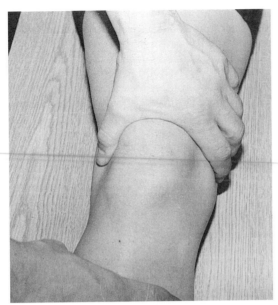

Figure 6–13. Clarke's sign for chondromalacia patella. The examiner cups the hand over the superior patellar pole as the athlete contracts the quadriceps. This test elicits a great deal of pain and elicits a positive result in otherwise asymptomatic knees.

wounds, the suprapatellar bursa is rarely injured by direct trauma. It may, however, become inflamed or enlarged secondary to effusion in, or inflammation of, the knee's joint capsule.

○ **Prepatellar bursa:** The examiner should ensure that the skin over the patella moves freely and is not painful. The prepatellar bursa may become irritated and inflamed from overuse, from a contusing force to the anterior patella, or from prolonged periods of time kneeling, as is seen with wrestlers. This bursa is also a common site of bacterial or staphylococcal infection.

○ **Subcutaneous infrapatellar bursa:** The mechanism of injury for the subcutaneous infrapatellar bursa is similar to that of the prepatellar bursa. Likewise, this structure should be palpated for tenderness, swelling, and the skin's ability to glide freely over the tibial tuberosity.

○ **Patellar tendon:** Palpate the tendon at the level of the infrapatellar pole moving distally to the tendon's midsubstance on through to its insertion at the tibial tuberosity. Pain elicited at the infrapatellar pole through the midsubstance is indicative of patellar tendinitis; pain localized in the midsubstance may reflect a strain of this structure or tendinitis; while pain isolated

to the tibial tuberosity may be traced to Osgood-Schlatter disease in adolescent athletes, a contusion, or patellar tendinitis.

○ **Fat pads and deep infrapatellar bursa:** Placing the knee in extension squeezes the fat pads beneath the patellar tendon out to either side, masking the deep infrapatellar bursa from palpation. These fat pads should be palpated as they exit behind, medially and laterally to the patellar tendon for signs of inflammation. Because these structures are highly innervated, they are prone to hypersensitivity during inflammatory conditions.

○ **Neuroma:** Hypersensitivity of one or more nerves can result in pain radiating through the knee and lower extremity. Neuroma most commonly occurs secondary to laceration of nerves during surgery involving the infrapatellar branch of the saphenous nerve and may be confirmed via a test for Tinel's sign over the medial aspect of the tibial flare.

○ **Related structures:** The examiner palpates the insertion of the pes anserine muscle group and its associated bursae in the area of the medial tibial flare. These are common sites of inflammation. The flexibility of the ITB must be determined because tightness of this structure serves to increase the amount of lateral patellar tracking. **Trigger points** can be found in the ITB, causing tightness along its entire length.

○ **Areas of scars:** Any scars from previous injury such as lacerations or abrasions or prior surgeries for MCL, LCL, meniscal, or cruciate ligament trauma should be thoroughly examined. These areas may develop a **keloid** or result in the formation of a neuroma, each of which may serve as the source of the athlete's pain.

Functional Testing

Unrestricted movement of the patella is required for the lower leg to achieve its full range of motion. This section discusses the normal and abnormal movement of the patella as the knee moves from flexion to extension. The complete range of motion testing of the knee joint is described in Chapter 5.

• **Active range of motion:** As the knee moves from flexion into extension, the patella should glide superiorly and track somewhat laterally. Tightness of the lateral structures accentuates the lateral displacement of the patella. During flexion the patella glides inferiorly and medially as it situates itself in the femoral trochlea.

Trigger point: A pathological condition characterized by a small, hypersensitive area located within muscles and fasciae.
Keloid: Hypertrophic scar formation secondary to excessive collagen.

- **Resisted range of motion:** Pain associated with the lateral aspect of the patella during movement may indicate a malalignment, resulting in soft tissue stretch as well as compressive forces on the articular facets. Resistive range of motion should be performed in both the open and closed kinetic chain to determine the effect of the introduction of the athlete's body weight on the motion of the patella. Isokinetic testing of athletes suffering from acute patellofemoral pain is not recommended because of the increased compressive forces placed on the patella at slower speeds.[15]

Ligamentous Testing

All major ligaments of the knee joint should be evaluated for normal integrity as described in Chapter 5. Laxity of the knee joint can result in abnormal patellar tracking secondary to uniplanar or rotatory shifting of the tibia or femur, causing patellofemoral pain.

The ligamentous and capsular stability of the patella is based on the presence of patellar tilt and the amount of glide available to the patella. Glide tests are performed to assess the laxity or tightness of the retinacula by measuring how far the patella can be passively moved from its resting position in the trochlea.

The following descriptions of assessing the amount of patellar glide and tilt have been adapted from the guidelines established by the American Association of Orthopaedic Surgeons.[16]

- **Patellar glide:** To determine the amount of glide, the patella is visualized as having four quadrants. The knee is placed on a **bolster** so that it is flexed to 30 degrees and the athlete must be fully reclined to relax the quadriceps muscles (Fig. 6–14). To ensure accuracy during the measurements the clinician must avoid tilting the patella as it is glided medially and laterally.

  ○ **Medial glide:** Moving the patella medially as it sits in the femoral trochlea stresses the lateral patellar retinaculum and the other soft tissue restraints. Normally, the patella should glide one to two quadrants (roughly half of its width) medially. Movement of one quadrant or less is described as being **hypomobile** and is caused by tightness of the lateral retinaculum or ITB tightness.[17] Movement of three or more quadrants is a **hypermobile patella**, indicating laxity of the lateral restraints (Fig. 6–15).
  ○ **Lateral glide:** Lateral patellar motion is restrained by the medial patellar retinaculum, the VMO, and the knee's medial joint capsule. Normal lateral motion is defined as 0.5 to 2 quadrants of glide. Less than that is described as a **hypomobile lateral glide**, indicating tightness of the medial restraints. Greater than three quadrants of motion reflects a **hypermobile lateral glide**, indicating incomplete medial restraint and predisposing the athlete to a laterally subluxating or dislocating patella (Fig. 6–16). It should be noted that the athlete may be apprehensive during measurement of lateral glide, indicating fear of the patella's subluxating or dislocating.

- **Patellar tilt:** Patellar tilt, the rotation of the patella about its midsagittal axis, evaluates the tension within the lateral retinaculum, lateral capsule, ITB, and vastus lateralis tendon. The evaluation is performed with the athlete lying supine, the knee extended, and the femoral condyles parallel to the table.

  ○ **Evaluation of patellar tilt:** The evaluation of patellar tilt is referenced to an axis passing through the femoral condyles. The patella is grasped with the forefinger and thumb, elevating its lateral border while depressing the medial border (Fig. 6–17). The degree of tilt is referenced by the amount of rise of the

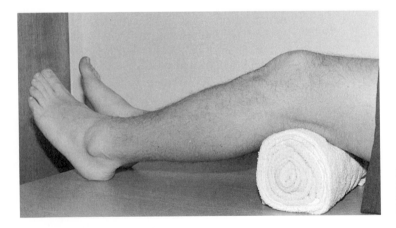

Figure 6–14. Positioning of the athlete during the patellar glide tests. The knee is flexed to 30° and the athlete is encouraged to keep the quadriceps musculature relaxed.

Bolster: A support used to maintain the position of a body part.

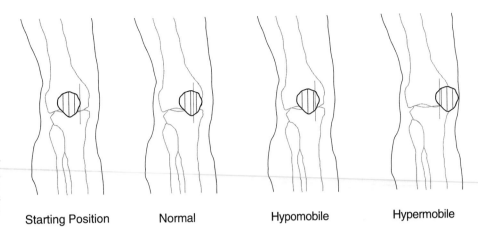

Figure 6–15. Test for medial patellar glide. Normally the patella should glide 1 to 2 quadrants medially. Movement of less than 1 quadrant is termed hypomobile; movement of 3 or more quadrants, hypermobile.

Starting Position   Normal   Hypomobile   Hypermobile

lateral border in the coronal patellar axis (Fig. 6–18). A positive tilt is considered to be between 0 and 15 degrees. A negative tilt of less than 0 degrees is indicative of significant tightness of the lateral restraints and often occurs in the presence of a hypomobile medial glide.[18]

• **Synthesis of findings:** The relationship between patellar glide and patellar tilt needs to be considered to determine the functional limitations of the patellofemoral articulation and subsequently to determine a rehabilitation regimen. A hypomobile medial glide in the presence of a positive tilt test result tends to respond favorably to conservative treatment. A negative patellar tilt test result combined with a hypomobile medial glide may require the surgical release of the lateral retinacular structures to permit proper glide within the trochlea. A negative preoperative patellar tilt has been positively correlated with a successful outcome of the release of the lateral structures.[19]

Neurological Testing

The assessment of the sensory, motor, and reflex function for the patellofemoral joint is the same as described for the knee in Chapter 5.

Pathologies and Related Special Tests

The terms "patellofemoral dysfunction" and "patellofemoral pain syndrome" are used to describe a wide range of symptoms occurring around the knee and patella. These symptoms range from pain being described as dull to sharp and in locations including the anterior (prepatellar) and posterior (retropatellar) portions of the patella, as well as its four borders. The onset of symptoms may occur during periods of inactivity, especially when sitting (theater sign) as well as during or after activity. This section describes the possible causes for this wide range of symptoms so that an adequate treatment and rehabilitation plan may be constructed not only to relieve the pain but also to correct the cause of the symptoms (Table 6–2).

Pain and dysfunction arising from the patellofemoral complex often mimic the symptoms of meniscal trauma. Table 6–3 presents subjective findings that may be used to differentiate injury between the two structures.

Patellar Maltracking

The onset of patellofemoral dysfunction has historically been attributed solely to an increased Q

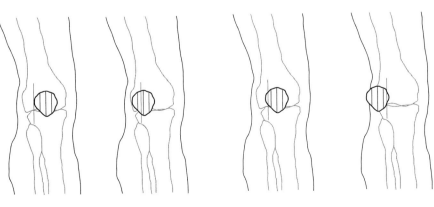

Figure 6–16. Test for lateral patellar glide. Normal lateral glide ranges from 0.5 to 2 quadrants. Less than 0.5 is indicative of hypomobility; greater than 3 quadrants represents hypermobility of the patella.

Starting Position   Normal   Hypomobile   Hypermobile

Table 6-3. Subjective Factors in the Differentiation of Meniscal and Patellar Pain

History	Meniscus	Patella
Onset	Usually acute twisting injury with recurrence	Occasionally direct anterior knee blow but usually insidious onset related to overuse and training errors
Symptom site	Localized medial or lateral joint line	Diffuse, anterior
Locking	Frank transient locking episodes with the knee unable to fully terminally extend	Grating ratcheting, stiffness after immobility, but not true locking
Weight bearing	Pain sharp and simultaneous with loaded weight bearing	Pain possibly coming on during weight bearing but often continues into the evening and night
Cutting sports	Pain with loaded twisting maneuvers	Some pain possible, but not sharp and clearly related to cuts
Squatting	Pain at full squat; inability to "duck walk"	Pain when extensors are used to rise from a squat
Kneeling	Not painful because meniscus is not weight loaded	Pain from patellar compression
Jumping	Weight loaded without torque or twist is tolerated	Extensors heavily stressed, causing pain on descent impact
Stairs or hills	Pain often going upstairs with loaded knee flexion, causing squatlike meniscal compression	More patellar loading and pain going downstairs because gravity-assisted impact increases patellofemoral stress
Sitting	No pain	Stiffness and pain from lack of the distraction-compression effect on abnormal articular cartilage
Quadriceps exercises	Helpful before and after surgery but not the real solution	Primary treatment for patellar pain, along with correction of training and gait abnormalities

From Bloom, MH,[19a] with permission.

reaction to a forced lateral movement of the patella (Fig. 6-20). The athlete may be apprehensive during the general palpation of the patella or during tests for medial and lateral patellar glide. The examiner may wish to perform this test before palpation of the patella and patellar articulating surfaces and before performing tests for medial and lateral patellar glide.

Apprehension Test for Patellar Dislocation (Fig. 6-20)

Position of athlete	Lying supine with the knee extended.
Position of examiner	Standing lateral to the involved side.
Evaluative procedure	The examiner attempts to move the athlete's patella as far laterally as possible, taking care not to cause it to actually dislocate.
Positive test results	The athlete forcefully contracts the quadriceps to guard against dislocation of the patella. The athlete may also demonstrate apprehension verbally or through facial expression.
Implications	Laxity of the medial patellar retinaculum, predisposing the athlete to patellar subluxations and/or dislocations.

Patellar Tendinitis

Common in jumping activities, running sports, and weight lifting, patellar tendinitis has an insidious onset. Acute cases of tendinitis can occur secondary to a blow to the patellar tendon. The most common site of pain associated with this condition is at the inferior pole of the patella, although pain may be described at the superior pole in the case of quadriceps tendinitis (jumper's knee), in the midsubstance of the tendon, or at the tendon's attachment to the tibial tuberosity (Table 6-6).

While pain in one of the aforementioned areas is the primary complaint of the athlete, other physical findings are common. Resisted knee extension usually increases pain in the area to the point that the athlete is inhibited by the pain. Passive knee flexion performed with the athlete in the prone position not

Table 6–4. Structural Abnormalities and Their Resultant Forces and Biomechanical Changes

Alignment	Resulting Forces and Biomechanical Changes
Genu varum	Increased compressive forces on the lateral tibiofemoral articulating surfaces Tensile forces on the medial tibiofemoral ligaments Medial tracking of the patella Compressive forces on the odd and medial facets Stretching of the lateral patellar restraints
Genu valgum	Increased compressive forces on the medial tibiofemoral articulating surfaces Tensile forces on the lateral tibiofemoral ligaments Lateral tracking of the patella Compressive forces on the lateral facet Stretching of the medial patellar restraints
Increased Q angle or lax medial restraints	Lateral tracking of the patella Compressive forces on the lateral facet Stretching of the medial patellar restraints
Decreased Q angle or lax lateral restraints	Medial tracking of the patella Compressive forces on odd and medial facets Stretching of the lateral patellar restraints

only elicits pain in the patellar tendon but may also cause the athlete to have decreased flexibility. Commonly, the athlete should be able to passively flex the knee so that the heel of the foot can touch, or almost touch, the buttocks. Crepitus can be palpated in tendons during active or resisted movements.

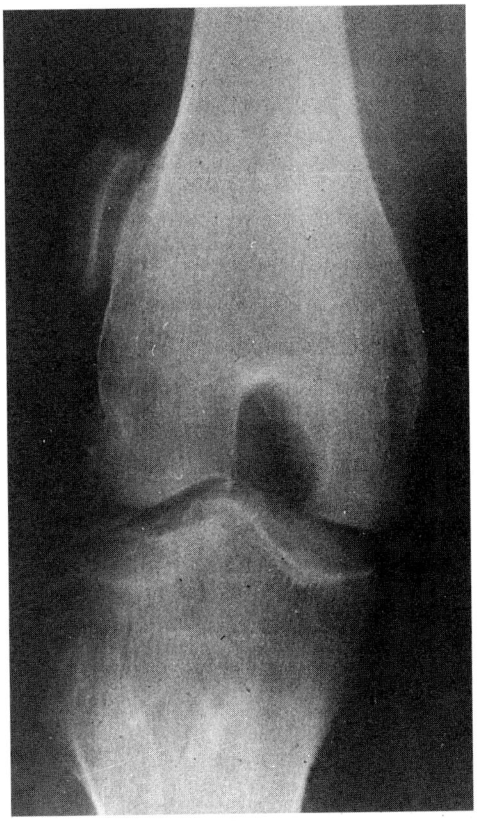

Figure 6–19. An x-ray view of a laterally dislocated patella. This view, taken from the knee's posterior aspect, shows the patella resting on the lateral femoral condyle.

Pain that is elicited from either side of the patellar tendon indicates **fat pad syndrome**.

Patellar Bursitis

The extensor mechanism's bursa may be inflamed secondary to a single traumatic force, repeated low-intensity blows, overuse, or infection (e.g., staphylococcus). The superficial prepatellar bursa and the subcutaneous infrapatellar bursa are most often injured secondary to direct trauma and results in localized swelling (Fig. 6–21). The suprapatellar and deep infrapatellar bursae tend to become inflamed secondary to overuse. Pain caused by bursitis tends to remain localized and the infrapatellar fat pads often become sympathetically tender (Table 6–7). Those conditions with a sudden onset and no history of trauma or overuse with associated redness and warmth about the knee should be referred to a physician to rule out infection.

Synovial Plica

A synovial plica is a fold of the fibrous membrane that projects into the joint cavity. This congenital abnormality is a remnant of folds formed during the embryologic stage of development. During maturation these folds are absorbed into the joint capsule but, in the majority of the population, leave either a thickened area or a crease within the membrane.[24] Normally a synovial plica remains asymptomatic until it is traumatized by a direct blow to the capsule or is inflamed secondary to friction caused by the plica bow-stringing across the femoral condyle during flexion, resulting in two reservoirs for synovial fluid: a suprapatellar reservoir and the cavity of the knee joint itself.[25,26] Although the onset of symptoms tends to occur in adolescent athletes, pli-

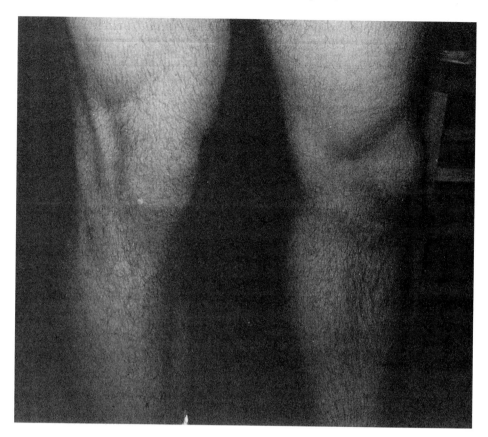

Figure 6–21. Photograph of a grossly swollen prepatellar bursa of the athlete's left knee.

Osgood-Schlatter Disease

Osgood-Schlatter disease is an adolescent inflammatory condition that strikes the tibial tuberosity's growth plate where the patellar tendon attaches. Its onset is traced to repeated avulsion fractures of the tendon from its attachment and is caused by rapid growth and/or increased strength of the quadriceps. These forces result in osteochondritis of the tubercle (Fig. 6–24). The symptoms of Osgood-Schlatter disease are similar to those of patellar tendinitis, but it is differentiated by the athlete's age (adolescent) and the pain's being localized to the tibial tuberosity

Table 6–7. Evaluative Findings of Patellar Bursitis

Examination Segment	Clinical Findings	
History	Onset:	Acute or chronic.
	Location of pain:	Localized to a specific bursa and possibly the infrapatellar fat pads.
	Mechanism:	Direct trauma to the bursa or overuse.
Inspection	Localized swelling may be seen if a superficial bursa is involved.	
Palpation	Point tenderness may be experienced when directly palpating the bursa or the area over the bursa. The athlete may also describe tenderness over the infrapatellar fat pads.	
Functional tests	AROM:	In chronic or severe cases, pain may be described as pain within a specified range or pain throughout the entire range of motion.
	PROM:	Pain is experienced at a specific point in the range of motion.
	RROM:	Decreased strength and pain occur throughout the range of motion.
Ligamentous tests	Not applicable.	
Neurological tests	Not applicable.	
Special tests	None.	
Comments	The specific bursa involved is based on the location of pain. Athletes with no relevant history for the onset of bursitis should be referred to a physician to rule out the possibility of infection.	

Table 6–9. Evaluative Findings of Osgood-Schlatter Dise[...]

Examination Segment	Clinical Findings	
History	Onset:	Insidious.
	Location of pain:	Over the tibial tu[...]
		patellar tendon[...]
	Mechanism:	Onset often assoc[...]
Inspection	Swelling over the tibial tuberosity an[...]	
Palpation	Tenderness and perhaps crepitus ove[...]	
Functional tests	AROM:	Pain may be experienced ov[...]
		especially when weight b[...]
	PROM:	Pain occurs over the tibial tu[...]
		secondary to strain place[...]
	RROM:	Pain and weakness during k[...]
Ligamentous tests	Not applicable.	
Neurological tests	None.	
Special tests	None.	
Comments	The signs and symptoms of Osgood-S[...]	
	but the symptoms are localized to t[...]	
	These findings in post-adolescent ath[...]	

of injury, and any associated sounds or other descriptors of the injury must be established. Initially it may be difficult to differentiate trauma to the patellofemoral joint from tibiofemoral injury.

The patella should be inspected to ensure that it assumes its normal position on the femur and has a normal shape. The patellar tendon should be visible

Table 6–10. Evaluative Findings of a Patellar Tendon Ru[...]

Examination Segment	Clinical Findings	
History	Onset:	Acute.
	Location of pain:	Patellar tendon[...]
	Mechanism:	Dynamic overl[...]
		the knee aga[...]
	Predisposing factor:	Disease states s[...]
		knee, or rece[...]
Inspection	Gross deformity is caused by the pate[...]	
	condyles.	
	Obvious anterior soft tissue swelling[...]	
Palpation	A palpable defect in the patellar tend[...]	
Functional tests	AROM:	The athlete is able to contra[...]
		gravity.
		The athlete is unable to perf[...]
		about the knee.
	PROM:	There is an empty end-feel [...]
		approximation of the ha[...]
	RROM:	This is not advised.
Ligamentous tests	These are not performed, although da[...]	
Neurological tests	Lower leg dermatome is checked to r[...]	
Special tests	Not applicable.	
Comments	Patellar tendon ruptures tend to occu[...]	
	population is susceptible.	

Table 6–8. Evaluative Findings of Synovial Plica Syndromes

Examination Segment	Clinical Findings	
History	Onset:	Acute or insidious.
	Location of pain:	Anterior portion of the knee. The athlete may describe clicking, popping, pseudolocking of the knee, or the knee "giving away." Symptoms are often described as being worse in the morning, with a gradual decrease as the day progresses.
	Mechanism:	Blow to the anterior joint capsule or friction caused by the plica rubbing across a femoral condyle.
Inspection	Swelling and redness may be localized to the involved side of the joint capsule.	
Palpation	Symptomatic plica may be felt as a thickened, bandlike structure that is tender to the touch. Plica tends to affect the anteromedial capsule more so than the anterolateral capsule.	
Functional tests	AROM:	Pain is experienced as the plica crosses the femoral condyle, with possible clicking or "catching" described by the athlete. A snapping may be heard by the examiner and may be felt by palpating the joint capsule.
	PROM:	A clicking or pseudolocking may be experienced as the knee is flexed and extended over the point at which the plica rubs or catches on the femoral condyle.
	RROM:	Pain is described for active range of motion.
Ligamentous tests	None. Lateral patellar glide, as described in the text of this chapter, may be decreased.	
Neurological tests	None.	
Special tests	Positive medial synovial plica test and/or stutter test result.	
Comments	The symptoms of synovial plica may mimic that of a meniscal tear, ACL injury, chondromalacia, or patellofemoral dysfunction.	

and distal portion of the patellar tendon (Table 6–9). A history of Osgood-Schlatter disease may lead to residual enlargement of the tibial tuberosity (see Fig. 5–17). In the adult population, enlargement of the tibial tuberosity may be caused by apophysitis.

Patellar Tendon Rupture

Resulting from a dynamic overload of the quadriceps musculotendinous unit, patellar tendon ruptures are uncommon in otherwise healthy individuals. Diseases such as rheumatoid arthritis,

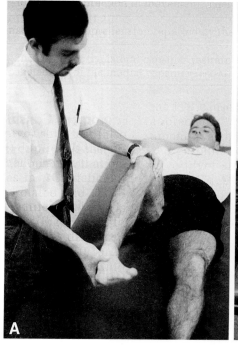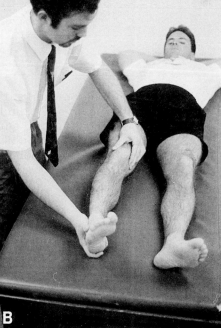

Figure 6–22. Test for medial synovial plica. (*A*) The athlete flexes the knee to 90° and internally rotates the tibia. The examiner applies a medial force to the patella. (*B*) The knee is extended and flexed while the anteromedial joint capsule is palpated. A positive test reproduces the athlete's symptoms and the examiner may feel the plica as it crosses the medial femoral condyle.

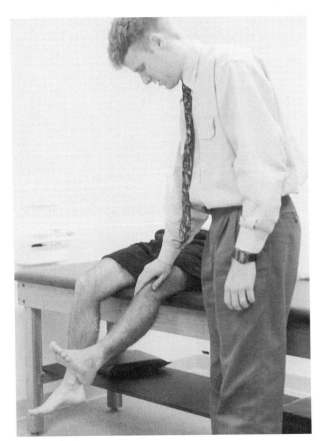

Figure 6–23. Stutter test for a medial synovial plica. The examiner palpates the patella for irregular movement (stutter) as the athlete extends the knee.

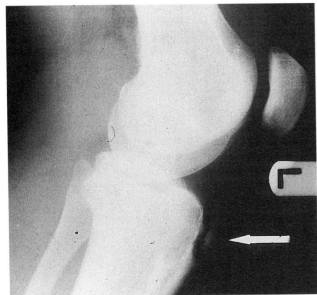

Figure 6–24. X-ray view of Osgood-Schlatter disease showing the bony outgrowth.

Lupus: A systemic disease affecting the internal organs, ski
Corticosteroid: A substance that permits many biochemica
   tissue healing).

lupı
mat
mec
set.
  P
defo
the
thro
trau
athl
leg
on
qua
thou
mis
test
the
Ath
sho
por

Patı

B
pla
frac
ture
sae
the
Act
flex
ten
onc

**ON
PA**

A
ticı
ing
on
tra
kne

Eqı

T
dis

Or

U
vic

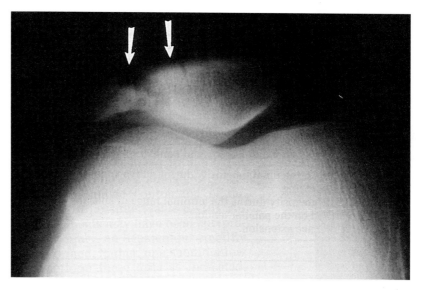

Figure 6–25. A "sunrise" x-ray view of a fractured patella.

process should be confirmed through palpation. Any indication of a patellar dislocation, fracture, or patellar tendon rupture should warrant the termination of the evaluation and immediate immobilization and transportation for further medical evaluation.

- **Soft tissue palpation:** The examiner begins by palpating the patellar tendon for tenderness, indicating a possible strain or aggravation of existing inflammation, from the tibial tuberosity to its insertion on the infrapatellar pole. He or she continues upward to palpate the quadriceps muscles, paying close attention to the tone of muscle and tenderness over the VMO. Spasm of the quadriceps muscle may indicate a patellar dislocation, especially if the knee remains flexed. Tenderness may be elicited over the VMO secondary to tearing of the fibers during lateral dislocation of the patella.

From the VMO palpate inferiorly to locate the medial joint capsule, which is tender after a lateral patellar dislocation. Likewise, the lateral joint capsule should be palpated for tenderness, indicating possible medial displacement of the patella.

On-Field Functional Tests

Once the possibility of major disruption to the patellofemoral joint has been ruled out, an assessment of the athlete's functional status may begin. Some of these movements may have been voluntarily performed by the athlete during the earlier portions of the examination.

- **Willingness to move the involved limb:** The athlete is asked to fully flex and extend the involved limb. An unwillingness or inability to complete this task is a sign that the athlete should be assisted off the field or court. If the athlete is able to complete the full range of motion, break pressure may be applied with the knee near full extension and again in partial flexion to obtain a gross determination of muscular strength.

- **Willingness to bear weight:** If these tests are normal or near normal, the athlete may be allowed to bear weight. This is performed by assisting the athlete to the standing position, bearing weight on the uninvolved limb. The athletic trainer then assumes a position under the involved side to help support the athlete's body weight if needed.

INITIAL MANAGEMENT OF ON-FIELD INJURIES

The primary concerns for the on-field management of patellofemoral injuries involve the rupture of the patellar tendon, fractures of the patella, or an unreduced patellar dislocation. The following protocol is suggested for the initial management of these conditions. It should be noted that the management of a fractured patella and that of a patellar tendon rupture are essentially the same.

Patellar Tendon Rupture

Sudden overloading of the musculotendinous unit of the quadriceps can result in a rupture of the tendon in its midsubstance or an avulsion from its attachment on the patella's inferior pole or the tibial tuberosity. This injury results in immediate loss of function and gross deformity as the quadriceps contracts, possibly pulling the patella to the midshaft of the femur. The knee should be splinted in extension and the athlete immediately transported for further medical attention.

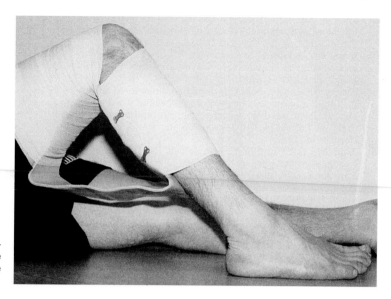

Figure 6–26. Splinting of the leg for an acutely dislocated patella, using a moldable aluminum splint. Note that part of the splint serves as a truss to maintain the current position of the knee.

Dislocated Patella

Dislocation of the patella is marked by obvious deformity where the patella is shifted laterally. Onfield reduction of a dislocated patella should not be attempted. However, spontaneous reductions may occur if the athlete relaxes the quadriceps group and gravity causes the knee to extend. All cases of patellar dislocation should be referred to a physician so that fractures to the patella's and femur's articulating surfaces may be ruled out.

Known patellar subluxation or patellar dislocation that has spontaneously reduced should be splinted with the knee fully extended or slightly flexed. An unreduced dislocation must be splinted in the position in which the knee was found. This is most easily accomplished using a long moldable aluminum splint, bending one end to serve as a truss between the femur and lower leg (Fig. 6–26).

REFERENCES

1. Goodfellow, J, Hungerford, DS, and Zindel, M: Patellofemoral joint mechanics and pathology: Functional anatomy of the patellofemoral joint. J Bone Joint Surg Br 58:287, 1976.
2. D'Agata, S, et al: An in vitro analysis of patellofemoral contact areas and pressures following procurement of the central one-third patellar tendon. Am J Sports Med 21:212, 1993.
3. Hubert, HH, and Hayes, WC: Patellofemoral contact pressures: The influence of Q-angle and tibiofemoral contact. J Bone Joint Surg Am 66:715, 1984.
4. Hubert, HH, et al: Force ratios in the quadriceps tendon and ligamentum patellae. J Orthop Res 2:49, 1984.
5. Rintala, P, and Lic, P: Patellofemoral pain syndrome and its treatment in runners. Athletic Training: Journal of the National Athletic Trainers Association 25:107, 1990.
6. Reilly, DT, and Mantens, M: Experimental analysis of the quadriceps muscle force and patellofemoral joint reaction force for various activities. Acta Orthop Scand 43:126, 1972.
7. Insall, J, Goldberg, V, and Saluati, ER: Recurrent dislocation and the high-riding patella. Clin Orthop 88:67, 1972.
8. Lieb, FJ, and Perry, J: Quadriceps function: An anatomical and mechanical study using amputated limbs. J Bone Joint Surg Am 50:1535, 1968.
9. Brownstein, BA, Lamb, RL, and Mangine, RE: Quadriceps torque and integrated electromyography. Journal of Orthopedic and Sports Physical Therapy 6:309, 1985.
10. Hanten, WP, and Schultheis, SS: Exercise effect on electromyographic activity of the vastus medialis oblique and vastus lateralis muscles. Phys Ther 70:561, 1990.
11. Voight, M, and Weider, D: Comparative reflex response times of vastus medialis oblique and subjects with extensor mechanism dysfunction. Am J Sports Med 19:131, 1991.
12. Spencer, JD, Hayes, KC, and Alexander, IJ: Knee joint effusion and quadriceps reflex inhibition in man. Arch Phys Med Rehabil 65:171, 1984.
12a. Ficat, P, and Hungerford, DS: Disorders of the Patello-Femoral Joint. Williams & Wilkins, Baltimore, 1977.
13. Tomaro, JE: Prevention and treatment of patellar entrapment following intra-articular ACL reconstruction. Athletic Training: Journal of the National Athletic Trainers Association 26:11, 1991.
14. Fulkerson, JP: Patellofemoral pain disorders: evaluation and management. Journal of the American Academy of Orthopedic Surgeons 2:124, 1994.
15. Bennett, G, and Stauber, W: Evaluation and treatment of anterior knee pain using eccentric exercise. Med Sci Sports Exerc 18:526, 1986.
16. Kolowich, P, et al: Lateral release of the patella: Indications and contraindications. Am J Sports Med 18:359, 1990.
17. Puniello, MS: Iliotibial band tightness and medial patellar glide in patients with patellofemoral dysfunction. Journal of Orthopedic and Sports Physical Therapy 17:144, 1993.
18. Fulkerson, J, et al: 1991 AAOS Instructional Course Lecture on Patellofemoral Pain, American Academy of Orthopaedic Surgeons, 1991.
19. Kolowich, P, et al: Lateral release of the patella: Indications and contraindications. Am J Sports Med 18:359, 1990.
19a. Bloom, MH: Differentiating between meniscal and patellar pain. Physical and Sportsmedicine 17:95, 1989.
20. Caylor, D, Fites, R, and Worrell, TW: The relationship between quadriceps angle and anterior knee pain syndrome. Journal of Orthopedic and Sports Physical Therapy 17:11, 1993.

21. Shelton, GL, and Thigpen, LK: Rehabilitation of patellofemoral dysfunction: A review of literature. Journal of Orthopedic and Sports Physical Therapy 14:234, 1991.
22. Moss, RI, DeVita, P, and Dawson, ML: A biomechanical analysis of patellofemoral stress syndrome. Journal of Athletic Training 27:64, 1992.
23. Clancy, WG, and Bosanny, JJ: Functional treatment and rehabilitation of quadriceps contusions, patellar dislocations and "isolated" medial collateral ligament injuries. Athletic Training: Journal of the National Athletic Trainers Association 17:249, 1982.
24. Hardaker, TW, Whipple, TL, and Bassett, FH: Diagnosis and treatment of the plica syndrome of the knee. J Bone Joint Surg Am 62:221, 1980.
25. Patel, D: Plica as a cause of anterior knee pain. Orthop Clin North Am 17:273, 1986.
26. Amatuzzi, MM, Fazzi, A, and Varella, MH: Pathologic synovial plica of the knee. Results of conservative treatment. Am J Sports Med 18:466, 1990.
27. Kurosaka, M, et al: Lateral synovial plica syndrome. A case report. Am J Sports Med 20:92, 1992.
28. Johnson, DP, et al: Symptomatic synovial plicae of the knee. J Bone Joint Surg Am 75:1485, 1993.

29. Noble, BA, Hajek, MR, and Porter, M: Diagnosis and treatment of iliotibial band tightness in runners. Physician and Sportsmedicine 10:67, 1982.
30. Podesta, L, Sherman, MF, and Bonamo, JR: Bilateral simultaneous rupture of the infrapatellar tendon in a recreational athlete. A case report. Am J Sports Med 19:325, 1991.
31. Rosenberg, JM, and Whitaker, JH: Bilateral infrapatellar tendon rupture in a patient with jumper's knee. Am J Sports Med 19:94, 1991.
32. Exler, Y: Patellar fracture: Review of the literature and five case presentations. Journal of Orthopedic and Sports Physical Therapy 13:177, 1991.
33. Casscells, W: Gross pathological changes in the knee joint of the aging individual. A study of three hundred cases. J Bone Joint Surg Am 57:1033, 1975.
34. Bentley, G, and Dowd, G: Current concepts of etiology and treatment of chondromalacia patella. Clin Orthop 189:209, 1984.
35. Metcalf, R: An arthroscopic method for lateral release of the subluxating or dislocating patella. Clin Orthop 167:9; 1982.
36. McGinty, J, et al: 1991 AAOS Instructional Course Lecture on Patellofemoral Pain. American Academy or Orthopaedic Surgeons, Chicago, 1991.

7

The Pelvis and Thigh

The pelvic girdle forms the structural base of support between the lower extremity and the trunk. A relatively immobile configuration, the pelvis is formed by pairs of three fused bones joined anteriorly at the pubic symphysis. The posterior portion is formed by the sacrum's wedging itself between the two halves of the pelvis. The hip articulation, formed by the femoral head and the acetabulum, is the strongest and most stable of the body's joints, but this benefit is gained at the expense of decreased mobility.

CLINICAL ANATOMY

The pelvis is formed by two innominate bones, each consisting of the **ilium**, the **ischium**, and the **pubis** (Fig. 7–1). On the lateral border of the pelvis a downwardly and outwardly directed depression, the **acetabulum**, accepts the femoral head. The acetabulum's superior wall is formed by the ilium, the inferior wall by the ischium, and the internal (medial) wall by the pubis. Centered in this fossa is a depression for the ligamentum teres. Lining the outer rim of the acetabulum is the **labrum**, a thick ring of fibrocartilage that deepens the articular area. The labrum is thicker and stronger superiorly than inferiorly (Fig. 7–2).

The posterior junction of the pelvic girdle is formed by its articulation with the sacrum (Fig. 7–3). Molded by five fused vertebrae, the sacrum is a broad, thick bone that fixates the spinal column to the pelvis and is responsible for stabilizing the pelvic girdle. Through the sacroiliac joints the weight of the torso and skull is transmitted to the lower extremity and ground reaction forces from the foot are transmitted up the spinal column.

The sacrum's laterally projecting articular surfaces have an irregular shape that, when matched to the iliac's facets, form the very stable **sacroiliac (SI) joint**. Its anterior and posterior surfaces are roughened to permit firm attachment of muscles acting on the femur and pelvis. Four pairs of *foramina* perforate the bone to permit the passage of the dorsal and ventral primary divisions of the sacral nerves from their posterior origin into the pelvic cavity.

The inferior end of the spinal column is formed by the **coccyx**. A structure formed by the fusion of three or four rudimentary bony pieces, the coccyx provides an attachment site for some of the muscles of the pelvic floor and, sometimes, portions of the gluteus maximus.

The **femoral head** is globular, being slightly over half a hemisphere in diameter. Its articulating surface is thickly covered with hyaline cartilage except at the central depression for the ligamentum teres. Connected to the femur's shaft by the femoral neck, the head is angled at approximately 125-degrees in the frontal plane (Fig. 7–4). This relationship, known as the **angle of inclination**, changes through an individual's development and is somewhat decreased in women (Fig. 7–5). In the transverse plane the relationship between the femoral head and femoral shaft is the **angle of torsion**, having a normal angle of 15 degrees (Fig. 7–6).

Distal to the femoral neck on the shaft the femur is the laterally projecting greater trochanter and the medially projecting lesser trochanter, which serve primarily as attachment sites for the pelvic and hip musculature.

Articulations and Ligamentous Support

The pelvic bones articulate anteriorly at a relatively immobile joint, the **pubic symphysis** (see Fig. 7–1). Formed by the fibrocartilaginous interpubic disk, a small degree of spreading, compression, and rotation between the two halves of the pelvic girdle occurs here.

Posteriorly, each ilium articulates with the sacrum at the **SI joints**. This combination of synovial and syndesmotic joints varies considerably in their shapes and sizes. The surfaces of each bone are a collection of concave and convex areas with the concavities of one bone corresponding to con-

---

Foramen (pl. *Foramina*): An opening in a bone or organ through which other structures pass.

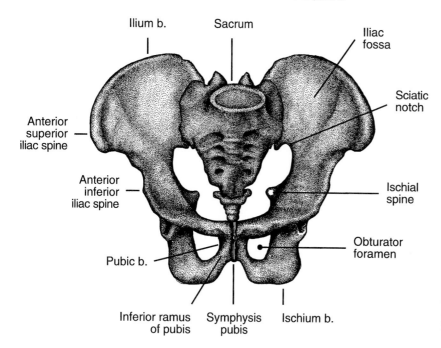

Ilium b.

Sacrum

Iliac fossa

Anterior superior iliac spine

Sciatic notch

Anterior inferior iliac spine

Ischial spine

Obturator foramen

Pubic b.

Inferior ramus of pubis

Symphysis pubis

Ischium b.

Figure 7–1. Anterior view of the bony pelvis. A total of seven bones form the pelvis: Two ischial, two pubic, and two ilial bones form each half, and the posterior border is formed by the sacrum.

vexities of the opposing bone. The resulting articulation is very sturdy with a limited range of motion.

A series of ligaments serve to bind the sacrum to the pelvis. The **interosseous sacroiliac ligaments** are formed by strong fibers spanning the anterior portion of the ilium and the posterior portion of the sacrum, filling the void behind the articular surfaces of these bones (Fig. 7–7). The anterior and posterior surfaces of the articulation are strengthened by the **dorsal and ventral sacroiliac ligaments**. The dorsal SI ligament is made of fibers that run transversely to join the ilium to the upper portion of the sacrum and vertical fibers connecting the lower sacrum to the posterior superior iliac spine (PSIS). Lining the anterior portion of the pelvic cavity, the ventral SI ligaments attach to the anterior portion of the sacrum. Two accessory ligaments assist in maintaining the stability of the SI joint. The **sacrotuberous ligament**

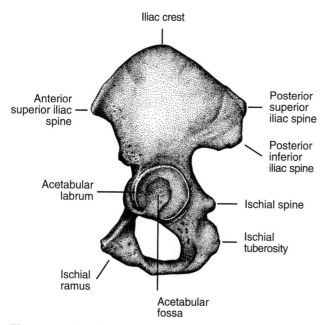

Iliac crest

Anterior superior iliac spine

Posterior superior iliac spine

Posterior inferior iliac spine

Acetabular labrum

Ischial spine

Ischial tuberosity

Ischial ramus

Acetabular fossa

Figure 7–2. Lateral view of the pelvis showing the acetablum. The acetabular fossa is lined by the fibrocartilaginous glenoid labrum.

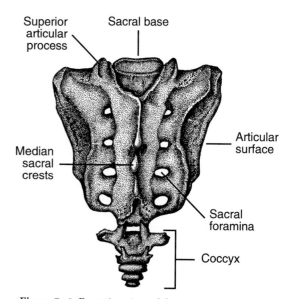

Superior articular process

Sacral base

Median sacral crests

Articular surface

Sacral foramina

Coccyx

Figure 7–3. Posterior view of the sacrum and coccyx.

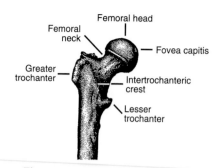

Figure 7–4. Femoral neck and head.

arises from the ischium to blend with the inferior fibers of the dorsal SI ligaments. Indirectly supporting the sacrum, the **sacrospinous ligament** originates from the ischial spine and attaches to the coccyx.

The SI joints are more mobile in the younger athlete, becoming less mobile with age. In the *postpartum* athlete, the stresses of athletics can injure the structurally weakened SI joints. At the time of birth the hormone **relaxin** is released into the mother's system to aid in the relaxation and to increase the extensibility of the ligamentous structures in and around the birth canal.[1] These hormones affect the ligaments of the SI joint, resulting in increased pelvic motion.

The hip articulation, the coxofemoral joint, is a ball-and-socket joint possessing three degrees of freedom of movement: flexion/extension, abduction/adduction, and internal/external rotation. The depth of the acetabulum, the relative strength of the ligaments, and the strong muscular support limit the hip's range of motion in all planes.

Surrounding the joint, a strong, dense synovial joint capsule arises from the acetebular rim and runs to the distal aspect of the femoral neck. Associated with the capsule are accessory bands, or ligaments, that reinforce the joint (Fig. 7–8).

The Y-shaped **iliofemoral ligament** (also referred to as the "Y ligament of Bigelow") originates from the anterior inferior iliac spine. Its central fibers split, with one band inserting on the distal aspect of the anterior intertrochanteric line and the other band on the proximal aspect of the anterior intertrochanteric line and the femoral neck. This strong structure reinforces the anterior portion of the joint capsule and limits hyperextension. Its superior fibers limit adduction and its inferior fibers limit abduction. The fibrous arrangement of the iliofemoral ligament allows us to stand upright with a minimum of muscular support. Also reinforcing the anterior capsule is the **pubofemoral ligament**. Emerging from the pubic *ramus* and inserting on the anterior aspect of the intertrochanteric fossa, this ligament limits abduction and hyperextension of the hip.

Posteriorly the joint is augmented by the **ischiofemoral ligament**. This triangular ligament has a spanning origin from the posterior acetabular rim with upwardly spiraling fibers attaching to the joint capsule and the inner surface of the greater trochanter. The spiraling nature of this ligament causes it to limit extension of the hip.

Within the joint the **ligamentum teres** (also referred to as the "ligament of the head of the femur") serves as a conduit for the medial and lateral circumflex arteries and has little function in stabilizing the hip (Fig. 7–9).[2] However, trauma to this structure through axial compression of the femoral head or dislocation of the joint may result in disruption of these arteries.

The **inguinal ligament** originates off the anterior superior iliac spine (ASIS) and inserts at the pubic symphysis and serves to contain the soft tissues as they course anteriorly from the trunk to the lower extremity. This structure demarcates the superior border of the femoral triangle.

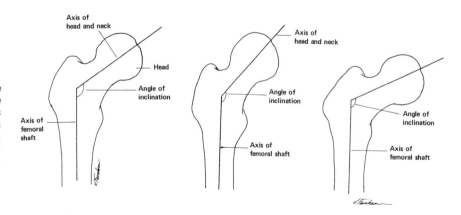

Figure 7–5. Deviations of the hip in the frontal plane. The femoral head normally assumes a 125° angle with the long axis of the femur (slightly higher in females). An increase in this angle is termed coxa valga; a decrease, coxa vara. (From Norkin, CC, and Levangie, PK,[2] p 305, with permission.)

Postpartum: Following childbirth.
Ramus: A division of a forked structure.

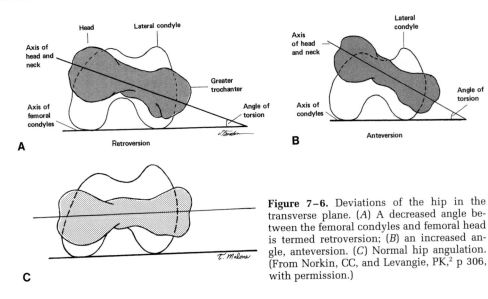

Figure 7–6. Deviations of the hip in the transverse plane. (*A*) A decreased angle between the femoral condyles and femoral head is termed retroversion; (*B*) an increased angle, anteversion. (*C*) Normal hip angulation. (From Norkin, CC, and Levangie, PK,[2] p 306, with permission.)

Muscular Anatomy

No muscles act directly to affect the movement at the SI joint, but movement can be indirectly influenced through two means: (1) the muscles originating in the sacrum that function to control the hip joint and (2) any musculature attaching to the pelvic bones that can cause rotation of the pelvis.

Movements of the hip joint are controlled by groups of large extrinsic muscles and groups of small intrinsic muscles. The large muscle groups act primarily to flex, extend, and internally rotate the hip, whereas the smaller intrinsic hip muscles serve to externally rotate it. The muscles acting on the hip, along with their origins, insertions, and innervations, are presented in Table 7–1.

Anterior Musculature

Crossing the anterior portion of both the knee joint and the hip, the **rectus femoris**, part of the quadriceps femoris group, is a powerful flexor of the hip, providing the greatest contribution to hip flexion when the knee is also flexed. It is also a

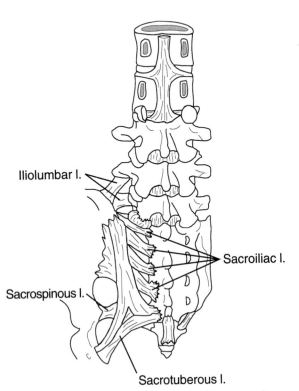

Figure 7–7. Posterior sacroiliac ligaments. The strong ligamentous configuration of the sacroiliac joint permits only slight movement.

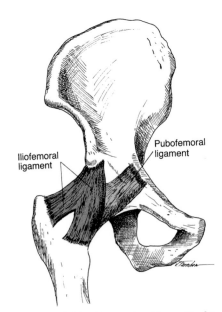

Figure 7–8. External hip ligaments. (From Norkin, CC, and Levangie, PK,[2] p 308, with permission.)

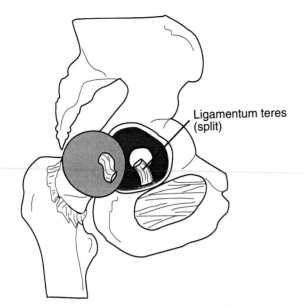

Figure 7–9. Ligamentum teres (shown split). This structure serves little, if any, role in supporting the hip. It serves primarily as a conduit for the passage of the medial and lateral circumflex arteries.

strong extensor of the knee as it crosses that joint. The **sartorius**, in addition to flexing the knee, contributes to flexion, abduction, and external rotation of the hip. The psoas major, psoas minor, and iliacus, collectively known as the **iliopsoas group**, are the primary hip flexors when the knee is extended and work in concert with the rectus femoris when the knee is flexed (Fig. 7–10).

The rectus femoris, sartorius, and iliacus can all rotate the pelvis at the SI joint as they contract. Tightness in these muscles can cause increased stress on the sacroiliac joint, also causing the pelvis to rotate anteriorly on the sacrum.

Medial Musculature

The medial muscles acting on the hip joint adduct and internally rotate it. The bulk of the inner thigh is formed by the adductor group, consisting of the adductor longus, adductor magnus, and adductor brevis. This muscle group's action is supplemented by the **pectineus** (Fig. 7–11). One additional adductor, the **gracilis**, is described in Chapter 5.

Lateral Musculature

The most superficial of the lateral muscles are the **gluteus medius** and the **tensor fasciae latae** (Fig. 7–12). A prime abductor of the hip joint, the gluteus medius is also important in maintaining the torso's posture during gait. Weakness of this muscle results in the torso's bending toward the afflicted side when the opposite leg is non–weight bearing. This compensating movement is termed Trendelenburg's gait pattern. Through its insertion on the ili-

otibial tract, the tensor fasciae latae is an abductor and internal rotator of the hip.

Six intrinsic muscles form a posterolateral cuff around the femoral head (Fig. 7–13). The **piriformis, quadratus femoris, obturator internus, obturator externus, gemellus superior,** and **gemellus inferior** all have the primary function of externally rotating the hip.

Posterior Musculature

The mass of the buttocks is formed by the **gluteus maximus**, a powerful extensor of the hip, especially when the knee is flexed (see Fig. 7–12). When the knee is extended, the hamstring muscle group also acts as an extensor of the hip. The hamstring group is also responsible for decelerating knee extension and hip flexion during running, through an eccentric contraction. The hamstrings can also cause posterior rotation of the pelvis on the sacrum from their attachment on the ischial tuberosity.

Femoral Triangle

Formed by the inguinal ligament superiorly, the sartorius laterally, and the adductor longus medially, the femoral triangle represents a clinically significant landmark (Fig. 7–14). Portions of the femoral nerve, femoral artery, and femoral vein are located within this area. The femoral pulse is palpable as it crosses the crease between the thigh and abdomen. Likewise, the triangle may also contain palpable lymph nodes if there is an infection or active inflammation in the lower extremity.

Bursae

Three primary bursae are found in the hip and pelvic region, each serving to decrease friction between the gluteus maximus and its adjacent bony structures. The **trochanteric bursa** lubricates the site at which the gluteus maximus passes over the greater trochanter. The **gluteofemoral bursa** separates the gluteus maximus from the origin of the vastus lateralis. The **ischial bursa** serves as a weight-bearing structure when an individual is seated, as it cushions the ischial tuberosity where it passes over the gluteus maximus.

CLINICAL EVALUATION OF THE PELVIS AND THIGH

Serving as the mechanical interface between the lower extremity and spinal column, the pelvis both influences and is influenced by these areas. A complete evaluation of the pelvis, thigh, and SI joint may also include a thorough evaluation of the lower extremity and spinal column (Table 7–2).

Table 7–1. Muscles Acting on the Hip

Muscle	Action	Origin	Insertion	Nerve	Root
Adductor brevis	Hip adduction Hip internal rotation	• Pubic ramus	• Pectineal line • Medial lip of linea aspera	Obturator	L2, L3, L4
Adductor longus	Hip adduction Hip internal rotation	• Pubic symphysis	• Middle one-third of medial linea aspera	Obturator	L2, L3, L4
Adductor magnus	Hip adduction Hip internal rotation	• Inferior pubic ramus • Ramus of ischium • Ischial tuberosity	• Line spanning from the gluteal tuberosity to the adductor tubercle of the medial femoral condyle	Obturator Sciatic	L2, L3, L4 L4, L5, S1

Biceps femoris	Long head
	  Hip extension
	  Hip external rotation
	  Knee flexion
	  External rotation of the tibia
		Long head
		• Ischial tuberosity
		• Sacrotuberous ligament
		Short head
		• Lateral lip of the linea aspera
		• Upper two-thirds of the supracondylar line
			• Lateral fibular head
			• Lateral tibial condyle
				Long head
				  Tibial
				Short head
				  Common peroneal
					Long head
					S1, S2, S3
					Short head
					L5, S1, S2

Gemellus inferior	Hip external rotation	• Tuberosity of ischium	• Greater trochanter of femur via the obturator internus tendon	Sacral plexus	L4, L5, S1
Gemellus superior	Hip external rotation	• Spine of ischium	• Greater trochanter of femur via the obturator internus tendon	Sacral plexus	L5, S1, S2
Gluteus maximus	Hip extension Hip external rotation Hip adduction (lower fibers) Hip abduction (upper fibers)	• Posterior gluteal line of ilium • Posterior sacrum • Posterior coccyx	• Gluteal tuberosity of femur • Through a fibrous band to the iliotibial tract	Inferior gluteal	L5, S1, S2

Gluteus medius	Hip abduction
	Anterior fibers
	  Hip flexion
	  Hip internal rotation
	Posterior fibers
	  Hip extension
	  Hip external rotation
		• External surface of superior ilium
		• Anterior gluteal line
		• Gluteal aponeurosis
			• Greater trochanter of femur	Superior gluteal	L4, L5, S1

Gluteus minimus	Hip abduction Hip internal rotation Hip flexion	• Lower portion of ilium • Margin of greater sciatic notch	• Greater trochanter of femur	Superior gluteal	L4, L5, S1

Muscle	Actions	Origin	Insertion	Nerve	Nerve root
Gracilis	Hip adduction Knee flexion	• Symphysis pubis • Inferior pubic ramus	• Medial tibial flare	Obturator	L3, L4
Iliacus	Hip flexion	• Superior surface of the iliac fossa • Internal iliac crest • Sacral ala	• Lateral to the psoas major, distal to the lesser trochanter	Lumbar plexus	L1, L2, L3, L4
Obturator externus	Hip external rotation	• Pubic ramus • Obturator membrane	• Trochanteric fossa of femur	Obturator	L3, L4
Obturator internus	Hip external rotation	• Margin of obturator foramen • Pelvic surface of ischium	• Greater trochanter of femur	Sacral plexus	L5, S1, S2
Pectineus	Hip adduction Hip external rotation	• Superior symphysis pubis	• Pectineal line of femur	Obturator	L3, L4
Piriformis	Hip external rotation	• Pelvic surface of sacrum • Rim of greater sciatic foramen	• Greater trochanter of femur	Sacral plexus	S1, S2
Psoas major and minor	Hip flexion	• Transverse process of T12 and all lumbar vertebrae	• Lesser trochanter of femur	Lumbar plexus	L1, L2, L3, L4
Quadratus femoris	Hip external rotation	• Tuberosity of ischium	• Intertrochanteric crest of femur	Sacral plexus	L4, L5, S1
Rectus femoris	Hip flexion Knee extension	• Anterior inferior iliac spine • Groove located superior to the acetabulum	• To the tibial tubercle via the patella and patellar ligament	Femoral	L2, L3, L4
Sartorius	Hip flexion Hip abduction Hip external rotation Knee flexion Internal rotation of the tibia	• Anterior superior iliac spine	• Proximal portion of the anteromedial tibial flair	Femoral	L2, L3
Semimembranosus	Hip extension Hip internal rotation Knee flexion Internal rotation of the tibia	• Ischial tuberosity	• Posteromedial portion of the medial condyle of the tibia	Tibial	L5, S1
Semitendinosus	Hip extension Hip internal rotation Knee flexion Internal rotation of the tibia	• Ischial tuberosity	• Medial portion of the tibial flair	Tibial	L5, S1, S2
Tensor fasciae latae	Hip flexion Hip internal rotation Knee extension	• Anterior superior iliac spine • External lip of the iliac crest	• Iliotibial tract	Superior gluteal	L4, L5, S1

Muscle actions, origins, and insertions adapted from Kendall and McCreary[20]; innervations adapted from Daniels and Worthingham.[21]

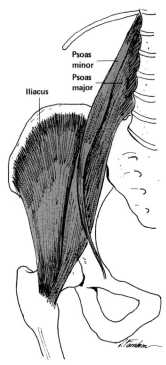

Figure 7–10. Iliopsoas group formed by the iliacus, psoas major, and psoas minor muscles. (From Norkin, CC, and Levangie, PK,[2] p 319, with permission.)

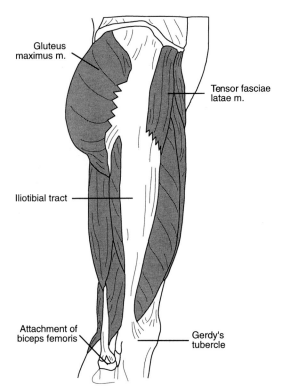

Figure 7–12. Superficial lateral and posterior hip muscles. The tensor fasciae latae muscle attaches to Gerdy's tubercle via the iliotibial tract. The remaining lateral muscles, the gluteus medius and gluteus minimus, lie hidden beneath the gluteus maximus, tensor fasciae latae, and iliotibial tract.

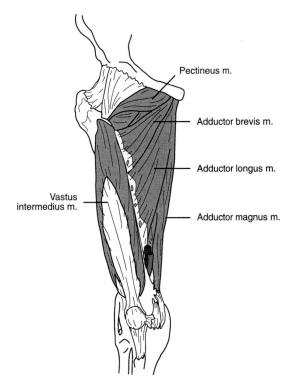

Figure 7–11. Adductors of the hip. The only muscle of this group that is uniquely identifiable is the adductor longus, which becomes visible during resisted adduction.

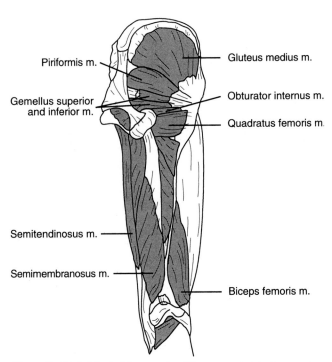

Figure 7–13. Intrinsic hip muscles. The upper intrinsic muscles serve primarily to externally rotate the hip.

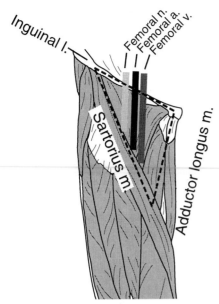

Figure 7–14. Femoral triangle. This anatomical area is formed by the sartorius muscle laterally, the adductor longus medially, and the inguinal ligament superiorly. The femoral neurovascular bundle passes through this area.

To permit the complete examination of these areas the athlete should be dressed in shorts and a tee shirt. Discretion must be used when evaluating areas around the genitalia. The descriptions presented in this section do not represent an endorsement of these procedures in every case, and the examiner should use prudent judgment when deciding to palpate this area. Whenever necessary an evaluator of the same gender as the athlete should be recruited to perform the evaluation in the presence of a witness.

History

The majority of pelvic girdle and hip injuries in athletics tend to be of a chronic or overuse origin, increasing the importance of a complete and accurate history of the injury.

- **Location of symptoms:** The location of the symptoms must be ascertained as specifically as possible. Sacroiliac pathology almost always manifests some type of pain around the PSIS of the affected side. Deep hip joint pain can originate in the hip joint itself or be referred from the lumbar spine and/or the sacroiliac joint. A strain to the hip adductors or hip flexors causes pain in the pubic region or anterior hip, respectively. Greater trochanteric bursitis is a common hip

pathology that almost always manifests pain in the posterior aspect of the greater trochanter (Table 7–3).

- **Onset:** As stated in the introduction to this section, most pelvic girdle and hip pathology tends to be chronic or caused by overuse. The date of onset of the athlete's symptoms should be correlated to any changes in training techniques such as surface changes, different footwear, or alterations in training techniques or intensity.

- **Training techniques:** Recent changes in training techniques can lead to overuse injuries including greater trochanteric bursitis or hip flexor tendinitis, especially if the history of the athlete's running regimen includes training on a banked surface. Development of stress fractures may be related to recent increases in training intensity, frequency, or duration.

- **Mechanism of injury:** A direct blow to the iliac crest usually leads to a contusion or **hip pointer**. Blows to the buttocks, such as may occur from a fall on the ice, can lead to a contusion of the coccyx or ischium or to sacroiliac pathology. A sudden pain, especially during an eccentric contraction of a muscle, usually indicates a strain of that muscle. Pain that gradually builds over time may indicate a stress fracture or tendinitis.

- **Prior medical conditions:** Congenital or childhood abnormalities of the hip can result in altered biomechanics of the hip, knee, and/or ankle during adulthood. ***Legg-Calvé-Perthes disease*** can lead to residual flattening of the proximal femoral epiphysis, resulting in decreased hip internal rotation and abduction.[3] A ***slipped capital femoris*** can lead to pathological external rotation of the hip and restricted or painful internal rotation.[4]

The history-taking process may be expanded based on the athlete's responses in the preceding categories.

Inspection

The bony, muscular, and ligamentous arrangement of the hip and pelvis make the inspection of most acute injuries difficult. With the exception of contusions to the iliac crest and hip dislocations, most trauma to this area cannot be visualized. The focus of the inspection phase of this area is to identify secondary signs of pathology or determine the presence of conditions that may alter the biomechanics of the hip and lower extremity, predisposing the athlete to injury.

Legg-Calvé-Perthes disease: Avascular necrosis occurring in children age 3 to 12 years, causing osteochondritis of the proximal femoral epiphysis.

Slipped capital femoris: Displacement of the femoral head relative to the femoral shaft; common in children age 10 to 15 years and especially prevalent in boys.

Table 7–2. Clinical Evaluation of the Hip and Pelvis

History	Inspection	Palpation	Functional Tests	Ligamentous Tests	Neurological Tests	Special Tests
Location of symptoms	Hip angulations	Medial structures	Active range of motion	Capsular testing		Muscle strains
Onset	Angle of inclination	Pubic bone	Flexion	Flexion		Quadriceps contusion
Training techniques	Angle of torsion	Adductor muscle group	Extension	Extension		Bursitis
Mechanism of injury	Medial structures	Anterior structures	Adduction	Internal rotation		Trochanteric bursitis
	Adductor group	Anterior superior iliac spine	Abduction	External rotation		Ischial bursitis
	Anterior structures	Anterior inferior iliac spine	Internal rotation			Degenerative hip changes
	Hip flexors	Sartorius	External rotation			Hip scouring
	Lateral structures	Rectus femoris	Passive range of motion			Sacroiliac dysfunction
	Iliac crest	Lateral structures	Flexion			Long sit test
	Nélaton's line	Iliac crest	Extension			Sacroiliac compression
	Posterior structures	Greater trochanter	Adduction			Sacroiliac distraction
	Gluteus maximus	Gluteus medius	Abduction			Fabere (Patrick's) test
	Posterior superior iliac spine	Tensor fasciae latae	Internal rotation			Gaenslen's test
	Median sacral crests	Posterior structures	External rotation			Piriformis syndrome
	Leg length discrepancy	Median sacral crests	Resistive range of motion			
	Functional leg length discrepancy	Posterior superior iliac spine	Flexion			
	True leg length discrepancy	Ischial tuberosity	Iliopsoas			
	Apparent leg length discrepancy	Gluteus maximus	Rectus femoris			
		Hamstring muscles	Sartorius			
		Ischial bursa	Extension			
		Sciatic nerve	Hamstrings			
			Gluteus maximus			
			Adduction			
			Abduction			
			Internal and external rotation			
			Thomas test for tightness of the hip flexors			
			Trendelenburg's test			

Table 7–3. Possible Trauma Based on the Location of Pain (Excluding Gross Injury)

| | *Location of Pain* | | | |
	Lateral	Anterior	Medial	Posterior
Soft tissue	Trochanteric bursitis (posterior portion of the greater trochanter) Gluteus medius strain Gluteus minimus strain	Rectus femoris strain Iliopsoas strain Symphysis pubis strain Rectus femoris/iliopsoas tendinitis Iliofemoral bursitis Lymphatic edema	Adductor strain Gracilis strain	Ischial bursitis Hamstring strain Gluteus maximus strain
Bony	Iliac crest contusion Hip joint dysfunction	Pubic bone fracture	Adductor avulsion fracture Stress fracture	Sacroiliac pathology

Inspection of Hip Angulations

- **Angle of inclination:** The angular relationship of the femoral head and the femoral shaft may be roughly determined by observing the relationship between the femur and tibia (see Fig. 5–16). An increase in the angle of inclination, **coxa valga**, may be manifested through either genu varum or laterally positioned patellae. Decreases in this angle, **coxa vara**, may lead to genu valgum or medially positioned "squinting" patellae (see Fig. 6–9). In each case the mechanical advantage of the gluteus medius is reduced by altering its line of pull on the femur. X-ray examination is necessary to definitively determine the angle of inclination.

- **Angle of torsion:** Like the angle of inclination, the angle of torsion must be definitively measured through the use of radiographs. However, increases greater than 15 degrees, **anteversion**, cause external femoral rotation and are characterized by a toe-out (duck-footed) gait. When the angle is decreased, **retroversion**, the femur internally rotates, resulting in a toe-in (pigeon-toed) position of the feet. The following technique has been found to be a reliable method of clinically determining the presence of femoral anteversion (Fig. 7–15)[5]:

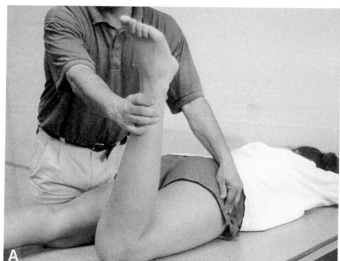
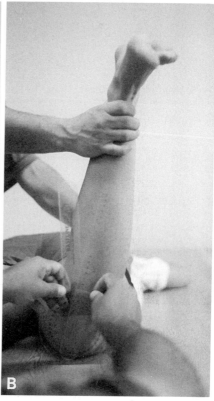

Figure 7–15. Clinical determination of femoral anteversion or retroversion. This procedure is most easily performed by two clinicians: (*A*) one to manipulate the leg and (*B*) the other to goniometrically measure the angle of the lower leg perpendicular to the table.

Gross Determination of the Angle of Inclination (Fig. 7–15)

Position of athlete	Prone with the knee of the leg being evaluated flexed to 90°.
Position of examiner	The use of two examiners is recommended. Examiner I: On the **contralateral** side to that being tested; one hand palpates the greater trochanter while the other hand manipulates the lower extremity. Examiner II: Holding a goniometer distal to the flexed knee; the stationary arm is perpendicular to the tabletop.
Evaluative procedure	Examiner I internally rotates the femur by moving the lower leg inward and outward until the greater trochanter is maximally prominent. This represents the point at which the femoral head is parallel with the tabletop. Examiner II then measures the angle formed by the lower leg while the knee remains flexed to 90°.
Positive test results	Angles below 15° represent femoral retroversion; angles above 15° represent anteversion.
Implications	As described in Positive Test Results above.

Inspection of the Medial Structures

• **Adductor group:** The examiner observes the area overlying the adductor muscle group for signs of swelling or ecchymosis, indicating a strain of these structures or a contusion to the area.

Inspection of the Anterior Structures

• **Hip flexors:** The area of the hip flexors distal to the ASIS should be observed for swelling or ecchymosis indicating a strain of these structures.

Inspection of the Lateral Structures

• **Iliac crest:** Located immediately beneath the skin, the iliac crest is vulnerable to contusions that set off a very active inflammatory process. These contusions, or **hip pointers**, result in great pain, disability, and discoloration (Fig. 7–16).

• **Nélaton's line:** An imaginary line from the ASIS to the ischial tuberosity, this is a quick screen that assists in the determination of coxa vara (Fig. 7–17).[6] If the greater tuberosity is located well superior to this line, it is an indication of coxa vara. As with all tests, the results should be compared with those of the uninvolved side.

Nélaton's Line (Fig. 7–17)

Position of athlete	Supine.
Position of examiner	At the side of the athlete.
Evaluative procedure	An imaginary line from the ASIS to the ischial tuberosity is visualized. The greater trochanter is then located.
Positive test results	The greater trochanter rides above the line formed between the ASIS and the ischial tuberosity.
Implications	Acute injury: hip dislocation. Chronic injury: coxa vara.

Inspection of the Posterior Structures

• **Gluteus maximus:** The gluteals should be inspected for bilateral symmetry. Any atrophy of the muscle group should be noted, as this could indicate an L5–S1 nerve root pathology.

• **Posterior superior iliac spine:** If visible, the skin indentations should be compared bilaterally for symmetry. This should include height of the PSIS from the floor and identification of localized swelling.

• **Sacral crests:** Although injury to this area is rare, **pilonidal cysts**, an infection over the posterior aspect of the **median** sacral crests, cause severe pain and disability. As the cyst matures it protrudes from the gluteal crease and appears vio-

---

Contralateral: Pertaining to the opposite side of the body or the opposite extremity.
Median: Along the body's midline.

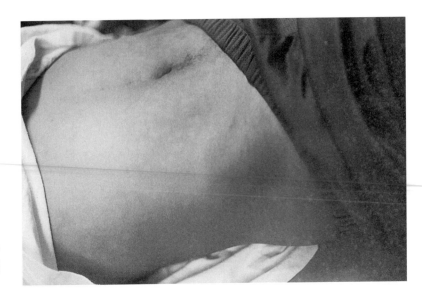

Figure 7–16. Contusion to the iliac crest. This injury, the so-called "hip pointer," results in gross discoloration, swelling, pain, and loss of function.

lently red. Athletes suspected as suffering from a pilonidal cyst should be immediately referred to a physician.

Inspection of Leg Length Discrepancy

Pain emanating from the foot, lower leg, knee, hip, and spine, or deficits in the athlete's gait may be caused by unequal leg lengths. Although the most accurate method for determining unequal leg lengths is through the use of x-ray evaluations, several methods are used clinically.

- **Functional leg length discrepancy:** The athlete is positioned standing, feet shoulder-width apart, and weight evenly distributed between the two legs. The examiner observes the ASIS and greater trochanters to determine whether they are an equal level from the floor (see Fig. 6–11). Inequality of these structures indicates rotation of the pelvic girdle, leg length discrepancy, or arch pathologies (e.g., pes cavus, pes planus).

- **True leg length discrepancy:** This test evaluates the athlete for a structural difference in the lengths of the femur and/or tibia (Fig. 7–18). The use of a tape measure has proved to be a valid and reliable method of determining leg length discrepancies,[7] especially when the average of two separate measurements is used.[8]

Determination of True Leg Length Discrepancy (Fig. 7–18)

Position of athlete	Supine with the legs positioned symmetrically.
Position of examiner	Standing lateral to the athlete. The ASIS and the crest of the medial malleolus are identified.
Evaluative procedure	The distance is measured from the medial malleolus to the ASIS on each leg.
Positive test results	A difference of greater than ¼ inch in distance between the two legs.
Implications	A structural (true) leg-length difference.
Modification	The lateral malleolus may be used as the distal reference point to minimize the effect of leg contour caused by hypertrophied or atrophied muscle.

Hoppenfeld[9] describes a method for determining which of the two bones is longer. The feet are placed flat and equal on the examining table with the knees flexed to 90°. The level of the knees is observed from in front of and to the side of the athlete. Anteriorly, a knee that appears higher indicates a long tibia on that side. Laterally, a knee that projects anteriorly relative to the opposite knee indicates an increased femoral length (Fig. 7–19).

- **Apparent leg length discrepancy:** Tests for apparent leg length discrepancies are meaningful only when the results for true leg length differences are negative (Fig. 7–20). This test is used to determine the presence of pelvic obliquity or an adductor contraction.

Determination of Apparent Leg Length Discrepancy (Fig. 7–20)

Position of athlete	Supine with the legs positioned symmetrically.
Position of examiner	Standing lateral to the athlete.
Evaluative procedure	The distance from the medial malleolus to the umbilicus is measured on each leg.
Positive test results	A difference in distance of greater than ¼ inch between the two legs.
Implications	Pelvic obliquity or a flexion and/or adduction contracture of the hip joint.
Comment	This test is meaningful only when the result for a true leg length discrepancy is negative (less than ¼ inch difference).

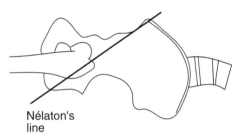

Nélaton's
line

Figure 7–17. Nélaton's line. This clinical test is used to determine the presence of coxa vara. An imaginary line is drawn from the anterior superior iliac spine to the ischial tuberosity. If the greater tuberosity is located superior to this line, coxa vara should be suspected.

Palpation

The hip and thigh are characterized by areas of subcutaneous bone and other areas of large muscle mass. The injured area must be carefully palpated to identify areas of underlying trauma and determine causes of referred pain. Palpation must be performed with discretion and with the athlete's modesty taken into account.

Palpation of the Medial Bony and Ligamentous Structures

• **Pubic bone:** Discretion must be used when deciding to palpate this area and should be performed only in the presence of a witness. The examiner follows the femoral creases downward toward the pubic bone, located under the pubic fat pad (mons pubis) superior to the genitalia. These bones, as well as the symphysis pubis, may be injured secondary to a blunt force such as a gymnast's striking the pubic bone against the horse, beam, or bars.

Palpation of the Medial Muscles and Related Soft Tissue

• **Adductor muscle group:** Abducting the hip places the adductor muscles on stretch, making the adductor longus muscle visibly prominent at the point that it arises from the symphysis pubis. Using discretion, the examiner palpates close to the origin of the adductor group for any tenderness or defect indicating an avulsion fracture. The examiner continues to palpate along the length of the adductor group for signs of tenderness or muscle spasm indicating a strain.

Palpation of the Anterior Bony and Ligamentous Structures

• **Anterior superior iliac spine:** The examiner follows the iliac crest anteriorly to locate the ASIS. This structure is easily palpable in thin athletes but may become obscured in muscular or obese individuals. With the athlete standing, the ASISs should be palpated bilaterally. These structures should be of equal height; any difference is indicative of a leg length discrepancy.

• **Anterior inferior iliac spine:** From the ASIS, the examiner continues to palpate downward to locate the anterior inferior iliac spine (AIIS). This structure is not always identifiable in many athletes.

Palpation of the Anterior Muscles and Related Soft Tissue

• **Sartorius:** The sartorius is palpable from its insertion on the ASIS to where it crosses the femoral crease. In some athletes it may be palpable along its entire length.

• **Rectus femoris:** Both heads of the rectus femoris lie under the sartorius and therefore are not palpable. However, when the knee is flexed and the hip forced into extension, the resulting

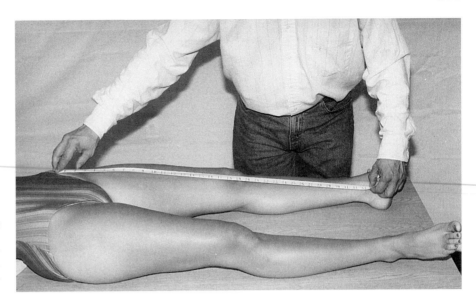

Figure 7–18. Test for the presence of a true leg length discrepancy. Measurements are taken from the anterior superior iliac spine to the medial malleolus. Discrepancies greater than ¼ inch are considered significant.

(A)

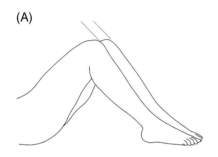

(B)

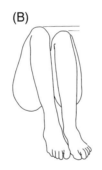

Figure 7–19. Clinical discrimination between femoral and tibial leg length differences. (*A*) When viewing the athlete from the side, an increased anterior position of one knee indicates a discrepancy in the lengths of the femurs. (*B*) When viewing the knees from the front, a difference in height indicates a discrepancy in the lengths of the tibias. Adapted from Hoppenfeld,[9] p 165.

Figure 7–20. Test for the presence of an apparent leg length discrepancy. Measurements are taken from each medial malleolus to the umbilicus. This test is meaningful only if the test for true leg length discrepancy is negative.

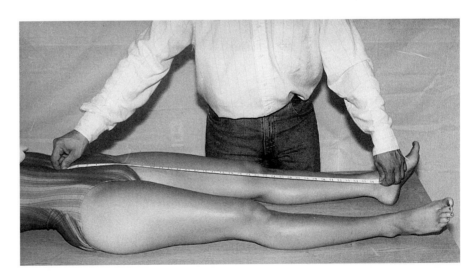

tension may cause a strain of the rectus femoris or an avulsion of its origin. The length of the muscle belly should be palpated to its insertion on the patella.

Palpation of the Lateral Bony and Ligamentous Structures

• **Iliac crest:** The iliac crest is easily located on most athletes and may be palpated along its length from the ASIS to the PSIS. Following a contusion, the iliac crest becomes swollen and tender to the touch, and crepitus may be present.

• **Greater trochanter:** Locate the greater trochanter at approximately the midline on the lateral thigh 4 to 6 inches below the iliac crest. The greater trochanter becomes more identifiable as the femur is internally and externally rotated and its posterior aspect becomes exposed. This area becomes tender secondary to tendinitis of the gluteus medius or iliotibial band tightness.

Palpation of the Lateral Muscles and Related Soft Tissue

• **Gluteus medius:** To isolate the gluteus medius, the athlete is positioned side-lying with the upper hip actively abducted 10 to 15 degrees. The

length of the muscle is palpable from its origin just inferior to the iliac crest to its insertion on the superior portion of the greater trochanter (Fig. 7–21). The inability of the athlete to maintain this position during the examination may indicate gluteus medius weakness, which should be confirmed through **Trendelenburg's test.**

• **Tensor fasciae latae:** Located below the anterior one-third of the iliac crest, the tensor fasciae latae is not easily distinguished from the gluteus medius.

• **Trochanteric bursa:** Overlying the posterior aspect of the greater trochanter, the trochanteric bursa is not directly palpable. Inflammation of this bursa causes it to feel thick and elicits pain at the posterior aspect of the greater trochanter.

Palpation of the Posterior Bony and Ligamentous Structures

• **Median sacral crests:** The fused remnants of the sacral spinous processes may be palpated from below the L5 vertebra to the midportion of the gluteal crease.

• **Posterior superior iliac spine:** The PSIS is located at the inferior portion of the gluteal dimples (Fig. 7–22). Under normal circumstances, these bony landmarks are palpable and align at the

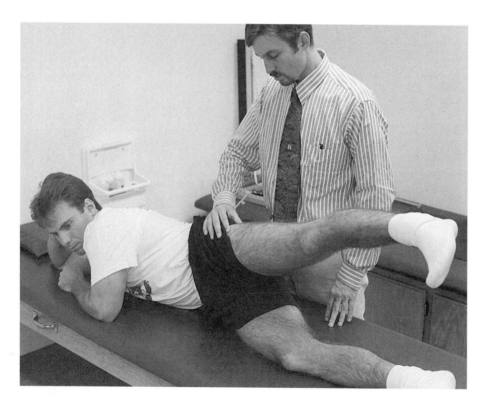

Figure 7–21. Positioning of the athlete to isolate the gluteus medius during palpation. Slightly abducting the hip makes the gluteus medius palpable.

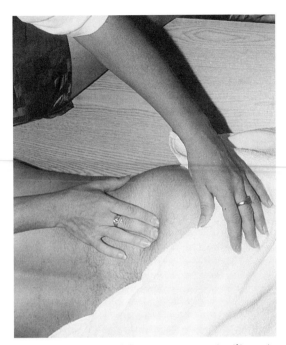

Figure 7–22. Location of the posterior superior iliac spine.

same level. Tenderness may indicate sacroiliac pathology.

- **Ischial tuberosity:** The athlete is positioned side-lying with the non–weight-bearing hip flexed. The ischial tuberosity can be identified by locating the gluteal fold and palpating deeply at approximately the midline of the gluteal fold (Fig. 7–23). Tenderness at this site may indicate an avulsion fracture or hamstring tendinitis.

Palpation of the Posterior Muscles and Related Soft Tissues

- **Gluteus maximus:** The bulk of the gluteus maximus is easily palpable and may be made more identifiable by having the athlete squeeze the buttocks together or extend the hip.

- **Hamstring muscles:** The common origin of the hamstring group is located on the ischial tuberosity. The semitendinosus and semimembranosus are palpated down the medial side of the posterior femur and the biceps femoris down the lateral border, noting for the presence of tenderness, spasm, defects, or pain.

- **Ischial bursa:** Palpation of this area is similar to that of the ischial tuberosity. Like the trochanteric bursa, the ischial bursa cannot be identified unless it is inflamed, at which time it is tender to the touch.

- **Sciatic nerve:** Although the sciatic nerve is not explicitly palpable, its approximate course can be palpated for tenderness. The examiner begins palpation of this structure by locating the ischial tuberosity and the greater trochanter. The sciatic nerve should be found as a cord midway between these two structures. An irritated sciatic nerve is exquisitely tender as compared with the contralateral side.

Functional Testing

The range of motion available to the hip joint is limited by its bony and soft tissue restraints and can be further limited by the position of the knee. A fully flexed knee can limit the amount of extension at the hip as the rectus femoris is stretched to its limits. An extended knee with stretched hamstrings can limit the amount of hip flexion available. The muscles acting on the hip in each of its motions are presented in Table 7–4.

There is no true active range of motion at the sacroiliac joints. Any motion is accessory in nature and is minimal in the absence of pathology.

Active Range of Motion

- **Flexion and extension:** The arc of motion available to the hip with the knee flexed ranges from 130 to 150 degrees. The majority of this motion

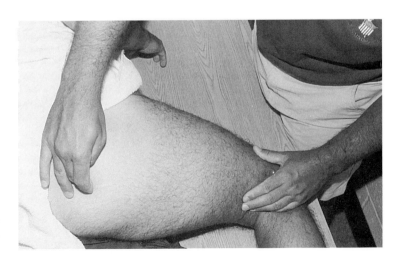

Figure 7–23. Positioning the athlete to palpate the ischial tuberosity. When inflamed, the ischial bursa may be felt during palpation of the ischial tuberosity.

Table 7–4. Muscles Acting on the Hip

Flexion	Abduction	Internal Rotation
Gluteus medius (anterior fibers)	Gluteus maximus (lower fibers)	Adductor brevis
Gluteus minimus	Gluteus medius	Adductor longus
Iliacus	Gluteus minimus	Adductor magnus
Psoas major	Sartorius	Gluteus medius (anterior fibers)
Psoas minor		Gluteus minimus
Rectus femoris		
Sartorius		

Extension	Adduction	External Rotation
Biceps femoris	Adductor brevis	Biceps femoris
Gluteus maximus	Adductor longus	Gemellus inferior
Gluteus medius (posterior fibers)	Adductor magnus	Gemellus superior
Semimembranosus	Gluteus maximus (upper fibers)	Gluteus maximus
Semitendinosus	Gracilis	Gluteus medius (posterior fibers)
	Pectineus	Obturator externus
		Obturator internus
		Piriformis
		Quadratus femoris
		Sartorius

(120 to 130 degrees) occurs during flexion (Fig. 7–24). Extending the knee greatly limits the amount of flexion available to the hip by placing the hamstring muscle group on stretch.

• **Adduction and abduction:** Active range of motion for abduction of the hip is approximately 45 degrees from the neutral position and for adduction, 20 to 30 degrees once the oppo-

site limb is cleared from the movement (Fig. 7–25).

• **Internal and external rotation:** With the hip in the flexed position, such as when the athlete is sitting with legs bent at the end of a table, exter-

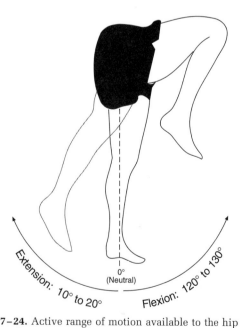

Figure 7–24. Active range of motion available to the hip during flexion and extension. The range for hip flexion is decreased when the knee is extended secondary to tightness of the hamstring muscles and is limited during extension when the knee is flexed because of tightness of the rectus femoris.

(A)

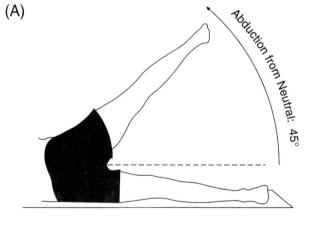

(B)

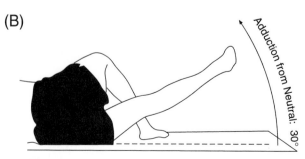

Figure 7–25. Active hip abduction and adduction.

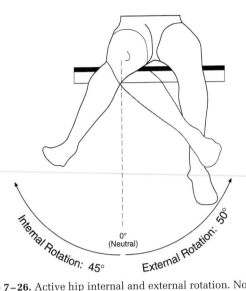

Figure 7–26. Active hip internal and external rotation. Note that, in the seated position, the lower leg moves in a direction opposite that of the femur (e.g., during internal femoral rotation the lower leg rotates outwardly).

nal rotation ranges from 40 to 50 degrees from the neutral position. Internal rotation is slightly less, 35 to 40 degrees from the neutral position (Fig. 7–26). Extending the hip reduces the range of motion available in each direction.

Passive Range of Motion

• **Flexion and extension:** To measure passive flexion of the hip, the athlete is supine. To eliminate compensation by pelvic rotation, the pelvis is stabilized by either grasping the iliac crest or placing the hand under the lumbar spine. As the hip is flexed, the knee is allowed to flex from tension placed on the hamstring muscles and gravity. With pressure applied proximal to the knee joint (i.e., without forcing knee extension), the normal end-feel for hip flexion is soft owing to the approximation of the quadriceps group with the abdomen. When the knee is forced to remain in extension during hip flexion, the end-feel is firm because of the stretching of the hamstring muscle groups (Fig. 7–27).

During passive hip extension range of motion measurements, the athlete is prone and the knee kept extended. The pelvis is stabilized to prevent it from being lifted off the table. The normal end-feel for hip extension is firm because of the stretching of the anterior joint capsule and the iliofemoral, ischiofemoral, and pubofemoral ligaments. If extension is measured with the knee flexed, a firm end-feel is obtained from tension within the rectus femoris muscle (Fig. 7–28).

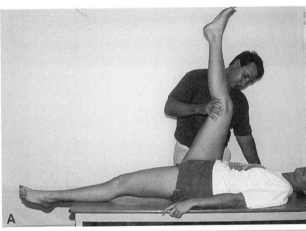

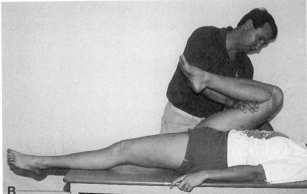

Figure 7–27. Passive hip flexion: (*A*) knee extended; (*B*) knee flexed.

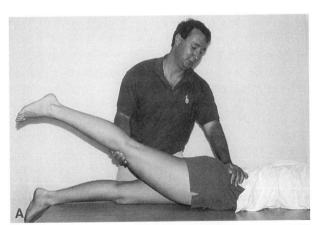

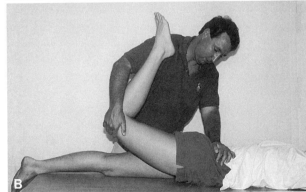

Figure 7–28. Passive hip extension: (*A*) knee extended; (*B*) knee flexed.

• **Adduction and abduction:** The athlete is positioned supine with the knee extended for the measurement of both passive adduction and abduction. The leg opposite that being tested is abducted to permit unrestricted adduction of the extremity being tested. To isolate the hip joint, the pelvis is stabilized to prevent lateral tilting during the motion (Fig. 7–29). The normal end-feel during adduction is firm owing to tension produced in the lateral joint capsule, the ITB, and the gluteus medius muscle. During abduction a firm end-feel is obtained because of the tightness in the medial joint capsule and in the pubofemoral, ischiofemoral, and iliofemoral ligaments.

• **Internal and external rotation:** At the end of a table, the athlete is positioned seated so that the hip and knees are flexed to 90 degrees and the arms are extended on either side to stabilize the torso. A rolled towel is used to bolster the knee, keeping the femur level with the tabletop (Fig. 7–30).

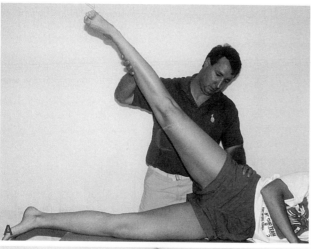

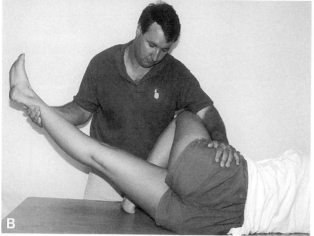

Figure 7–29. (*A*) Passive hip abduction. (*B*) Passive hip adduction.

When the athlete is seated and the knees are flexed, the lower leg rotates in the direction opposite that of the femur (e.g., when the femur is internally rotated the lower leg rotates outwardly). In both directions the end-feel is firm. Internal femoral rotation is limited by tension in the posterior joint capsule and the intrinsic external hip rotators. External femoral rotation is limited by the anterior joint capsule, the iliofemoral, and the pubofemoral ligaments.

Resistive Range of Motion

• **Flexion:** Resisted hip flexion should be performed once with the knee extended and then again with the knee flexed to differentiate pain and/or weakness in the iliopsoas muscle group from that arising from the rectus femoris (Fig. 7–31).

  ○ **Iliopsoas:** The athlete is positioned supine with the knee extended. Stabilization is provided over the ASIS while the motion is resisted on the anterior aspect of the femur, just proximal to the knee. This test may be modified to the sitting position to minimize movement during this portion of the examination.

  ○ **Rectus femoris:** With the athlete seated and the knee bent at the edge of the table, the anterolateral portion of the pelvis is stabilized by the examiner while he or she applies resistance to the distal femur.

  ○ **Sartorius:** The sartorius may be isolated by resisting knee flexion and flexion, external rotation, and abduction of the hip (see Fig. 5–25). This motion is performed by the athlete's running the heel of the leg to be tested up the anterior tibial border of the opposite leg while the clinician resists this movement.

• **Extension:** To isolate the contribution of the gluteus maximus from that of the hamstring muscle group (Fig. 7–32), resistive range of motion is again performed with the knee flexed and extended.

  ○ **Hamstring muscle group:** With the athlete lying prone and the knee extended, the examiner stabilizes the posterior portion of the pelvis while providing resistance just proximal to the popliteal fossa.

  ○ **Gluteus maximus:** The knee is flexed to a minimum of 90 degrees to eliminate the contribution of the hamstring muscle group during resisted extension. The clinician stabilizes the posterior pelvis while providing resistance on the posterior aspect of the distal femur.

• **Adduction:** The recommended position for testing resisted adduction is with the athlete lying on the involved side and the knee extended

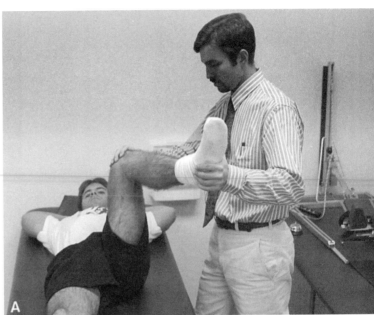

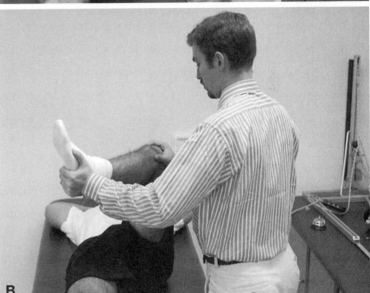

Figure 7–30. (*A*) Passive hip rotation, internal, and (*B*) passive hip rotation, external.

in a slightly abducted position. The opposite (upper) leg is supported by the examiner. The involved leg is adducted to touch the supported leg. Resistance is provided over the medial femoral condyle of the leg being tested. An alternative method of resisting hip adduction has the athlete lying supine and both hips abducted. Resistance is applied on the medial femur proximal to the knee (Fig. 7–33). The advantage of this technique is that adduction occurs with the muscle initially on stretch and resistance may be provided during the entire range of hip adduction.

• **Abduction:** With the athlete lying on the side opposite that being tested, the knee of the bottom leg is slightly flexed to provide stabilization and the knee of the extremity being tested remains fully extended. The pelvis and torso are stabilized over the iliac crest while resistance is provided over the lateral femoral condyle.

• **Internal and external rotation:** The athlete is placed in the seated position over the edge of the table with the arms extended on either side to provide stabilization to the torso. For movement in either direction, stabilization is provided on the thigh opposite the application of resistance on the lower leg. To resist internal femoral rotation, stabilization is provided on the medial distal thigh and resistance placed on the lateral aspect of the lower leg. To resist external femoral rota-

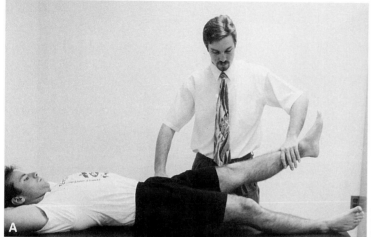

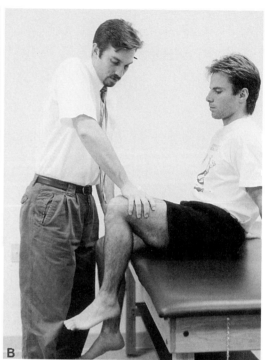

Figure 7–31. Resisted hip flexion. (*A*) With the knee extended to isolate the iliopsoas (in the presence of knee pathology, resistance to this motion should be applied proximal to the knee) and (*B*) with the knee flexed, allowing the rectus femoris to contribute to the movement.

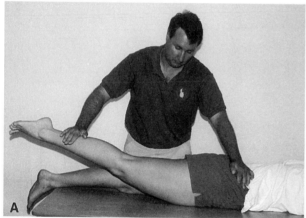

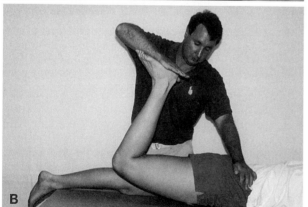

Figure 7–32. Resisted hip extension. (*A*) With the knee extended to allow for contribution from the hamstring group and (*B*) with the knee flexed to isolate the gluteus maximus.

tion, stabilization is provided on the medial distal thigh while resistance is provided to the medial aspect of the lower leg (Fig. 7–34).

Thomas Test for Tightness of the Hip Flexors

The Thomas test is used to differentiate between tightness of the iliopsoas muscle group and tightness of the rectus femoris muscle (Fig. 7–35). Tightness of the hip flexors results in an increased lordotic curve. As the hip is flexed, the lumbar spine flattens as the muscles are placed on slack, stabilizing the pelvis. The remaining motion represents true hip flexion (see bottom of page 219).

Trendelenburg's Test

During gait, athletes suffering from weakness of or trauma to the gluteus medius list the pelvis to the side opposite the insufficiency, displaying Trendelenburg's gait. Weakness of the gluteus medius muscle is manifested through the use of Trendelenburg's test (Fig. 7–36). Trendelenburg's gait is discussed in detail in Chapter 8 (see top of page 220).

Ligamentous Testing

No specific tests exist to determine the integrity of the hip's ligaments. Any dysfunction in the mechanics of these structures is determined through testing

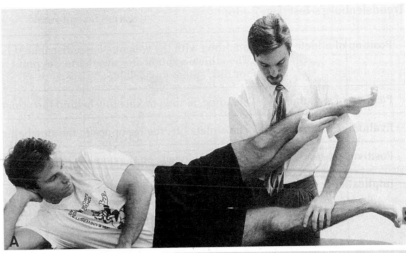
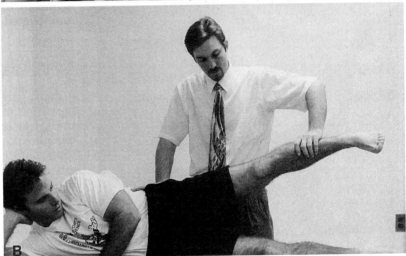

Figure 7–33. (*A*) Resisted hip adduction and (*B*) resisted hip abduction.

Thomas Test for Hip Flexor Tightness (Fig. 7–35)

Position of athlete	Lying supine with the knees bent at the end of the table.
Position of examiner	Standing beside the athlete.
Evaluative procedure	The examiner places one hand between the lumbar lordotic curve and the tabletop. One leg is passively flexed to the athlete's chest, allowing the knee to flex during the movement. The opposite leg (the leg being tested) rests flat on the table.
Positive test results	1. The involved knee rests at less than 90° of flexion. 2. The involved leg rises off the table.
Implications	1. Inability to flex the knee to 90°: tightness of the rectus femoris. 2. Leg rising off the table: tightness of the iliopsoas muscle group.
Modification	This test may be performed with the athlete lying flat on the table. The athlete may passively flex the hip and knee by using the arms to pull the leg to the chest. The amount of lumbar flattening can be determined by placing a hand under the lumbar spine.

Table 7–6. Evaluative Findings of Trochanteric Bursitis

Examination Segment	Clinical Findings
History	Onset: Acute or insidious. Location of pain: Over the greater trochanter, radiating posteriorly to the buttock; pain increased when the athlete climbs stairs. Mechanism: Acute: Direct blow to the greater trochanter. Chronic: Irritation from the ITB passing over the bursa.
Inspection	The area over the greater trochanter is usually unremarkable. The examiner measures the Q angle. Increased Q angles (above the norm for the athlete's gender) may predispose him or her to overuse forces being placed on the trochanteric bursa.
Palpation	Palpation reveals tenderness over the trochanteric bursa. Crepitus may also be experienced during active movement of the hip.
Functional tests	Flexion and extension and internal and external rotation, either actively or passively, cause pain as the ITB passes over the greater trochanter, resulting in decreased range of motion. RROM: Pain occurs during resisted hip extension. Pain occurs during resisted hip adduction.
Ligamentous tests	Not applicable.
Neurological tests	Not applicable.
Special tests	Ober's test for iliotibial band tightness.
Comments	Chronic trochanteric bursitis may result in "snapping hip" syndrome.

teric bursa may lead to "snapping hip" syndrome, in which an audible snap occurs as the ITB passes over the greater trochanter. The athlete with greater trochanteric bursitis tends to lose range of motion of the hip, especially in flexion/extension and internal/external rotation secondary to pain located directly posterior to the greater trochanter.

Ischial Bursitis

Movement of the buttocks while the athlete is weight bearing in the seated position, such as the rocking motion associated with rowing or biking, can cause friction to irritate the ischial bursa. Also, these structures can be traumatized secondary to a direct blow, such as a fall (Table 7–7). Ischial bursitis can be further irritated by prolonged periods of sitting, as occurs in a bus or airplane trip. The athlete is specifically point tender at the ischial tuberosity. A careful history must be taken to rule out the possibility of a hamstring strain or an avulsion of its attachment, which has signs and symptoms similar to those of ischial bursitis. Athletes may be given an inflatable doughnut pad on which to sit during periods of prolonged sitting to lessen the weight-bearing forces placed on these structures.

Degenerative Hip Changes

Age, repetitive trauma, acute trauma, or improper bony arrangements of the hip may all result in degeneration of the articular surfaces of the femur and acetabulum. In the athletic population these conditions most commonly include arthritis, osteochondritis dissecans, acetabular labrum tears, and *avascular necrosis*. All have the common characteristic of further degeneration if left undetected and untreated. Chronic hip degeneration occurs with age and tends to strike athletes over the age of 50. Younger athletes may develop degenerative hip changes secondary to acute trauma.

Athletes in the early stages of hip degeneration present with pain that occurs only during weight bearing. As the degeneration continues, the pain becomes more constant. The location of this pain may lead to the suspicion of lumbar spine or sacroiliac pathology, as many times the pain not only involves the hip but also is referred to the low back and distally into the thigh.

Physical evaluation reveals a loss of motion in all of the hip's planes. Strength assessment with manual muscle testing may be inconclusive secondary to pain. Scouring the hip causes the two articular surfaces to compress and rub over one another, resulting in pain. X-ray evaluation by a physician provides conclusive evidence of deterioration of the hip's articular surfaces.

Avascular necrosis: Death of cells secondary to lack of an adequate blood supply.

Table 7–7. Evaluative Findings of Ischial Bursitis

Examination Segment	Clinical Findings
History	Onset: Acute or insidious. Location of pain: Over the ischial tuberosity in the vicinity of the gluteal fold. Mechanism: Acute: Direct blow to the ischial tuberosity, such as falling on it. Chronic: Repeated shifting and moving while weight bearing in the seated position (e.g., rowing).
Inspection	Unremarkable.
Palpation	Tenderness over the ischial tuberosity. The bursa feels thick, and crepitus may be present.
Functional tests	AROM: Pain occurs during active hip flexion. PROM: Pain occurs during passive hip flexion. RROM: Pain occurs during resisted hip extension with the knee flexed to isolate the gluteus maximus.
Ligamentous tests	Not applicable.
Neurological tests	Prolonged irritation of the ischial bursa may place pressure on the sciatic nerve, requiring the evaluation of the sensory and motor nerves of the posterior lower leg.
Special tests	None.
Comments	Prolonged periods of sitting may cause an increase in symptoms.

Hip Scouring

The hip joint is scoured back and forth in external and internal rotation while the joint is compressed (Fig. 7–38). This movement causes compression of the joint surfaces and consequent tenderness with lesions of the articular cartilage or the joint surface, including osteochondral defects or arthritis.

Hip Scouring Test (Fig. 7–38)

Position of athlete	Supine.
Position of examiner	At the side of the athlete, fully flexing the athlete's hip and knee.
Evaluative procedure	The examiner applies pressure downward along the shaft of the femur while repeatedly externally and internally rotating the hip with multiple angles of flexion.
Positive test results	The athlete describes pain or reproduction of symptoms at the hip.
Implications	A possible defect in the articular cartilage of the femur or acetablum.

Sacroiliac Dysfunction

Although the SI joints are relatively immobile, a slight amount of accessory movement, rotation, and/or translation of the ilium on the sacrum occurs here. When these motions become extreme, the ilium rotates to the point that it subluxates on the sacrum. The resulting pain and dysfunction often resemble those associated with lumbar nerve root compression (Table 7–8). Single tests for sacroiliac dysfunction are not reliable measures of the presence of pathology in this region.[12] Combining the results of a series of these tests, however, does improve reliability.[13]

Long Sit Test

When viewed from its lateral aspect, the ilium may rotate clockwise with respect to the sacrum, producing an anterior motion. Tightness of the hip flexors is usually found in the athlete stressing the ilium, causing rotation to occur. The anterior rotation is typified by the involved lower extremity appearing to be longer than the contralateral limb with the athlete supine. As the athlete assumes a long sit position, the rotated ilium causes the limb to move from a relatively longer position to a shorter position, so that the limb now appears shorter. Such an occurrence is a positive long sit test result, indicating an anterior rotation of the SI joint on the **ipsilateral** side.

Ipsilateral: Pertaining to the same side of the body.

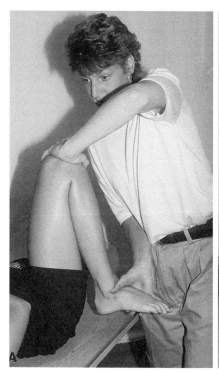
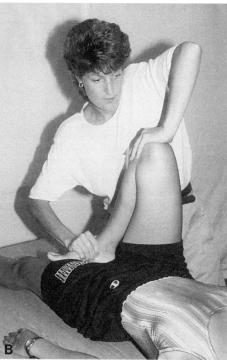

Figure 7–38. Hip scouring test. Compression of the hip's articular surfaces produces pain while passively rotating the hip in the presence of pathology such as osteochondral defects or arthritis.

Alternatively, when viewed from its lateral aspect, the ilium may rotate clockwise with respect to the sacrum, producing a posterior rotation (Fig. 7–39). Tightness of the hamstrings is usually found in the athlete as a contributory cause of this rotation. The posterior rotation is typified by the involved lower extremity appearing to be shorter than the contralateral limb with the athlete supine. As the athlete assumes a long sit position, the rotated ilium causes the limb to move from a relatively shorter position to a longer one, causing the limb to appear longer. This occurrence is a positive long sit test result, indicating a posterior rotation of the SI joint on the ipsilateral side as the leg moves from a shorter to a longer position.

Table 7–8. Evaluative Findings of Sacroiliac Dysfunction

Examination Segment	Clinical Findings	
History	Onset:	Acute or insidious.
	Location of pain:	Over one or both SI joints; pain possibly radiating to the buttock, groin, or thigh.
	Mechanism:	No one mechanism leads to the onset of SI joint dysfunction, but it may be related to prolonged stresses placed across the sacroiliac joint by soft tissues.
Inspection	The levels of the iliac crests and the PSIS are observed.	
Palpation	The athlete may describe tenderness over the SI joint and the PSIS.	
Functional tests	Forward flexion of the trunk, either actively or passively, with the knees extended may cause sufficient movement of the sacrum on the ilia to cause pain.	
Ligamentous tests	See special tests.	
Neurological tests	A complete lower quarter screen of the sensory, motor, and reflex distributions to rule out lumbar nerve root involvement.	
Special tests	Long sit test; SI compression and distraction; straight leg-raising, fabere test; Gaenslen's test.	
Comments	The pain distribution may mimic lumbar nerve root involvement. A combination of findings from multiple special tests is more reliable than the results of a single test.	

Long Sit Test (Fig. 7–39)

Position of athlete	Supine with the heels off the end of the table.
Position of examiner	Holding the feet of the athlete with the thumbs placed over the medial malleoli.
Evaluative procedure	The examiner provides slight traction on the legs while the athlete arches and lifts the buttocks off the table. The athlete then rests supine on the table. The athlete then moves from a supine to a long sit position. The examiner must pay close attention to the position of the malleoli at all times throughout the test. This test should be done actively if possible, without assistance provided by the upper extremities.
Positive test results	The movement of the medial malleoli is observed. If the involved leg (painful side) goes from a longer to a shorter position, there is an anterior rotation of the ilium on that side. If the involved side goes from a shorter to a longer position, posterior rotation of the ilium on the sacrum is indicated.
Implications	Rotated ilium as noted above.

Sacroiliac Compression and Distraction Tests. In the presence of an inflamed SI joint, compression or distraction of the two halves of the pelvis causes motion at the SI joint, resulting in a duplication of the athlete's symptoms (Fig. 7–40). A positive compression or distraction test result does not indicate the nature of the pathology, but only that a form of pathology is present.

Sacroiliac Compression Test (Fig. 7–40)

Position of athlete	Supine.
Position of examiner	At the side of the athlete with the hands placed over the opposite ASIS bilaterally.
Evaluative procedure	The examiner applies pressure to spread the ASIS, thus compressing the SI joints.
Positive test results	Pain arising from the SI joint.
Implications	Sacroiliac pathology.

Sacroiliac Distraction Test (Fig. 7–40)

Position of athlete	Side-lying.
Position of examiner	Behind the athlete with both hands over the lateral aspect of the pelvis.
Evaluative procedure	The examiner applies pressure down through the anterior portion of the ilium, spreading the SI joints.
Positive test results	Pain through the SI joint.
Implications	Sacroiliac pathology.

Fabere Sign (Patrick's) Test:

The fabere sign or Patrick's test is used to elicit pain in the SI joints as well as the hip. The term fabere is used as a mnemonic describing the position of the hip during testing: **f**lexion, **ab**duction, **e**xternal **r**otation, and **e**xtension (Fig. 7–41) (see top of page 229).

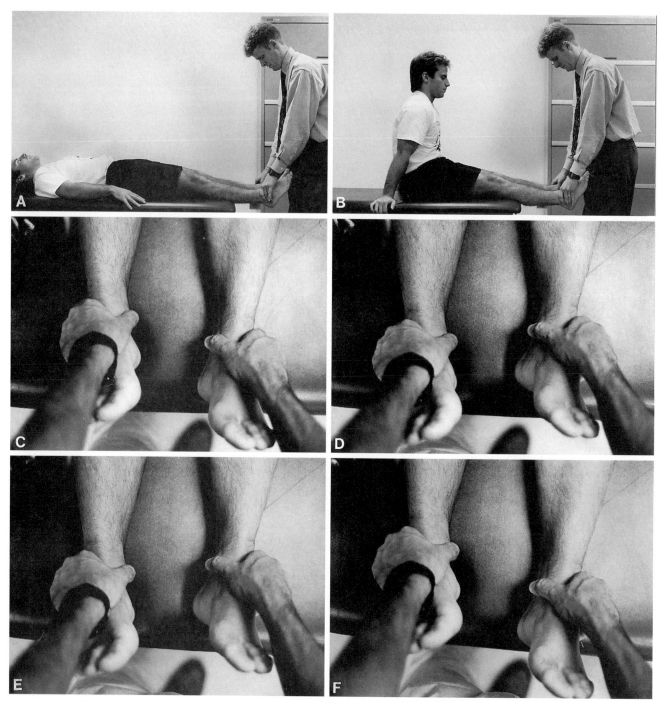

Figure 7–39. Long sit test for sacroiliac dysfunction. (*A* and *B*) While the examiner places the thumb over the malleoli, the athlete moves from a supine to a seated position. (*C* and *D*) The athlete's left leg moves from a long position to a short position, indicating anterior rotation of the left ilium on the sacrum. (*E* and *F*) The athlete's left leg moves from a short position to a longer position, indicating posterior rotation of the left ilium on the sacrum.

Fabere Sign (Fig. 7–41)

Position of athlete	Supine, with the foot of the involved side crossed over the opposite thigh.
Position of examiner	At the side of the athlete to be tested. One hand is on the opposite ASIS, the other on the medial aspect of the flexed knee.
Evaluative procedure	The extremity is allowed to rest into full external rotation. The examiner then applies *overpressure* at the knee and ASIS.
Positive test results	Pain in the sacroiliac joint or hip.
Implications	Pain in the inguinal area anterior to the hip may be indicative of hip pathology. Pain during the application of overpressure in the SI area may indicate SI joint pathology..

Gaenslen's Test

A modification of the Thomas test, Gaenslen's test is used to place a rotatory stress on the SI joint by forcing one hip into hyperextension (Fig. 7–42).

Gaenslen's Test (Fig. 7–42)

Position of athlete	Supine, lying close to the side of the table.
Position of examiner	Standing lateral to the athlete.
Evaluative procedure	The examiner slides the athlete close to the edge of the table and allows the near leg to hang over. The athlete pulls the far knee up to the chest. While stabilizing the athlete, the examiner applies pressure to the near leg, forcing it into hyperextension.
Positive test results	Pain in the SI region.
Implications	SI joint dysfunction.

Piriformis Syndrome

The reader should recall that the sciatic nerve passes under or through the piriformis muscle as the nerve travels across the posterior pelvis. Spasm or hypertrophy of the piriformis places pressure on the sciatic nerve, mimicking the signs and symptoms of lumbar nerve root compression or sciatica in the buttock and posterior leg. The resulting clinical manifestation of symptoms, piriformis syndrome, is six times more common in women than men.[14] Improved diagnostic tests for lumbar nerve root impingement and intervertebral disk disease have decreased the frequency and popularity of the diagnosis of piriformis syndrome.[15]

The signs and symptoms of piriformis syndrome are similar to those caused by other lumbopelvic maladies. Complaints include burning, pain, numbness, and/or paresthesia. However, there is little commonality in the factors leading to these symptoms.[16] Symptoms may be heightened by the straight leg-raising test on the involved side, passive hip internal rotation, and resisted external rotation with the athlete seated (Table 7–9). Resisted hip abduction with the athlete seated may also increase the symptoms (Fig. 7–43). These same symptoms may be caused by entrapment of the sciatic nerve by the hamstring muscles, termed **hamstring syndrome**.[17]

Overpressure: A force that attempts to move a joint beyond its normal range of motion.

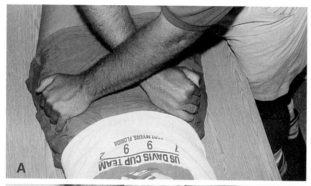

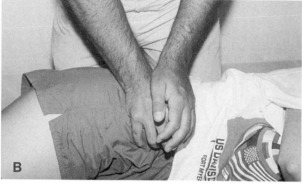

Figure 7–40. (*A*) Sacroiliac compression test. (*B*) Sacroiliac distraction test.

ON-FIELD EVALUATION OF PELVIS AND THIGH INJURIES

Trauma to the hip articulation is rare in sports; however, when it does occur, it tends to be of significant magnitude. More commonly, injuries to this region tend to involve muscular strains, contusions, and sprains of the SI joint. The bony and muscular anatomy is normally well padded in collision sports, such as football and ice hockey, which mandate the use of protective padding over the anterior thigh, ilium, and sacrum.

Upon arrival at the scene, the clinician should note whether the athlete is moving the involved leg. If the leg is moving, a gross dislocation of the hip or fracture of the femur may be ruled out, although a subluxation of the hip should still be considered. A fixed, immobile, awkwardly positioned, or noticeably shortened leg may indicate a dislocation of the hip joint or a fracture of the femoral neck. The shaft of the femur should be inspected for normal contour.

The mechanism of injury and other factors surrounding the onset of the injury should be ascertained as soon as possible in the history-taking process. Relevant questions include the determination of the injurious force, associated sounds and sensations, and any pertinent past history.

Once a hip dislocation or subluxation and femoral fracture has been ruled out, active range of motion of both the knee and the hip should be initiated. This is easily performed by having the athlete flex the thigh to the chest and straightening the leg back out again. This procedure is then repeated for passive and resisted motion. If the athlete is unable to fully bear weight a decision needs to be made on how to remove the athlete from the playing arena. These techniques are described in Chapter 1.

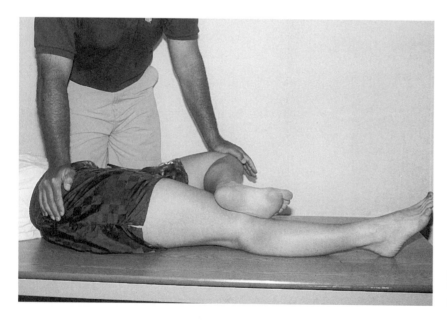

Figure 7–41. Fabere (flexion, abduction, external rotation, and extension) test for hip or sacroiliac pathology.

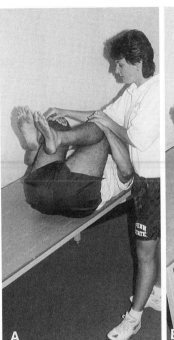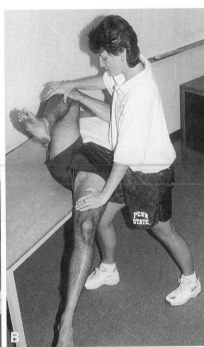

Figure 7–42. Gaenslen's test, placing a rotatory stress on the sacroiliac joint.

Table 7–9. Evaluative Findings of Piriformis Syndrome

Examination Segment	Clinical Findings	
History	Onset:	May be acute onset secondary to trauma. Insidious onsets may be related to hypertrophy of the piriformis or biomechanical changes in the hip, pelvis, and/or sacrum. In most cases time of onset is not discernible.
	Location of pain:	Pain is deep in the posterior aspect of the hip, radiating into the buttock and down the posterior aspect of the leg. It increases upon standing and often decreases when the athlete lies supine with the knees flexed.
	Mechanism:	Few common traits are associated with the onset of piriformis syndrome. Factors such as a blow to the buttock, hyperinternal rotation of the femur, or other trauma may cause spasming of the piriformis muscle.
Inspection	The athlete may present with an antalgic gait. In chronic conditions, atrophy of the gluteus maximus may be noted.	
Palpation	There is tenderness during palpation of the sciatic notch. An associated increase in symptoms may also be reported.	
Functional tests	AROM:	Pain may be experienced during external rotation owing to the piriformis muscle's contracting and placing pressure on the sciatic nerve.
	PROM:	Passive internal rotation of the hip with the athlete in the supine position increases the symptoms.
	RROM:	Pain is elicited or symptoms are increased during resisted external hip rotation with the athlete in the seated position (see Fig. 7–23). Pain may also be produced during resisted hip abduction.
Ligamentous tests	Not applicable.	
Neurological tests	The L2 through L4 dermatomes should be evaluated for numbness and/or paresthesia.	
Special tests	Positive straight leg-raise test result and/or resisted hip abduction in the seated position.	
Comments	The signs and symptoms of piriformis syndrome closely replicate those of other lumbopelvic disorders. A definitive diagnosis should be made by a physician.	

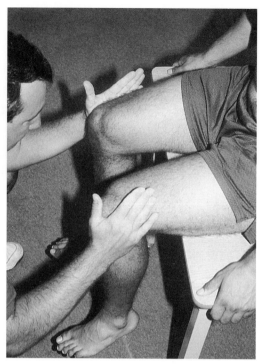

Figure 7–43. Resisted hip abduction with the athlete seated to duplicate pain caused by piriformis syndrome.

INITIAL MANAGEMENT OF ON-FIELD INJURIES

On-field management of hip and thigh injuries is needed mostly for contusions or muscle strains. However, hip dislocations and femur fractures represent medical emergencies that must be astutely managed to limit the scope of trauma and increase the athlete's chances for a full recovery.

Iliac Crest Contusions or "Hip Pointers"

Contusions to the iliac crest, "hip pointers," result in a seemingly disproportionate amount of pain, swelling, discoloration, and subsequent loss of function (see Fig. 7–16). The key to reducing the amount of time lost due to this injury lies in the recognition of its signs and symptoms (Table 7–10) and its immediate management.

Athletes suspected of sustaining a significant contusion of the iliac crest should be immediately removed from competition, treated with ice packs, and placed on crutches to avoid weight-bearing stresses. If the injury is minor and occurs during a game situation, the athlete may be allowed to return to competition, provided that full lower extremity and torso function is demonstrated. In this case the injured area should be padded to protect against further injury and the athlete must be treated immediately following the game.

Quadriceps Contusions

Critical to the long-term management and rehabilitation of athletes suffering from quadriceps contusions is the first 24 hours after the injury. Athletes who describe pain during active knee and/or hip

Table 7–10. Evaluative Findings of an Iliac Crest Contusion (Hip Pointer)

Examination Segment	Clinical Findings	
History	Onset:	Acute.
	Location of pain:	Iliac crest, possibly radiating into the internal and external oblique muscles.
	Mechanism:	Direct blow to an unprotected ilium.
Inspection	Swelling and redness have a rapid onset; ecchymosis sets in over time.	
Palpation	Pain and crepitus are felt during palpation of the iliac crest. Spasm of the associated muscles may also be present.	
Functional tests	All muscles having an origin or insertion along the iliac crest are liable to be affected. In most cases, the internal and external obliques elicit pain when the trunk is flexed away from the involved side. In more severe instances, hip flexion and abduction and movement of the trunk in any direction also cause pain.	
Ligamentous tests	None.	
Neurological tests	A complete sensory and vascular check of the involved lower leg must be performed to rule out trauma to the neurovascular structures about the hip.	
Special tests	None.	
Comments	Radiography may be required to rule out the possibility of an iliac fracture.	

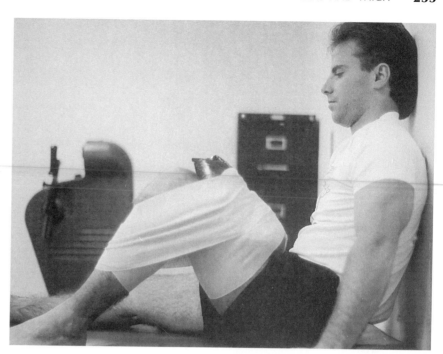

Figure 7–44. Method of managing a quadriceps contusion. The quadriceps is flexed to the point that pain is experienced and then extended to the point that the pain disappears. Ice is applied and the process is repeated when the athlete reports numbness.

extension and who have a noticeable deficit during manual muscle testing of these motions should be removed from competition and their injury immediately managed. Once the determination of the injury has been made, ice packs should be applied to the area and as much flexion of the knee joint as pain allows should be encouraged. As the treated area becomes numb, the amount of knee flexion is gradually increased to the athlete's tolerance (Fig. 7–44).

Hip Dislocations

Because of the hip's strong ligamentous and bony arrangement, dislocations are rare, but their occurrence represents a medical emergency requiring immediate care. The majority of hip dislocations result in the femoral head's being displaced posteriorly. Fractures to the femoral neck and/or the acetabulum may also result. Most dislocations occur when the hip is in flexion and adduction and a force is delivered to the femur, displacing it posteriorly and causing the head to be driven through the posterior capsule.[18]

Athletes suffering from a hip dislocation complain of immediate, intense pain within the joint and buttock and may describe the sensation of the hip "going out." The femur and lower leg are often positioned in internal rotation and adduction so that the involved knee rests against the knee of the opposite side (Fig. 7–45).[19] Active range of motion is impossible or results in severe pain. Although no attempt should be made at an on-field reduction of the dislocation, the examiner should perform a sensory and vascular check of the involved extremity.

This documentation should be noted for reference by the emergency room staff. The athlete should be immediately immobilized and transported to an emergency facility to allow rapid reduction of the dislocation with the athlete anesthetized.

Femoral Fractures

Resulting from a torsional or shear force to the shaft, femoral fractures occur relatively rarely in athletics. This fact is based on the "weak link" prin-

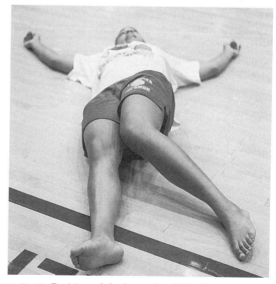

Figure 7–45. Position of the lower leg following a posterior hip dislocation: adduction and internal rotation of the hip.

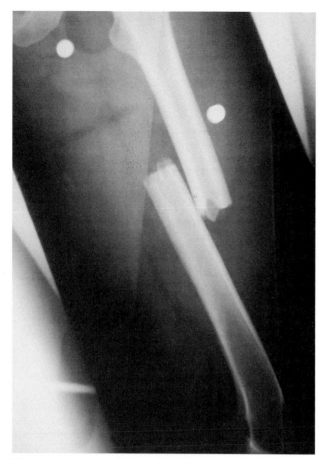

Figure 7–46. X ray of a complete fracture of the femoral shaft. This type of injury results in obvious deformity of the thigh.

ciple, in which these forces are more likely to result in trauma to the ankle, lower leg, or knee. Because they result in immediate loss of function, pain, and deformity, complete fractures of the femur are easily recognizable (Fig. 7–46).

The femoral shaft and neck may also be the site of a stress fracture, a pathology that is difficult to diagnose because of the similarity in symptoms to those of a chronic hip flexor strain or tendinitis of the muscles in the area. The athlete initially complains of pain only during activity and may then progress to pain at rest. A definitive diagnosis is made through a bone scan. The most commonly prescribed treatment is rest to prevent the stress fracture from progressing to full-fledged femoral fracture.

REFERENCES

1. MacLennan, AH: The role of the hormone relaxin in human reproduction and pelvic girdle relaxation. Scand J Rheumatol 20(Suppl 88):7, 1991.
2. Norkin, CC, and Levangie, PK: The hip complex. In Norkin, CC, and Levangie, PK: Joint Structure and Function: A Comprehensive Analysis, ed 2. FA Davis, Philadelphia, 1992, p 310.
3. Fisher, R: An epidemiological study of Legg-Perthes disease. J Bone Joint Surg Am 54:769, 1972.
4. Jacobs, B: Diagnosis and history of slipped capital femoral epiphysis. In American Academy of Orthopaedic Surgeons: Instructional Course Lectures, Vol 21. CV Mosby, St Louis, 1972.
5. Ruwe, PA, et al: Clinical determination of femoral anteversion: A comparison with established techniques. J Bone Joint Surg Am 74:820, 1992.
6. Adams, MC: Outline of Orthopaedics. London: E and S Livingstone, 1968.
7. Beattie, P, Rothstein, JM, and Kopriva, C: The clinical reliability of measuring leg length (abstr). Phys Ther 68:588, 1988.
8. Beattie, P, et al: Validity of derived measurements of leg length differences obtained by the use of a tape measure. Phys Ther 70:150, 1990.
9. Hoppenfeld, S: Physical examination of the hip and pelvis. In Hoppenfeld, S: Physical Examination of the Spine and Extremities. Appleton-Century-Crofts, New York, 1976, p 165.
10. Johnson, GE: Personal communication. August 19, 1994.
11. Clancy, WG, and Bosanny, JJ: Functional treatment and rehabilitation of quadriceps contusions, patellar dislocations and "isolated" medial collateral ligament injuries. Athletic Training: Journal of the National Athletic Trainers Association 17:249, 1982.
12. Potter, NA, and Rothstein, JM: Intertester reliability for selected clinical tests of the sacroiliac joint. Phys Ther 65:1671, 1985.
13. Cibulka, MT, Delitto, A, and Koldehoff, RM: Changes in innominate tilt after manipulation of the sacroiliac joint in patients with low back pain: An experimental study. Phys Ther 68:1359, 1988.
14. Keskula, DR, and Tamburell, M: Conservative management of piriformis syndrome. Journal of Athletic Training 27:102, 1992.
15. Hughes, SS, et al: Extrapelvic compression of the sciatic nerve. An unusual cause of pain about the hip: Report of five cases. J Bone Joint Surg Am 74:1553, 1992.
16. Carter, AT: Piriformis syndrome: A hidden cause of sciatic pain. Athletic Training: Journal of the National Athletic Trainers Association 23:243, 1988.
17. Woodhouse, ML: Sciatic nerve entrapment: A cause of proximal posterior thigh pain in athletes. Athletic Training: Journal of the National Athletic Trainers Association 25:351, 1990.
18. Gieck, J, et al: Fracture dislocation of the hip while playing football. Athletic Training: Journal of the National Athletic Trainers Association 21:124, 1986.
19. O'Donoghue, DH: Injuries of the pelvis and hip. In O'Donoghue, DH: Treatment of Injuries to Athletes, ed 3. WB Saunders, Philadelphia, 1976, p 497.
20. Kendall, FP, and McCreary, EK: Muscles: Testing and Function, ed 3. Williams & Wilkins, Baltimore, 1983.
21. Daniels, L, and Worthingham, C: Muscle Testing: Techniques of Manual Examination, ed 5. WB Saunders, Philadelphia, 1986.

8

Gait

Gait analysis is the functional evaluation of an athlete's walking or running style.[1] An organized approach to this analysis provides a systematic method of identifying specific deviations in the gait pattern and determining their cause and implications.

Dysfunction in the lower extremity or spine often manifests itself in an athlete's running or walking pattern. Consider, for example, an athlete limping off a basketball court after suffering an ankle sprain. In this case the trauma to the ankle's ligaments, combined with pain, prohibits the ankle from normal weight bearing. The foot compensates for this dysfunction by altering the weight-bearing surfaces, which, in turn, alters the mechanics of the knee, the hip, and possibly the lumbar spine. When an acute injury heals, normal gait should return. Chronic injuries or congenital abnormalities can alter the gait pattern, further influencing the stresses placed on the joint surfaces, bone, and soft tissue and predisposing the athlete to further injury.

Abnormal gait caused by improper or irregular lower extremity biomechanics redistributes the forces across the joint surfaces, potentially resulting in injury. In this case, the biomechanics must be corrected as a part of the athlete's rehabilitation program to prevent a recurrence of the condition.

THE GAIT CYCLE

The gait cycle represents the combined function of the lower extremity, pelvis, and spinal column. An understanding of each segment of the gait cycle, its role in the absorption and distribution of forces, and its relationship to the other phases of gait is needed to fully comprehend the information gained during the analysis of gait.

The articulations of the foot and toes, ankle, knee, hip, pelvis, and spine compose a kinetic chain though which gait occurs.[2] The position and movement of one joint influences the position and movement at the other joints. When the limb is weight bearing a **closed kinetic chain** is established, in which movement of a distal joint influences the position of the joints proximal to it.[3] When the extremity is non−weight bearing, an **open kinetic**

chain is formed, in which movement of a proximal joint influences the position of the joints distal to it (Fig. 8−1).[4]

Defining the Gait Cycle

This chapter uses the terminology established by the Rancho Los Amigos Medical Center.[5] This terminology is more descriptive of the actions that take place in the gait cycle than the traditional terminology. A comparison between traditional terminology and that used by the Rancho Los Amigos method is presented in Table 8−1. When walking, the gait cycle begins with the initial contact of the heel as it strikes the ground and ends when that heel contacts the ground again. The Rancho Los Amigos system of gait analysis addresses two distinct phases: the **stance phase**, when the foot is in contact with the ground and the **swing phase**, when the foot is off the ground. The stance phase begins with the initial contact of the heel on the ground and ends as the toe breaks contact with the surface (toe-off). The period between toe-off and initial contact is termed the swing phase, the open kinetic chain period during which the limb repositions itself. During walking, while one leg is in the stance phase, the other is in the swing phase.

Stance Phase

Constituting 62 percent of the gait cycle, the stance phase provides support of the body weight during forward movements as the lower extremity is in a closed kinetic chain, allowing the forces to be transmitted proximally from the trunk or distally from the ground.[6] Abnormal biomechanics along this chain cause the forces to be abnormally distributed, placing increased stress on the tissues and potentially causing overuse injuries.[7] In the case of acutely injured tissues, forces placed on the structures are beyond their tolerance level. Five distinct periods occur during the stance phase: Initial contact, loading response, midstance, terminal stance, and preswing (Fig. 8−2).

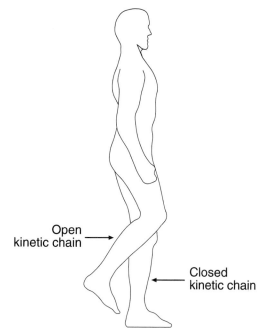

Figure 8–1. Open and closed kinetic chains of the lower extremity. The weight-bearing limb represents a closed kinetic chain; the non–weight-bearing limb is in an open kinetic chain.

Table 8–1. Comparison of Gait Terminology

Traditional	Rancho Los Amigos
Heel strike	Initial contact
Heel strike to foot flat	Loading response
Foot flat to midstance	Midstance
Midstance to heel-off	Terminal stance
Toe-off	Preswing
Toe-off to acceleration	Initial swing
Acceleration to midswing	Midswing
Midswing to deceleration	Terminal swing

From Norkin, CC, and Levangie, PK,[6a] p 456, with permission.

The **initial contact** period of the stance phase begins with the heel striking the ground as the stance phase of the opposite limb is ending with toe-off. During this period both limbs are in contact with the ground at the same time, representing 22 percent of the total gait cycle (Table 8–2). Immediately following initial contact the **loading response** occurs. This period lasts until the opposite extremity has left the ground and the double limb support has ended (Table 8–3).

As the loading response is completed, the **midstance** period occurs as the body weight passes directly over the support limb and concludes when the center of gravity is directly over the foot (Table 8–4). The **terminal stance** period begins as the center of gravity passes over the foot and ends just before the contralateral limb makes initial contact with the ground (Table 8–5). In this period of the gait cycle the heel has left the ground in preparation

for the beginning of the swing phase. The final period of the stance phase, **preswing**, begins with the initial contact of the opposite limb and ends with toe-off of the stance limb (Table 8–6). This is the second of the two periods with double limb support in a normal gait cycle.

Swing Phase

The non–weight-bearing phase of gate, the swing phase, begins as soon as the toes leave the ground and terminates when the limb makes contact with the ground. The swing phase represents 38 percent of the gait cycle.[6] Three distinct periods occur during the swing phase: initial swing, mid-swing, and terminal swing (Fig. 8–2).

The **initial swing** period begins at the point when the toes leave the ground and continues until the knee reaches its maximum range of flexion, approximately 60 degrees (Table 8–7). **Midswing** is the second period of the swing phase of the gait cycle. During midswing the knee extends from the point of maximum flexion to the point at which the tibia reaches a vertical position perpendicular to the ground (Table 8–8). The final period of the swing phase is the **terminal swing**. This occurs from the end of the midswing to the initial contact period of the stance phase (Table 8–9).

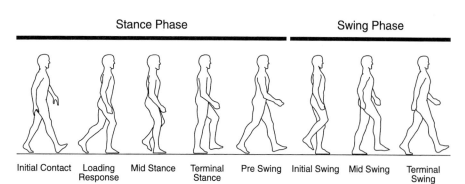

Stance Phase					Swing Phase		
Initial Contact	Loading Response	Mid Stance	Terminal Stance	Pre Swing	Initial Swing	Mid Swing	Terminal Swing

Figure 8–2. Phases of the gait cycle. With the right (facing) limb as an example, two distinct phases occur—the weight-bearing stance phase and the non–weight-bearing stance phase. With the exception of the dual phases of double limb support, one limb is in the stance phase when the other is in the swing phase, and vice versa. (Adapted from Norkin, CC, and Levangie, PK,[6a] with permission.)

Table 8–6. Preswing

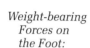

*Weight-bearing
Forces on
the Foot:*

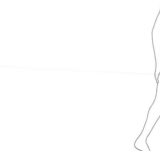

Joint Angles
  Subtalar joint:
  Talocrural joint:
  Knee:

  Hip:

Muscle Actions
  Foot intrinsics:
  Ankle plantarflexors:
  Ankle dorsiflexors:
  Quadriceps femoris mus
    group:
  Hamstring muscle group
  Hip adductors:
  Gluteus maximus:
  Gluteus medius and
    minimus:
  Iliopsoas:

Table 8–2. Initial Contact

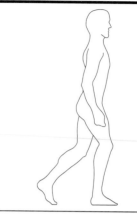

*Weight-bearing
Forces on
the Foot:*

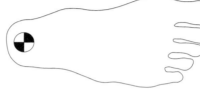

Joint Angles	
Subtalar joint:	5° of supination
Talocrural joint:	Neutral to dorsiflexion
Knee:	0° of flexion: tibia is internally rotated
Hip:	30° of flexion: femur is internally rotated

Muscle Actions	
Foot intrinsics:	No activity
Ankle plantarflexors:	No activity
Ankle dorsiflexors:	Eccentric
Quadriceps femoris muscle group:	Concentric/eccentric
Hamstring muscle group:	Eccentric
Hip adductors:	Eccentric
Gluteus maximus:	Isometric to eccentric
Gluteus medius and minimus:	Eccentric
Iliopsoas:	No activity

Table 8–3. Loading Response

*Weight-bearing
Forces on
the Foot:*

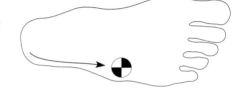

Joint Angles	
Subtalar joint:	10° pronation
Talocrural joint:	15° plantarflexion
Knee:	15° flexion: tibia internally rotates, begins to externally rotate
Hip:	30° flexion: femur moves from internal rotation to neutral

Muscle Actions	
Foot intrinsics:	No activity
Ankle plantarflexors:	No activity
Ankle dorsiflexors:	Eccentric
Quadriceps femoris muscle group:	Concentric
Hamstring muscle group:	No activity
Hip adductors:	Eccentric
Gluteus maximus:	Concentric
Gluteus medius and minimus:	Isometric
Iliopsoas:	No activity

the loading response and
through the rest of the st:
  The talocrural joint is
range of 25 degrees at t
The subtalar joint, altho
initial contact, then pron
to uneven surfaces. As
midstance to preswing,
tarflexes and the subtala
rigid lever for the athlete
  The swing phase clea:
limb over the ground an
cept weight bearing, allo
as efficiently as possibl

BIOMECHANICAL CONSIDERATIONS IN THE GAIT CYCLE

During the stance phase, from the time of initial contact through the period of loading response, a number of important biomechanical events are initiated. At initial contact the subtalar joint is supinated and the talocrural joint dorsiflexed. As the gait cycle proceeds through the loading response, the talocrural joint plantarflexes while the subtalar joint pronates, resulting in calcaneal eversion.[8] Subtalar pronation unlocks the midtarsal joints, allowing the foot to become flexible and accommodate uneven surfaces. During this time, the tibialis posterior eccentrically contracts, decelerat-

ing the rate of pronation.[6] Tibial internal rotation results because of the subtalar pronation and slightly flexes the knee. The hip maintains a flexed position during this time.

As the gait cycle continues through midstance, the talocrural joint dorsiflexes and the subtalar joint remains pronated. As the gait cycle proceeds on to terminal stance the talocrural joint continues to dorsiflex, but the subtalar joint now supinates, increasing calcaneal inversion. The supination of the subtalar joint locks the midtarsal joints, stiffening the foot into a rigid lever and making the limb more efficient during propulsion at toe-off. External rotation of the tibia occurs as the knee and hip joints move into extension.

Table 8–4. Midstance

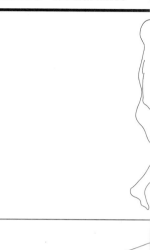

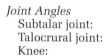

Weight-bearing Forces on the Foot:

Joint Angles
  Subtalar joint:
  Talocrural joint:
  Knee:

  Hip:

Muscle Actions
  Foot intrinsics:
  Ankle plantarflexors:
  Ankle dorsiflexors:
  Quadriceps femoris muscle group:
  Hamstring muscle group:
  Hip adductors:
  Gluteus maximus:
  Gluteus medius and minim
  Iliopsoas:

At terminal stance the to
ing weight with the subt
knee and hip begin to fl
swing phase of gait. Durin
tact of the contralateral
weight bearing is taking pl
ties.

During the swing phase
siflexed and the knee and
the foot to clear the grou
The subtalar joint initi
supinates in the latter asp
it prepares the limb fo
stance.

Table 8–8. Mid-Swing

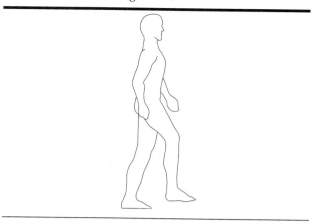

Weight-bearing Forces on the Foot:

	Non−weight bearing
Joint Angles	
Subtalar joint:	Neutral
Talocrural joint:	Neutral
Knee:	30° to 0° flexion: tibia internally rotates
Hip:	20° to 30° flexion: femur internally rotates
Muscle Actions	
Foot intrinsics:	Isometric
Ankle plantarflexors:	Concentric
Ankle dorsiflexors:	Isometric
Quadriceps femoris muscle group:	Concentric
Hamstring muscle group:	Eccentric
Hip adductors:	Isometric
Gluteus maximus:	Eccentric
Gluteus medius and minimus:	Isometric
Iliopsoas:	Concentric

degrees of plantarflexion but proceeds rapidly to 10 degrees of dorsiflexion, where it remains until initial contact during the stance phase.

Walking Versus Running Gait

During walking gait there is a wider base of support than there is during running, in which the width of the step narrows secondary to the increased velocity and length of the stride (Fig. 8–3). The foot lands forward to the center of gravity in the walking gait, whereas in the running gait it lands directly under the center of gravity, increasing the ground reaction forces to approximately 275 percent of the athlete's body weight.[1] Running increases the joint reaction forces to between six and eight times the actual body weight, whereas walking increases them to only three times the body weight.[9]

Table 8–9. Terminal Swing

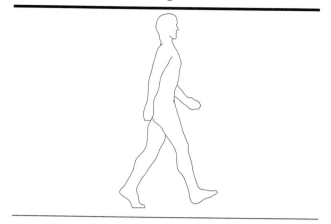

Weight-bearing Forces on the Foot:

	Non−weight bearing
Joint Angles	
Subtalar joint:	5° supination
Talocrural joint:	Neutral
Knee:	0°: tibia internal rotation
Hip:	30° flexion: femur internal rotation
Muscle Actions	
Foot intrinsics:	No activity
Ankle plantarflexors:	Isometric
Ankle dorsiflexors:	Isometric
Quadriceps femoris muscle group:	Concentric
Hamstring muscle group:	Eccentric
Hip adductors:	Eccentric
Gluteus maximus:	Eccentric
Gluteus medius and minimus:	Isometric
Iliopsoas:	Isometric

In contrast to walking, the running gait includes a period when both limbs are non−weight bearing, thus decreasing the percentage of time that the athlete spends in the stance phase. During walking, the stance phase accounts for 62 percent of the total gait cycle; during running, it accounts for 33 percent.[1] As each phase of gait occurs faster during running and the feet are in contact with the ground for a shorter length of time, an increase in the speed and strength of muscular function is necessary, particularly with the eccentric contractions required to achieve control of pronation and initiate supination prior to toe-off.[10]

Muscle Function During Running

When running, the frequency and length of each stride increase relative to the walking gait, causing the swing phase to constitute 67 percent of the cy-

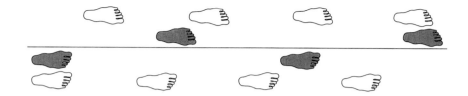

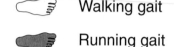

Walking gait

Running gait

Figure 8–3. Comparison of strides between walking and running gaits. Running requires a greater range of motion, balance, and strength compared with walking. Notice the increased stride length and decreased stride width associated with running.

cle. During the entire gait cycle, the muscles of the anterior compartment are active 70 percent of the time, producing concentric and eccentric contractions. The anterior compartment musculature is active in clearing the foot over the surface as the leg swings forward. The gastrocnemius-soleus complex is active at the late stages of the swing phase and remains active for approximately 70 percent of the stance phase.

The quadriceps femoris muscle group works in an eccentric fashion during the early stages of the stance phase, controlling the amount of knee flexion. The quadriceps begins concentric contractions in the later stages of the swing phase as it actively extends the knee from approximately 125 degrees of flexion to 40 degrees of flexion just before initial contact.

The hamstrings provide motion at the knee as well as at the hip. At the knee, the hamstrings are active late in the swing phase and continue to be active early in the stance phase. During late swing and into early stance, the hamstrings contract eccentrically to control knee extension. At the hip, the hamstrings contract in unison with the gluteus maximus to create extension during the stance phase.

The hip flexor group is active beginning in late stance and continuing throughout the swing phase as these muscles position the extremity forward. The hip abductors are active throughout stance as they contract to keep the pelvis as level as possible during unilateral weight bearing. The hip adductors are active during the late stance through the early swing phase.

GAIT ANALYSIS AS AN EVALUATIVE TOOL

An analysis of gait provides the examiner with a means of objective assessment of dynamic function. Gait deviations may occur secondary to inherent biomechanical irregularities in the athlete or as a result of unconscious compensation. Analysis of the gait provides the examiner with relevant informa-

tion regarding the nature of the athlete's present condition, as well as demonstrating predisposing factors that may have contributed to the injury mechanism or that may inhibit recovery (Fig. 8–4).

Several significant variations in gait patterns may be noted in athletes, and these can be observed by the examiner when analyzing the various phases of walking and/or running gait. Detailed observation is best obtained by using stop-action video. The speed of the video can be decreased and replayed, allowing the examiner to carefully break down the phases of the gait cycle. The video can be used to quantify the position of the limb, determine the amount and speed of motion, and assess the timing of each particular event of the gait cycle. Video analysis is also useful because it is a permanent record of the athlete's gait that can be used for future comparison to assess the progress of the athlete's condition.

The examiner must be careful to note several factors when performing gait analysis. The athlete should be encouraged to use the footwear that is normally worn for practice and competition. If a treadmill is used to analyze the gait, it is important that the athlete be familiar with walking or running on this device. The examiner must be aware of the subtle differences between ambulation on a treadmill versus a regular playing surface and consider these differences when making any conclusions. Although it is beneficial to use video equipment and a treadmill to analyze gait, gait is more commonly evaluated with the naked eye with the athlete running along a flat surface. It is essential that the examiner take the time needed to thoroughly analyze the gait and observe the detail and timing of motion.

The observation of an athlete's running gait begins when the foot makes initial contact. Approximately 5 degrees of supination is desired at the subtalar joint at the initiation of this period, and contact is made on the plantar surface of the heel. A variation in this may include pronation in the subtalar joint as the heel strikes the ground, increasing the stress applied to the medial structures of the foot and leg. In some cases the initial contact is

OXFORD PHYSICAL THERAPY & REHABILITATION

LOWER EXTREMITY BIOMECHANICAL EVALUATION

I. HISTORY

Name _____ Age _____ Date _____ Diagnosis _____

Occupation _____

Chief Complaint _____

Onset of Symptoms_____ When Does Pain Occur _____

Amount of Participation _____

Physical History _____

II. PRONE

A. STJ	R	L	B. Forefoot	R	L	C. Flexibility	R	L
Valgus	___	___	Valgus	___	___	Gastroc	___	___
Varus	___	___	Varus	___	___	Soleus	___	___
Neutral	___	___				Rectus femoris	___	___
Inversion	___	___				Hip flexors	___	___

D. Callus Formation   E. PSIS   R   L   F. Palpation _____

_____   Med/Lat   Med/Lat   _____

_____   Inf/Sup   Inf/Sup   G.   Resistive Testing _____

                                  Post/Ant Post/Ant   _____

                                  Level

III. SUPINE

A. 1st Ray

   R   Plantarflex   Dorsiflex   Neutral
   L   Plantarflex   Dorsiflex   Neutral

B. 1st Ray ROM

   R ↑ Plantarflex   ↑ Dorsiflex   Equal
   L ↑ Plantarflex   ↑ Dorsiflex   Equal

C. MTP ROM	R	L
Dorsiflexion	_____	_____
Plantarflexion	_____	_____

D. Midtarsal ROM (O-oblique/L-longitudinal)

_____

_____

E. Talar Rock   R   +   -   L   +   -

F. Passive Spring Test   R   +   -   L   +   -

G. Superior Tibiofibular Joint   R ↓ Anterior ↓ Posterior   Equal
                                        L ↓ Anterior ↓ Posterior   Equal

H. Femoral Torsion Test   R   Neutral   IR/ER   IR____ ER ____
                                         L   Neutral   IR/ER   IR____ ER ____

I. ASIS   R   L
                                      Med/Lat   Med/Lat   equal
                                       Inf/Sup   Inf/Sup
                                       Post/Ant   Post/Ant

A

Figure 8–4. (*A*) Documentation used during the physical evaluation of gait. (Courtesy of Oxford Physical Therapy & Rehabilitation, Oxford, OH, with permission.)

III. **SUPINE** (Continued)

J. Piriformis Flexibility   R   Tight   Normal   L   Tight   Normal

K. Hamstring Flexibility   R   Tight   Normal   L   Tight   Normal

IV. **SITTING**

A. Resistive Testing _____

B. Palpation _____

C. Tibial Torsion   R _____   L _____

V. **STANDING**

A. Toe Raise
   R ↓ Rearfoot Supination   Rearfoot Supination
   R ↓ Forefoot Pronation   Forefoot Pronation

   L ↓ Rearfoot Supination   Rearfoot Supination
   L ↓ Forefoot Pronation   Forefoot Pronation

B. 1/4 Squats
   R ↓ Rearfoot Pronation   Rearfoot Pronation
   R ↓ Forefoot Pronation   Forefoot Supination

   L ↓ Rearfoot Pronation   Rearfoot Pronation
   L ↓ Forefoot Pronation   Forefoot Supination

C. Standing Rotation _____

D. Tib/fib Rotation Test   R   L
   Anterior Glide   ___ ___
   Posterior Glide   ___ ___

E. Rearfoot Position   R   L
   Pronated   ___ ___
   Supinated   ___ ___
   Neutral   ___ ___

F. Supro Test_____   G. Knee Position _____

H. Iliac Crest   Level   R Low   L Low   I. Marh Test   R +   -   L   +   -

J. Gait _____

VII. **ASSESSMENT** _____

VIII. **TODAY'S TREATMENT**

A. Modalities_____

B. Orthotics/Shoe Lift _____

C. Pelvic Girdle _____

D. Cross Friction Massage _____

IX. HOME EXERCISE PROGRAM

	SETS	REPS	TIME		SETS	REPS	TIME
Heel Raises	___	___	___	Gastroc/soleus	___	___	___
Toe Raises	___	___	___	Hamstring	___	___	___
Windshield Wiper	___	___	___	IT Band	___	___	___
Theraband inversion	___	___	___	Piriformis	___	___	___
eversion	___	___	___	Plantar fascia	___	___	___
dorsiflexion	___	___	___				
plantarflex	___	___	___				

X. **PLAN** _____

XI. **NEXT MD VISIT** _____ PT/ATC

B

Figure 8–4. (*B*) *Continued.*

made with increased supination, which increases the amount, and possibly the speed, of motion required at the subtalar joint to move into loading response. Supinated feet are usually high-arched and often inflexible, with initial contact possibly occurring on the lateral border of the foot or the forefoot.

Early in the loading response the subtalar joint begins to pronate and the midtarsal joints become unlocked to allow for accommodation to irregular surfaces. Factors such as bony foot abnormality, tightness of the tricep surae muscle group, and/or decreased motion at the first MTP joint can all contribute to increased weight-bearing pronation. Pronation may also occur very rapidly, which can increase the stress to the medial structures of the foot and leg. If the initial contact or loading response periods demonstrate increased supination, the amount and speed of pronation may be excessive as the foot adapts to the ground beneath it. Internal tibial rotation may be increased, which causes increased rotational forces to occur at the leg, knee, and patellofemoral joints.

Progressing through the loading response to midstance, maximal pronation of the subtalar joint should be achieved. Now the foot must prepare to become a more rigid lever by returning to a neutral position through the initiation of supination at the subtalar joint. Ideally, the tibia has begun to externally rotate. Frequently the subtalar joint continues to pronate further during this period or does not initiate supination. This necessitates continued internal tibial rotation and creates increased medial forces at the foot, leg, and knee. An irregular foot configuration or weakness of the extrinsic musculature, particularly the posterior tibialis and flexor hallucis longus, is a possible cause of this prolonged pronation.

At terminal stance the tibia should be externally rotated, the subtalar joint in approximately 5 degrees of supination, and the midtarsal joint locked, with the weight-bearing forces on the first MTP joint. Inefficient variations from this positioning may include the foot's still moving from prolonged pronation and the midtarsal joints unlocked and unprepared for generating propulsion forces.

The examiner must be aware of the normal components of motion in each period of the stance phase in order to assess variance and its relevance to injury mechanism and resulting compensatory changes. The position of the foot and leg, the amount and speed of motion, the timing of the occurrence of motion, and the patterns of weight and force distribution are critical to determining causes and effects of pathology. This determination depends on a thorough static assessment of relevant anatomy as well as a complete and detailed history of the onset and symptoms present. As always, a bilateral comparison is required to make meaningful observation of individual characteristics particular to the athlete.

PATHOLOGIES AFFECTING THE GAIT CYCLE

Various conditions may predispose an athlete to injury or, once an injury has occurred, may inhibit recovery or cause further injury. Many athletes experience the frustration of allowing for sufficient recovery from an injury only to have the symptoms return once they return to functional activity. This dilemma can be better managed by including a comprehensive assessment of observable gait patterns that may need correction to prevent injury.

The findings relevant to predisposing conditions that may be identified during the athlete's physical examination are correlated with gait changes particular to each period during the stance phase (Table 8–10). Observation of gait variations must be correlated with clinical evaluation results, as there are many individual gait patterns that, although not typical, do not result in pathology. This determination is very important, as it is not prudent to make alterations in a functional gait unless it is warranted by the athlete's signs and symptoms.

When determining the correlation of the evaluation findings with gait variation, the examiner must determine whether a relationship exists between the forces occurring in each phase of gait and the pathology present for the athlete. Once a static assessment has been completed and the examiner has determined the particular structures that may be involved, the relationships between etiologic factors in anatomical structure, alignment, and function should be identified. Table 8–11 lists common lower extremity injuries defined by etiologic factors.

Deviations in the Gait Cycle

The athlete's gait cycle may be altered to compensate for pain experienced during the normal gait or it may be altered secondary to a mechanical or neurological deficit. Gait deviations may also arise from central nervous system dysfunction, a topic that is outside the scope of this text.

After lower extremity injury, gait deviations occur frequently. The most common of these is an **antalgic gait**, in which the weight is removed as rapidly as possible from the affected limb, shortening the stance phase. This gait pattern is accompanied by a shift in the upper extremity as it attempts to provide a counterbalance to the uneven weight distribution in the lower extremity. The affected limb may be externally rotated to relieve pain during weight bearing, resulting in a unilateral toe-out. The types of injury that result in an antalgic gait are summarized in Table 8–12. The observed deviations in gait occur without conscious effort by the

Table 8–10. Effects of Predisposing Conditions on the Gait Cycle

	Initial Contact	Loading Response	Midstance	Terminal Stance
Decreased dorsiflexion		Increased subtalar pronation		Decreased force at toe-off
		Forefoot abduction	Increased midtarsal joint pronation	
Decreased motion: 1st MTP joint	Altered foot position			Decreased ability to toe-off
Extrinsic leg/thigh muscle weakness			Increased subtalar joint pronation / Increased tibial rotation	Incomplete resupination
			Inability to supinate	Decreased ability to toe-off
		Toe-out		
Hip rotator muscle weakness		Increased rotation of femur and tibia		
Neurological impairment	Inability to dorsiflex		Multiple compensatory changes	Inability to plantarflex
Rearfoot valgus	Increased subtalar pronation		Excessive pronation	Incomplete resupination
	Increased medial foot/leg stresses		Impaired resupination	
Rearfoot varus	Decreased shock absorption	Decreased subtalar pronation	Decreased ability to accommodate	

continued

Table 8–10. Effects of Predisposing Conditions on the Gait Cycle—*Continued*

	Initial Contact	Loading Response	Midstance	Terminal Stance
Hypomobile 1st ray	Altered midfoot and forefoot position	Instability in midtarsal joints and forefoot	Altered distribution of ground reaction forces	Pain and/or decreased force at toe-off
1st ray plantarflexed	1st ray contacts the ground	Decreased subtalar pronation	Decreased ability to absorb shock	Increased force on 1st ray
Forefoot varus		Toe-out / Increased pronation at midtarsal joints		
Forefoot valgus		Decreased ability to absorb shock		Decreased force at toe-off
Tarsal coalition		Decreased subtalar joint motion		
Tibial torsion		Increased compensatory subtalar joint pronation		
Femoral torsion		Toe-in gait / Increased subtalar joint pronation (internal tibial rotation)		
Leg length discrepancy		Compensatory pronation of longer leg / Compensatory supination of shorter leg		
Rapid or prolonged pronation of subtalar joint		Increased medial foot/leg forces / Increased tibial rotation		Decreased ability to toe-off

Table 8–11. Etiologic Factors in Common Lower Extremity Injuries

	Decreased Strength or Neurological Function	Decreased Range of Motion	Variations in Foot Structure and Function	Other Lower Extremity Biomechanical Variations
1st MTP joint pain		Joint motion restriction	1st ray plantarflexed; increases force	
2nd through 5th MTP joint pain	Nerve pressure or entrapment		Forefoot valgus; alters weight-bearing pattern	
Sesamoid fracture		Joint motion restriction	1st ray plantarflexed	
Sesamoiditis				
Metatarsal fracture			Increased midtarsal rigidity and/or foot pronation	
Midtarsal joint pain		Tarsal coalition	Increased metatarsal and/or forefoot motion	
Tarsal tunnel syndrome	Direct trauma to nerve		Excessive pronation	Tibial varum
Plantar fasciitis	Medial extrinsic muscle weakness	Ankle dorsiflexion limited	Rearfoot valgus / Forefoot varus	
Peroneal tendinitis		Ankle dorsiflexion limited	Rearfoot varus / Forefoot valgus	Tibial varum / Genu valgum
Medial tibial stress syndrome	Medial extrinsic muscle weakness	Ankle dorsiflexion limited	Rearfoot valgus / Forefoot varus	Tibial varum
Tibialis posterior tendinitis	Tibialis posterior weakness	Ankle dorsiflexion limited	Rearfoot valgus / Forefoot varus / Navicular subluxation	
Anterior compartment syndrome		Ankle dorsiflexion limited	Flexible: pes planus / Rigid: pes cavus	Hypertrophy of posterior leg musculature / Tibial varum
Tibial stress fracture	Extrinsic leg muscle weakness	Ankle dorsiflexion limited	Hypermobile rear foot, midfoot, forefoot	Tibial varum
Patellofemoral pain	Extrinsic leg and thigh muscle weakness	Tightness in lateral patellofemoral restraints	Rearfoot valgus / Forefoot varus	Tibial torsion / Femoral torsion
Pes anserine bursitis	Extrinsic leg and thigh muscle weakness		Rearfoot valgus / Forefoot varus	Femoral torsion / Genu varum
Patellar tendinitis	Extrinsic leg and thigh muscle weakness	Tightness in lateral patellofemoral restraints	Rearfoot valgus / Forefoot varus	Tibial varum
ITB friction syndrome	Hip rotation weakness	Lack of tensor fasciae latae/iliotibial band flexibility	Rearfoot valgus / Forefoot varus	Tibial varum

Table 8–12. Examples of Antalgic Gait Deviations

Type of Injury	Limitation	Examples
Bone/joint disruption	Pain with weight bearing	Leg, ankle, or foot fractures or dislocations
Ligament injury	Decreased joint stability	Ankle, knee sprains
	Pain with movement	
Overuse syndromes	Pain with function	ITB syndrome, medial tibial stress syndrome, Achilles tendinitis
Muscular weakness	Lack of strength and function	Quadriceps, hip rotators
Muscle tightness	Decreased range of motion	Plantarflexors, hamstring, hip flexors
Periods of immobilization	Decreased strength and range of motion; pain with movement	Ankle immobilization

athlete; rather, they represent the body protecting itself after an injury.

Other conditions, such as muscular weakness or neurological inhibition, may result in characteristic compensatory gait changes. These are defined by their unique deviations in gait (Table 8–13).

Table 8–13. Compensatory Gait Deviations

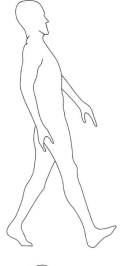

Gluteus Maximus Gait
At initial contact the thorax is thrust posteriorly to maintain hip extension during the stance phase, often causing a lurching of the trunk.
Cause: Weakness or paralysis of the gluteus maximus muscle.

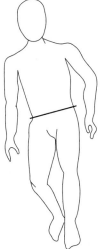

Trendelenburg's Gait (Gluteus Medius Gait)
During the stance phase of the affected limb, the thorax lists toward the uninvolved limb. This serves to maintain the center of gravity and prevent a drop in the pelvis on the affected side.
Cause: Weakness of the gluteus medius muscle.

continued

Table 8–13. Compensatory Gait Deviations—*Continued*

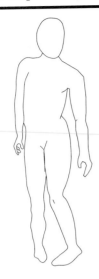

Psoatic Limp
To compensate during the swing phase, lateral rotation and flexion of the trunk occurs with hip adduction. The trunk and pelvic movements are exaggerated.
Cause: Weakness or ***reflex inhibition*** of the psoas major muscle (Legg-Perthes disease).

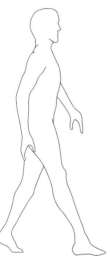

Steppage Gait (Dropfoot)
The foot slaps at initial contact, owing to foot drop. During the swing phase the affected limb demonstrates increased hip and knee flexion to avoid toe dragging, producing a "high-step" pattern.
Cause: Weakness or paralysis of the dorsiflexors.

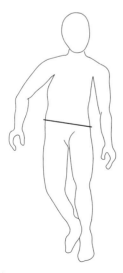

Stiff Knee/Hip Gait
In the swing phase the affected extremity is lifted higher than normal to compensate for knee or hip stiffness. The uninvolved extremity demonstrates increased plantarflexion to accomplish this.
Cause: Knee or hip pathology that results in a decrease in the range of motion.

continued

Reflex inhibition: The inability of a muscle to actively contract secondary to sensory impulses.

Table 8–13. Compensatory Gait Deviations—*Continued*

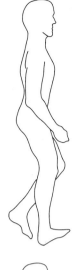

Calcaneal Gait

During the stance phase, increased dorsiflexion and knee flexion occur on the affected side, resulting in a decreased step length.

Cause: Paralysis or weakness of the plantarflexors or painful weight bearing on the forefoot or toes.

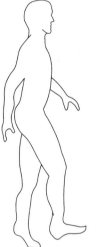

Short Leg Gait

Increased pronation occurs in the subtalar joint of the long leg, accompanied by a shift of the trunk toward the longer extremity.

Cause: True (anatomical) leg length discrepancy. The right (facing) leg is longer.

REFERENCES

1. Nuber, GW: Biomechanics of the foot and ankle during gait. Clin Sports Med 7:1, 1988.
2. Murray, MP: Gait as a total pattern of movement. Am J Phys Med 21:290, 1987.
3. Voight, M, and Tippett, S: Closed-kinetic chain. Presented at the 41st Annual Clinical Symposium of the National Athletic Trainers' Association, Indianapolis, June 12, 1990.
4. Magee, DJ: Lower leg, ankle, and foot. In Magee, DJ: Orthopaedic Physical Assessment, ed 2. WB Saunders, Philadelphia, 1992, p 450.
5. Normal and Abnormal Gait Syllabus. Physical Therapy Department, Rancho Los Amigos Hospital, Downey, CA, 1989.
6. Root, ML, Orient, WP, and Weed, JH: Normal and abnormal function of the foot. Clinical Biomechanics—Vol II. Clinical Biomechanics Corp, Los Angeles, 1977.
6a. Norkin, CC, and Levangie, PK: Joint Structure and Function: A Comprehensive Analysis, ed 2. FA Davis, Philadelphia, 1992.
7. Greenfield, B: Evaluation of overuse syndromes. In Donatelli, R: The Biomechanics of the Foot and Ankle. FA Davis, Philadelphia, 1990, p 153.
8. Donatelli, R, et al: Biomechanical foot orthotics: A retrospective study. Journal of Orthopedic and Sports Physical Therapy 10:205, 1988.
9. Mann, RA: Biomechanics of running. Symposium on the Foot and Leg in Running Sports. CV Mosby, St Louis, 1982, p 1.
10. Donatelli, R: The Biomechanics of the Foot and Ankle, ed 2. FA Davis, Philadelphia, 1996.

9

The Spine

Formed by 33 vertebral segments and divided into four distinct portions, the spinal column provides postural control to the torso and skull, while also protecting the length of the spinal cord. The contradictory needs for range of motion versus protection of the spinal cord are met in varying degrees among the various spinal segments (Fig. 9–1). To provide proper posture, these segments maintain curvatures in the frontal plane.

The cervical spine provides the greatest range of motion, but here the spinal cord is the most vulnerable. The thoracic spine provides the greatest protection of the spinal cord but at the expense of range of motion. The lumbar spine provides an equal balance between protection and range of motion but at the cost of stable muscular balance. The sacrum and coccyx are composed of fused bone. At this level the spinal cord has exited the column and the sacrum's primary function is to affix the spinal column to the pelvis.

Injury to the spine during athletic competition accounts for an estimated 10 to 15 percent of all injuries, with 6 to 10 percent resulting in trauma to the spinal cord or spinal nerve roots.[1] This chapter discusses those conditions affecting the spine that are most likely to be evaluated away from practice and competition. On-field recognition and management of spinal injuries are discussed in Chapter 16, Head and Neck Injuries.

CLINICAL ANATOMY

Figure 9–2 compares the relative sizes of the cervical (n = 7), thoracic (n = 12), and lumbar (n = 5) vertebrae and identifies the bony landmarks. The body's weight is mostly transmitted along the column via the vertebral body, whose size depends on the amount of force it transmits. Carrying only the weight of the head, the vertebral bodies of the cervical vertebrae are much smaller than those of the lumbar vertebrae, which are required to transmit and absorb the weight of the entire torso.

The neural arch, formed by the pedicle and lamina, serves as the protective tunnel through which the spinal cord passes. The laterally projecting **transverse processes** provide an attachment site for the spine's intrinsic muscles, increasing their mechanical advantage. The prominent posterior projections, the **spinous processes**, act as attachment sites for muscles and ligaments. Their angulation relative to the other vertebrae serves to limit extension of the spine.

Arising from the superior and inferior surfaces of the lamina are two sets of articular processes. The superior facets articulate with the inferior facets of the vertebrae immediately above, forming synovial *facet joints* (zygapophyseal joints). The bony arrangement of these joints is such that the lateral portion of the superior facet articulates with the medial portion of the inferior facet. These joints decrease the weight-bearing stress through the vertebral body and disk by widening its base, transmitting 20 percent of the weight-bearing forces through the facet joints.[2] The area connecting the superior and inferior facets, the **pars interarticularis**, is a common site of stress fractures in the lumbar spine.

The anterior portion of the pedicles contains the vertebral notches, concave depressions on the anterior and inferior surfaces of the vertebrae. When matched with contiguous vertebrae, these depressions align to form the **intervertebral foramen**, the space where spinal nerve roots exit the vertebral column (Fig. 9–3).

The relative sizes of the vertebral body and the transverse and spinous processes vary according to their function at each of the spinal levels (Table 9–1). The first two vertebrae of the cervical spine are unique. The first cervical vertebra, the **atlas**, supports the weight of the skull through two concave articular surfaces, forming the **atlanto-occipital joint**. The primary movement at the junction between the atlas and the skull (the C0-C1 articulation) is that of flexion and extension, as when nodding the head "yes." At the C1 level, the transverse processes are exceptionally long and no true spinous process exists. The second cervical vertebra, **the axis**, has a small body with a superior projection, **the dens**. The articulation between the anterior arch

---

Facet joint: An articulation of the facets between each contiguous part of vertebrae in the spinal column.

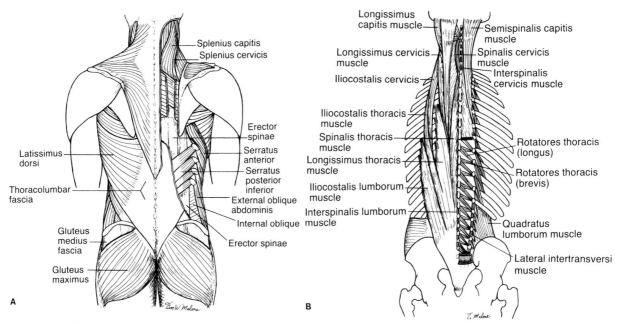

Figure 9–13. Muscles of the spinal column: (A) superficial muscles, (B) deep muscles. (From Norkin, CC, and Levangie, PK,[2a] pp 159–160, with permission.)

Table 9–4. Intrinsic Muscles Acting on the Spinal Column

Muscle	Action	Origin	Insertion	Nerve	Root
Splenius capitis Splenius cervicis	Lateral bending of the cervical spine Rotation of the face toward the same side Extension of the cervical spine	• Lower half of the ligamentum nuchae • Spinous processes of C7 through T6 vertebrae	• Mastoid process of the temporal bone and adjacent occipital bone (capitis portion) • Transverse processes of C2 through C4 vertebrae (cervicis portion)	Branches of cervical nerves (CN)	C4–C8
Iliocostalis lumborum		• Iliac crest	• Inferior angles of ribs 6 through 12	Branches of CN	C4–C8
Iliocostalis thoracis		• Ribs 6 through 12	• Ribs 1 through 6 • Transverse process of C7	Branches of CN	C4–C8
Iliocostalis cervicis		• Ribs 3 through 6	• Transverse processes of C4 through C6	Branches of CN	C4–C8
Longissimus thoracis	Extension of spinal column Lateral bending of spinal column	• Common erector spinae tendon	• Transverse process of T3 through T21 • Ribs 3 through 12	Branches of CN	C4–C8
Longissimus cervicis	Extension of spinal column Lateral bending of spinal column	• Transverse processes of T1 through T5	• Transverse processes of C2 through C6	Branches of CN	C4–C8
Longissimus capitis	Extension of skull and cervical spine Rotation of the face toward the same side	• Articular processes of C5 through C7	• Mastoid process of skull	Branches of CN	C4–C8

Table 9–4. Intrinsic Muscles Acting on the Spinal Column (*Continued*)

Muscle	Action	Origin	Insertion	Nerve	Root
Spinalis thoracis	Extension of the spine Lateral bending of the spine	• Common erector spinae tendon	• Spinous processes of upper thoracic spine	Branches of CN	C4–C8
Spinalis cervicis	Extension of the spine Lateral bending of the spine	• Upper thoracic and lower cervical spinous processes	• Ligamentum nuchae	Branches of CN	C4–C8
Spinalis capitis	Extension of the spine Lateral bending of the spine	• Upper thoracic and lower cervical spinous processes	• Ligamentum nuchae	Branches of CN	C4–C8
Semispinalis thoracis	Extension of thoracic and cervical spine Rotation to the opposite side	• Transverse process	• Travel upwardly and medially to attach to a spinous process 5 or 8 vertebrae above the origin	Deeper stratum of CN	C4–C8
Semispinalis cervicis	Extension of thoracic and cervical spine Rotation to the opposite side	• Transverse process	• Travel upwardly and medially to attach to a spinous process 5 or 8 vertebrae above the origin	Deeper stratum of CN	C4–C8
Semispinalis capitis	Extension of skull Rotation of the opposite side	• Transverse process	• Travel upwardly and medially to attach to a spinous process 5 or 8 vertebrae above the origin	Deeper stratum of CN	C4–C8
Multifidus (or multifidi)	Rotation of spine to the opposite side Stabilization of vertebral column	Lumbar region • Superior aspect of sacrum Thoracic region • Transverse processes Cervical region • Articular processes	• Spinous process	Deeper stratum of CN	C4–C8
Rotatores	Extension of spine Rotation of spine Stabilization of vertebral column	• Transverse process	• Spinous process of the vertebra immediately above the origin	Deeper stratum of CN	C4–C8

trapezius (discussed in Chapter 11) acts to extend and rotate the cervical spine and skull. The **sterno-cleidomastoid** is responsible for rotating the skull to the opposite side and for lateral bending of the cervical spine to the same side (Fig. 9–14). Divided into anterior, middle, and posterior portions, the **scalene** muscle laterally flexes the cervical spine and, when the cervical spine is fixated, elevates the rib cage to assist in inspiration. The scalene is also of importance in that the brachial plexus passes between its anterior and middle portions. Spasming of this muscle can therefore place pressure on the neurovascular structures of the upper extremities.

CLINICAL EVALUATION OF THE SPINE

Because of its important role in protecting the spinal cord and spinal nerve roots, injury to the vertebrae can have catastrophic results. In the event of acute trauma, the primary role of the athletic trainer is to rule out the presence of bony trauma that has, or can, jeopardize the integrity of the spinal cord. Chapter 16 discusses these evaluative procedures. The techniques presented in this chapter assume that vertebral fractures and/or dislocations have been ruled out (Table 9–6).

Table 9–5. Muscles Acting on the Cervical Spinal Column

Muscle	Action	Origin	Insertion	Nerve	Root
Trapezius (upper one-third)	Elevation of scapula Upward rotation of scapula Rotation of the scapula to the opposite side	• Occipital protuberance • Nuchal line of the occipital bone • Upper portion of the ligamentum nuchae • Spinous process of C7	• Distal/lateral one-third of clavicle • Acromion process	Accessory	Cranial nerve XI
Levator scapulae	Elevation Downward rotation Extension of cervical spine	• Transverse processes of cervical vertebrae C1 through C4	• Superior medial angle of scapula	Dorsal subscapular	C3, C4 C5
Sternocleidomastoid	Rotation of the skull to the opposite side Lateral bending of the cervical spine Elevation of the clavicle and sternum	• Medial clavicular head • Lateral border of the sternum	• Mastoid process of the skull	Spinal accessory	CR 11 C2, C3
Scalene, anterior	Lateral bending of the cervical spine Elevation of the rib cage	• Anterior portion of the transverse processes of C3 to C6	• Sternal attachment of the 1st rib	Cervical branches	C6, C7, C8
Scalene, middle	Lateral bending of the cervical spine Elevation of the rib cage	• Anterior portion of the transverse processes of C2 to C7	• Lateral to the insertion of the anterior scalene	Cervical branches	C6, C7, C8
Scalene, posterior	Lateral bending of the cervical spine Elevation of the rib cage	• Anterior portion of the transverse processes C5 and C6	• Medial portion of the 2nd rib	Cervical branches	C6, C7, C8

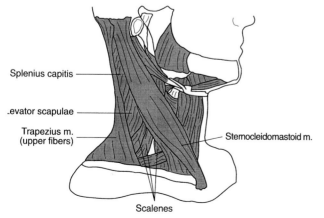

Figure 9–14. Cervical musculature.

History

A good history-taking process is essential to coming to a purposeful evaluation of the athlete with a spinal injury. The onset and identification of functional activities bringing on the athlete's symptoms help determine the underlying pathology.

• **Location of the pain:** Is the pain centralized or does it radiate through the torso or extremities? One must be mindful of the fact that pain radiating through the extremity is the result of impingement or pressure on a nerve anywhere proximal to the area of identified pain.

Table 9–6. Evaluation of the Spine

History	Inspection	Palpation	Functional Tests	Ligamentous Tests	Neurological Tests	Special Tests
Location of the pain	General Inspection	Cervical Spine	Cervical Spine	Spring test for intervertebral disk mobility	Upper Motor Neuron Lesions	Cervical Spine
Onset of the pain	Sagittal curvature	Hyoid bone	Active range of motion		Babinski's test	Brachial plexus pathology
How the spine was injured	Test for scoliosis	Thyroid cartilage	Flexion		Oppenheim's test	Brachial plexus traction test
Consistency of the pain	Frontal curvature	Cricoid cartilage	Extension			Cervical nerve root
Activities or positions that alter the level of symptoms	Observance of gait	Sternocleidomastoid	Lateral flexion		Lower Motor Neuron Lesions	Impingement
	Cervical Spine	Carotid artery	Rotation		Upper quarter screen	Compression test
	Position of the head on the shoulders	Lymph nodes	Passive range of motion		Lower quarter screen	Distraction test
	Bilateral soft tissue parison	Occiput	Flexion			Spurling test
Bowel or bladder signs		Spinous processes	Extension			Shoulder abduction test
Prior history of spinal injury	Level of the shoulders	Transverse processes	Lateral flexion			Vertebral artery test
		Trapezius	Rotation			
	Thoracic Spine	Thoracic Spine	Resisted range of motion			Thoracic and Lumbar Spine
	Breathing patterns	Bony palpation	Flexion			Muscle strain
	Bilateral comparison of skinfolds	Spinous processes	Extension			Sciatica
		Costovertebral junction	Lateral flexion			Straight leg-raise test
	Lumbar Spine	Soft tissue palpation	Rotation			Tension sign
	General movement and posture	Trapezius	Trunk			Intervertebral disk lesions
	Lordotic curve	Lumbar Spine	Active range of motion			Well straight leg-raising test
	Standing posture	Paravertebrals	Flexion			Valsalva's test
		Spinous processes	Extension			Milgram test
		Step-off deformity	Lateral bending			Kernig's test
		Soft tissue palpation	Rotation			Beevor's sign
		Sacrum and Pelvis	Passive range of motion			Femoral nerve stretch
		Posterior superior iliac spine	Flexion			Hoover test
		Iliac crests	Extension			Spondylopathies
		Pubic symphisis	Rotation			Spondylolysis
		Greater trochanter	Side gliding			Spondylolisthesis
		Ischial tuberosity	Resisted range of motion			Single-leg stance test
		Gluteals	Flexion			
		Sciatic nerve	Extension			
			Rotation			
			Lateral bending			

• **Onset of the pain:** Does the athlete describe an acute, chronic, or insidious onset of pain and other symptoms?

• **How was the spine injured?** The examiner should determine the mechanism of injury—flexion, extension, lateral bending, or rotation—in order to identify the structures possibly involved. A direct blow to the lumbar or thoracic area may cause a contusion of the involved structures or lead to a contusion of the kidneys.

• **Consistency of the pain:** Is the athlete's pain constant or intermittent? Constant pain is indicative of chemical and/or mechanical forces being placed on the intervertebral disk or spinal nerve root, with pain of chemical origin decreasing in proportion to the decrease in inflammatory response. Pain arising from a mechanical force varies with different positions and movements but never completely subsides. Intermittent pain is relieved by placing the spine in different anatomical positions, suggesting relief of an impingement on the neurological structures.

• **Activities or positions that alter the level of symptoms:** Pain produced during the activities of daily living provides valuable evidence of the cause of the athlete's pain and other activities that may reproduce the pain (Table 9–7).

• **Bowel or bladder signs:** Increased frequency or *incontinence* (cauda equina syndrome) is suggestive of lower nerve root lesions. These signs warrant the immediate referral to a physician.

• **Prior history of spinal injury:** The examiner should identify any pertinent past history that may lead to structural degeneration or predispose the athlete to chronic problems. The athlete's current symptoms may be the result of the build-up of scar tissue that is impinging and/or restricting other structures.

Inspection

A general inspection of the entire spinal column should be made for all problems involving this area to determine alignment in the sagittal and frontal planes. The muscles of the spinal column and torso should be inspected to determine the presence of spasm or atrophy, each indicating a possible irritation of one or more spinal nerve roots. Last, finite inspection of each spinal segment as well as the individual vertebra may provide an indication of a malalignment of one vertebra relative to the ones above and below it.

• **General inspection**
  ◦ **Sagittal curvature:** The alignment of the lumbar, thoracic, and cervical vertebrae should be inspected with the athlete lying prone and while weight bearing. Normally this alignment should be straight. Lateral curvature of the spinal column, **scoliosis**, generally afflicts the thoracic and/or lumbar spine (Fig. 9–15). Scoliosis may be visible when the athlete is weight bearing, non–weight bearing, or both. Subtle scoliosis may be detected by having the athlete flex the spine while weight bearing (Fig. 9–16). Athletes suspected of having previously undiagnosed scoliosis should be referred to a physician for further evaluation.

Table 9–7. Ramifications of Spinal Pain Exhibited During the Activities of Daily Living

Activity	Ramifications
Bending	Pain is worsened with flexion exercises.
Sitting	Pain may be worsened with flexion exercises.
Rising from sitting	This motion causes changes in the interdiskal forces. Sharp pain suggests derangement of the disk.
Standing	The spine is placed in extension. Pain worsens as the spine is further extended.
Walking	The amount of spinal extension increases as the speed of gait increases.
Lying prone	The spine is placed in, or near, full extension.
Lying supine	When lying supine on a hard surface the amount of extension is maintained. When lying on a soft surface the spine falls into flexion.

Test for Scoliosis (Fig. 9–16)

Position of athlete	Standing. The hands are held in front with the arms straight.
Position of examiner	Seated in front of or behind the athlete.
Evaluative procedure	The athlete bends forward with the hands together.
Positive test results	An asymmetrical hump is observed along the lateral aspect of the thoracolumbar spine.
Implications	Spinal scoliosis is suggested.

Incontinence: A loss of bowel and/or bladder control.

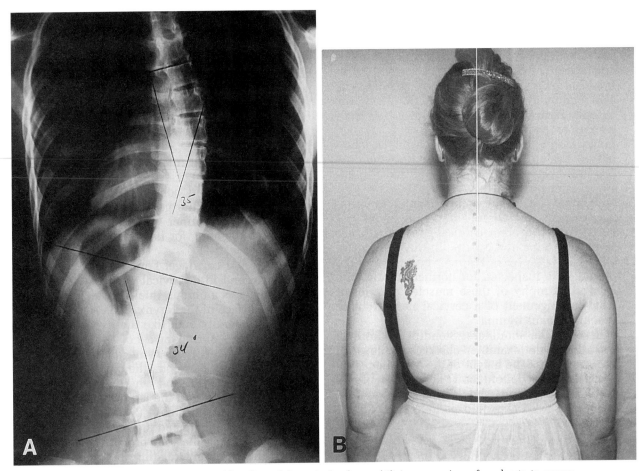

Figure 9–15. Scoliosis, lateral bending of the spinal column. (*A*) An x-ray view of moderate to severe scoliosis. (*B*) Subtle scoliosis. Dots have been placed over the spinous processes.

○ **Frontal curvature:** While viewing the athlete from the side, the examiner watches for the normal presence of the lordotic cervical curvature, the kyphotic thoracic curve, and a lordotic curve in the lumbar area. Changes in any of these curves may produce stress on spinal structures, leading to pain and dysfunction.

○ **Observation of gait:** Spinal pain may grossly influence the athlete's walking and running gait. Common gait deviations resulting from spinal pain include a "slouched," shuffling, or shortened gait. Chapter 8 provides detailed discussion regarding gait analysis. Additionally, the athlete may display an unwillingness to move the body as a whole.

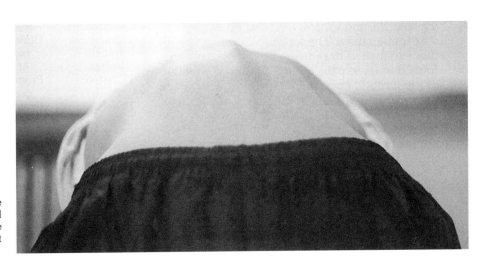

Figure 9–16. Test for the presence of scoliosis. View the flexed spinal column from the rear. Note the hump formation of the athlete's left side, indicating scoliosis.

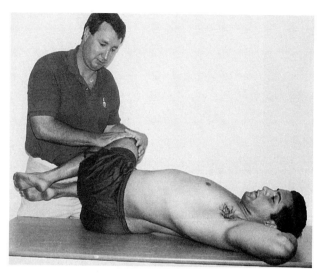

Figure 9–32. Passive trunk rotation.

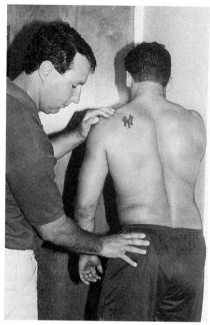

Figure 9–33. Passive lateral glide of the trunk. The athlete's shoulder is stabilized against the wall while the examiner forces the pelvis laterally.

- **Resisted range of motion**
  ○ **Flexion:** To determine the strength of the abdominal muscles, the athlete lies supine with the knees flexed and the feet flat on the table. With the athlete's hands interlocked behind the head, resistance is provided to the chest as the athlete attempts to lift the scapula off the table (Fig. 9–34A).
  ○ **Extension:** The strength of the spinal erector muscles is determined with the athlete prone, arms outstretched above the head or with the hands interlocked behind the head. While stabilizing the lower lumbar region, resistance is provided to the upper portion of the thoracic spine as the athlete attempts to lift the head, chest, and arms off the table (Fig. 9–34B).
  ○ **Rotation:** The position and procedure for testing the abdominal obliques are the same as for the trunk flexors, except the athlete attempts to lift one shoulder off the table and bring it toward the contralateral knee (Fig. 9–35).
  ○ **Lateral bending:** Resisted testing of flexion and rotation also checks the integrity of those muscles responsible for lateral bending.

Ligamentous Tests

There are no tests to check the integrity of single isolated ligaments. Clues to the presence of ligamentous pathology arise during the passive testing of the spine's range of motion (Table 9–9). However, these results may easily be confused with pain caused by intervertebral disk lesions or pathology to the nerve roots or peripheral nerves.

Sprains to the spinal ligaments are relatively rare events and tend to occur more frequently in the cervical spine because of its increased range of motion. The conclusion of a ligamentous sprain is generally derived by excluding the possibility of other pathologies. If all other pathology has been ruled out and pain is localized along the spinal column, it may be assumed that a sprain has occurred.

While it is impossible to check the amount of motion that occurs at each individual spinal segment, the accessory movement of the segment can be grossly determined. Each vertebral junction should have a small amount of movement, or "spring," to it. Hypomobility or hypermobility of these joints can potentially cause pain along the spinal column.

Test for Intervertebral Disk Mobility

The total range of motion available to the spinal column is equal to the sum of the motions between any two contiguous vertebrae. In order for the full range of motion to be available to the spinal column, each pair of vertebrae must have the full range of motion. The spring test for intervertebral disk mobility is used to determine adhesions of the vertebrae (Fig. 9–36).

Spring Test for Intervertebral Disk Mobility

Position of athlete	Prone.
Position of examiner	Standing over the athlete with the thumbs placed over the spinous processes to be tested.
Evaluative procedure	The examiner carefully pushes the spinous process anteriorly, feeling for the springing of the vertebrae.
Positive test results	The vertebrae do not move or spring.
Implications	Hypomobility of the vertebrae, especially at the facet joints.

Neurological Examination

Because of the close involvement of the spinal column to the spinal cord and its nerve roots, many of the maladies affecting the spine may result in decreased neurological function in the extremities as well as the trunk. Clinically, this involvement can be determined through the use of manual muscle tests, deep tendon reflexes, and sensory testing. Any

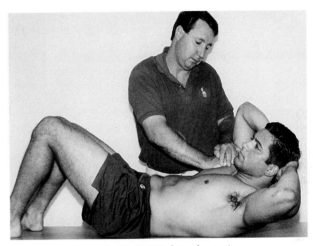

Figure 9–35. Resisted trunk rotation.

positive test results elicited during the neurological examination warrant the termination of the evaluation and the immediate referral of the athlete to a physician. Chapter 16 discusses the management of acute spinal injuries.

Table 9–9. Spinal Ligaments Stressed During Passive Range of Motion Testing

Motion	Ligaments Stressed
Flexion	Posterior longitudinal ligament
	Supraspinous ligament (thoracic and lumbar spine)
	Ligamentum nuchae (cervical spine)
	Interspinous ligament
	Ligamentum flavum
Extension	Anterior longitudinal ligament
Rotation	Interspinous ligament
	Ligamentum flavum
Lateral bending (these tests are usually inconclusive)	Interspinous ligament
	Ligamentum flavum

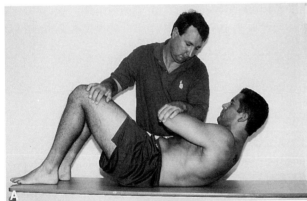

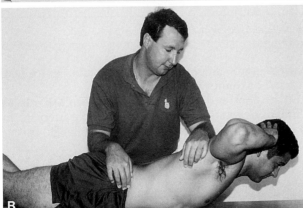

Figure 9–34. Resisted trunk (A) flexion and (B) extension.

Upper Motor Neuron Lesions

Trauma such as closed head injury or disease states of the brain or spinal cord above the anterior horn can result in *hyperreflexia*, spasticity, and hypertonicity of muscles, weakness of the muscles innervated distal to the lesion, and ataxia. Other clinical findings of this condition may include muscle tremor and uncontrollable involuntary movement. In the athletic population, upper motor neuron lesions most often are the result of head injury, and Babinski's and Oppenheim's tests are used to determine their presence.

Babinski's Test

Used to determine the presence of upper motor neuron lesions, especially in the pyramidal tract, Babinski's test involves a blunt object stroked along the lateral aspect of the foot's plantar surface to elicit a response (Fig. 9–37). A negative, or normal, Babinski's test result causes flexion of the great toe. In the presence of an upper motor neuron lesion, the great toe extends and the lateral four toes spread, deeming the test result positive. This test yields a positive result in newborns but rapidly diminishes shortly after birth.

Babinski's Test (Fig. 9–37)

Position of athlete	Supine.
Position of examiner	At the foot of the athlete. A blunt device, such as the handle of a reflex hammer or the handle of a pair of scissors, is needed.
Evaluative procedure	The examiner runs the device up the plantar aspect of the foot, making an arc from the calcaneus to the ball of the great toe.
Positive test results	The great toe extends while the other toes splay.
Implications	Upper motor neuron lesion. This may be caused by brain trauma or pathology.
Comments	Babinski's reflex occurs normally in newborns and should spontaneously disappear shortly after birth.

Oppenheim's Test

Oppenheim's test is used to determine the hypersensitivity of nerve endings by running the fingernail along the tibial crest (Fig. 9–38). In the presence of an upper motor neuron lesion, the athlete describes an inordinate amount of pain and a toe response resembling Babinski's test.

Oppenheim's Test (Fig. 9–38)

Position of athlete	Supine.
Position of examiner	At the athlete's side.
Evaluative procedure	The examiner's fingernail is run along the crest of the anteromedial tibia.
Positive test results	The great toe extends while the other toes splay or the athlete reports hypersensitivity to the test.
Implications	Upper motor neuron lesion. This may be caused by brain trauma or pathology.

Lower Motor Neuron Lesions

Lower motor neuron trauma to the cells of the anterior horn of the spinal cord, spinal nerve roots, or the peripheral nervous system results in *hyporeflexia*, flaccidity of the muscles, and deinnervation atrophy. In athletics, this condition most often results from compression or stretching of the nerves.

Lower motor neuron injuries may include neurapraxia, axonotmesis, or neurotmesis.

The upper and lower quarter screens provide an efficient evaluation for neurological function in the extremities. The screens use manual muscle testing, sensory testing, and deep tendon reflexes to assess neurological function.

Hyperreflexia: Increased action of the reflexes.
Hyporeflexia: A diminished or absent reflex response.

Upper Quarter Neurological Screen

Nerve Root Level	Sensory Testing	Motor Testing	Reflex Testing
C5	Axillary n.	Axillary n.	Biceps brachii
C6	Musculocutaneous n.	Musculocutaneous n.(C5 & C6)	Brachioradialis
C7	Radial n.	Radial n.	Triceps brachii
C8	Ulnar n. (mixed)	Median & palm. interosseous n.	None
T1	Med. brachial cutaneous n.	None	None

Lower Quarter Neurological Screen

Nerve Root Level	Sensory Testing	Motor Testing	Reflex Testing
L1		Lumbar plexus	None
L2		Femoral n.	Partial
L3		Femoral n.	Partial
L4		Femoral n.	Patellar t.
L5		Semitendinosus Semimembranosus - Tibial n.	None
S1		Biceps femoris - Tibial n.	None

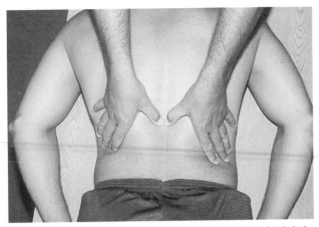

Figure 9–36. Spring test for mobility of the intervertebral disks. This test is positive when the examiner fails to elicit vertebral movement.

Pathologies and Related Special Tests

The structure and function of the spinal column exposes it and its supportive structures to almost constant stress. In addition to the contact forces re-

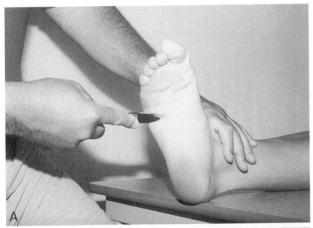

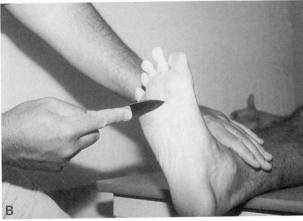

Figure 9–37. Babinski's test for upper motor neuron lesions. (*A*) A negative Babinski's test results in toe flexion. (*B*) A positive Babinski's test results in extension of the great toe and spreading of the lateral four toes. This test should be used for suspected brain trauma.

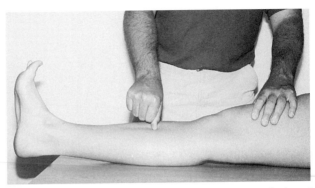

Figure 9–38. Oppenheim's test for upper motor neuron lesion. A positive test results in splaying of the toes as described for Babinski's test.

lated to athletic competition, movement of the torso results in shear forces across the column, while sitting or standing upright places an axial load on these structures. Even lying down can result in dysfunction if the surface is too hard or too yielding.

These facts notwithstanding, the spinal column displays an enormous capability to adapt to the forces placed on it. When the spinal column is unable to adapt, injury occurs. This section describes noncatastrophic injury to the cervical, thoracic, and lumbar spine. The tests presented in this section should be performed only after having ruled out the presence of a vertebral fracture or dislocation.

Cervical Spine Pathologies

Acute injuries to the cervical spine occur with relative frequency in contact and collision sports by being compressed or forced past its normal range of motion. The "whiplash" type of injury occurs as the athlete's head is moving in one direction and the cervical muscles eccentrically contract to counter this motion. Chronic conditions develop from poor postural habits, repetitive movements, decreased flexibility, and muscular insufficiency. These conditions worsen with time secondary to the adaptive shortening of tissues, resulting in increased pain and spasm. Certain disease states such as viral infections, allergic reactions to medication, and other diseases may mimic the symptoms of traumatic injury to the cervical spine.[8]

In evaluating cervical pathologies, the presence of any potentially catastrophic injuries must first be ruled out. The examiner must be thorough in evaluating the local cervical structures as well as determining any effect the pathology may be causing distally through the radiation of signs and symptoms.

Brachial Plexus Pathology

Acute trauma to the brachial plexus, often referred to as a "burner" or "stinger," is common in contact sports. The onset of this injury may be

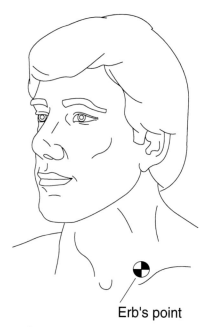

Erb's point

Figure 9–39. Erb's point, representing the most superficial passage of the brachial plexus. Pressure to this area can result in pain and paresthesia radiating into the upper extremity.

caused by a traction force placed on the brachial plexus itself (**brachial plexus stretch**) or an impingement of the cervical nerve roots (**brachial plexus pinch**). With football players, the brachial plexus may be traumatized by compression of the brachial plexus between the shoulder pad and the superior medial scapula and is more common in defensive players.[9,10] This site, **Erb's point**, is located 2 to 3 cm above the clavicle in front of the transverse process of the sixth cervical vertebra and represents the most superficial passage of the brachial plexus (Fig. 9–39).

Stretching of the brachial plexus occurs when the head is forced laterally while the opposite shoulder is depressed, such as when tackling in football (Fig. 9–40). The resulting force places traction on the nerves on the side opposite the lateral bending of the neck. A brachial plexus pinch occurs on the side toward the bending of the neck when the nerve roots are impinged between the vertebrae.

The signs and symptoms of any type of brachial plexus pathology are similar. The athlete suffers immediate pain, often described as "burning" or "an electrical shock" radiating through the upper extremity. Characteristically, the athlete leaves the field with the involved arm dangling limply at the side. Manual muscle testing reveals decreased strength on the involved side (Table 9–10). These signs and symptoms may subside within minutes or take days and even weeks to resolve.

Athletes must not be allowed to return to competition until all symptoms have cleared. A bilateral handshake is used to make a gross determination of the athlete's grip strength (Fig. 9–41). Athletes suffering from chronic brachial plexus trauma display a dropped shoulder and atrophy of the shoulder and cervical musculature on the involved side and note a decrease in bench press weight.[9]

The likelihood of the impingement mechanism (brachial plexus pinch) is increased in athletes having a narrowing of the intervertebral foramen (spinal stenosis).[12] A positive Spurling test result (described later in this chapter) is evidence of spinal stenosis, degenerative disk disease, or an asymmetric disk bulge as displayed with an MRI.[12]

Despite the presence of a common set of symptoms, the examiner must not become complacent to the possibility of more severe cervical trauma. A thorough examination of the cervical spine must be undertaken to rule out the presence of a cervical fracture or dislocation. Once these conditions have been ruled out, the brachial plexus traction test may be used to duplicate the mechanism of injury and reproduce the athlete's symptoms. Additionally, many of the special tests described in the following Cervical Nerve Root Impingement section also produce positive results for the presence of brachial plexus pathology.

Brachial Plexus Traction Test

This test attempts to duplicate the traction force placed on the athlete's brachial plexus by laterally bending the cervical spine and depressing the opposite shoulder (Fig. 9–42). Symptoms may be reproduced in the arm opposite the direction of the bending of the cervical spine, indicating a brachial plexus stretch. Reproduction of pain on the side toward the lateral bending represents a duplication of the mechanism for a brachial plexus pinch (see top of page 281).

Cervical Nerve Root Impingement

Degenerative disk changes, acute disk trauma, or exostosis of the cervical nerve root foramina and/or inflammation can result in pressure being placed on one or more cervical nerve roots. This pressure results not only in pain and spasm in the cervical region but also pain, paresthesia, muscular weakness, altered reflexes, and atrophy in the region supplied by the involved root (Table 9–11).

The following special tests are not to be used in the evaluation of an acute cervical injury until the possibility of a fracture or dislocation has been ruled out.

Compression Test

Pressure being placed on a cervical nerve root from degeneration or narrowing of the neural foramen can be detected through the compression test. The exam-

Brachial Plexus Traction Test (Fig. 9–42)

Position of athlete	Seated.
Position of examiner	Standing behind the athlete. One hand is placed on the side of the athlete's head; the other hand is placed over the acromioclavicular joint.
Evaluative procedure	The cervical spine is laterally bent and the opposite shoulder is depressed.
Positive test results	Pain radiating through the upper arm.
Implications	Pain on the side opposite the lateral bending: stretching of the brachial plexus. Pain on the side toward the lateral bending: pinching of the cervical nerve roots between two vertebrae.
Comments	This test should not be performed until the possibility of a cervical fracture or dislocation has been ruled out.

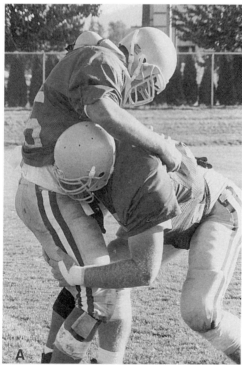

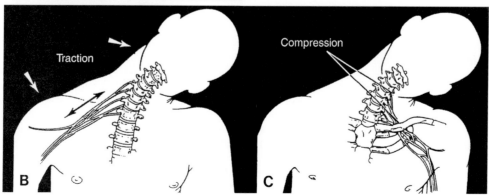

Figure 9–40. Mechanism for a brachial plexus injury. (*A*) The cervical spine is forced laterally and the opposite shoulder is depressed, resulting in elongation of the trapezius and brachial plexus. (*B*) Elongation of the trapezius muscle with concurrent depression of the shoulder can result in a traction injury to the brachial plexus. (*C*) Compression (impingement) of the brachial plexus can result on the side toward which the head is tilted. (Figures *B* and *C* from Vereschagin, KS,[10] with permission.)

Table 9–10. Evaluative Findings of Brachial Plexus Trauma

Examination Segment	Clinical Findings		
History	Onset:	Acute.	
	Location of pain:	Trapezius and deltoid, radiating through the arm.	
	Mechanism:	Brachial plexus stretch: Lateral bending of the cervical spine and depression of the opposite shoulder, resulting in tension on the brachial plexus. Symptoms occur on the side opposite the lateral bend.	
		Brachial plexus pinch: Lateral bending of the cervical spine, resulting in the entrapment of the cervical nerve roots. Symptoms occur on the side toward the lateral bend.	
Inspection	The involved arm hangs limply at the athlete's side.		
	The cervical spine should be inspected for signs of a cervical fracture or dislocation.		
Palpation	Cervical spine, to rule out the possibility of a vertebral fracture or dislocation.		
Functional tests	Initially, active range of motion is diminished and the athlete is unable to complete a manual muscle test. Motor function should begin to return minutes after the onset of injury.		
	Resisted range of motion should be equal in both arms prior to allowing the athlete to return to competition. The dual handshake may be used to measure upper body strength.		
Ligamentous tests	Not applicable.		
Neurological tests	A complete upper quarter screen should be performed to identify the involved cervical nerve roots.		
	All sensory, motor, and reflex test results should be normal and equal prior to allowing the athlete to return to competition.		
Special tests	Brachial plexus stretch tests; cervical compression and distraction tests and Spurling test.		
Comments	The presence of a cervical fracture or dislocation must be ruled out before initiating the tests for brachial plexus pathology.		

iner attempts to compress the cervical vertebrae together by applying a downward force on the skull, placing pressure on one or more cervical nerve roots (Fig. 9–43). In the presence of pathology, the athlete's pain is duplicated. The distribution of the pain pattern is then used to identify the level of the nerve root involved (see bottom of this page).

Distraction Test

This test is used in cases when the athlete has constant cervical pain as well as pain radiating from the cervical spine. Manual traction to the skull separates the cervical vertebrae, relieving any pressure placed on the nerve roots (Fig. 9–44). The distraction is also used as a gross determinant of an individual's response to traction therapy (see top of page 283).

Spurling Test

The Spurling test is a modification of the cervical compression test. The athlete's head is laterally flexed and extended to one side and a compressive force is placed along the cervical spine (Fig. 9–45). A positive test result causes pain to radiate into the arm of the flexed side. This test is very useful in differentiating symptoms that radiate to the upper extremity from local pathology to that extremity (see middle of page 283).

Shoulder Abduction Test

Athletes suffering from cervical nerve root compression or **herniation** of a cervical disk describe a decrease in the symptoms when performing the shoulder abduction test[13] (Fig. 9–46) (see bottom of page 283).

Cervical Compression Test (Fig. 9–43)

Position of athlete	Sitting.
Position of examiner	Standing behind the athlete with hands interlocked over the top of the athlete's head.
Evaluative procedure	The examiner presses down on the crown of the athlete's head.
Positive test results	The athlete experiences pain in the upper cervical spine and/or upper extremity.
Implications	Compression of the facet joints and/or neural foramina, causing pain.

Herniation: The protrusion of a tissue through the wall that normally contains it.

Cervical Distraction Test (Fig. 9–44)

Position of athlete	Supine to relax the postural muscles of the cervical spine.
Position of examiner	Seated at the head of the athlete with one hand under the occiput and the other on top of the forehead, stabilizing the head.
Evaluative procedure	The examiner applies traction on the head, causing distraction of the cervical spine.
Positive test results	The athlete's symptoms are relieved or reduced.
Implications	Compression of the cervical facet joints and/or stenosis of the neural foramina.

Spurling's Test (Fig. 9–45)

Position of athlete	Seated.
Position of examiner	Standing behind the athlete with the hands interlocked over the crown of the athlete's head.
Evaluative procedure	The athlete extends and laterally bends the cervical spine. A compressive force is then placed along the cervical spine.
Positive test results	Pain radiating down the athlete's arm.
Implications	Nerve root impingement by narrowing of the neural foramina.

Shoulder Abduction Test (Fig. 9–46)

Position of athlete	Seated.
Position of examiner	Standing in front of the athlete.
Evaluative procedure	The athlete actively abducts the arm so that the hand is resting on top of the head.
Positive test results	Decrease in the athlete's symptoms.
Implications	Herniated disk or nerve root compression.

Vertebral Artery Test

A test for *patency* of the vertebral artery, the vertebral artery test determines whether there is potential for *claudication* and interruption of the blood flow to the brain (Fig. 9–47). Dizziness or an uncontrolled side-to-side movement of the eyes (nystagmus) indicates an impingement of the cervical arteries.[14] A positive test result precludes further evaluation and treatment of the cervical spine until the athlete is properly evaluated by a physician for occlusion of the vertebral arteries (see top of page 284).

Thoracic and Lumbar Spine Pathologies

Thoracic and lumbar spine injuries historically have not received much attention in the evalua-tion and treatment of athletic injuries. In part this is because of a low incidence of these injuries as well as the fact that most athletic injuries in this area are strains and tend to be self-limiting.[15] The majority of lumbar injuries tend to occur during conditioning and practice and initially may go unreported by the athlete. Although catastrophic injury is possible with any spinal injury, catastrophic injuries involving the lumbar spine are rare.

The evaluation of back injuries relies on a thorough, accurate history that provides the examiner with a reasonable expectation of any pathology that is present in the athlete. A standardized physical evaluation is used to corroborate the findings from the athlete's history.

Patency: The state of being freely open.
Claudication: Intermittent lameness and limping.

Vertebral Artery Test (Fig. 9–47)

Position of athlete	Supine.
Position of examiner	Seated at the head of the athlete. One hand is placed under the occiput and the other stabilizes the forehead.
Evaluative procedure	The examiner passively extends and laterally flexes the cervical spine. The head is then rotated toward the laterally flexed side. During this procedure the examiner should monitor the athlete's pupillary activity.
Positive test results	Dizziness or nystagmus.
Implications	Occlusion of the cervical vertebral arteries.
Comments	Athletes with a positive test result should be referred to a physician before any other evaluative tests are performed or a rehabilitation plan is implemented and before being allowed to return to competition.

Muscle Strain

The athlete suffering from a strain of the spine's intrinsic musculature describes pain and stiffness but is often unable to identify a single incident that caused the injury. The pain caused by this injury tends to be localized without the symptoms radiating into the extremities, and results of the special tests for disk involvement and the neurological examination are negative. The athlete is observed as functioning with stiff, deliberate movements. Active and passive range of motion is limited by pain during flexion, and active movement back to extension also produces pain. Resisted range of motion results in decreased strength and, potentially, an increase in the athlete's symptoms.

Sciatica

Sciatica is a general term for any inflammation involving the sciatic nerve. The term does not speak to the actual pathology that is insulting the nerve and causing the inflammation. Whenever possible, this term should be avoided and the cause of the irritation should be determined. The evaluation of the athlete with sciatica should center on determining the cause of the inflammatory condition so that an adequate treatment plan can be developed.

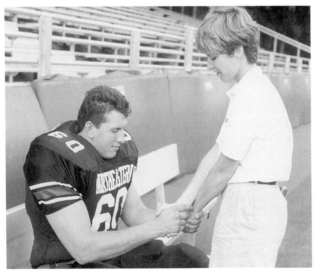

Figure 9–41. Method for determining gross bilateral strength of the upper extremity. The examiner checks the grip strength while the athlete resists extension of the arms.

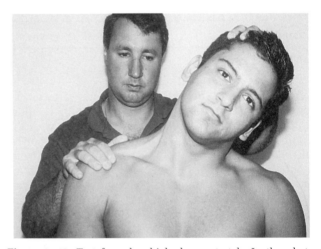

Figure 9–42. Test for a brachial plexus stretch. In the photograph, the examiner attempts to duplicate the mechanism of injury and replicate the athlete's symptoms. Pain radiates down the athlete's right shoulder when a traction injury exists and down the athlete's left shoulder when a compression injury exists. This test should be duplicated in each direction and should not be performed until the possibility of bony trauma has been ruled out.

Table 9–11. Evaluative Findings of Lumbar Nerve Root Compression/Disk Degeneration

Examination Segment	Clinical Findings
History	Onset: A single acute episode or insidious onset. Location of pain: Low back and buttocks; may radiate to the thigh, calf, heel, and foot. Mechanism: Stressful flexed position of lumbar spine or a high load change in position.
Inspection	The gait is slow. The lumbar spine is flattened Changes in position are guarded and painful.
Palpation	Spasm of the musculature may be revealed.
Functional tests	Range of motion is limited by pain in all directions. The athlete may list to one side during spinal flexion. The examiner should determine if motion in one direction increases the symptoms in the lower extremity. Motion that decreases symptoms may be useful in the treatment of the athlete.
Ligamentous tests	Not applicable.
Neurological tests	Lower quarter screen may produce muscular weakness, paresthesia, and diminished deep tendon reflexes in the involved nerve root distribution.
Special tests	Straight leg raising, well straight leg raising, Milgram test, sciatic and femoral nerve tension tests.

Straight Leg-Raise Test

One of the most commonly used special tests for sciatic nerve pathology, the straight leg-raise test (also referred to as Lasègue's test) is used to deter-mine whether tension of, or pressure on, the sciatic nerve is the cause of pain (Fig. 9–48).[16–21]

Straight Leg-Raise Test (Fig. 9–48)

Position of athlete	Supine.
Position of examiner	At the athlete's side that is to be tested. One hand grasps under the heel while the other is placed on the anterior knee to keep it in full extension during the examination.
Evaluative procedure	While keeping the knee in extension the examiner raises the leg by flexing the hip until discomfort is experienced or the full range of motion is obtained.
Positive test results	The athlete complains of pain prior to the end of the normal range of motion (80°). The pain may be described as radiating distally along the tested leg, usually in the posterior thigh, radiating into the calf, and perhaps the foot.
Implications	Sciatic nerve irritation.
Modification	After pain is experienced, the leg is lowered to the point at which the pain stops. The examiner passively dorsiflexes the ankle and/or has the athlete flex the cervical spine. Serving to stretch the dura mater, the spinal cord's outer layering, this flexion recreates the athlete's symptoms. If the athlete's prior pain was caused by tight hamstrings, this modification does not elicit pain.

Tension Sign

This test attempts to duplicate the pain caused by traction on the sciatic nerve. The examiner passively flexes the athlete's hip and passively extends the knee, putting tension on the sciatic nerve (Fig. 9–49). In the presence of sciatic nerve irritation, pain is reproduced in the lower extremity (see top of page 286).

Femoral Nerve Stretch

The femoral nerve stretch test determines impingement of the L2, L3, or L4 nerve roots and should be used when the athlete complains of upper lumbar pain with symptoms radiating through the dermatomes of these nerve roots (Fig. 9–56).

Femoral Nerve Stretch Test (Fig. 9–56)

Position of athlete	Prone with a pillow under the lumbar spine or side-lying.
Position of examiner	At the side of the athlete.
Evaluative procedure	The examiner passively extends the hip while keeping the knee flexed to 90°.
Positive test results	Pain is elicited in the anterior and lateral thigh.
Implications	Nerve root impingement at the L2, L3, or L4 level.
Comments	The examiner should attempt to fully flex the knee with the hip in the neutral position to determine any strain of the quadriceps muscle.

The Hoover Test

By their very nature, lumbopelvic disorders are difficult to objectively evaluate, forcing the clinician to rely on subjective data from the athlete. On occasion an athlete may overstate the quantity of pain and dysfunction associated with an injury. The Hoover test[26-28] is a classic procedure used to determine whether an athlete is malingering during the performance of functional and special tests (Fig. 9–57).

Hoover Test (Fig. 9–57)

Position of athlete	Supine.
Position of examiner	At the feet of the athlete. The evaluator's hands are cupping the calcaneus of each leg.
Evaluative procedure	The athlete attempts an active straight leg raise on the involved side.
Positive test results	The athlete does not attempt to lift the leg and/or the examiner does not sense pressure from the uninvolved leg pressing down on the hand as should instinctively happen.
Implications	The athlete probably is not attempting to perform the test (i.e., malingering).

Spondylopathies

Bony disorders of the spinal column, spondylopathies, can afflict athletes of any age and sport. The etiology may be traced to overmobility of the spine, disease states, or acute trauma, but a stress reaction leading to a fracture is the most prevalent bony injury to the spine in athletes.[29] These defects, caused by repetitive forced hyperextension such as that experienced by football linemen, gymnasts, and cheerleaders, most commonly occur at the L4-L5 or L5-S1 levels but may occur anywhere along the spinal column. Table 9–13 presents an encapsulated description of the most frequently seen spondylopathies in athletes.

Spondylolysis

Spondylolysis is a defect in the pars interarticularis, the area of the vertebral arch between the inferior and superior articular facets, usually brought on by repetitive stress and occurring bilaterally or unilaterally. Bilateral defects in the pars interarticularis result in the posterior portion of the vertebra's becoming separated from the vertebral body, with the posterior fragment consisting of the laminae, inferior articular surfaces, and spinous process.[30] This defect, when seen on a posterior oblique x-ray view, appears as a "collared Scotty dog" deformity, with the area of the stress fracture representing the dog's collar (Fig. 9–58).

The athlete presents with localized low back pain that is increased during and after activity. On observation there is usually normal spinal alignment. Active range of motion is normal for flexion, but pain restricts extension. Results of special tests and neurological tests are normal. The evaluative findings of advanced spondylolysis resemble those of spondylolisthesis.

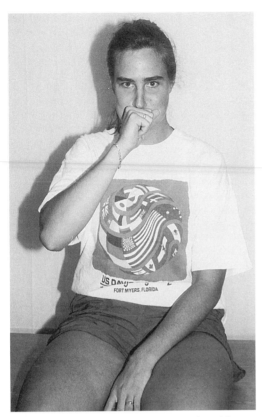

Figure 9–52. Modification of Valsalva's test. The athlete attempts to blow air into a closed fist.

Spondylolisthesis

Spondylolysis may progress to spondylolisthesis, in which the defects in both elements of the pars interarticularis result in the separation of the vertebra into two uniquely identifiable structures. The fixation between the affected vertebra and the one below it is lost, resulting in the superior vertebra sliding anteriorly, and possibly inferiorly, on the one below it (Fig. 9–59). An x-ray examination of this condition reveals a "decapitated Scotty dog" deformity, in which the head of the dog, the anterior element of the vertebra, has become detached from the body, the posterior element (Fig. 9–60).

Age and gender appear to have a strong predisposing influence to the onset of spondylolisthesis. Also, young gymnasts have an incidence of pars interarticularis defects that is four times higher than that of the average population.[23] The athlete with spondylolisthesis has a history and physical presentation that is very similar to that of an athlete with spondylolysis. The pain may be more intense and is likely to be more constant. On observation and with palpation, an actual "step-off" deformity may be identified, as the normal continuity of the lumbar spine is lost when the vertebra shifts forward. More severe cases of spondylolisthesis result in a flattening of the buttocks when viewed laterally and more severe limitations in

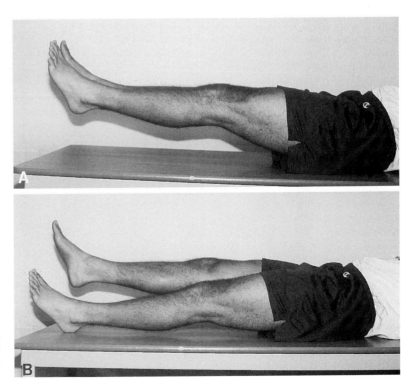

Figure 9–53. (A) The Milgram test attempts to increase intrathecal pressure, increasing the pressure placed on the spinal cord secondary to a herniated disk. (B) A positive test results in the inability to hold both legs off the table for a 30-second period.

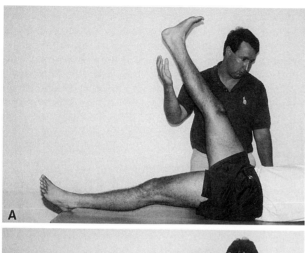

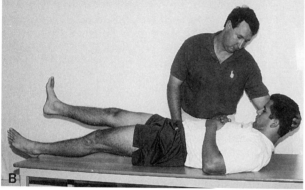

Figure 9–54. Kernig's test for entrapment or irritation of the spinal cord. (*B*) Modification of Kernig's test.

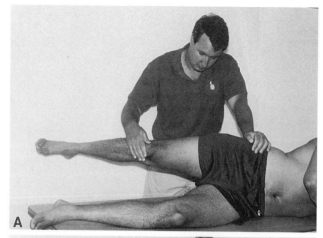

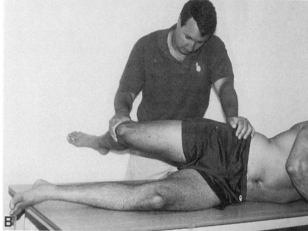

Figure 9–56. Femoral nerve traction test. The hip is extended while the knee is flexed to 90°. This test may also be performed with the athlete prone.

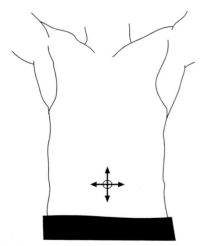

Figure 9–55. Beevor's sign. Observe the umbilicus as the patient performs an abdominal curl. With a positive test the umbilicus moves up, down, left, or right, indicating inhibition of the nerves innervating the rectus abdominis.

range of motion. Results of special tests and neurological tests may become positive if the slippage of the vertebra is great enough to impinge on the neurological structures (Table 9–14). Although not a definitive test, a suspicion of spondylolysis or spondylolisthesis may be reinforced by the single-leg stance test.

Single-Leg Stance Test

Strain is placed on the pars interarticularis by having the athlete stand on one leg and move the lumbar spine into extension, a movement that may be assisted by the examiner (Fig. 9–61). Extension of the spine compresses the spinous process, and the contraction of the iliopsoas tends to pull the vertebra anteriorly, resulting in a shear force being placed on the pars interarticularis. Pain, weakness, or both are elicited in the presence of pathology.

Single-Leg Stance Test (Fig. 9–61)

Position of athlete	Standing with the body weight evenly distributed between the two feet.
Position of examiner	Standing behind the athlete, ready to provide support if the athlete begins to fall.
Evaluative procedure	The athlete lifts one leg, then places the trunk in hyperextension. The examiner may assist the athlete during this motion. The procedure is then repeated for the opposite leg.
Positive test results	Pain in the lumbar spine area.
Implications	Compressive forces are placed on the pars interarticularis, resulting in pain.
Comments	When the lesion to the pars interarticularis is unilateral, pain is evoked when the opposite leg is raised. Bilateral pars fractures result in pain when each leg is lifted.

ON-FIELD EVALUATION AND MANAGEMENT OF SPINAL INJURIES

All injuries to the spinal column requiring an on-field evaluation must be treated as being catastrophic in nature until ruled out. Bilateral symptoms in the upper extremities or symptoms in the lower extremities should alert the examiner to the potential of spinal cord involvement. Chapter 16 discusses the evaluation and management of potentially catastrophic spinal cord injuries.

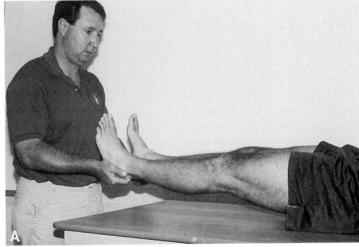

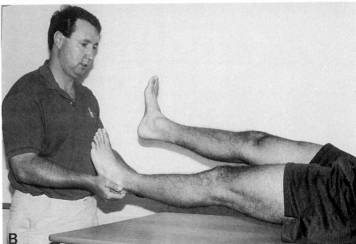

Figure 9–57. The Hoover test to identify malingering patients. With the examiner cupping both of the patient's heels, the individual is asked to lift the right (or left) leg. If an effort is being made, the examiner feels pressure in the opposite hand. No pressure in the opposite hand suggests that an effort is not being made.

Table 9–13. Classification of Spondylopathies

Term	Description
Spondylalgia	Pain arising from the vertebrae
Spondylitis	Inflammation of the vertebrae
Spondylizema	Downward (inferior) displacement of a vertebra, caused by the degeneration of the one below it
Spondylolisthesis	Forward slippage of a vertebra on the one below it (may occur secondary to spondylolysis, in which the fracture of the pars interarticularis results in the anterior displacement of the vertebral body)
Spondylolysis	Degeneration of a vertebral structure, most commonly affecting the pars interarticularis but with no displacement of the vertebral body
Spondylopathy	Any disorder of the vertebrae
Spondylosis	Arthritis or osteoarthritis of the cervical or lumbar vertebrae; results in pressure being placed on the vertebral nerve roots

Brachial Plexus Injury

Typically, athletes with a brachial plexus injury leave the field of play under their own power, with the involved arm dangling limp at the side. The head may be held in a manner to relieve any compression placed on the brachial plexus as the result of spasm of the trapezius muscle. The athlete's signs and symptoms (see Table 9–10) are usually transient in nature. After a thorough evaluation to rule out the possibility of trauma to the cervical vertebrae, the cervical spine should be treated with ice packs to decrease pain and spasm.

The athlete should demonstrate a normal neuro-

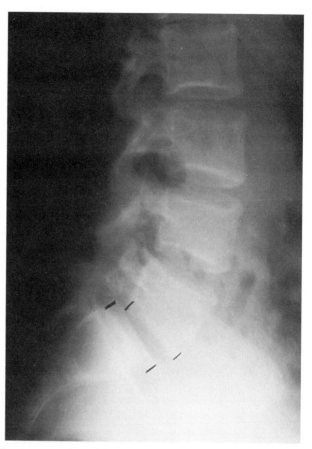

Figure 9–59. Spondylolisthesis of the L5-S1 junction. Notice that the L5 vertebra is anteriorly displaced relative to S1.

logical examination without weakness and with full pain-free range of motion before returning to activity. Any continuation of the signs and symptoms precludes further participation until the athlete is cleared to return to play by a physician. Repeated episodes of brachial plexus trauma may

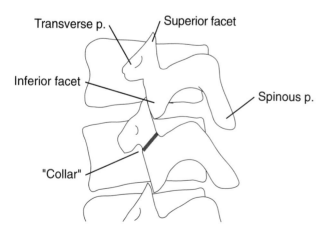

Figure 9–58. "Collared Scotty dog" deformity. On an x ray, the presence of a collar on the Scotty dog indicates a nondisplaced stress fracture on the pars interarticularis.

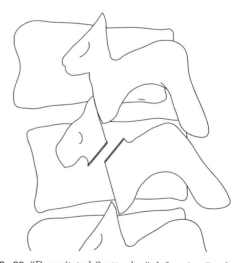

Figure 9–60. "Decapitated Scotty dog" deformity. Further degeneration of the pars interarticularis can lead to a displaced fracture. Here the "collared Scotty dog" loses its head as the superior vertebra slides anteriorly

Table 9–14. Evaluative Findings of Spondylolysis and Spondylolisthesis

Examination Segment	Clinical Findings
History	Onset: Insidious; the pain begins as an ache and evolves to constant pain. Location of pain: Lumbar spine, possibly radiating into the buttocks and upper portion of the legs. Mechanism: Current thought suggests that the pars interarticularis suffers a stress fracture secondary to repetitive stress caused by the spine's going into extension.
Inspection	Gross inspection of the spinal curvatures may reveal hyperlordosis in the lumbar spine. A "step-off" deformity of the anteriorly shifted vertebra may be seen.
Palpation	A palpable "step-off" deformity may be detected at the involved lumbar level. Spasm of the paraspinal muscles may be noted.
Functional tests	AROM: Range of motion during trunk flexion is restricted but pain-free. Pain is described as the athlete returns to an upright posture and during active extension of the spine. Pain may also be elicited during lumbar rotation and lateral rotation. PROM: Hip flexion may indicate tightness of the hamstring muscles. PROM: Weakness of the spinal erector muscles is due to decreased efficiency secondary to a fracture of the insertion site.
Ligamentous tests	Not applicable.
Neurological tests	Lower quarter screen to rule out involvement of one or more lumbar nerve roots. Results of this are typically negative.
Special tests	Single leg stance. Straight leg raises may produce a pain that is more extreme than that normally caused by tightness of the hamstring group.
Comments	An x-ray examination or MRI is required to differentiate between spondylolysis and spondylolisthesis.

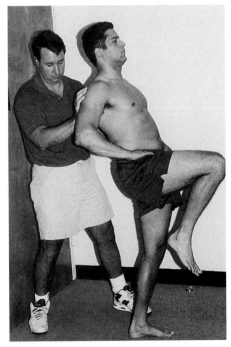

Figure 9–61. Single-leg stance test. This position places stress on the pars interarticularis, resulting in pain, thus leading to the suspicion of spondylolysis or spondylolisthesis.

result in scar tissue forming over one or more nerve roots or may cause a pathological narrowing of the foramen.

Lumbar Spine

Catastrophic injury to the lumbar spine is relatively rare owing to the decreased range of motion of this area and the extremely high forces needed to cause this injury. However, this fact should not allow the athletic trainer to become complacent during the evaluation process. As with all spinal injuries, the evaluation of the lumbar spine must be approached as if a catastrophic injury exists until it has been ruled out.

The athlete must be questioned for a history of symptoms including pain and paresthesia. Pain localized over a spinous process could indicate a compression or burst fracture, and this alone is reason for immediate referral. Any symptoms suggesting neurological involvement must be investigated. An athlete reporting bilateral symptoms should be treated as having a spinal cord injury, immobilized on a spine board, and properly transported to a medical facility.

Direct blows to the lumbar or thoracic region may result in trauma to the kidneys, ribs, or other internal organs. The evaluation of these conditions is discussed in Chapter 10.

REFERENCES

1. Tall, RL, and DeVault, W: Spinal injury in sport: Epidemiologic consideration. Clin Sports Med 12:441, 1993.
2. Nachemson, A, and Eifstrom, G: Intravital dynamic measurements in lumbar discs. Scand J Rehabil Med 1(Suppl):1, 1960.
2a. Norkin, CC, and Levangie, PK: Joint Structure and Function: A Comprehensive Analysis, ed 2. FA Davis, Philadelphia, 1992.
3. Oegema, TR: Biochemistry of the intervertebral disc. Clinics in Sports Medicine 12:419, 1993.
4. Carrigg, SY, and Hillemeyer, LE: The effect of running-induced intervertebral disc compression on thoracolumbar vertebral column mobility in young, healthy males. Journal of Orthopedic and Sports Physical Therapy 16:19, 1992.
5. Hollinshead, WH, and Jenkins, DB: The organs and organ systems. In Hollinshead, WH, and Jenkins, DB: Functional Anatomy of the Limbs and Back. WB Saunders, Philadelphia, 1981, p 55.
5a. Rothstein, JM, Roy, SH, and Wolf, SL: The Rehabilitation Specialist's Handbook. FA Davis, Philadelphia, 1991.
6. Moore, KL: The back. In Moore, KL: Clinically Oriented Anatomy, ed 2. Williams & Wilkins, Baltimore, 1985, p 599.
7. McKenzie, RA: The lumbar spine: Mechanical diagnosis and therapy. Spinal Publications, Waikanae, New Zealand, 1981.
8. Yang, SS, and Hershman, EB: Idiopathic brachial plexus neuropathy: A review. Critical Reviews in Musculoskeletal Medicine 5:193, 1993.
9. Markey, KL, Di Benedetto, M, and Curl, WW: Upper trunk brachial plexopathy: The stinger syndrome. Am J Sports Med 21:650, 1993.
10. Vereschagin, KS, et al: Burners. Don't overlook or underestimate them. The Physician and Sportsmedicine 19:96, 1991.
11. Meyer, SA, et al: Cervical spinal stenosis and stingers on collegiate football players. Am J Sports Med 22:158, 1994.
12. Reilly, PJ, and Torg, JS: Athletic injury to the cervical nerve roots and brachial plexus. Operative Techniques in Sports Medicine 1:231, 1993.
13. Davidson, RI, Dunn, EJ, and Metzmaker, JN: The shoulder abduction test in the diagnosis of radicular pain in cervical extradural compressive monoradiculopathies. Spine 6:441, 1981.
14. Maitland, GD: Vertebral manipulation. Budderworth Publishing, London, 1973.
15. Keene, JS, et al: Back injuries in college athletes. J Spinal Disord 2:190, 1989.
16. Charnley, J: Orthopedic signs in the diagnosis of disc protrusion with special reference to the straight-leg-raising test. Lancet 1:156, 1951.
17. Edgar, MA, and Park, WM: Induced pain patterns on passive straight-leg-raising in lower lumbar disc protrusion. J Bone Joint Surg Br 56:658, 1974.
18. Goddard, BS, and Reid, JD: Movements induced by straight-leg-raising in the lumbo-sacral roots, nerves, and plexus and in the intrapelvic section of the sciatic nerve. J Neurol Neurosurg Psychiatry 28:12, 1965.
19. Urban, LM: The straight-leg-raising test: A review. Journal of Orthopedic and Sports Physical Therapy 2:117, 1981.
20. Scham, SM, and Taylor, TKF: Tension signs in lumbar disc prolapse. Clin Orthop 75:195, 1971.
21. Wilkins, RH, and Brody, IA: Lasegue's sign. Arch Neurol 21:219, 1969.
22. Jensen, MC, et al: Magnetic imaging of the lumbar spine in people without back pain. N Engl J Med 331:69, 1994.
23. Tertti, M, et al: Disc degeneration in young gymnasts: A magnetic resonance imaging study. Am J Sports Med 18:206, 1990.
24. Hudgens, WR: The crossed-straight-leg-raising test. N Engl J Med 297:1127, 1977.
25. Woodhall, R, and Hayes, GJ: The well-leg-raising test of Fajersztajn in the diagnosis of ruptured lumbar intervertebral disc. J Bone Joint Surg Am 32:786, 1950.
26. Hoover, CF: A new sign for the detection of malingering and functional paresis of lower extremities. JAMA 51:746, 1908.
27. Archibald, AC, and Wiechec, F: A reappraisal of Hoover's test. Arch Phys Med Rehabil 51:234, 1970.
28. Arieff, AJ, et al: The Hoover sign: An objective sign of pain and/or weakness in the back or lower extremities. Arch Neurol 5:673, 1961.
29. Jackson, D, et al: Stress reactions involving the pars interarticularis in young athletes. Am J Sports Med 9:305, 1981.
30. Moore, KL: The perineum and pelvis. In Moore, KL: Clinically Oriented Anatomy, ed. Williams & Wilkins, Baltimore, 1985, p 389.

10

The Thorax and Abdomen

The internal organs responsible for constantly maintaining the body's homeostasis, the heart, lungs, spleen, kidneys, and liver, lie well protected within the thorax. However, extraordinary forces can result in damage to these structures, endangering the athlete's life. The digestive system and lower portion of the urinary tract, although less well protected as they lie within the abdominal region of the torso, are more resilient to trauma because of their relatively hollow nature.

Injury to the body's visceral organs can range from the mundane to the catastrophic. The athletic trainer must have a keen awareness of the internal systems of the body, the factors predisposing these organs to injury, and the signs and symptoms of trauma to these structures. The progressive nature of the symptoms makes early suspicion and repeated examination and evaluation the critical part of the health care of the athlete.

CLINICAL ANATOMY

With the sternum anteriorly, the vertebrae posteriorly, and the ribs connecting the two, the thorax forms a protective shell around the torso's upper internal organs (Fig. 10–1). The **sternum** consists of three sections, the **manubrium** superiorly, the central **body**, and the inferiorly projecting **xiphoid process**. The sternal body and the manubrium are connected by a fibrocartilaginous joint in young athletes that fuses during the maturation process to form a single, solid piece of bone.

The upper seven ribs are classified as **true ribs** because they articulate with the sternum through their own **costal cartilages**. As ribs 8 through 10 articulate with the sternum through a conjoined costal cartilage, they are termed **false ribs**. Ribs 11 and 12 do not have an anterior articulation and are considered to be **floating ribs**. An anomalous **cervical rib** may project off the seventh cervical vertebra. Although this structure is often benign, it can be a source of compression on the brachial plexus, the subclavian artery, or the subclavian vein, leading to **thoracic outlet syndrome** (see Chapter 11).

The abdominal region has no anterior or lateral bony protection and receives only slight protection on its posterior surface from the thoracic and lum-

bar vertebrae and the floating ribs. The inferior portion of the abdomen is protected by the sacrum posteriorly and the ilia laterally.

Muscular Anatomy

Many of the muscles acting on the thorax and abdomen have been previously discussed and are only superficially presented in this chapter. Additionally, those muscles arising from the thorax to act on the scapula and humerus also influence the thorax (these muscles are discussed in Chapter 11).

Muscles of Inspiration

The **diaphragm** is a muscular membrane partitioning the thoracic cavity from the abdominal cavity. Innervated by the **phrenic nerve**, contraction of the diaphragm causes it to move downward, creating a vacuum in the thorax that pulls air into the lungs. At several points the diaphragm is interrupted by portals through which the major vessels pass into the torso and lower legs.

The rib cage's intrinsic skeletal muscles are collectively referred to as the **intercostal muscles**. Spanning from rib to rib, these muscles assist in the respiratory process. Also assisting in respiration by elevating the thorax are the **scalene** and the **sternocleidomastoid** muscles.

Muscles of Expiration

The abdominal muscles, the **rectus abdominis, internal oblique**, and **external oblique** (discussed in Chapter 9), are supported across the abdomen by the **transverse abdominis**. In addition to flexing and rotating the lumbar and thoracic spine, the contraction of these muscles creates a positive pressure gradient across the diaphragm, resulting in the expiration of air.

Internal Organs

Many of the internal organs come in pairs. Reference to these organs is relative to the athlete, thus the right kidney is on the examiner's left side when facing the athlete from the front.

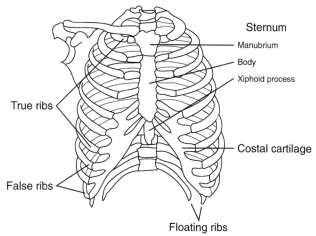

Figure 10–1. Illustration of the thorax. The rib cage formed by the true ribs (1 through 7), false ribs (8 through 10), and floating ribs (11 and 12); the sternum (manubrium, body, and xiphoid process); and the costal cartilage. The posterior margin of the thorax is formed by the thoracic and vertebrae.

Organs of Respiration

The **trachea**, connecting the larynx to the bronchioles, is a membranous tube formed by muscle and connective tissue. Its anterior border is protected from crushing forces by a series of cartilaginous semicircular rings. The trachea diverges into two principal **bronchi**. The left bronchus divides into two **segmental bronchi** while three segmental bronchi are formed on the right side (Fig. 10–2). Each segmental bronchus then subdivides into the **bronchioles**.

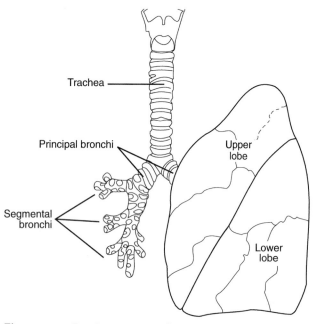

Figure 10–2. Respiratory tract. The trachea, principal bronchi, the segmental bronchi, and the right lung. The left lung has been removed to view the bronchial segments. The right lung is formed by two lobes, whereas the left lung has a third, or middle, lobe between the upper and lower ones.

Carbon dioxide is exchanged for oxygen in the **lungs**. The left lung has three lobes (upper, middle, and lower), whereas the right lung has only an upper and lower lobe, each matching with a segmental bronchus. The thoracic cavity is encased with pleural linings. A **visceral pleura** lines the thoracic wall and a **parietal pleura** surrounds the lungs, forming a **pleural cavity** between the two. As the chest cavity expands during inspiration, a negative pressure is formed within the pleural cavity, causing an expansion of the lungs and the subsequent entry of air for breathing.

The actual exchange of gases occurs at the level of the **alveoli**, the terminal branches of the bronchioles. The alveolar walls contain the capillary system carrying deoxygenated blood from the right side of the heart. Following the transfer of gases, the oxygenated blood returns to the left side of the heart via the **pulmonary veins**.

The trachea and its conducting airways are lined with **mucosal cells**. Mucus is formed in the submucosa by glands and is excreted to the mucosal lining. Here, the mucus acts as a filtration system, working like millions of little sponges absorbing airborne pollutants, dust, and other unwanted substances. Normally the mucus is routed by **ciliary cells** to the pharynx, where it is unconsciously swallowed. When an excess demand is placed on the mucosal system, the mucus is routed up, through, and out the nasal passage.

The upper portions of the respiratory system, the nose, mouth, larynx, and pharynx, are discussed in Chapter 15.

Cardiovascular Anatomy

Of course, the **heart** is the cardiovascular system's hub. Under normal circumstances the heart beats at a rate that equals the metabolic needs of the body, delivering oxygen and nutrients to the body's tissues. As the tissues' demands for these nutrients increase, so does the heart rate.

The heart is divided into four chambers, with the right-side chambers handling deoxygenated blood and the left-side chambers handling oxygenated blood (Table 10–1). The **aorta** exits the heart, carrying oxygenated blood to the body. Soon after leaving the heart the aorta takes a sharp bend inferiorly, forming the **aortic arch**. From this arch many other arteries diverge from the aorta: the **brachiocephalic trunk**, the **left common carotid artery**, and the **left subclavian artery**. After exiting its arch the aorta forms the **descending aorta**, supplying blood to the torso and lower extremity (Fig. 10–3). The brachiocephalic trunk forms the **right subclavian** and **right common carotid arteries**, delivering blood to the right upper extremity and brain.

Despite the fact that the heart is responsible for supplying the rest of the body with fresh blood, it must still pump blood to itself through the right and left **coronary arteries**. The right coronary artery

Table 10-1. The Chambers of the Heart

Heart Chamber	Function
Right atrium	Receives deoxygenated blood via: Superior vena cava from the head, neck, and upper extremity. Inferior vena cava from the trunk and lower extremity. Delivers blood to the right ventricle through the tricuspid valve.
Right ventricle	Receives deoxygenated blood from right atrium. Through the semilunar valves, delivers blood to the lungs via the left and right pulmonary arteries.
Left atrium	Receives oxygenated blood from the lungs via the right and left pulmonary veins. Delivers blood to the left ventricle through the mitral valve.
Left ventricle	Delivers oxygenated blood through the semilunar valves to the aorta.

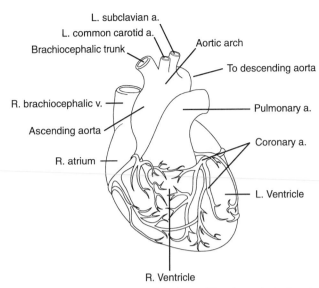

Figure 10-3. Anterior view of the heart. Blood supply to the viscera, extremity, and brain is delivered through the aorta. The left atrium is hidden in this view.

branches into the right marginal artery and the posterior **interventricular artery**. The left coronary artery branches into the anterior interventricular artery and the **circumflex artery**, which then leads to the left marginal artery.

Digestive Tract Anatomy

Solids and liquids enter the digestive tract through the mouth and travel through the **esophagus** to enter the stomach. Once in the stomach, the ingested food substances form a **bolus**, which is routed into the **small intestine** through the **pylorus** portion of the stomach. The small intestine is divided into the **duodenum, jejunum,** and **ileum**. After passing through the small intestine, the bolus enters the **large intestine** (colon) to travel a meandering route through the **ascending colon, transverse colon, descending colon,** and **rectum** to its final exit from the body via the **anus** (Fig. 10-4).

Lymphatic Organs

Toxic substances and cellular wastes are filtered from the bloodstream by the liver and spleen (Fig. 10-5). The **liver**, the largest organ in the body, takes up the entire right side of the torso inferior to the diaphragm and is protected by the lower ribs and the costal arch of the false ribs (see Fig. 10-4). The liver functions to filter poisons out of the blood and

produce mediators for blood clotting. Through its connection with the bile duct the liver introduces **bile** into the stomach to assist in the digestion of fats. The liver also acts as a warehouse for storing glucose, the body's immediate fuel system, and is a repository for the metabolism of intrinsic and extrinsic chemical substances. The liver's many tasks require a large blood supply. Injury to this organ results in massive amounts of blood being lost into the abdominal cavity.

Located on the left side of the body at the level of the 9th through 11th ribs, the **spleen** is a solid, fragile organ that is supported by ligaments attaching it to the kidney, colon, stomach, and diaphragm (Fig. 10-6). The largest of the lymphatic organs, its primary function is to produce and destroy blood cells during times of systemic infection. During certain disease states, such as *mononucleosis*, the spleen becomes engorged with blood, causing it to bulge below the ribs' protective bony cover, increasing the risk of injury. When the spleen is traumatized, surgical removal may be necessary, at which time its functions are assumed by the liver and bone marrow.

Urinary Tract Anatomy

The kidneys too are responsible for filtering toxins from the blood, but they also regulate the body's *electrolyte* level by maintaining the balance of wa-

---

Mononucleosis: A disease state caused by an abnormally high number of mononuclear leukocytes in the bloodstream.
Electrolyte: Ionized salts including sodium, potassium, and chlorine in blood, tissue fluid, and cells.

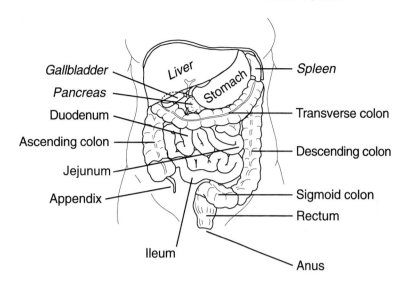

Figure 10–4. Stomach and intestine. Although not directly involved with the digestive tract, the liver, gallbladder, pancreas, and spleen are presented for reference purposes.

ter, sodium, and potassium. The kidneys lie on each side of the vertebral column at the level of the T12 to L3 vertebrae, with the right kidney lying slightly lower than the left. The lower portion of each kidney is unprotected by the ribs, making them susceptible to bruising secondary to direct blows to the low back (Fig. 10–7).

The kidney's filtrate, **urine**, exits through small, muscular tubes, the **ureters**. Well protected by the posterior wall of the abdomen, these structures are rarely injured. Both ureters deposit their contents into a central **urinary bladder**, located posterior to the pubic symphysis, outside of the abdominal cavity. As the bladder fills, the smooth muscle reacts to parasympathetic stimuli, triggering the urge to urinate. From the bladder, urine exits the body through the **urethra**.

Reproductive Anatomy

The essential organs of reproduction are located in the lower abdomen in both men and women. The male **testes** have the dual function of producing sperm and the male sex hormone, testosterone. The **epididymis** is a coiled tube on the posterior aspect of the testes that stores sperm (Fig. 10–8). The extrinsic location of the male reproductive organs increases the incidence of injury, most often occurring secondary to a direct blow.

The female organs of reproduction, the paired **ovaries** and a singular hollow **uterus**, are attached by ligaments to the pelvic wall and sit relatively well protected. The ovaries are endocrine glands that are the source of estrogen and progesterone, the female sex hormones (Fig. 10–9). Dysfunction of

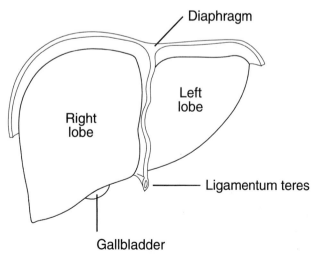

Figure 10–5. Anterior view of the liver. This structure is supported by ligaments arising from the inferior surface of the diaphragm.

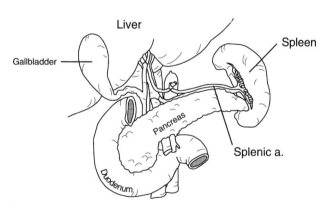

Figure 10–6. Spleen. During illness the spleen may become enlarged, causing it to become vulnerable to injury.

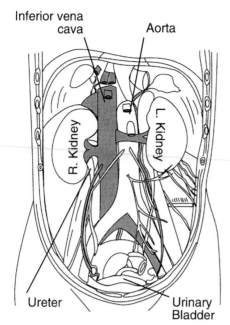

Figure 10–7. Relative location of the kidneys. Note that the right kidney is located inferior to the left kidney, exposing its inferior border to direct trauma from blows to the posterolateral thorax.

the female reproductive system is rarely the result of trauma but may occur in athletes in the form of **amenorrhea** or **dysmenorrhea**. These conditions warrant referral for further assessment of their etiology by a physician.

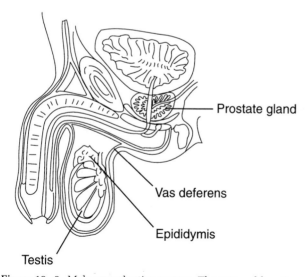

Figure 10–8. Male reproductive system. The external location of the testicles predisposes them to injury from direct blows.

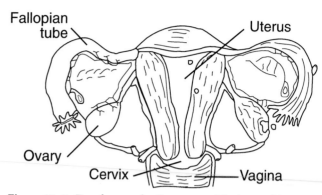

Figure 10–9. Female reproductive system. The internal location of these organs provides excellent protection against most traumatic forces.

EVALUATION OF THORACIC AND ABDOMINAL INJURIES

Injuries to the internal organs and ribs usually follow a high-velocity blow to the affected area, resulting in trauma in the area beneath the impact or across the cavity as those structures rebound off bony structures. These conditions may not be clearly evident immediately following the injury but can quickly progress to life-threatening conditions, thereby necessitating frequent re-examination.

The thoracoabdominal region is referenced on a quadrant system, dividing the torso into left and right upper and lower quadrants relative to the umbilicus (Fig. 10–10). The evaluation process is somewhat eased by the clinician's awareness of the organs housed in each of these quadrants and their normal function. Additionally, as discussed in the Neurological Testing section of this chapter, pain of visceral origin may be referred to the body's periphery. Table 10–2 presents the sequential evaluation of thoracoabdominal injuries.

History

All individuals who are responsible for the medical coverage of athletic practices and games should be acutely aware of the early signs and symptoms of internal injury. These conditions may not be clearly evident immediately following the injury but can quickly progress to a life-threatening condition.

• **Location of pain:** The exact location of the pain should be determined as closely as possible. Musculoskeletal injuries to the ribs, costal cartilage,

Amenorrhea: Absence of the menstrual period.
Dysmenorrhea: Pain during menstruation.

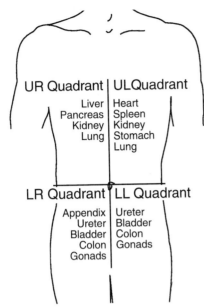

Figure 10–10. Abdominal quadrant reference system. The sagittal quadrants are relative to the athlete. Therefore, the right kidney is on the athlete's right-hand side.

or abdominal muscles are usually tender at the site of the injury. Injury to the internal organs may result in a more diffuse pain at rest but can be more specifically localized as the athlete moves or the area is palpated. Blows to the low back may result in a kidney contusion, especially on the athlete's right side (see Fig. 10–7). Cutaneous pain in the thorax, abdomen, shoulder, or arm can be referred from the visceral organs. Actual physical trauma may occur either at the site of the blow or on the side opposite the impact, a **contrecoup injury.**

• **Onset of symptoms:** The onset of pain with an internal injury may take hours to develop as internal bleeding accumulates within the cavity. Musculoskeletal injury can be acute or may initially go unnoticed or undernoticed. When the rib cage or abdominal muscles are injured, pain may be provoked by breathing, coughing, or sneezing.

Distance runners may be affected by stomach or abdominal cramping during competition. Causes of this condition may be irregular breathing patterns, gastrointestinal upset, bloating, gas, nausea, heartburn, dehydration, constipation, or dysmenorrhea.[1]

• **Mechanism of injury:** Injury to the thoracic, abdominal, and pelvic organs almost always results from a direct blow to the area. The athlete may have been hit by a competitor or may have collided with a piece of equipment or the ground. Suspicion of trauma to the ribs or internal organs is increased when the blow is received to an unprotected area.

• **Symptoms:** The athlete's chief complaint may include pain or difficulty breathing, diffuse abdominal pain, nausea, dizziness, or vomiting of blood. The athlete should also be questioned regarding the presence of blood in the urine or stool. Because of the associated metabolic changes, injury to the abdominal organs increases the athlete's thirst beyond that which is expected following competition.

• **Previous history:** Because of the acute nature of these injuries, the athlete typically does not have a previous history. With certain asthmatic conditions, a history of disease may be documented, but athletes with *exercise-induced asthma* may not have been previously diagnosed nor documented. Other illnesses may predispose the athlete to acute internal injury. For example, mononucleosis can enlarge the spleen and expose it to an increased incidence of injury.

• **General medical health:** The use of medications and other medical treatments now allows athletes to compete with conditions that once would have excluded them from competition. Athletes may now compete with cystic fibrosis, asthma, spastic colitis, renal disease, hypertension, and undescended testicles. The presence of these conditions should be identified during the preparticipation physical examination, but a prudent evaluation involves questions regarding the existence of any underlying medical conditions.

Inspection

The inspection process begins with observation of the overall posture of the athlete. Leaning the thorax to one side may indicate that the athlete is stretching spasming muscle; flexing of the trunk may indicate cramping. The athlete may also be splinting the painful area by grasping the torso or abdomen. An athlete suffering from a significant internal injury is unwilling to move, preferring to remain in the fetal position or lie supine with the knees bent.

• **Breathing pattern:** Any abnormalities in the athlete's breathing pattern should be noted. Difficulty in breathing may have many causes including asthma, allergies, cardiac contusion, injury to the ribs or costal cartilage, lung trauma (pneumothorax or hemothorax), or other injury to the internal organs.

Respiration should be observed for its rate and quality. Athletes with an internal injury breathe rapidly and shallowly, as deep breaths may cause pain. The chest wall should be observed in those

---

Exercise-induced asthma: Bronchospasm caused by exercise in a cold, dry climate.

Table 10–2. Evaluation of the Thorax and Abdomen

History	Inspection	Palpation	Functional Tests	Ligamentous Tests	Neurological Tests	Special Tests
Location of pain	Breathing pattern	Rib cage	Heart rate	Not applicable	Referred pain patterns	Rib fracture
Onset of symptoms	Guarding pattern	Sternum	Respiratory rate			Rib compression test
Mechanism of injury	Discoloration of skin	Costal cartilage and rib	Blood pressure			Costochondral injury
Symptoms	Vomiting	Abdomen				Cardiac contusions
Previous history	Hematuria	Muscle guarding				Solar plexus injury
General medical health	Auscultation	Areas of pain				Pneumothorax
		Rebound tenderness				Hemothorax
		Percussion				Injury to the spleen
		Quadrant analysis				Appendicitis
						Hollow organ rupture
						Testicular contusion
						Spermatic cord torsion

having trouble breathing. The ribs should rise and fall in a symmetrical pattern; any deviations in this pattern could be the result of fractured ribs or a pneumothorax.

• **Guarding pattern:** The rigidity of the abdomen should be observed. As time progresses the injured area may become distended secondary to bleeding.

• **Discoloration of skin:** The location of contusions, wounds, or abrasions serve to warn of possible injury to the underlying internal organs.

• **Vomiting:** The athlete should be observed for and questioned regarding any vomiting after the injury, as is common following many internal injuries or injury to the male genitals. Blood in the vomitus may signify injury to the stomach or esophagus.

• **Hematuria:** The athlete should be questioned regarding the presence of blood in the urine, or hematuria. This symptom denotes significant injury to the kidneys and warrants immediate referral to a physician. The athlete who has not urinated since the injury or did not pay attention to the color of the urine should be instructed to do so with the next voiding. Immediately following the injury blood may not be visible to the unaided eye but can be detected through the use of a microscope or chemical analysis with chemical strips that are dipped into the urine. It should be noted that hematuria may normally be present after certain athletic events such as long-distance running or in *menstruating* female athletes.

• **Auscultation:** Auscultation, listening to sounds with the stethoscope, is helpful in establishing the presence of internal injury in the athlete (Fig. 10–11). The abdomen typically makes an occasional "gurgling" sound as *peristalsis* occurs. Following injury the peristaltic mechanism may be inhibited or may sympathetically shut down. In either case the bowel sounds are absent. The exact placement of the stethoscope over specific portions of the bowel is not crucial, as these sounds resound throughout the cavity.

Palpation

The findings of the history-taking process are reinforced and supplemented by the findings obtained during the palpation phase. Because there are few special tests for assessing thoracic and abdominal injuries, the examiner must have a keen knowledge of the underlying anatomy so that a specific palpation assessment may be performed.

Palpation of the Rib Cage

• **Sternum:** The palpation of the rib cage is begun at the sternum. Here the manubrium, body, and xiphoid process should be palpated for tenderness and deformity. Injury to the upper sternum may involve the sternoclavicular joint (see Chapter 11).

• **Costal cartilage and rib:** The costal cartilage and ribs can be palpated as a whole, with the

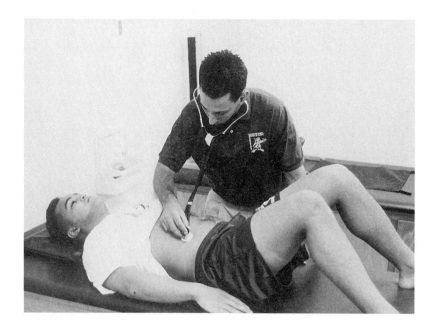

Figure 10–11. Auscultation of the abdomen. The integrity of the abdomen and its hollow organs can be assessed through listening to the bowel sounds. Although the abdomen typically makes a gurgling sound, abdominal trauma reduces or eliminates this noise.

Menstruation: The period of bleeding during the menstrual cycle.

Peristalsis: A progressive smooth muscle contraction producing a wavelike motion that moves matter through the intestines.

specific areas of tenderness being isolated. The costal cartilage and rib should be palpated from anterior to posterior, noting any pain, crepitus, and deformity. Any suspicion of a rib fracture should be fully evaluated by a physician. Rib pain arising insidiously may indicate a stress fracture.

Palpation of the Abdomen

The athlete should be in the hook-lying position to relax the abdominal muscles (Fig. 10–12). The abdomen should be palpated relative to the four quadrants depicted in Figure 10–10.

- **Muscle guarding:** The athlete may display abdominal rigidity secondary to muscle guarding. Abdominal rigidity may also be caused by the accumulation of blood in the abdomen. Its presence alone should lead to the suspicion of internal injury necessitating further evaluation by a physician.

- **Areas of pain:** Pain caused by palpation is another cause of concern. An awareness of the approximate location of the organs within the abdomen should assist in detecting possible injury.

- **Rebound tenderness:** An inflamed peritoneum is sensitive to stretching. Pressure applied over the injured site gradually stretches the peritoneum in a relatively pain-free manner. However, pain experienced when the pressure is suddenly released indicates inflammation of the peritoneum.

- **Percussion:** With practice, skill can be acquired in percussing over specific organs to determine the density of the underlying tissues. The exam-iner lightly places one hand palm down over the area to be assessed, using the index and middle fingers of one hand to tap the DIP joints of the hand placed over the athlete's abdomen (Fig. 10–13). Areas over solid organs have a dull thump associated with them. Hollow organs make a crisper, more **resonant** sound. Internal bleeding may fill the abdominal cavity, causing the abdomen to feel and sound solid.

- **Quadrant analysis:** The abdomen is palpated in the quadrant format presented in Figure 10–10. Correlations of tenderness include the following:

	Quadrant Segment	
	Right	**Left**
Upper	**Liver:** Pain is associated with ***cholecystitis*** or liver laceration. **Gallbladder:** Pain without the history of trauma indicates gallbladder disease.	**Spleen:** Rigidity under the last several ribs indicates a ruptured spleen.
Lower	**Appendix:** Rebound tenderness indicates appendicitis. **Pelvic inflammation** results in diffuse tenderness.	**Colon:** Colitis or diverticulitis may cause pain. **Pelvic inflammation** results in diffuse tenderness.

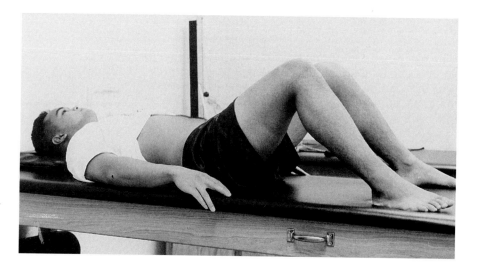

Figure 10–12. Positioning of the athlete during palpation of the abdomen. The "hook-lying" position relaxes the abdominal muscles, easing palpation of the underlying structures.

Resonant: Producing a vibrating sound or percussion.
Cholecystitis: Inflammation of the gallbladder.

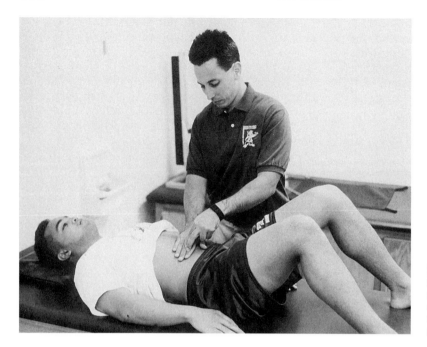

Figure 10–13. Abdominal percussion. Abdominal percussion is performed by striking the dorsal fingers of one hand with the fingertips of the other. The resulting sound should be hollow, but the build-up of fluids can result in a solid-sounding echo.

Other, less specific symptoms include pain in the upper abdomen arising from the pancreas, heart, diaphragm, or esophagus or pain in the lower middle abdomen in the area of the femoral creases from bladder or **gonad** pathology. The low back may be painful and have increased tenderness with palpation owing to kidney contusions, **kidney stones**, or infection.

Functional Tests—Vital Signs

Previous chapters have examined a joint's range of motion as an indicator of its functional ability. This chapter uses the vital signs to assess the function of the internal abdominal and thoracic organs. The examiner should have prior skill, practice, and knowledge in assessing the vital signs and interpreting the significance of these findings. This assessment is important for any injury that the athlete may suffer, especially in the event of internal injury or shock (Table 10–3). *During the evaluation and management of an injury or illness, the values obtained for each of these tests should be recorded and periodically retaken to note trends in the vital signs.*

- **Heart rate:** The heart rate is determined by identifying the athlete's pulse over the carotid

artery, although the radial, femoral, or brachial pulses may be used as well. An athlete's resting heart rate should be in the range of 60 to 100 beats per minute (bpm). Highly conditioned athletes have a lower heart rate, whereas older or recreational athletes have a heart rate at the higher end of the scale. When assessing the heart rate of an athlete who has just stopped exercising, an increased heart rate caused by the demands of exercise should be considered. *Following an internal injury, the athlete displays a rapid heart rate.*

Table 10–3. Signs and Symptoms of Shock

Rapid, weak pulse
Decreased blood pressure
Rapid, shallow breathing
Excessive thirst
Nausea and vomiting
Pale, bluish skin
Restlessness or irritability
Drowsiness or loss of consciousness

Gonad: An organ producing gender-based reproductive cells; the ovaries or testicles.
Kidney stones: A crystal mass formed in the kidney that is passed through the urinary tract.

Determination of the Carotid Pulse (Fig. 10–14)

Position of athlete	The athlete should be seated or lying down.
Position of examiner	Using the index and middle fingers, the examiner locates the thyroid cartilage and moves the fingers laterally in either direction to find the common carotid artery between the thyroid cartilage and the sternocleidomastoid muscle.
Evaluative procedure	The examiner counts the number of pulses in a 15-sec interval and multiplies that number by 4 to determine the number of beats per minute. The examiner should also attempt to determine the quality of the pulse: strong (bounding) or weak.
Positive test results	Not applicable.
Implications	The quality and quantity of the athlete's heart rate is established.
Comments	The baseline heart rate should be recorded and rechecked at regular intervals.

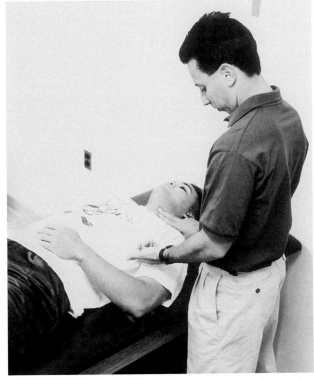

Figure 10–14. Palpation of the carotid pulse. The pulse is calculated by counting the number of beats within 15 seconds and multiplying that number by four.

• **Respiratory rate:** At rest, normal respiration ranges from 12 to 20 breaths per minute, with well-conditioned athletes falling on the low end of the range. Abnormal breathing patterns and the possible causes of their onset include:

  ○ **Rapid, shallow breaths:** internal injury; shock.
  ○ **Deep, quick breaths:** pulmonary obstruction; asthma.

Any *sputum* that may be produced as the injured athlete coughs should be checked for the presence of blood. Pink or bloody sputum indicates internal bleeding and should be treated as a medical emergency.

• **Blood pressure:** A measurement of the pressure exerted by the blood on the arterial walls, blood pressure is affected by a decrease in blood volume (severe bleeding or dehydration), a decreased capacity of the vessels (shock), or a decreased ability of the heart to pump blood (cardiac arrest). Decreased blood pressure indicates a decreased ability to deliver blood, with its nutrients and oxygen, to the organs of the body. Organs are highly susceptible to anoxia and can be severely damaged secondary to a decrease in blood pressure.

High blood pressure, or hypertension, is commonly seen in the general population. A dangerous precursor to cardiac problems in the athletic population, high blood pressure can exert extreme pressure on the blood vessels, particularly in the smaller vasculature of the brain. Excessive pressure causes these vessels to rupture, resulting in a cerebrovascular accident (CVA) or "stroke." The presence of high blood pressure in the athletic population warrants referral to a physician for further evaluation.

The blood pressure consists of two numbers: a **systolic pressure**, representing the pressure within the arteries when the heart is contract-

---

Sputum: A substance formed by mucus, blood, or pus that is expelled by coughing or clearing the throat.

ing, and a **diastolic pressure**, the pressure within the arteries when the heart is relaxed. The normal systolic pressure is between 100 and 140 millimeters of mercury (mm Hg) and the diastolic pressure ranges between 65 and 90 mm Hg.

Blood Pressure Assessment (Fig. 10–15)

Position of athlete	Seated or lying supine.
Position of examiner	In front of or beside the athlete in a position to read the gauge on the blood pressure cuff.
Evaluative procedure	The cuff is secured over the upper arm. Many cuffs have an arrow that must be aligned with the brachial artery. The examiner places the stethoscope over the brachial artery. The cuff is inflated to 180 to 200 mm Hg. The air is slowly released from the cuff. While reading the gauge, the examiner notes the point at which the first pulse sound, the systolic pressure, is heard. Continuing to slowly release the air from the cuff, the examiner notes the value at which the last pulse, the diastolic value, is heard.
Positive test results	1. A systolic value below 100 mm Hg or above 140 mm Hg. 2. A diastolic value below 65 mm Hg or above 90 mm Hg.
Implications	1. Low blood pressure may indicate shock or internal injury. 2. High blood pressure indicates hypertension.
Comments	The athlete's baseline blood pressure should be obtained annually during the preparticipation physical examination and should be compared with the current readings. Larger athletes may require the use of a larger blood pressure cuff. A cuff that is too small erroneously increases the blood pressure.

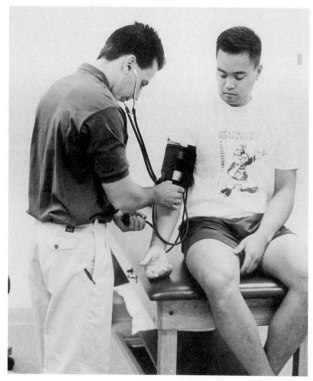

Figure 10–15. Assessment of blood pressure. The blood pressure cuff must be of adequate size for the athlete's arm. Too small a cuff can cause erroneously high readings.

Neurological Tests

Illness and trauma to the internal organs often manifest themselves by radiating symptoms in the upper extremity, chest, and low back. These patterns of referred pain from the viscera tend to radiate to the part of the body served by the somatic sensory fibers associated with the segment of the spinal cord receiving sensory information (Fig. 10–16).

Pathologies and Related Special Tests

Almost all injuries to the thorax and abdomen have an acute onset, although an underlying disease state or illness may predispose an organ to trauma. Many of these conditions have no apparently visible signs or symptoms, causing the conclusion to be based on the findings obtained during the history and palpation section of the examination. When the nature of the athlete's condition is in doubt, it is best to err on the side of safety and refer the athlete to a physician.

Rib Fractures

The fifth through ninth ribs are most commonly fractured in athletics. The upper two ribs are pro-

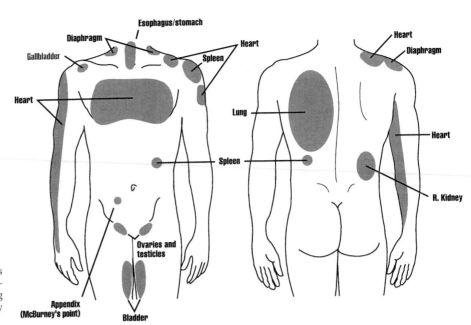

Figure 10–16. Referred pain patterns from the viscera. Pain from the internal organs tends to radiate along the corresponding somatic sensory fibers.

tected by the clavicle and the mass of the pectoralis major, and the upper six or seven ribs are protected on their posterior aspect by the scapula, lessening the incidence of rib trauma in these areas. The floating ribs have only a posterior attachment on the vertebrae, allowing them to bend and absorb the force of an impact. Additionally, in sports such as football the upper ribs are protected by shoulder pads and the lower ribs by a "flak jacket" type of padding (Fig. 10–17).

In cases of a rib fracture, the athlete's chief complaint is pain directly at the fracture site, which worsens and radiates with deep inspirations, coughing, sneezing, and movement of the torso. The ath-

lete may assume a comfortable posture by leaning toward the side of the fracture and may actively splint the fracture site by holding the painful area to limit the amount of chest wall movement during inspiration. Respirations are usually shallow and rapid to minimize the amount of chest movement. Palpation of the area produces pain over the site of the injury, and deformity of the bone or crepitus may also be noted (Table 10–4). The suspicion of a rib fracture can be confirmed through the **rib compression test.**

A blow in the anteroposterior plane tends to result in an outward dispersion of forces along the ribs, forcing the fractured rib segments outward as well. Blows to the lateral rib cage have a higher incidence of inwardly projecting fractures, possibly leading to a pneumothorax or hemothorax.[2] Unrecognized rib fractures can result in a nonunion, seriously impairing the athlete's ability to compete.[3] Sports such as crew (rowing) and golf have a higher incidence of rib stress fractures than do other sports.[4] The possible complications warrant that all suspected rib fractures be referred to a physician for further evaluation and a definitive diagnosis.

Rib Compression Test

An athlete with an injury to the ribs themselves or to the costal cartilage has increased pain as the thorax changes dimension. A quick check for rib trauma can be performed by compressing the thorax and then suddenly releasing it (Fig. 10–18). This procedure is contraindicated in the presence of an obvious fracture or lung trauma (see top of page 312).

Costochondral Injury

A costochrondral strain or separation from the ribs is usually caused by overstretching the costo-

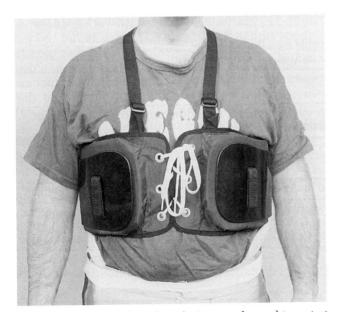

Figure 10–17. Flak jacket. These devices may be used to protect the ribs, kidneys, and spleen from traumatic forces.

lapse. If this condition goes unchecked, the subsequent pressure affects the opposite lung, the heart, and the major arteries, leading to death.

The common trait in these conditions is respiratory distress. The athlete may complain of pain and shortness of breath but may be unable to speak at all. Labored and shallow respirations accompany a rapidly decreasing blood pressure. The athlete may appear to be *cyanotic* and, in extreme cases, the tissues between the ribs and clavicle are distended (Table 10–5).

Penetrating wounds through the chest wall and into the pleural cavity from a foreign object or a rib fracture result in an **open pneumothorax.** Air is allowed to leak in and out of the pleural cavity, disabling the normal respiratory mechanism. This injury is also referred to as a "sucking chest wound" because of the sound made when the athlete inhales.

Hemothorax

A hemothorax is similar to a pneumothorax except that the respiratory distress is caused by a collection of blood in the pleural cavity. Bleeding oc-

curs from an internal chest wound (e.g., a fractured rib lacerating a lung) or from the rupture of a blood vessel within the chest cavity. The signs and symptoms of a hemothorax are very similar, if not identical, to those of a pneumothorax, and it is not uncommon for these two conditions to occur concurrently (Table 10–5). An athlete who is suffering from a hemothorax may also cough up bloody sputum.

Injury to the Spleen

The spleen is injured when the athlete collides with another player, strikes a stationary object, or is hit by an object traveling at a high velocity. The subsequent force delivered to the spleen can result in its being contused or lacerated. An inflamed spleen, which can occur during mononucleosis or systemic infection, is predisposed to injury because of the organ's increased mass and decreased elasticity.

The signs and symptoms of shock are soon seen in athletes suffering from acute spleen trauma. The telltale indicator of a ruptured spleen is the **Kehr's sign,** pain in the upper left quadrant and left shoul-

Table 10–5. Evaluative Findings of a Pneumothorax

Examination Segment	Clinical Findings	
History	Onset:	Acute or insidious.
	Location of pain:	Upper left or right quadrant; diaphragm. In some cases the athlete is unable or unwilling to speak.
	Mechanism:	Rupture of a bleb, causing air to enter the pleural cavity or an object or rib puncturing the pleural cavity.
Inspection	The athlete may be seen having difficulty breathing. A guarding posture is noted and the athlete may be clutching the chest and ribs. In an acute spontaneous pneumothorax, no visible signs are present over the rib cage. Acute traumatic pneumothorax may show trauma at the point of impact. The athlete may become cyanotic. A traumatic pneumothorax may progress to the point that the tissue between the clavicle and ribs and the neck veins becomes distended.	
Palpation	If of a traumatic onset, the affected area is tender secondary to a contusion, fracture, or costal-cartilage separation. Percussion of the affected side of the chest produces a hollow sound when compared with the opposite lung.	
Functional tests	Respiration is labored and shallow. Blood pressure drops rapidly.	
Ligamentous tests	Not applicable.	
Neurological tests	Not applicable.	
Special tests	Not applicable.	
Comments	An open pneumothorax is characterized by a penetrating wound into the chest cavity. Air can be heard rushing in and out of the wound during respirations. Oxygen may be administered to decrease the amount of respiratory distress.	

Cyanotic: Dark blue or purple tint to the skin and mucous membranes caused by a decreased oxygen supply.

der. These symptoms are aggravated by movement and the athlete may vomit or describe nausea (Table 10–6).

Appendicitis

Although the onset of appendicitis is rarely attributed to athletic competition, blows to the lower right quadrant may accelerate an existing inflammatory process or cause the inflamed appendix to rupture. Acute appendicitis commonly occurs in the age range of 15 to 25 years and is more common in men than in women. The outward symptoms of lower abdominal tenderness, fever, nausea, and vomiting occur approximately 2 days after the initial inflammation of the appendix. A pus-filled abscess forms 1 to 3 days following the onset of the symptoms. Athletes suffering from appendicitis prefer lying supine with the right leg flexed at the hip and knee to lessen the amount of pressure on the lower right quadrant (Table 10–7). Athletes suspected of suffering from appendicitis should be immediately referred to a physician.

Kidney Injury

Injuries to the kidneys, either contusions or lacerations, are associated with high-velocity impact forces to the upper lumbar and lower thoracic area. The kidneys sit well protected behind the lower ribs, and forces of sufficient magnitude to traumatize the kidneys are often associated with concurrent injury to the lower ribs, lower thoracic vertebrae, upper lumbar vertebrae, or other internal organs. Any penetrating wounds most likely involve some of these structures as well.

Athletes suffering from kidney trauma have a history of blunt trauma to the upper lumbar and lower thoracic region. The only outward signs of a kidney contusion or laceration may be bruising or bleeding over the area of contact. The athlete may complain of rib pain that increases in intensity during deep inspiration. Cases of severe internal bleeding also produce the signs and symptoms of shock. Palpation of the area generally reveals diffuse tenderness unless a rib is concurrently injured, at which time a more focused pain and crepitus are demonstrated (Fig. 10–19). With severe bleeding, guarding of the abdomen may reflexively occur because of pain (Table 10–8).

A diagnostic sign of an injured kidney is hematuria. Except in the case of severe bleeding within the kidney, the urine may not seem noticeably discolored to the unaided eye and bleeding can be detected only through laboratory analysis. Urine should be collected from an athlete suspected of suffering from a kidney injury so that it may be further analyzed. The absence of blood in the urine immediately following the injury does not rule out the potential of kidney trauma, and the use of CT scans or contrast imaging of the urinary tract may be required for a definitive diagnosis.[6] The potential loss of a kidney warrants that athletes demonstrating any of these signs and symptoms be immediately referred to a physician.

Hollow Organ Rupture

The rupture of a hollow organ is very rare in athletics. As an athlete receives a blow to the abdomen, the hollow organs are able to absorb the forces, deforming and returning to their initial shape without

Table 10–6. Evaluative Findings of Spleen Injury

Examination Segment	Clinical Findings	
History	Onset:	Acute, although the onset of symptoms may take hours.
	Location of pain:	Pressure experienced in the upper left quadrant, discrete area of referred pain in the anterior and posterior portions of the lower left quadrant, and the upper left shoulder (Kehr's sign).
	Mechanism:	Blow to the abdomen or thorax, compressing or jarring the spleen.
Inspection	The impact site may show signs of a contusion or rib fracture. The athlete may show signs of nausea and vomiting.	
Palpation	The athlete feels cold and clammy with the onset of shock. The area over the impact site may be tender. The abdomen's upper left quadrant may feel distended.	
Functional tests	Pain in the upper left quadrant and shoulder is aggravated by movement. Blood pressure is low.	
Ligamentous tests	Not applicable.	
Neurological tests	Not applicable.	
Special tests	Not applicable.	
Comments	Athletes suffering from mononucleosis or other systemic infection are predisposed to spleen injury secondary to the enlargement and hardening of this organ.	

Table 10–7. Evaluative Findings of Appendicitis

Examination Segment	Clinical Findings		
History	Onset:		Rapid. Males between the ages of 15 and 25 years are most prone to this condition.
	Location of pain:		Diffuse in the abdomen, tender and rigid in the lower right quadrant. The athlete describes nausea and may vomit. Bowel function is altered to its dichotomy of function: diarrhea or constipation.
	Mechanism:		Infection of the appendix, causing it to inflame and eventually rupture.
Inspection	The athlete has a sickly appearance and prefers to lie supine with the right hip and knee flexed to reduce pressure in the lower right quadrant.		
Palpation	Tenderness in the lower right quadrant, especially in the area of McBurney's point (see Fig. 10–16). Rebound tenderness occurs. As the appendicitis progresses, the athlete displays a fever in the range of 99° to 101° F. The athlete's pulse is rapid.		
Functional tests	The athlete describes pain with movement. Urination and bowel movements increase pressure within the abdominal cavity, increasing the pain experienced by the athlete.		
Ligamentous tests	Not applicable.		
Neurological tests	Not applicable.		
Special tests	Not applicable.		
Comments	Athletes suspected of suffering from appendicitis must immediately be transported to an emergency room. In female athletes, the signs and symptoms of appendicitis are similar to those of *pelvic inflammatory disease*, ruptured *ectopic pregnancy*, and painful ovulation.		

permanent injury. When a hollow organ is ruptured, the outcome is extremely dangerous and potentially fatal secondary to hemorrhage and/or to peritoneal contamination.

Upon hollow organ rupture, the athlete reports a blow to the abdomen as well as pain and possible nausea. On further evaluation the athlete has guarding, abdominal rigidity and tenderness, and shock. Bowel sounds are absent when evaluated with a stethoscope.[7]

Because the onset of symptoms associated with hollow organ trauma is gradual, the symptoms may resemble those of a contusion, costal-cartilage sprain, or similar injury. The athlete with a seemingly benign abdominal injury should be cautioned to report increased symptoms and should visually inspect the stool for blood, as hemorrhage may leak into the feces.[8] As with all internal organ injuries, the athlete with suspected rupture of a hollow organ should be referred for evaluation at an appropriate medical facility. Although the liver is not a hollow organ, its location and relative rigidity predispose it to injury as well.

Injury to the Reproductive Organs

The female reproductive organs are well protected within the abdominal cavity. When trauma occurs to these organs, the signs and symptoms tend to duplicate those of appendicitis or trauma to the hollow organs but may be accompanied by untimely, irregular, or increased menstrual flow. Injury to the pubic symphysis is discussed in Chapter 7.

Because of their external location, the male reproductive organs much more commonly experience trauma. In a direct impact to the genitals, the resulting contusion or lacerations are often embarrassing, especially for younger athletes. These conditions must be professionally managed, not only to comfort the athlete but also to preserve the integrity of these organs.

Testicular Contusion
Direct blows to the testicles result in immediate pain, often at an intensity sufficient to cause vomiting, speech inhibition, breathing hindrance,

---

Pelvic inflammatory disease: An infection of the vagina that spreads to the cervix, uterus, fallopian tubes, and broad ligaments.
Ectopic pregnancy: The formation of a fetus outside of the uterine cavity.

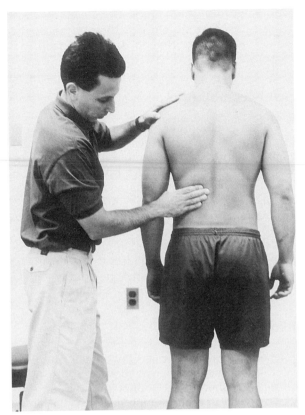

Figure 10–19. Palpation of the left kidney. Following an injury, the area overlying the kidneys may become tender to the touch or reveal crepitus secondary to a rib fracture.

and prevention of meaningful movement (the athlete may assume the fetal position). Additionally, the athlete may clutch the painful area. The priority in managing this condition is to comfort the athlete. This may be performed by assisting the athlete with breathing by instructing him to breathe deeply and slowly in through the nose and out through the mouth. Lifting the athlete's belt and waistband on the pants may reduce the feeling of pressure on the testicles and lower abdomen. The efficacy of other anecdotal techniques, such as lifting and dropping the athlete on his buttocks, has never been established.

Once the athlete's pain has been controlled, he should be instructed to feel the testicles for normal size and consistency. The trauma may cause the testicle to rupture, giving it a relatively soft, inconsistent texture. Swelling may occur within the testicles and may involve the collection of fluids within the scrotum. Either condition warrants follow-up examination by a physician.

Spermatic Cord Torsion

Torsion of the spermatic cord occurs as the testicle and spermatic cord are twisted within the scrotal sac. This injury can be prevented with the use of an athletic supporter. Unsupported, the testicle and spermatic cord are susceptible to injury from a direct blow or from the simple jarring movements that occur with athletic activity.

An onset due to acute trauma is associated with intense testicular pain, nausea, and possible vomiting. Symptoms of spermatic cord torsion may develop as gradually increasing pelvic or testicular pain. In this case the athlete may not be able to pinpoint a mechanism of injury. Inspection reveals a localized swelling of the testicle and tenderness during palpation. The athlete should be referred for further evaluation, as delayed treatment could lead to loss of the testicle.

Table 10–8. Evaluative Findings of a Contused or Lacerated Kidney

Examination Segment	Clinical Findings	
History	Onset:	Acute.
	Location of pain:	Posterolateral portion of the upper lumbar and lower thoracic region.
	Mechanism:	Blunt trauma or penetrating injury to the kidney (e.g., contusive forces, fractured rib impaling the kidney).
Inspection	The impacted area may reveal a contusion or laceration. Inspection of the urine may reveal hematuria. The signs and symptoms of shock may also be present.	
Palpation	There is tenderness over the impact site. Abdominal rigidity may occur.	
Functional tests	Pain may be described during urination.	
Ligamentous tests	Not applicable.	
Neurological tests	Not applicable.	
Special tests	Laboratory findings of hematuria.	
Comments	The traumatic forces may also result in a rib fracture or costochondral injury. Athletes suspected of suffering from a kidney injury should immediately be referred to a physician.	

ON-FIELD MANAGEMENT OF THORAX AND ABDOMINAL INJURIES

Because trauma to the thorax and abdomen is most often the result of acute, high-velocity impact, the need for on-field evaluation of these conditions is commonplace. At first, injuries to the internal organs may produce only the signs and symptoms of a contusion overlying the impact area. As blood collects within the viscera, outward symptoms of the underlying condition are produced.

Rib Fractures

Typically, athletes suffering a rib cage injury leave the area of athletic activity under their own power. In the case of a frank rib fracture or multiple rib fractures, the athlete may not be able to move and must be evaluated on the field. If the presence of a rib fracture is established, further evaluation must be performed to rule out the presence of a pneumothorax or hemothorax. If the absence of these conditions, the athlete should be calmed and the area stabilized before the athlete can be assisted from the field. The area may be stabilized by the use of a rib belt or, more commonly, by wrapping the ip-

silateral arm to the side of the athlete with a swathe (Fig. 10–20). The athlete can then be assisted off the field and transported to a medical facility for further evaluation.

Open Pneumothorax

An open pneumothorax can result from an open rib fracture that also pierces the pleural cavity or from a puncture resulting from the impalement by a sharp object (e.g., javelin). An open pneumothorax is characterized by a sucking sound as the athlete attempts to inhale air.

No attempt should be made to remove an object that has impaled the athlete. The opening should be covered with a sterile dressing and sealed with a nonporous material (e.g., a plastic bag) to prevent the passage of air. Oxygen may be administered to decrease the amount of respiratory distress.[9]

Hollow Organ Injury

Suspected injury to a hollow organ should be treated as a medical emergency and the athlete managed for shock. For comfort, the athlete's legs may be placed in a hook-lying position. The athlete

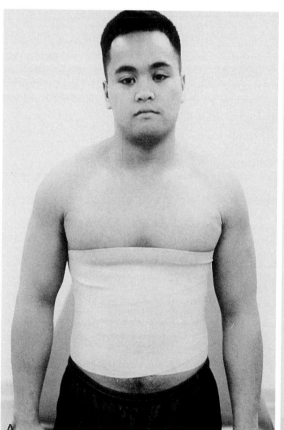
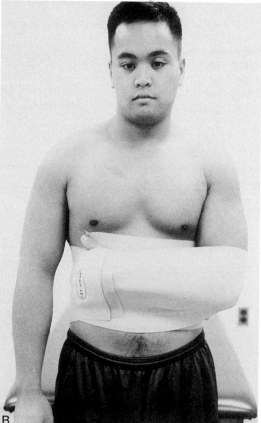

Figure 10–20. Immobilization of the rib cage through the use of a swath. (*A*) Compression of the ribs to minimize movement. (*B*) The arm of the involved side may be immobilized to reduce pain that is secondary to movement of the shoulder.

should be covered with a blanket to maintain body temperature if warranted. Vital signs should be continuously monitored and recorded, including the time they are taken. These readings should be given to the medical transport team to be delivered with the athlete to the medical facility.

Under no circumstances should the athlete be given anything by mouth. Oral ingestion of fluids or liquids may induce vomiting, further injuring the athlete, or it may complicate the task of anesthetizing the athlete for any surgical procedure that may be needed.

REFERENCES

1. Anderson, CR: Case Report: A runner's recurrent abdominal pain. One simple solution. The Physician and Sportsmedicine 20:81, 1992.
2. Vacarro, PS: Thoracic and vascular injuries in athletes. Athletic Training: Journal of the Nathonal Athletic Trainers Association 22:290, 1987.
3. Proffer, DS, Patton, JJ, and Jackson, DW: Nonunion of a first rib fracture in a gymnast. Am J Sports Med 19:198, 1991.
4. Wasik, M, and McFarland, M: Rib stress fractures: An overview (poster presentation). Journal of Athletic Training 27:156, 1992.
5. Yates, MT, and Aldrete, V: Case report. Blunt trauma causing aortic rupture. The Physician and Sportsmedicine 19:96, 1991.
6. Freitas, JE: Renal imaging following blunt trauma. The Physician and Sportsmedicine 17:59, 1989.
7. Baker, B: Jeunal perforation occurring in contact sports. Am J Sports Med 6:403, 1978.
8. Dauneker, DT, et al: Case report: Intra-abdominal injury to a gymnast. The Physician and Sportsmedicine 7:119, 1979.
9. Moore, S: Management of a pneumothorax in a football player. Athletic Training: Journal of the National Athletic Trainers Association 19:129, 1984.

11

The Shoulder and Upper Arm

The shoulder girdle is perhaps the most complex of the body's articulations because it is required to provide a large range of motion in many anatomical planes. The relationship between the glenohumeral joint and the scapula allows the humerus to be placed in 16,000 positions that can be differentiated in 1-degree increments.[1]

Relying on its musculature to provide much of its stability, the shoulder complex in general, and specifically the glenohumeral joint, is inherently unstable. Injury to this complex may occur from a direct force or from secondary forces transmitted proximally along the upper extremity. The glenohumeral joint is prone to overuse conditions, especially in sports requiring repeated overhead movements.

CLINICAL ANATOMY

The shoulder girdle is connected to the axial skeleton by a single joint. This configuration results in a mechanism in which the upper extremity is suspended from the torso by muscular attachments that secure it to the rest of the body. The motions provided by the upper extremity arise from the intricate interactions of the four bones that form the shoulder girdle and the four articulations that provide movement. The great range of motion provided by the shoulder complex, especially the glenohumeral (GH) joint, is achieved at the expense of joint stability. Unlike the hip joint, which gains its stability through a deep ball-and-socket joint and strong ligamentous support (at the expense of mobility), the GH joint is characterized by shallow articular surfaces receiving much of its support from a musculature arrangement that is augmented by bony struts.

Bony Anatomy

The shoulder girdle, formed by the sternum, clavicle, scapula, and humerus, may be likened to a series of hinges, pulleys, and levers working in unison to choreograph intricate motions in many anatomical planes (Fig. 11–1). A fine degree of coordination must be maintained between these bones to ensure the proper biomechanics and, therefore, strength and range of motion of the upper extremity.

The sternum's **manubrium** serves as the site of attachment for each clavicle. Projecting above the body of the sternum, the manubrium's superior surface is indented by the **jugular (suprasternal) notch**. Projecting off each side of the jugular notch is the **clavicular notch**, which accepts the medial head of the clavicle (Fig. 11–2).

Serving as a "strut" between the sternum and scapula, the **clavicle** elevates and rotates to maintain the alignment of the scapula, allowing for additional motion when the arm is raised and preventing excessive anterior displacement of the scapula. The proximal two-thirds of the clavicle is characterized by a convex (forward) bend. The distal one-third begins to flatten while curving concavely to meet with the scapula (Fig. 11–3). The point at which the clavicle begins its lateral bend, approximately two-thirds along its shaft, is relatively weak and is a common site for fractures. The superior surface of the clavicle is not protected by muscle mass, making the bone susceptible to injury.

Having no direct bony or ligamentous attachment to the axial skeleton, the **scapula** gains its attachment to the torso by way of the clavicle. Its anterior surface is held against the torso by atmospheric pressure and muscle attachments. The scapula's unique form gives rise to its unique function of being a lever and a pulley.

Thin and triangular, the scapula's anterior costal surface is concave, forming the **subscapular fossa**. The **vertebral (medial) border** is marked by the **inferior** and **superior angles**. The posterior surface is distinguished by the horizontal **scapular spine** dividing the large **infraspinous** fossa below and the smaller **supraspinous** fossa above. On the lateral end of the scapular spine is the anteriorly projecting **acromion process**, allowing for the articulation with the clavicle. Projecting inferiorly and anteriorly to the acromion is the beak-shaped **coracoid process**. The infraspinous, supraspinous, and sub-

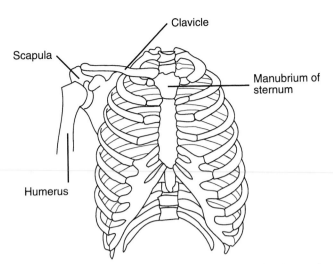

Figure 11–1. Bones of the shoulder girdle and glenohumeral joint.

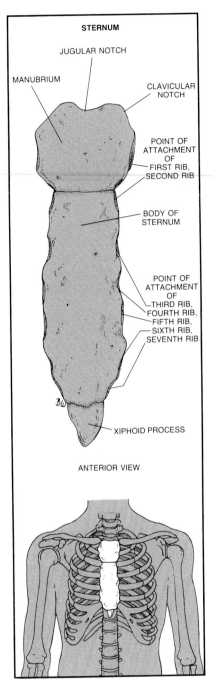

Figure 11–2. The sternum, formed by the manubrium, body, and xiphoid process. In preadolescents, the junction between the manubrium and sternal body is pliable, but it fuses with age. (From Thomas, CL [ed]: Taber's Cyclopedic Medical Dictionary, ed 17. FA Davis, Philadelphia, 1993, p 1875, by Beth Anne Willert, MS, medical illustrator, with permission.)

scapular fossae merge on the axial border to form the glenoid fossa. Located below the acromion, this fossa is designed to allow for articulation with the humeral head (Fig. 11–4).

When the scapula is placed in its anatomical position the glenoid fossa angles 30 degrees toward the midline of the body and its face assumes a downward direction (Fig. 11–5).[2] Known as the **plane of the scapula**, this angle provides a more functional plane for movement than is present in the cardinal planes. For example, when reaching for an item on an overhead shelf, it is more natural to lift the arm in the plane of the scapula rather than through the sagittal or frontal planes.

The proximal end of the **humerus** is characterized by the medially projecting **humeral head** (Fig. 11–6). Bisecting the upper one-quarter of the anterior surface of the humerus is the **bicipital groove**, or intertubercular groove, through which the long head of the biceps tendon passes. The lateral edge of the groove is formed by the **greater tuberosity**, and the medial border, by the **lesser tuberosity**. The inferior borders of the greater and lesser tuberosities mark an area known as the **surgical neck**. This name is given because fractures at this site generally require surgical intervention owing to the large number of nerves passing through this site. Laterally and slightly above midshaft is the attachment site for the deltoid muscle group, the deltoid tuberosity. The distal structures of the humerus are covered in Chapter 12.

The **angle of inclination** describes the relationship between the shaft of the humerus and the humeral head in the frontal plane, having a normal value of 130 to 150 degrees. In the transverse plane, the relationship between the shaft of the humerus and the humeral head is the **angle of torsion**, which varies greatly from individual to individual (Fig. 11–7).[3]

Joints of the Shoulder Girdle

The motion of the GH joint is augmented by the sternoclavicular and acromioclavicular joints and the movement between the scapula and the thorax. A decrease in the mobility or function at any of

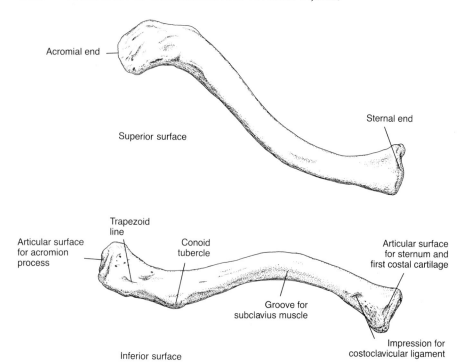

Figure 11–3. Clavicle, superior and inferior views. (From Rothstein, JM, Roy, SH, and Wolf, SL,[3a] p 23, with permission.)

these associated joints decreases the function at the GH joint.

The Sternoclavicular Joint

The shoulder girdle's only bony attachment to the axial skeleton occurs at the sternoclavicular (SC) joint. Here, the proximal portion of the clavicle meets the manubrium of the sternum and a portion of the first costal cartilage to form a gliding joint that allows 3 degrees of freedom of motion: elevation/depression, **protraction/retraction**, and internal/external rotation.

The articulation between the manubrium and clavicle is inherently incongruent as the proximal end of the clavicle extends one-half of its width above the manubrium (Fig. 11–8). The stability of this junction is enhanced by the presence of a fibrocartilaginous disk. Surrounded by a synovial membrane, the SC joint is supported by the anterior and

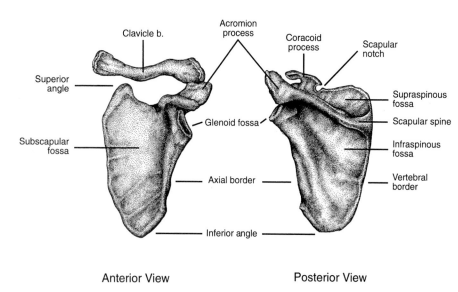

Figure 11–4. Bony anatomy of the scapula, anterior (costal), and posterior (dorsal) views, showing the relationship with the clavicle.

Protraction (scapular): Movement of the vertebral borders of the scapula away from the spinal column.
Retraction (scapular): Movement of the scapular vertebral borders toward the spinal column.

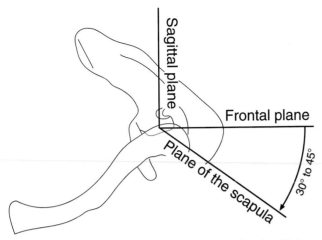

Figure 11-5. Plane of the scapula. The face of the glenoid fossa sits at a 30° angle toward the midline of the body. Movements within the plane of the scapula are more "natural" than movements in the cardinal plane.

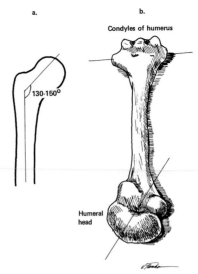

Figure 11-7. Angular alignment of the humerus. Angle of inclination representing the angle formed by the long axis of the humeral shaft and the axis of the humeral head. Angle of torsion representing the relationship between the humeral condyles and the humeral head in the transverse plane. (From Norkin, CC, and Levangie, PK,[3] p 219, with permission.)

posterior SC ligaments, the **costoclavicular ligament**, and the interclavicular ligament.

The **sternoclavicular disk** has qualities similar to the menisci found in the knee, functioning as a shock absorber and acting as the axis for clavicular rotation. Its upper portion is attached to the clavicle, its lower portion to the manubrium and first costal cartilage. The presence of this disk also serves to divide the joint into two articular cavities, one between the disk and the clavicle and a second between the disk and the manubrium.

The **anterior** and **posterior sternoclavicular ligaments** reinforce the synovial membrane. The anterior fibers resist posterior displacement of the clavicle on the manubrium while the posterior fibers resist anterior displacement. The costoclavicular ligament serves as an axis of clavicular elevation/depression and protraction/retraction. Its anterior fibers limit ele-

vation and lateral clavicular movement. Likewise, the posterior fibers check elevation and medial movement of the clavicle.

Both of the SC joints are joined by the **interclavicular ligament**. Attaching to the proximal ends of the left and right clavicles, the ligament has a common connection on the superior border of the sternum. The interclavicular ligament resists downward movement of the clavicle and assists in dissipating force across the entire upper extremity.

The Acromioclavicular Joint

The distal end of the clavicle meets the scapula's acromion process to form the acromioclavicular (AC) joint. This plane synovial joint allows a gliding articulation between the acromion and the clav-

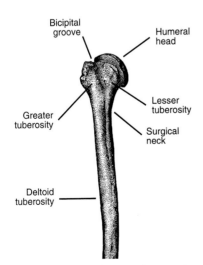

Figure 11-6. Upper humerus, showing the prominent bony landmarks.

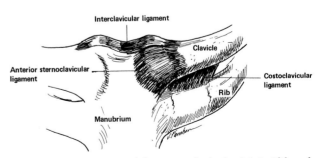

Figure 11-8. Ligaments of the sternoclavicular joint. Although the sternoclavicular joint does not have inherent bony stability, the ligamentous arrangement provides great strength to the joint. (From Norkin, CC, and Levangie, PK,[3] p 214, with permission.)

icle capable of 3 degrees of freedom of movement: (1) scapular rotation, (2) *scapular winging*, and (3) *scapular tipping*. This articulation allows for the motion necessary to maintain the relationship between the scapula and the clavicle in the early and late stages of the GH joint's range of motion.

Surrounded by a synovial membrane, the AC joint is supported by the **acromioclavicular ligament** and the **coracoclavicular ligament**, which suspend the scapula from the clavicle (Fig. 11–9). In the younger years a synovial disk is present between the clavicle and the acromion, but it disappears during adolescence and therefore may or may not be present in the athlete's shoulder.

Divided into two separate bands, the superior and inferior portions of the acromioclavicular ligament function jointly to maintain continuity between the articulating surfaces of the acromion and clavicle. With much of its restraint in the horizontal plane, this ligament maintains stability by preventing the clavicle from riding up and over the acromion process.

Most of the AC joint's intrinsic stability arises from the coracoclavicular ligament. This ligament is divided into two unique portions, the quadrilateral **trapezoid ligament** and the triangular **conoid ligament**. Separated by a bursa, the trapezoid limits lateral movement of the clavicle on the acromion and the conoid checks superior movement of the clavicle. Acting in concert, these ligaments jointly limit rotation of the scapula and provide some degree of horizontal stability. However, a horizontal dislocation of the AC joint can occur with the coracoclavicular ligament's remaining intact.

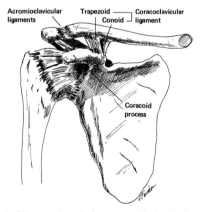

Figure 11–9. Ligaments of the acromioclavicular joint. The acromioclavicular ligament provides horizontal stability to the joint. The two portions of the coracoclavicular ligament prevent anterior/posterior displacement of the clavicle on the scapula. (From Norkin, CC, and Levangie, PK,[3] p 217, with permission.)

The Scapulothoracic Articulation

The articulation between the scapula and the posterior rib cage is not a true anatomical joint because it lacks the typical joint characteristics of connection by fibrous, cartilaginous, or synovial tissues. The movements associated with the scapulothoracic articulation are scapular elevation/depression, protraction/retraction, and upward/downward rotation. The motions rarely occur in an isolated manner but more typically occur in unison (e.g., protraction and upward rotation). Movement at the scapulothoracic, AC, or SC joint produces motion of the other two joints, creating a closed kinetic chain.

The Glenohumeral Joint

Formed by the head of the humerus and the scapula's glenoid fossa, the GH articulation is a ball-and-socket joint capable of 3 degrees of freedom of motion: flexion/extension, abduction/adduction, and internal/external rotation. Although not a true anatomical motion, the movement known as horizontal flexion and extension (or horizontal abduction and adduction) also occur at this joint. Because of its relevance to many athletic movements, it is considered as a unique movement throughout this chapter. Most athletic upper extremity motions do not occur in a single isolated plane but, rather, are a combination of movements in two or more planes.

The GH joint is inherently unstable because of the relationship in the sizes of the articular surfaces of the glenoid fossa and the humeral head, a loose joint capsule, and relatively weak ligamentous support. The articulating surface of the glenoid fossa is significantly smaller than that of the humeral head and only vaguely resembles the ball-and-socket joint of the hip. The socket is somewhat deepened by the **glenoid labrum**, which also slightly increases the articular surface. Traditionally thought of as a synovium-lined fibrocartilage, recent findings suggest that the glenoid labrum is actually a fold of dense fibrous connective tissue.[4] Disruption of the glenoid labrum is associated with chronic shoulder instability.

Possessing a volume twice the size of the humeral head, the joint capsule arises from the glenoid fossa and merges with the muscles of the rotator cuff. Studies on human cadavers indicate that the laxity of the capsular arrangement allows the humeral head to be distracted 2 cm or more from the glenoid fossa.[5] The capsule is reinforced by the **glenohumeral ligaments** and the **coracohumeral ligament** (Fig. 11–10).

The three glenohumeral ligaments—superior, middle, and inferior—are not distinct joint struc-

---

Scapular winging: The vertebral border of the scapula lifting away from the thorax.
Scapular tipping: The inferior angle of the scapula moving away from the thorax while its superior border moves toward the thorax.

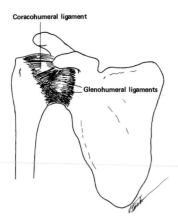

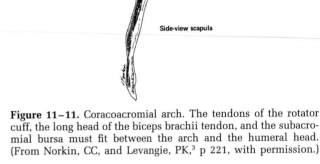

Figure 11–10. Ligaments of the glenohumeral joint: the coraco-humeral and glenohumeral ligaments. The glenohumeral ligament is divided into superior, middle, and inferior portions. To provide the necessary range of motion to the glenohumeral joint, these ligaments must be relatively lax. Much of the stability of this articulation is gained from its muscular arrangement. (From Norkin, CC, and Levangie, PK,[3] p 220, with permission.)

Figure 11–11. Coracoacromial arch. The tendons of the rotator cuff, the long head of the biceps brachii tendon, and the subacromial bursa must fit between the arch and the humeral head. (From Norkin, CC, and Levangie, PK,[3] p 221, with permission.)

tures but are actually thickenings in the joint capsule. As a group they limit external rotation of the humerus and check anterior displacement of the humeral head on the glenoid fossa. The inferior glenohumeral ligament possesses an anterior and posterior band with a hammocklike structure connecting the two. The area between the superior and middle glenohumeral ligaments, known as the **foramen of Weitbrecht**, is a weak site on the capsule that is often torn during anterior GH dislocations.

Emanating from the coracoid process, the coracohumeral ligament merges with the superior capsule and the supraspinous tendon to insert on the greater tuberosity. The anterior fibers of this ligament limit extension while the posterior fibers limit the amount of GH flexion.

When the humerus is hanging at rest in the anatomical position the articular surfaces of the GH joint have very little contact. Much of the weight of the arm is supported by the superior glenohumeral ligament and the inferior portion of the glenoid labrum. When the humerus is abducted to 90 degrees and externally rotated, the entire joint capsule is wound tight, placing the GH joint in its closed-packed position.

Superior to the humeral head is the coracoacromial arch, formed by the coracoacromial ligament that traverses from the inferior portion of the acromion process to the posterior portion of the coracoid process (Fig. 11–11). This structure protects the superior portion of the humeral head, the tendons of the rotator cuff muscles, and various bursae from trauma while also providing a restraint against superior and anterior GH dislocations. As is discussed later, this structure also plays a principal role in shoulder impingement syndrome.

Muscles of the Shoulder Girdle

The relationship between the muscles acting on the scapula and those acting on the humerus must be understood by the examiner. A complete explanation of the static and dynamic relationships of the forces placed on the scapula and humerus is beyond the scope of this text. The reader is encouraged to consult an anatomy or kinesiology text for a more detailed description of these forces.

Muscles Acting on the Scapula

The muscles acting on the scapula have two purposes: (1) to move the scapula and, thus, the glenoid fossa, to allow the arm increased range of motion, and (2) to fixate the scapula on the thorax in order to provide the arm with a fixed base of support during isometric contractions. The action, origin, insertion, and nerve supply for those muscles acting on the scapula are presented in Table 11–1.

Inserting on the scapula's vertebral border are the **rhomboid minor** and **rhomboid major**. These muscles retract the vertebral border toward the spine and elevate and downwardly rotate the scapula. The **levator scapulae** acts on the scapula to elevate and downwardly rotate it. The **serratus anterior**, inserting on the costal surface of the vertebral border, acts as a unit to upwardly rotate and protract the scapula. Working segmentally, its lower fibers depress the scapula and its upper fibers elevate it. Additionally, this muscle plays a primary function in fixating the scapula's vertebral border to the thorax. A weakness in this muscle or injury to the long thoracic nerve innervating it can result in **scapular winging**, in which the vertebral border lifts away from the thorax. The **pectoralis minor** serves to up-

Table 11–1. Muscles Acting on the Scapula

Muscle	Action	Origin	Insertion	Nerve	Root
Latissimus dorsi	Retraction Downward rotation	• Spinous processes of T6 through T12 and the lumbar vertebrae via the lumbodorsal fascia. • Posterior iliac crest	• Intertubercular groove of the humerus • Inferior portion of the scapula	Thoracodorsal	C6, C7, C8
Levator scapulae	Elevation Downward rotation Extension of C-spine	• Transverse processes of cervical vertebrae C1 through C4	• Superior medial angle of the scapula	Dorsal subscapular	C3, C4, C5
Rhomboid major	Retraction Elevation Downward rotation Fixation of T-spine	• Spinous processes of T2, T3, T4, and T5	• Vertebral border of scapula (lower two-thirds)	Dorsal scapular	C5
Rhomboid minor	Retraction Elevation Downward rotation Fixation of T-spine	• Inferior portion of the ligamentum nuchae • Spinous processes C7 and T1	• Vertebral border of scapula (upper one-third and superior angle)	Dorsal scapular	C5
Serratus anterior	Upward rotation Protraction Depression (lower fibers) Elevation (upper fibers) Fixes the scapula to the thorax	• Anterior portion of 1st through 8th or 9th ribs • Aponeuroses of the intercostal muscles	• Costal surfaces of the: • Superior angle of scapula • Vertebral border of scapula • Inferior angle of scapula	Long thoracic	C5, C6, C7
Trapezius (upper one-third)	Elevation of scapula Upward rotation of scapula Rotation of C-spine to the opposite side Extension of C-spine	• Occipital protuberance • Nuchal line of the occipital bone • Upper portion of the ligamentum nuchae • Spinous process of C7	• Distal/lateral one-third of clavicle • Acromion process	Accessory	Cranial nerve XI
Trapezius (middle one-third)	Retraction of scapula Fixation of thoracic spine	• Lower portion of the ligamentum nuchae • Spinous processes of the 7th cervical vertebra and T1 through T5	• Acromion process • Spine of the scapula (superior, lateral border)	Accessory	Cranial nerve XI
Trapezius (lower one-third)	Depression of scapula Retraction of scapula Fixation of thoracic spine	• Spinous processes and supraspinal ligaments of T8 through T12	• Spine of the scapula (medial portion)	Accessory	Cranial nerve XI
Pectoralis major	Depression of the shoulder girdle (clavicular fibers)	• Medial one-half of the clavical • Anterolateral portion of the sternum • Costalcartilages of ribs 6 through 7	• Greater tuberosity of the humerus	Medial and lateral pectoral	C5, C6, C7, C8, T1
Pectoralis minor	Upward rotation Forward tilting	• Anterior portion of 3rd through 5th ribs	• Coracoid process of scapula	Medial pectoral	C6, C7, C8, T1

Muscle actions, origins, and insertions adapted from Kendall and McCreary[5a]; innervations adapted from Daniels and Worthingham.[5b]

wardly rotate the scapula and tilt it forward so that the inferior angle lifts away from the thorax (Fig. 11–12).

The **trapezius** muscle can be divided into upper, middle, and lower segments (Fig. 11–13). Each of these three segments of the trapezius has a unique action on the scapula. The upper fibers elevate and upwardly rotate, the middle fibers retract, and the lower fibers retract and depress the scapula.

Two additional muscles have an indirect force on the scapula. The upper fibers from the **latissimus dorsi** act on the scapula to retract and downwardly rotate it. The clavicular portion of the **pectoralis major** depresses the scapula by its attachment to the clavicle at the AC joint.

Muscles Acting on the Humerus

Motion at the shoulder joint can occur as pure GH motion or, as in the case of sport-specific motions, can be the result of the motion provided by the entire shoulder complex. The action, origin, insertion, and nerve supply for those muscles acting primarily on the humerus are presented in Table 11–2.

Four muscles arising off the scapula form the musculotendinous or **rotator cuff** muscle group (Fig. 11–14). As a unit, the rotator cuff stabilizes the humeral head in the glenoid fossa and, during the later stages of abduction, provide a downward pull on the humeral head, allowing for its passage under the acromion. The **subscapularis muscle** is the only member of the rotator cuff group that internally rotates the humerus. The **supraspinatus** assists the deltoid group in abducting the arm. The

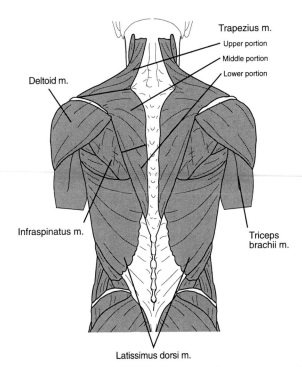

Figure 11–13. Superficial posterior muscles acting on the scapula and glenohumeral joint. The trapezius (upper, middle, and lower portions), latissimus dorsi, infraspinatus, posterior portion of the deltoid, and the triceps brachii.

remaining two members of the rotator cuff, the **infraspinatus** and **teres minor**, externally rotate the humerus and provide a degree of assistance during horizontal abduction. Additionally, the teres minor is an assistive mover during extension of the GH joint. The eccentric contractions of the infraspinatus and teres minor muscles have a major function in decreasing the velocity of overhand throwing motions. Closely associated with the muscles of the rotator cuff is the **teres major**, which assists with internal rotation, adduction, and extension of the humerus.

Although having a common insertion on the deltoid tuberosity of the humerus, each section of the **deltoid** muscle group should be considered independently. As a whole, the deltoid muscle group is the prime mover during abduction. Considered as individual units, the **anterior fibers** flex the GH joint and horizontally flex and internally rotate the humerus. The **middle fibers** serve to abduct the humerus. The **posterior fibers** act to extend, horizontally extend, and externally rotate the humerus. The deltoid group and the upper fibers of the trapezius merge at the AC joint and assume the role of secondary stabilizers of this articulation.

During abduction a ***force couple*** exists between

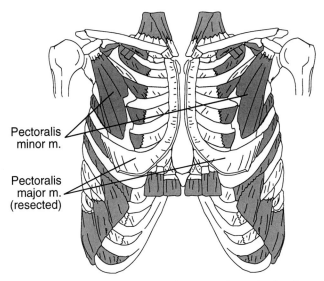

Figure 11–12. Pectoralis minor. The pectoralis major has been resected.

Force couple: Coordination between dynamic and static contractions of opposing muscle groups to perform a movement of a joint.

Table 11–2. Muscles Acting on the Humerus

Muscle	Action	Origin	Insertion	Nerve	Root
Biceps brachii	Flexion Abduction	• Long head: Supraglenoid tuberosity of scapula • Short head: Coracoid process of scapula	• Radial tuberosity	Musculocutaneous	C5, C6
Coracobrachialis	Flexion Adduction	• Coracoid process	• Medial shaft of the humerus, adjacent to the deltoid tuberosity	Musculocutaneous	C6, C7
Deltoid (anterior one-third)	Flexion Abduction Horizontal flexion Internal rotation	• Lateral one-third of the clavicle	• Deltoid tuberosity	Axillary	C5, C6
Deltoid (middle one-third)	Abduction Flexion	• Acromial process	• Deltoid tuberosity	Axillary	C5, C6
Deltoid (posterior one-third)	Extension Horizontal extension Abduction External rotation	• Spine of the scapula	• Deltoid tuberosity	Axillary	C5, C6
Infraspinatus	External rotation Horizontal extension Stabilizes humeral head	• Infraspinatus fossa of the scapula	• Greater tuberosity of the humerus • Glenohumeral joint capsule	Suprascapular	C5, C6
Latissimus dorsi	Extension Internal rotation Adduction	• Spinous processes of T6 through T12 and the lumbar vertebrae via the lumbodorsal fascia. • Posterior iliac crest	• Bicipital groove of the humerus • Inferior portion of the scapula	Thoracodorsal	C6, C7, C8
Pectoralis major	Adduction Horizontal flexion Flexion (clavicular segment) Internal rotation	• Medial one-half of the clavicle • Anterolateral portion of the sternum • Costalcartilages of ribs 6 through 7	• Greater tuberosity of the humerus	Medial and lateral pectoral	C5, C6, C7, C8, T1
Subscapularis	Internal rotation Stabilizes humeral head	• Anterior surface (subscapular fossa) and axillary border of the scapula	• Lesser tuberosity of the humerus • Ventral portion of the glenohumeral capsule	Superior and inferior subscapular	C5, C6
Supraspinatus	Abduction Stabilizes humeral head	• Supraspinatus fossa (medial two-thirds) of the scapula	• Greater tuberosity • Glenohumeral joint capsule	Suprascapular	C5
Teres major	Extension Internal rotation Adduction	• Inferior angle of the scapula • Lower one-third of the axillary border of the scapula	• Lesser tuberosity of the humerus	Inferior subscapular	C5, C6
Teres minor	External rotation Extension Horizontal extension Stabilizes the humeral head	• Lateral upper two-thirds of axillary border of the scapula	• Greater tuberosity of the humerus	Axillary	C5
Triceps brachii	Extension (long head) Adduction	• Long head: Infraglenoid tuberosity of scapula	• Olecranon process of ulna	Radial	C7, C8

Muscle actions, origins, and insertions adapted from Kendall and McCreary[5a]; innervations adapted from Daniels and Worthingham.[5b]

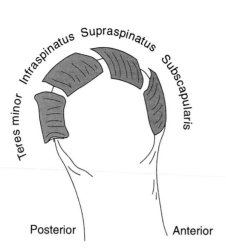

Figure 11–14. Muscles of the rotator cuff as they attach to the humeral head.

the line of pull between the rotator cuff and the deltoid muscle groups. The line of force created by the deltoid's contraction tends to pull the head of the humerus against the inferior portion of the acromion process and the coracoacromial ligament. In the early stages of abduction, the rotator cuff's angle of pull must be sufficient to hold the head of the humerus close against the glenoid fossa. Once the humerus moves past 90 degrees, the rotator cuff's angle of pull changes so that its force rolls the humeral head inferiorly on the glenoid fossa, creating clearance to pass under the acromion process and the coracoacromial ligament (Fig. 11–15). A damaged or weak rotator cuff group changes the dynamics of the force couple, resulting in the impingement of the rotator cuff and long head of the biceps brachii tendon between the humeral head and the acromion process.

The **pectoralis major** may be divided into two portions having a common insertion on the greater tuberosity: the clavicular portion and the sternal portion (Fig. 11–16). The action of this muscle as a whole is to adduct and internally rotate the humerus. The clavicular portion, in addition to adduction, serves to flex, internally rotate, and horizontally adduct the humerus.

The **latissimus dorsi** has a broad origin on the lumbar spine and iliac crest. Inserting on the intertubercular groove of the humerus, the actions of the latissimus dorsi on the humerus are adduction, internal rotation, and extension. Attaching to the infraglenoid tuberosity of the scapula, the **long head of the triceps brachii** is an adductor and extensor of the humerus, especially when the elbow is flexed.

The **coracobrachialis** acts on the humerus as a flexor and adductor. Both heads of the **biceps brachii** have an attachment on the scapula (Fig. 11–17). The short head attaches to the coracoid process while the long head passes through the bicipital groove to attach on the supraglenoid tuberosity. Stability within the bicipital groove is maintained by the transverse humeral ligament, which is lined by a capsular sheath emanating from the GH capsule. Both heads assist in GH flexion and, when the humerus is externally rotated, the long head assists in GH abduction.

The long head of the biceps enters the joint capsule through an invagination between the supraspinatus and subscapularis muscles. While the capsule is penetrated, the tendon does not enter the synovial membrane of the articulation. During the motions of flexion and abduction, the tendon must slide within the bicipital groove. Although the bi-

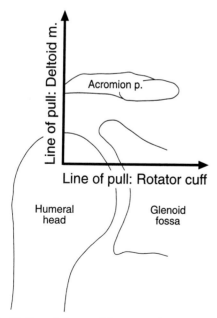

Figure 11–15. Scapulohumeral force couple. Contraction of the deltoid muscle pulls the humeral head upward. To prevent contact between the humeral head and the acromion process during abduction, the rotator cuff must hold the humeral head close to the glenoid fossa and, when the humerus approaches 90° of abduction, must serve to glide the humerus inferiorly.

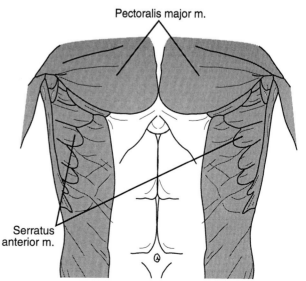

Figure 11–16. Pectoralis major and serratus anterior.

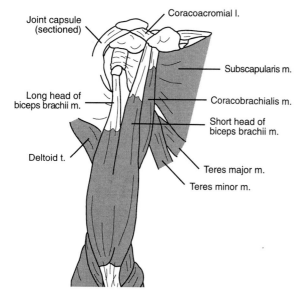

Figure 11-17. Coracobrachialis and attachment of the long and short heads of the biceps brachii muscle.

ceps produces little force during these motions, an inflammatory response or damage to the transverse humeral ligament results in pain and disrupts the normal mechanics of this joint.

Scapulothoracic Rhythm

For the hand to obtain its maximal arc of motion, the humerus and scapula must combine their individual ranges of motion. If the humeral head were rigidly fixated in the glenoid fossa in a manner eliminating GH movement, the humerus could still be elevated to 60 degrees through upward rotation of the scapula. For the humerus to be abducted to its maximum range of motion of 180 degrees, a minimum 2:1 ratio between GH abduction and upward scapular rotation must occur (120 degrees occurring from GH movement and 60 degrees through upward rotation of the scapula).

This ratio is not smooth or consistent. Early in the range of motion the movements of abduction and flexion occur primarily at the GH joint, with the scapula fixating to provide stability for the contracting muscles. During the intermediate stages of humeral elevation (whether abduction or flexion) the ratio between the GH joint and the scapula is approximately 1:1.[6] At the extremes of these movements, these motions again occur primarily at the GH joint. Maintenance of this rhythm is based on the coordination of the prime movers of the humerus as well as on the synergistic contractions of the scapular stabilizers.

Bursa of the Shoulder Girdle

The primary bursa of the GH joint is the subacromial bursa, although many references cite two bursae in this area: the subacromial and the subdeltoid.

However, these two bursae are often fused into one unit that is commonly referred to as the subacromial bursa. The bursa is located on the superior surface of the supraspinatus tendon and serves to lubricate the movement of the overlying fibers of the deltoid muscle, acting as a secondary joint cavity.[7] When the humerus is elevated, the bursa buffers the supraspinatus tendon against its contact with the acromion process and the coracoacromial ligament.

CLINICAL EVALUATION OF SHOULDER INJURIES

A strong understanding of the normal anatomy and biomechanics of the shoulder girdle is necessary so that the evaluation of this complex can be approached in a logical, systematic manner (Table 11-3). Because of the interrelationship of the shoulder complex to the cervical and thoracic spine, torso, abdomen, and elbow, the clinician should be prepared to undertake a thorough evaluation of these areas. Chapter 9 discusses pain that may be referred from the cervical spine, and Chapter 10 describes visceral pain that is referred into the shoulder and upper arm.

History

During the history-taking phase of the examination, the onset and duration of the condition must be ascertained and the location of the pain identified. Because the shoulder and upper arm are common sites for referred pain of orthopedic or visceral origins, a complete examination of the cervical spine, thorax, and abdomen may be indicated, particularly when the athlete presents a vague history of injury to the shoulder girdle (see Fig. 10-16). These conditions are covered in their corresponding chapters.

The following information should be obtained during history taking so that the mechanism of injury, prior injuries, the structures involved in the injury, and the nature of the pain can be localized:

- **Location of the pain:** The examiner should begin the examination by localizing the area of pain, the type of pain, and any dysfunction noted by the athlete.

- **Onset:** The duration of the pain experienced by the athlete is often indicative of the underlying pathology. Many inflammatory conditions of the shoulder complex, such as tendinitis, bursitis, or osteoarthritis, have an insidious onset. In these cases the athlete may first notice the pain after activity. This then progresses to pain during activity and, eventually, constant pain.

- **Activity and injury mechanism:** An external force applied to the shoulder girdle, such as a direct blow or joint force beyond normal limits, re-

Table 11–3. Clinical Evaluation of the Shoulder

History	Inspection	Palpation	Functional Tests	Ligamentous Tests	Neurological Tests	Special Tests
Location of the pain	General	Anterior Structures	Active Range of	Sternoclavicular laxity	Brachial plexus	Ligament Instability
Onset	The position of	Sternoclavicular	Motion	Acromioclavicular laxity	Cervical nerve root	SC joint sprains
Activity	the head	joint	Flexion	Glenohumeral laxity	Thoracic outlet	AC joint sprains
Injury mechanism	The position of	Clavicular shaft	Extension		syndrome	traction test
Symptoms	the arm	Acromion process	Abduction		Adson's test	AC compression
Prior injury	Anterior Structures	Acromioclavicular	Adduction		Allen test	test
	Level of the	joint piano key	Internal rotation		Military brace	GH instability
	shoulders	sign	External rotation		position	Apprehension
	Contour of the	Coracoid process	Horizontal flexion			test
	clavicles	Pectoralis major	Horizontal extension			Relocation test
	Symmetry of the	Pectoralis minor				Sulcus sign
	deltoid muscle	Coracobrachialis	Passive Range of			Posterior
	groups		Motion			apprehension
	Anterior humerus	Humerus	Flexion			test
	Biceps brachii	Humeral head	Extension			Posterior insta-
		Greater tuberosity	Abduction			bility in the
	Lateral Structures	Bicipital groove	Adduction			plane of the
	Deltoid muscle	Lesser tuberosity	Internal rotation			scapula
	group	Humeral shaft	External rotation			
	Acromion process	Deltoid group	Horizontal flexion			Rotator Cuff
	Step deformity	Biceps brachii	Horizontal extension			Pathology
	Position of the	Triceps brachii				Cuff impingement
	humerus	Rotator cuff	Resisted Range of			Impingement
		Teres major	Motion			test
	Posterior Structures	Latissimus dorsi	Flexion			Modified test
	Alignment of the		Extension			Rotator cuff ten-
	spinal vertebrae	Scapula	Abduction			dinitis
	Position of the	Spine of the	Adduction			Drop arm test
	scapula	scapula	Internal rotation			Empty can test
	Muscle tone	Superior angle	External rotation			
	Position of the	Inferior angle	Horizontal flexion			Biceps Tendon
	humerus	Axial border	Horizontal extension			Pathology
		Trapezius				Yergason's test
		Levator scapulae	Scapular Movements			Speed's test
		Rhomboids				Subacromial
						Bursitis
						Scapular Injuries
						Humeral Injuries

sults in acute soft tissue or bony injury. Repetitive motion such as that experienced in overhead sports activities, such as throwing, swimming, or tennis, are prone to overuse injuries.

- **Symptoms:** The symptoms to be noted are resting pain, pain with movement, and dysfunction of the shoulder girdle. The athlete may describe the shoulder as "going out of place," indicating glenohumeral instability, decreased velocity or accuracy when throwing, or discomfort when performing overhand motions indicative of inflammatory conditions. Table 11–4 presents the phases of the pitching motion and relates the structures involved with each.

- **Prior injury:** A history of previous injury to the acromioclavicular or GH joints can alter the biomechanics of the shoulder girdle. Because cervical spine pathology can result in referred pain to the upper extremity, the previous injury history of the cervical spine should be ascertained. If the athlete has a history of injury to the cervical spine or thorax, the exact diagnosis of the injury should be obtained so that its possible relationship to the existing condition can be determined.

The preceding list is not all-inclusive for the questions to be asked during the history-taking process. The scope of the questions expands for those cases involving an insidious onset. When an acute traumatic injury is being assessed, the history-taking process should become more focused based on the mechanism of injury.

Inspection

The inspection of the extremity begins during the history-taking process, at which time the examiner notes:

- **The position of the head:** The athlete's head normally assumes an upright position. A head that is tilted or rotated may indicate muscle spasm, pressure on a cervical nerve root, or stretching of the cervical nerves. Conditions relating to the cervical spine and its nerve network are discussed in Chapter 9.

- **The position of the arm and the athlete's willingness to move the involved limb:** One should note whether the athlete splints the arm alongside the body or whether it simply hangs limp at the side. Does the athlete gesture with the involved arm or duplicate the motion or position causing pain?

The athlete should remove any clothing that may inhibit the full inspection of both shoulders and the cervical, thoracic, and lumbar spine. If feasible, female athletes should be asked to wear a bathing suit (or similar clothing) during the clinical portion of the examination.

The athlete's willingness to move the involved limb should be observed throughout the examination. For instance, does the athlete raise the involved arm when removing the shirt or jacket or does the arm remain at the side with the clothing dropped down over it? Unwillingness to move the arm may indicate a chronic problem or an acute condition with mild to moderate symptoms.

When the athlete has appropriately disrobed, an observation of the following details should be performed while inspecting the skin for discoloration or signs of previous trauma. Generally there is no visible edema in the shoulder area.

Inspection of the Anterior Structures

- **Level of the shoulders:** When looking at the athlete from the front, the level of each shoulder girdle is noted. The height of the AC joints, the clavicle, and the SC joints should align with the opposite structure, although it is common for the dominant shoulder to appear slightly lower than the nondominant one (Fig. 11–18).

A painful shoulder is often held in an elevated position by the athlete.[8] Unilateral elevation may also indicate trapezius hypertrophy (upper fibers) on the raised side or atrophy on the depressed side. Another cause is the presence of scoliosis (see Inspection of the Posterior Structures).

Bilaterally raised shoulders may result from well-developed trapezius muscles or unwanted spasm in these muscle groups. Shoulders that are abnormally depressed bilaterally may occur as a result of decreased trapezius muscle tone. Bilaterally or unilaterally depressed shoulder girdles can place pressure on the arterial, venous, and nervous supply of the arm and can predispose an athlete to **thoracic outlet syndrome** (see Pathologies and Related Special Tests section of this chapter). Rounded shoulders can indicate tightness of the pectoralis major muscles.

- **Contour of the clavicles:** In thin athletes or athletes with well-defined upper body musculature the superior surface of the clavicle is easily visible. By comparing bilaterally, the SC joint, the shaft of the clavicle, and the clavicle's termination at the AC joint may be observed for symmetry.

Acute traumatic conditions involving the clavicle are typically identifiable during the inspection process. Sternoclavicular or acromioclavicular sprains may be marked by a gross deformity at the articulation, with one side having a more predominant protrusion than the other side. Any previous history involving these joints must be established because deformity may be residual from past trauma.

Complete clavicular fractures are indicated by a clear deformity of the shaft (Fig. 11–19). Al-

Table 11–4. Phases of the Pitching Motion

	Wind-up	Cocking	Acceleration	Deceleration	Follow-through
Glenohumeral joint position	Neutral	90° abduction Maximum external rotation	90° abduction Moving to internal rotation	90° abduction Internal rotation	Horizontal flexion Internal rotation Decreasing abduction
Glenohumeral joint stresses	Low joint stresses	Anterior joint capsule Inferior joint capsule	Anterior joint capsule	Posterior joint capsule Distraction of GH joint	Posterior joint capsule Distraction of GH joint
Elbow position	Some degrees of flexion	Approximately 90° flexion	90° flexion moving into extension	20° to 30° flexion moving into extension	Extension
Concentric muscle contraction	Muscular forces are mostly generated by the lower extremity	External rotators	Internal rotators Serratus anterior Upper trapezius Trunk and lower extremity	Internal rotators Triceps brachii	Internal rotators
Eccentric muscle contraction		Internal rotators	External rotators Rhomboids Trapezius	External rotators Biceps brachii Brachialis	External rotators
Center of gravity	Elevated over pivot foot	Over pivot foot	Between pivot foot and plant foot	Over plant foot	Forward of plant foot

Adapted from Fleisig, GS, Dillman, CJ, and Andrews, JR,[8a] p 355; and Souza, TA,[8b] p 71.

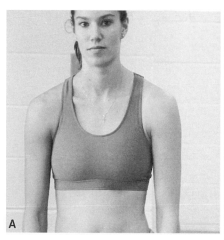

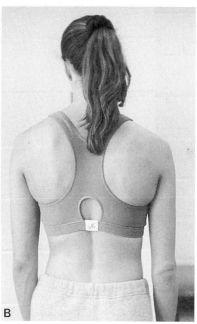

Figure 11–18. (*A*) Anterior and (*B*) posterior view of the shoulders. Note that the shoulder of the athlete's dominant right arm hangs lower than the shoulder of the nondominant arm.

though these fractures tend to occur at the juncture between the concave and convex bends (the distal one-third of the shaft), they can occur anywhere along the clavicle. Athletes suffering from a fractured clavicle tend to support the involved arm next to the body and rotate the head to the opposite side. If a fractured clavicle is suspected, the evaluation should be terminated at this point and the athlete referred to a physician.

• **Symmetry of the deltoid muscle groups:** The examiner notes the deltoid muscle tone bilaterally. Normally, this muscle group has a rounded contour. The deltoid of the dominant arm may

display a slight amount of hypertrophy when compared with the nondominant side. Atrophy of this muscle group may indicate a lack of use of the involved arm or may reflect pathology to the C5 and C6 nerve roots (axillary nerve involvement).

The presence of a dislocated GH joint disrupts the contour of the deltoid group by flattening the area passing over the head of the humerus (Fig. 11–20). In some instances the humeral head may be seen protruding anteriorly. If a dislocated GH joint is suspected, the evaluation should be terminated and the athlete immediately referred to a physician. The absence of a distal pulse indicates

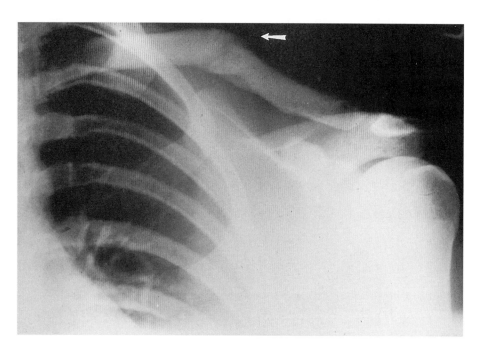

Figure 11–19. X-ray view of a fractured clavicle.

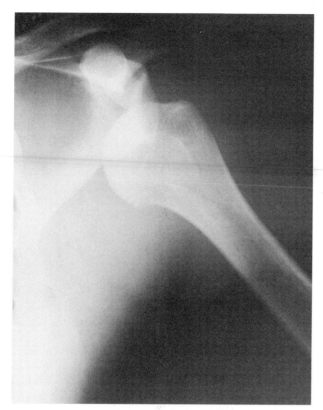

Figure 11–20. X-ray view of an anterior glenohumeral dislocation.

cle should be noted. A tendon rupture is characterized by the muscle's shortening away from the involved structure. A careful inspection of the entire muscle should be performed, as the distal tendon can rupture from its insertion, causing a unilateral deformity.

Inspection of the Lateral Structures

Each shoulder should be viewed from the side and compared with the opposite limb for symmetry.

• **Deltoid muscle group:** This portion of the inspection process is a continuation of the observation of the anterior portion of the deltoids. The contour of this group should be noted and compared with the lateral side, giving special attention to the roundness of the muscle as it passes over the humeral head.

• **Acromion process:** The junction between the clavicle and the acromion process should be smooth and even; in the absence of previous injury to this area, the joints should compare bilaterally. The presence of a **step deformity** must be noted. This condition involves the clavicle's riding above the acromion process, indicating an AC sprain (Fig. 11–21). This finding should be confirmed during the palpation phase (**piano key sign**) and during the special tests portion (**traction test**).

• **Position of the humerus:** The humerus should be hanging in the anatomical position. Adhesions within the GH joint, muscle spasm, or pain associated with bursitis and/or tendinitis may cause the athlete to splint the humerus to guard against motion.

As previously noted, an athlete suffering from a

potentially catastrophic impingement of the neurovascular bundle supplying the arm, wrist, and hand.

• **Anterior humerus and biceps brachii muscle group:** The shape and contour of the biceps brachii and any unilateral bulges within the mus-

Figure 11–21. X-ray view of a third-degree acromioclavicular sprain. The superior displacement of the clavicle's distal aspect creates a characteristic "step deformity."

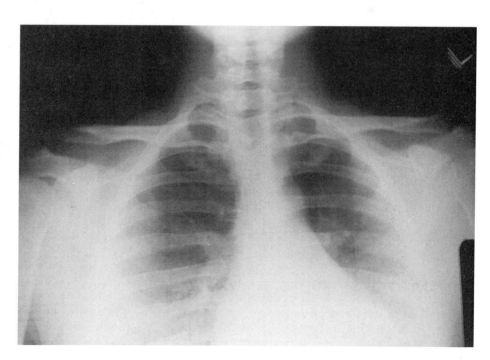

fractured clavicle splints the humerus along the lateral portion of the rib cage and supports the forearm across the chest. Athletes suffering from anterior GH dislocations tend to have the humerus fixed in a position of abduction and external rotation.

Inspection of the Posterior Structures

• **Alignment of the spinal vertebrae:** The alignment of the cervical, thoracic, and lumbar spine should be inspected as a unit to determine the presence of **scoliosis**. This malady may predispose the athlete to altered biomechanics of the shoulder girdle.

• **Position of the scapulae:** The vertebral borders of both scapulae should rest an equal distance from the spinous processes of the thoracic vertebrae. The superior angle normally sits at the level of the second rib and the inferior angle at the seventh rib. The most medial aspect of the scapular spine is located at the level of the third thoracic vertebra.

While the athlete is standing in the anatomical position, the scapula should be in full contact with the thorax. Presence of the vertebral border lifting away from the thorax (winging scapula) should be noted. The examiner should also check for the presence of any unilateral scapular protraction, retraction, or tilting.

Sprengel's deformity is the term for a congenitally undescended scapula. The high-riding scapula is indicative of poorly developed or malformed scapular elevators, and the deformity may occur on one scapula or both. The clinical ramifications of this condition vary from little or no dysfunction to extreme disability. In the athletic population, the clinician may expect to find a decreased range of motion in the involved extremity.

• **Muscle tone:** The examiner inspects the posterior musculature for symmetry on each side. The superficial muscles of well-developed athletes are usually easily identifiable, as are the prominent bony landmarks. Any spasm, deformity, or discoloration of the musculature and/or skin should be noted as well.

Observe the prominence of the scapular spine. Atrophy of the supraspinatus or infraspinatus muscles leads to the spine of the scapula's becoming more visible and palpable. Chronic rotator cuff tears are classically marked by the wasting of the infraspinatus muscle.[8]

• **Position of the humerus:** All athletes with acute shoulder injury should be checked for possible posterior GH dislocation, even though this condition is rare. The head of the humerus, when posteriorly dislocated, usually rests on the infraspinous fossa. This injury is associated with possible bony and articular surface injury as well as

neurovascular damage. If a posteriorly dislocated GH joint is suspected, the evaluation should be terminated and the athlete immediately referred to a physician.

Palpation

The purpose of palpation is to check the integrity of bony and soft tissue associated with the shoulder girdle. To rule out fractures, dislocations, and gross joint injury, the bony structures should be palpated before the soft tissue is palpated. If palpation reveals any gross deformity, the examination should be terminated and the athlete referred to a physician for a definitive diagnosis.

Palpation of the Anterior Bony Structures

• **Sternoclavicular joint:** The examiner begins the palpation process by locating the jugular notch on the manubrium (Fig. 11–22). Here, the common junction provided by the interclavicular ligament between the SC joints may be palpated. Proceed laterally to identify the SC joint, checking for point tenderness over the articulation. Dislocations of this joint tend to displace the clavicular head medial and superior to the clavicular notch. Posterior SC dislocations are considered a medical emergency because posterior displacement of the clavicle may jeopardize the integrity of the large vessels exiting the heart or may place pressure on the trachea and/or lung. Regardless of the relative displacement of the clavicle on the sternum, if an SC dislocation is suspected, the evaluation should be immediately terminated and the athlete referred to a physician.

• **Clavicular shaft:** From the SC joint, the examiner continues to palpate laterally along the shaft of the clavicle. The superior surface is generally easily palpable because of the absence of muscle attachments. The examiner palpates the entire length of the clavicle, noting any crepitus or pain that is caused. If the athlete has had a previous clavicular fracture, it is not uncommon to palpate nodules over the healed fracture site.

• **Acromion process and acromioclavicular joint:** As the clavicle extends laterally, it may become less palpable in those athletes having well-developed pectoralis major and deltoid musculature. The acromion process may be more easily located by palpating to the lateral end of the scapular spine.

If a step deformity is observed during the observation phase of the examination, the examiner should note for any bobbing of the clavicle when downward pressure is applied. Known as the **piano key sign**, this test checks the integrity of the coracoclavicular ligaments.

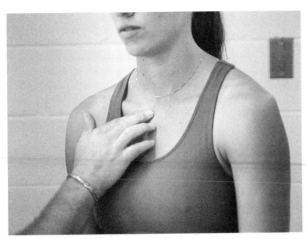

Figure 11–22. Palpation of the sternoclavicular joint and clavicle. The sternum's jugular notch is a good reference point from which to begin palpation. From here, the sternoclavicular joint, the length of the clavicle, and the acromioclavicular joint can be sequentially palpated.

- **Coracoid process:** From the acromion process, the examiner moves two fingers' breadths medially. From this point, the examiner's fingers should move approximately 1 inch below the clavicle, applying gentle pressure laterally. This bony prominence should be felt just above and behind the tendon of the pectoralis major. To confirm that the coracoid process has been located, the examiner may passively move the athlete's GH joint through 15 to 30 degrees of flexion/extension and abduction/adduction. No movement of the coracoid process should be felt within this range of motion. If movement is felt beneath the fingers, the humeral head is most probably being palpated; in this case, the examiner moves the fingers medially and attempts this procedure again.

The coracoid process serves as the point of insertion for the pectoralis minor and the short head of the biceps brachii and is the origin of the coracobrachialis muscle, in addition to providing a source of attachment for several ligaments. Pressure should be applied carefully when palpating this area because it is easily irritated.

Palpation of the Anterior Musculature

- **Pectoralis major:** The pectoralis major is easily located on the anterior thoracic cavity. The examiner should palpate this muscle as it flares into its tendon, noting the integrity and any point tenderness as it crosses the GH capsule and attaches on the greater tuberosity of the humerus.

- **Pectoralis minor:** Located beneath the pectoralis major, the bulk of the pectoralis minor is not palpable. Its tendon's insertion on the coracoid process may be palpable.

- **Coracobrachialis:** This muscle originates off the coracoid process and may be palpable at this

point. Its body and insertion lie deep in the superficial musculature of the humerus and are therefore difficult to palpate.

Bony Palpation of the Humerus

- **Humeral head:** Direct palpation of the humeral head may not be possible in athletes with well-developed shoulder musculature. Moving laterally from the acromion process, the anteromedial portion of the humeral head can be palpated in the axilla posterior to the tendon of pectoralis major. Moving posteriorly into and through the axilla, the inferior portion of the head may be felt.

The relationship of the humeral head to the glenoid fossa must be determined. An anteriorly or inferiorly displaced humeral head is easily palpable.

- **Greater tuberosity:** The greater tuberosity can be located in the anatomical position approximately one finger's breadth below the lateral edge of the anterior portion of the acromion process. This structure is more easily palpated by passively extending the athlete's humerus, causing the greater tuberosity to move from beneath the acromion process.

- **Bicipital groove:** The examiner externally rotates the humerus to make the bicipital groove more palpable. The groove is felt as an indentation in the bone just medial to the greater tuberosity. This area should be gently palpated along its length to elicit any tenderness caused by bicipital tendinitis or damage to the transverse ligament.

- **Lesser tuberosity:** The medial border of the bicipital groove is formed by the lesser tuberosity and is more easily palpated with the humerus externally rotated.

- **Humeral shaft:** The shaft of the humerus is more easily palpated along its medial and lateral borders under the belly of the biceps brachii and brachioradialis muscles.

Palpation of the Humeral Musculature

- **Deltoid group:** Each of three portions of the deltoid should be palpated from its unique origin to the common insertion on the humerus.

- **Biceps brachii:** From the belly of the biceps brachii, each of the two heads should be palpated. The long head may be felt through its passage in the bicipital groove until it passes beneath the anterior deltoid. The muscle's short head may be palpated along its length as it passes beneath the pectoralis major tendon and inserts on the coracoid process.

- **Triceps brachii:** The triceps' close association with the shoulder girdle is often overlooked. The examiner should palpate the long head of the triceps brachii's insertion on the scapula's infraglenoid tubercle.

- **Rotator cuff:** The mass of three of the four rotator cuff muscles can be palpated on the scapula. The supraspinatus, infraspinatus, and teres minor should be palpated along their lengths until they disappear beneath the mass of the deltoid. By passively extending the GH joint from the anatomical position, the greater tuberosity becomes prominent, allowing for the palpation of these muscles' insertions on the humerus. Although the individual tendons are not distinguishable from each other, any pain or tenderness elicited during palpation should be noted, as this could indicate rotator cuff tears or inflammation. The origin, mass, and tendinous insertion of the subscapularis muscle are not directly palpable.

- **Teres major:** The origin and body of the teres major muscle are located immediately inferior to the teres minor. The insertion of this muscle cannot be directly palpated. As this muscle is a common site for trigger points in athletes who throw and in swimmers, any hypersensitive areas should be noted.

- **Latissimus dorsi:** The latissimus dorsi tendon is located inferior to the teres major. The examiner follows this tendon through the axilla to its attachment on the floor of the bicipital groove.

Bony Palpation of the Scapula

- **Spine of the scapula:** The spine of the scapula can be located by finding the acromion process. The examiner palpates posteriorly along the bony surface of the acromion to meet with the scapular spine. Palpation continues medially along the length of the shaft to its termination along the scapula's vertebral border.

- **Superior angle:** From the vertebral border, the examiner palpates upward to find the superior angle of the scapula. This landmark may be obstructed by muscle mass of the upper portion of the trapezius, supraspinatus, and levator scapulae.

- **Inferior angle:** Moving inferiorly along the vertebral border, the apex of the inferior angle of the scapula can be felt. Asking the athlete to touch the inferior angle of the opposite scapula from below causes the scapula undergoing examination to wing, making the inferior angle and the lower portions of the vertebral and axial borders more easily palpable.

- **Axial border:** The examiner palpates upwardly and laterally from the inferior angle along the axial border of the scapula. While palpating up the axial border the bony structure is lost below the teres major, teres minor, infraspinatus, and latissimus dorsi muscles.

Palpation of the Scapular Musculature

- **Trapezius:** This muscle is the most superficial of the muscles acting on the scapula and therefore overlies the levator scapulae and the rhomboid muscle group. The trapezius muscle should be palpated relative to its upper, middle, and lower portions.

- **Levator scapulae:** Although largely covered by the upper band of the trapezius muscle, the origin of the levator scapulae can be palpated on the transverse processes of the first through the fourth cervical vertebrae.

- **Rhomboids:** Rhomboid major and rhomboid minor cannot be directly palpated and are indistinguishable from each other except for their relative location.

Functional Tests

The motion occurring at the GH, AC, and SC joints, as well as the motion of the scapula, is evaluated during functional testing. During the evaluation, the clinician should be mindful of the interrelationship among these articulations because a deficit at one joint affects the motion of the others. One should not attempt these functional tests when severe traumatic injuries such as fractures, joint dislocation, or complete muscle tears are suspected.

The amount of motion that the GH joint is capable of producing is dependent on the position of the greater and the lesser tuberosities relative to the scapula's bony structures. To achieve complete abduction, the humerus must be externally rotated to allow the greater tuberosity to clear the acromion process. When the GH joint is internally and externally rotated with the arm at the side, the range of motion is reduced, a result of the lesser tuberosity's contacting the glenohumeral fossa during internal rotation and the greater tuberosity's striking the acromion process during external rotation. The motion of flexion does not depend on relative internal or external rotation of the humerus because the greater tuberosity depresses inferiorly and passes beneath the acromion process.[9]

In normal, healthy athletes, isotonic strength should be equal in both extremities.[10] This relationship may vary among athletes involved in throwing and racquet sports. A study of collegiate tennis players indicates that the dominant shoulder produces a significantly greater amount of torque and power during internal rotation than the nondominant shoulder.[11] Professional baseball pitchers do not display a significant difference in the amount of peak torque produced during internal rotation when compared bilaterally, but a significant difference does arise at high speeds (greater than or equal to 300 degrees per second) during external rotation, with the dominant arm producing more torque.[12] The strength ratio of internal to external rotators has been described as 3:2 for concentric contractions and 3:4 for eccentric contractions.[13]

Active Range of Motion

The muscles acting on the scapula are presented in Table 11–5 and those acting on the humerus in

Table 11–6. The examiner must be familiar with these muscles' actions, origins, and insertions, as well as the nervous innervation, so that a definitive evaluation can be made.

An evaluation of the aggregate motion available to the shoulder girdle can be quickly determined through the **Apley's scratch test** (Fig. 11–23). Each

Apley's Scratch Test (Fig.11–23)

With the Athlete Standing or Sitting:	Motions Produced:
The examiner asks the athlete to touch the opposite shoulder from the front.	Glenohumeral adduction, horizontal flexion, and internal rotation; scapular protraction.
The examiner asks the athlete to reach behind the head and touch the opposite shoulder from behind.	Glenohumeral abduction and external rotation; scapular protraction, elevation, and upward rotation.
The examiner asks the athlete to reach behind the back and touch the opposite shoulder blade.	Glenohumeral adduction and internal rotation; scapular retraction and downward rotation.

of the three components of this test should be compared bilaterally to determine a decrease in the range of motion or the elicitation of any pain:

The following active glenohumeral and shoulder complex motions are also included in the functional testing process with the presence of any painful arcs of motion being noted:

- **Flexion and extension:** The shoulder girdle is capable of producing a total of 220 to 240 degrees of movement in the sagittal plane (Fig. 11–24). The majority of this range of motion, accounting for 170 to 180 degrees of motion from the anatomical position, is provided by flexion. The remaining 50 to 60 degrees occur from the limb moving from the anatomical position to extension.

Table 11–5. Muscles Contributing to Scapular Movements

Elevation	Protraction	Upward Rotation
Levator scapulae Rhomboid major Rhomboid minor Serratus anterior (upper fibers) Trapezius (upper fibers)	Serratus anterior	Serratus anterior Trapezius Pectoralis minor

Depression	Retraction	Downward Rotation
Serratus anterior (lower fibers) Trapezius (lower fibers) Pectoralis major (clavicular fibers)	Latissimus dorsi Rhomboid major Rhomboid minor Trapezius (middle fibers) Trapezius (lower fibers)	Latissimus dorsi Rhomboid major Rhomboid minor Levator scapulae

- **Abduction and adduction:** Occurring in the frontal plane, the normal range of motion for abduction is 170 to 180 degrees (Fig. 11–25). The motion of adduction is blocked in the anatomical position and any further movement requires that the GH joint be flexed or extended so that the humerus can pass in front of or behind the torso. The athlete's ability to control adduction should be noticed. An arm that falls uncontrollably from 90 degrees of abduction indicates a positive **drop arm test** for rotator cuff pathology (see Special Tests for Rotator Cuff Pathology section in this chapter).

The athlete may describe an area within the range of motion that elicits pain. This **painful arc** is often associated with impingement of the rotator cuff musculature between the humeral head and the coracoacromial arch and tends to occur between 60 and 120 degrees of abduction.

- **Internal and external rotation:** Internal and external rotation should be tested in both the neutral position and in 90 degrees of abduction. In the neutral position, the humeral head and the greater tuberosity are allowed to rotate beneath the acromion without interference. During internal rotation a block is presented by the torso.

The glenohumeral joint should be abducted to 90 degrees so that the greater and lesser tuberosities can clear the structures of the scapula (Fig. 11–26). In the transverse plane, the neutral position is considered to be 90 degrees of abduction with the elbow flexed to 90 degrees. The normal range of motion in this position is 80 to 90 degrees of external rotation and 70 to 80 degrees of internal rotation.

Another method of measuring internal rotation is to have the athlete reach behind and up the

Table 11–6. Muscles Contributing to Humeral Movements

Flexion	Adduction	Horizontal Flexion	Internal Rotation
Biceps brachii Coracobrachialis Deltoid (anterior one-third) Deltoid (middle one-third) Pectoralis major (clavicular fibers)	Coracobrachialis Latissimus dorsi Pectoralis major Teres major Triceps brachii	Deltoid (anterior one-third) Pectoralis major	Deltoid (anterior one-third) Latissimus dorsi Pectoralis major Subscapularis Teres major
Extension	**Abduction**	**Horizontal Extension**	**External rotation**
Deltoid (posterior one-third) Latissimus dorsi Teres major Teres minor Triceps brachii	Biceps brachii Deltoid (anterior one-third) Deltoid (middle one-third) Deltoid (posterior one-third) Supraspinatus	Deltoid (posterior one-third) Infraspinatus Teres minor	Deltoid (posterior one-third) Infraspinatus Teres minor

back (Fig. 11–27). This measurement is more representative of functional motion than standard goniometry. The measurement is taken from the spinal level where the thumb rests at maximal motion. The athlete should generally be capable of obtaining with the dominant hand a spinal level that is equal to or greater than that obtainable on the nondominant side.

- **Horizontal flexion and extension:** The neutral position for horizontal flexion and extension is 90

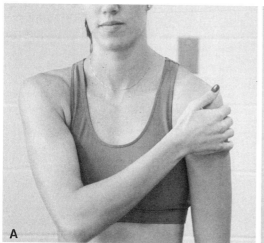

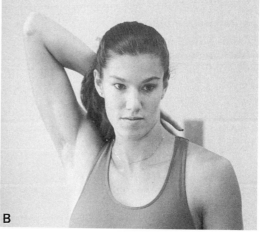

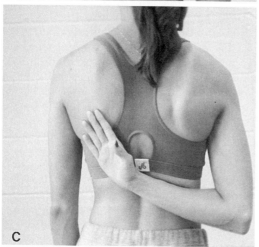

Figure 11–23. Photographic sequence of the Apley scratch test: (*A*) Reaching across the chest. (*B*) Reaching behind the head. (*C*) Reaching behind the back.

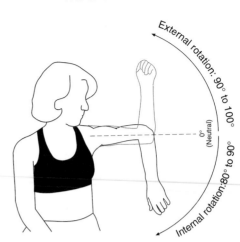

Figure 11–26. Range of motion for shoulder internal rotation and external rotation.

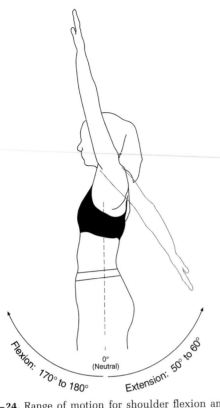

Figure 11–24. Range of motion for shoulder flexion and extension.

degrees of abduction with the arm flexed at a 30-degree angle from the torso in the plane of the scapula (see Fig. 11–5). Occurring in the horizontal plane, the expected range of motion is 45 degrees of horizontal extension and 120 degrees of horizontal flexion relative to the plane of the scapula.

Passive Range of Motion

• **Flexion and extension:** Passive range of motion may be isolated to the GH joint or may encompass the entire motion allowed by the shoulder girdle. To isolate the GH joint, the scapula must be stabilized to prevent its contribution to shoulder motion. When the entire motion provided by the shoulder girdle is evaluated, the thorax must be stabilized. Each of these two methods of stabilization is more easily accomplished with the athlete lying supine during flexion and prone during extension (Fig. 11–28).

Flexion should have a firm end-feel for both GH and shoulder girdle motions. During GH flexion, the terminal motion is checked by the tightening

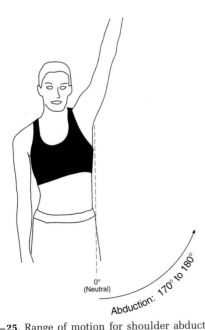

Figure 11–25. Range of motion for shoulder abduction and adduction.

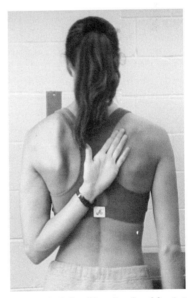

Figure 11–27. Method of checking for shoulder internal rotation as recommended by the American Academy of Orthopaedic Surgeons. The amount of internal glenohumeral rotation is determined by measuring the distance up the spinal column the athlete can reach and comparing this result to that of the opposite shoulder.

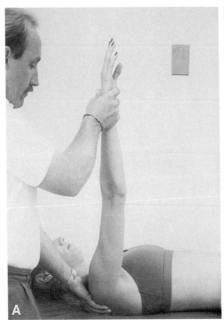

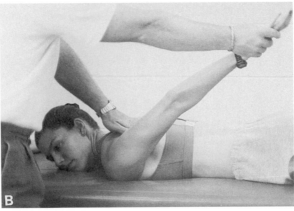

Figure 11–28. Passive range of motion testing for shoulder flexion and extension.

of the GH capsule (especially the coracohumeral ligament and the posterior capsular fibers) and the teres minor, teres major, and infraspinatus muscles. The muscles attaching to the anterior portion of the humerus, especially the pectoralis major and the latissimus dorsi, normally terminate flexion accomplished by the entire shoulder girdle.

The two types of passive extension should result in a firm end-feel. During isolated GH extension, the coracohumeral ligament and the anterior joint capsule become taut. During extension of the shoulder girdle, the pectoralis major (clavicular fibers) and serratus anterior muscles contribute to the end-feel.

Pain that occurs during passive flexion may indicate impingement of the supraspinatus tendon between the inferior portion of the acromion process and the humeral head. Pain during passive extension may result from damage to the anterior portion of the GH capsule or the coracohumeral ligament.

• **Abduction and adduction:** As in the case of flexion and extension, abduction is the result of motion arising from the shoulder complex or isolated to its pure GH movement. When attempting to isolate GH abduction, the scapula is stabilized to prevent its upward rotation and elevation. To restrict motion to the shoulder complex, the examiner stabilizes the thorax to eliminate lateral bending of the spine. Passive abduction may be examined with the athlete supine or sitting (Fig. 11–29).

The normal range of motion resulting from purely GH movement has a firm end-feel because of the stress placed on the glenohumeral ligaments (middle and inferior bands), the inferior capsule, and the pectoralis major and latissimus dorsi muscles. During abduction arising from the

entire shoulder complex, the rhomboids and the middle and lower fibers of the trapezius muscle contribute to the end-feel.

Passive range of motion measurements and end-feels are not normally taken for adduction because of the humerus striking the body, but hyperadduction may be measured by moving the arm in front of the torso. The examiner should note the presence of a painful arc, indicative of rotator cuff impingement, when passively moving the athlete's arm from abduction to adduction. Pain experienced during both passive abduction and passive adduction may indicate subacromial bursitis.

• **Internal and external rotation:** Passive range of motion for rotation of the humerus should be taken with the GH joint abducted to 90 degrees and the elbow flexed to 90 degrees. To isolate rotation at the GH joint, the examiner stabilizes the scapula to prevent elevation/depression and tilting. When measuring motion produced by the shoulder girdle, the thorax should be stabilized to prevent flexion or extension of the spine (Fig. 11–30).

The firm end-feel associated with normal internal rotation is due to tightening of the posterior fibers of the GH capsule and the infraspinatus and teres minor muscles. During internal rotation provided by the shoulder girdle, the rhomboid muscle group and the middle and lower fibers of the trapezius contribute to the end-feel.

During external rotation the GH ligaments, the coracohumeral ligament, and the joint capsule wind tight, resulting in a firm end-feel for both isolated GH movements and the shoulder girdle. Muscular contributions lending to the end-feel for GH motion are the subscapularis, pectoralis major, latissimus dorsi, and the teres major. During external rotation provided by the shoulder girdle,

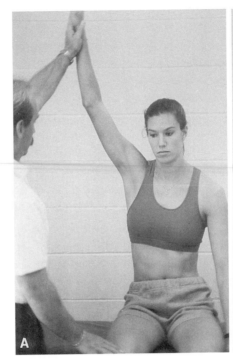
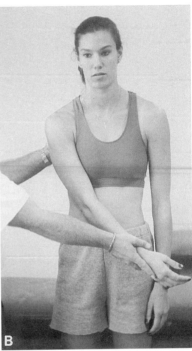

Figure 11–29. Passive range of motion testing for shoulder abduction and adduction.

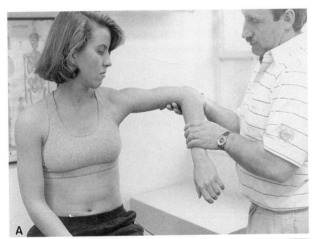
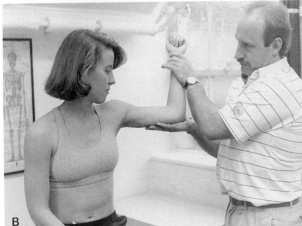

Figure 11–30. Passive range of motion testing for shoulder internal rotation and external rotation.

the serratus anterior and pectoralis minor muscles also provide tension.

Athletes who throw overhand, including baseball players, javelin throwers, tennis players, and quarterbacks, often have an increased range of external rotation and decreased internal rotation.

Examination of passive external rotation should be delayed until the end of the assessment procedure in those athletes suspected of suffering a GH dislocation, subluxation, or chronic instability, and the examination should proceed with great care. Passive external rotation of the GH joint is the same procedure as the **apprehension test**, discussed in detail in the Special Tests section of this chapter.

The examiner palpates the GH joint during passive internal and external rotation to determine the presence of crepitus, which may indicate rotator cuff or bicipital tendinitis, and subacromial bursitis, or "clicks," which may indicate a labral tear.

• **Horizontal flexion and extension:** To isolate GH motion the scapula must be stabilized to prevent protraction and retraction. During evaluation of the entire shoulder girdle, the examiner stabilizes the torso so that spinal motion does not contribute to motion of the shoulder (Fig. 11–31).

A firm end-feel is expected during horizontal extension owing to the tightening of the anterior GH capsule and the middle and inferior GH ligaments. Some tension may also be developed by the supraspinatus, infraspinatus, and teres minor muscles. During horizontal extension obtained through motions of the entire shoulder girdle, ad-

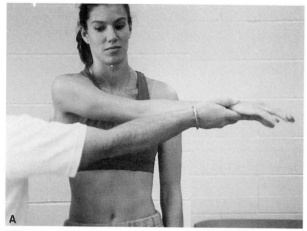

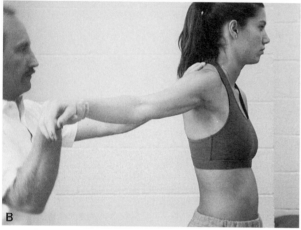

Figure 11–31. Passive range of motion testing for (*A*) shoulder horizontal flexion and (*B*) shoulder horizontal extension.

ditional tension is developed by the pectoralis major.

Horizonal flexion may have a soft end-feel because of soft tissue approximation in those athletes who have well-developed pectoralis major, biceps, and anterior deltoid musculature, or in obese individuals. If this is not the case, a firm end-feel is associated with stretching of the posterior GH capsule and tension developed by the rhomboid muscle group.

Resisted Range of Motion

• **Flexion and extension:** With the athlete in the sitting position, the examiner resists flexion by providing resistance on the humerus proximal to the elbow joint while stabilizing the joint on the superior surface of the shoulder girdle. Resistive extension may be more easily performed with the athlete lying prone, although it may be performed with the athlete sitting. Resistance is provided on the distal humerus while the joint is stabilized over the clavicle and scapula (Fig. 11–32).

• **Abduction and adduction:** With the athlete sitting, the examiner resists abduction and adduction by providing resistance on the humerus proximal to the elbow joint (Fig. 11–33).

• **Internal and external rotation:** Internal and external GH rotation may be performed with the GH joint abducted to 90 degrees or with the arm at the side and the elbow flexed to 90 degrees. Resistance is provided by firmly grasping the forearm just proximal to the wrist (Fig. 11–34).

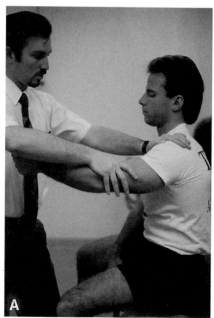

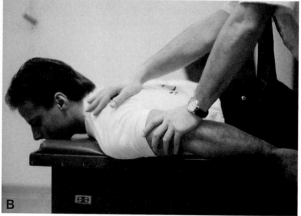

Figure 11–32. Resisted range of motion testing for (*A*) shoulder extension and (*B*) flexion. This motion may be tested with the athlete either seated or lying.

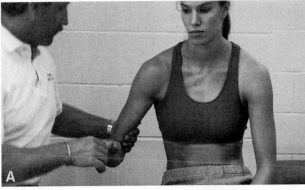

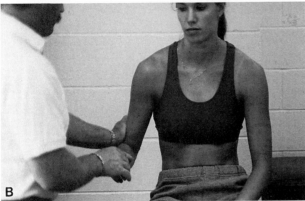

Figure 11–33. Resisted range of motion testing for (*A*) shoulder abduction and (*B*) adduction.

- **Horizontal flexion and extension:** The athlete should be sitting during resisted horizontal flexion and extension. These tests may also be conducted with the athlete lying supine or prone. Resistance to horizontal extension is provided at the distal humerus over the olecranon process (Fig. 11–35).

Scapular Movements

During the evaluation of active humeral movements, the motion of the scapula should be observed. The examiner should note any winging of the scapula and the scapulothoracic rhythm compared with the opposite side. Athletes suffering from GH instability, rotator cuff tendinitis, or impingement syndromes normally display dysfunction in the scapulothoracic mechanism.[8] In this event a greater than normal contribution to humeral elevation is provided by the scapulothoracic articulation.

During the examination of scapulothoracic movement in athletes suffering from GH instability, the clinician may note irregular movement of the scapula. Winging of the vertebral border may occur during elevation of the humerus and, more probably, during the movement back to the neutral position.[8]

Scapular winging may occur secondary to weakness of the serratus anterior muscle or inhibition of the long thoracic nerve. The most common clinical approach to determining the presence of a winging scapula is to have the athlete push against the wall

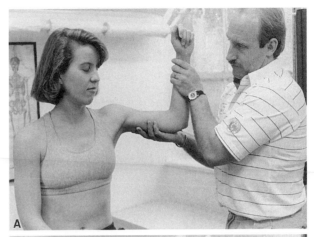

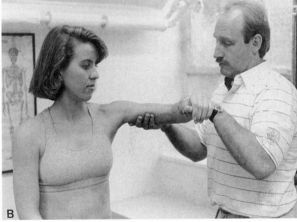

Figure 11–34. Resisted range of motion testing for shoulder (*A*) internal rotation and (*B*) external rotation. This test may also be performed with the glenohumeral joint in 0° abduction.

while observing the relative scapular alignment (Fig. 11–36).

The athlete performs active and resistive shoulder elevation to determine the integrity of the levator scapulae and upper fibers of the trapezius (Fig. 11–37). Scapular elevation is defined as shrugging the shoulders. Active protraction and retraction may also be assessed by having the athlete roll the shoulders forward and bring the shoulders back into the military "attention" position.

Ligamentous and Capsular Testing

The integrity of the ligaments and capsule of the SC, AC, and GH joints are determined through joint glide. Because of the relative difficulty in manipulating the clavicle, the tests for SC and AC instability are less discrete than the other joints in the body and generally test positive only in the more severe cases. These tests are contraindicated when a fracture or joint dislocation is suspected.

Sternoclavicular Laxity

The examiner firmly grasps the clavicle just distal to the medial clavicular head. The stability of the SC joint and the integrity of the ligaments are estab-

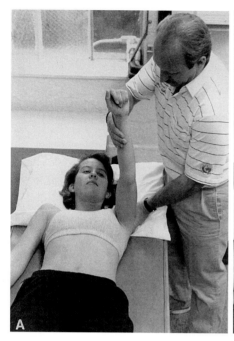
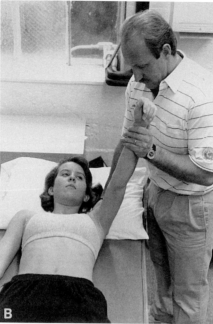

Figure 11–35. Resisted range of motion testing for (A) horizontal flexion and (B) extension.

lished by the examiner applying pressures that force the medial clavicle downward, upward, anteriorly, and posteriorly while noting any pain or bilateral laxity that is elicited:

Sternoclavicular Laxity

Clavicular Movement:	Structures Involved:
Downward	Interclavicular ligament
Upward	Anterior and posterior fibers of the costoclavicular ligament
Anterior	Sternoclavicular ligament (posterior fibers)
Posterior	Sternoclavicular ligament (anterior fibers)

Pain that is evoked during all movements may result from either damage to the SC joint disk or a complete disruption of the joint capsule, indicating a possible dislocation or subluxation of the joint.

Acromioclavicular Laxity

This articulation can be manipulated by grasping the clavicle along its distal one-third. The examiner should check the joint play movements in all planes

Acromioclavicular Laxity

Clavicular Movement:	Structures Involved:
Downward	Acromioclavicular ligament (superior fibers).
Upward	Coracoclavicular ligament (conoid fibers). Acromioclavicular ligament (inferior fibers). Coracoclavicular ligament (trapezoid fibers).
Anterior	Acromioclavicular ligament. Coracoclavicular ligament (in the absence of the acromioclavicular ligament).
Posterior	Normally a bony block is felt against the acromion process. A high-riding clavicle stresses the acromioclavicular ligaments.

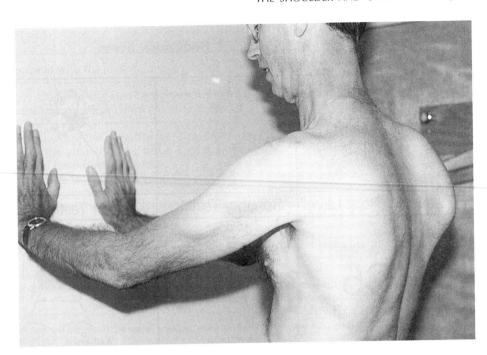

Figure 11–36. Test for winging scapula. In the presence of a weakened serratus anterior muscle, or long thoracic nerve injury, performing a "push-up" against a wall causes the vertebral border of the scapula to lift off the thorax.

and make note of any pain or laxity demonstrated during the test (see bottom of page 346).

Glenohumeral Laxity

This section discusses the measurement of pure GH glide, the sliding of the humeral head relative to the glenoid fossa. The ligaments tested during this procedure are also stressed during many of the special tests used to determine GH instability. However, it is important to understand that laxity and instability are not synonymous: a lax shoulder can still be stable and an unstable shoulder may not show any laxity during glide.

The glide tests are performed in three directions: anterior, posterior, and inferior, with the humerus in the neutral position and the scapula stabilized (Fig. 11–38). All motions occur relative to the plane of the scapula; therefore, anterior glide is not tested by drawing the humerus forward relative to the sagittal plane but, rather, forward relative to the face of the glenoid fossa.[14] The degree of instability is based on the amount of translation relative to the opposite limb. Any situation in which the humeral head can be displaced from the labral rim warrants further examination by a physician.

Superior glide is not tested because of the bony block formed between the humeral head and the acromion process. The Pathology and Related Special Tests section of this chapter discusses multiplanar instabilities. The results of the glide tests in each direction are compared with those of the opposite extremity to roughly determine their equality (see top of page 349).

Neurological Testing

As noted earlier, the shoulder and upper arm are common sites of referred pain. This section presents the upper quarter neurological screen for involvement of the cervical nerve roots or impingement of the portions of the brachial plexus. Chapter 9 describes the brachial plexus and the actual mechanisms and tests for cervical nerve root impingement; Chapter 10 discusses visceral origins of referred pain into this area (see Neurological Screen on page 348).

Pathologies and Related Special Tests

Because of the number of bones, muscles, articulations, ligaments, and other supporting structures associated with the shoulder girdle, this complex is susceptible to a wide range of injuries. This section presents major orthopedic and athletic injuries to each segment and describes the signs, symptoms, and special evaluative procedures used to reach the appropriate conclusions. The clinician should structure the examination approach to include only those special tests that are relevant to confirm or deny the suspected pathology.

Sternoclavicular Joint Sprains

Injuries to the sternoclavicular joint usually occur from a longitudinal force being placed on the clavicle. This mechanism most commonly occurs when the athlete falls on an outstretched arm or when a

Sulcus Sign for Inferior Glenohumeral Laxity (Fig. 11–43)

Position of athlete	Sitting. Arm hanging at the side.
Position of examiner	Standing lateral to the involved side. The athlete's arm is gripped at the elbow and midforearm.
Evaluative procedure	A downward traction is applied to the athlete's arm.
Positive test results	An indentation (sulcus) appears beneath the acromion process. To differentiate the results of this test from those of the traction test for acromioclavicular joint instability, in this test the movement of the humeral head is away from the scapula and clavicle, whereas in the traction test the humerus and scapula move away from the clavicle.
Implications	The humeral head slides inferiorly on the glenoid fossa, indicating laxity in the superior glenohumeral ligament or a tear of the inferior portion of the glenoid labrum.

Table 11–9. Evaluative Findings of Acromioclavicular Joint Sprains

Examination Segment	Clinical Findings	
History	Onset Location of pain: Mechanism: 	Usually acute. Localized to the acromioclavicular joint area. Pain may radiate down the deltoid muscle or along the clavicle. Force applied longitudinally to the clavicle, such as falling on an outstretched arm. Falling on the point of the shoulder.
Inspection	Displacement of the clavicle may be present. Step deformities indicate damage to the coracoclavicular ligament.	
Palpation	Anterior displacement of the clavicle demonstrates the piano key sign.	
Functional tests	AROM: There is pain with elevation of the humerus and during protraction and retraction of the scapula. PROM: Pain is produced during elevation of the humerus owing to movement at the AC joint. RROM: Decreased strength may be noted for all movements, especially with those muscles having an attachment on the acromion or clavicle.	
Ligamentous tests	Joint play movements reveal hypermobility of the AC joint.	
Neurological tests	Not applicable.	
Special tests	Traction test.	
Comments	Athletes with fractures of the distal clavicle may present with the clinical signs and symptoms of an acromioclavicular joint sprain.	

Tests for Posterior Glenohumeral Instability

Damage to the posterior GH capsule and/or weakness of the posterior rotator cuff musculature can result in excessive posterior displacement of the humeral head on the glenoid fossa.

Posterior Apprehension Test

This special test attempts to elicit apprehension in the athlete by exerting a posterior force on the humerus to drive the humeral head posteriorly on the glenoid fossa (Fig. 11–44). The examination may

be varied by altering the relative amount of humeral flexion and/or internal rotation (see top of page 355).

Test for Posterior Instability in the Plane of the Scapula

This evaluative technique somewhat replicates the posterior apprehension test, but the humerus is placed in the more functional plane of the scapula (Fig. 11–45). A force is applied to the humeral shaft or the humeral head, encouraging it to move posteriorly on the glenoid fossa (see middle of page 355).

Posterior Apprehension Test for Glenohumeral Laxity (Fig. 11–44)

Position of athlete	Sitting or supine. The shoulder is flexed to 90° and the elbow bent to 90°.
Position of examiner	Standing on the involved side of the athlete. One hand grasps the elbow at the olecranon process. The opposite hand stabilizes the posterior scapula.
Evaluative procedure	The examiner applies a longitudinal force to the humeral shaft, encouraging the humeral head to move posteriorly on the glenoid fossa. The examiner may choose to alter the amount of flexion and rotation of the humerus.
Positive test results	The athlete displays apprehension and produces muscle guarding to prevent the shoulder from subluxating posteriorly.
Implications	Laxity in the posterior glenohumeral capsule or weakness of the posterior rotator cuff muscle group.

Test for Posterior Instability in the Plane of the Scapula (Fig. 11–45)

Position of athlete	Lying supine. The shoulder is in 90° of abduction and horizontally flexed to approximately 30° to place the humerus in the plane of the scapula. The elbow is flexed to a comfortable position.
Position of examiner	One hand supports the weight of the arm at the elbow. The opposite palm or thumb is placed over the anterior portion of the glenohumeral capsule.
Evaluative procedure	Using the thumb or palm, a pressure is applied to the humeral head, attempting to drive it posteriorly on the glenoid fossa. Additional force may be used by applying a longitudinal force on the humerus by applying pressure from the elbow.
Positive test results	Pain or laxity in the posterior glenohumeral capsule or the athlete displaying apprehension of a posterior subluxation.
Implications	Laxity in the posterior glenohumeral capsule or weakness of the posterior rotator cuff muscle group.

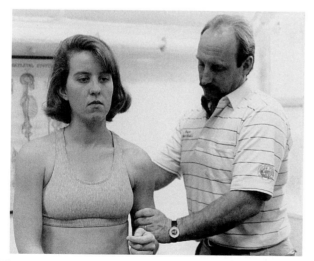

Figure 11–39. Traction test for acromioclavicular joint injury. Applying a downward force to the humerus separates the scapula from the clavicle if significant trauma exists within the acromioclavicular and coracoclavicular ligaments.

Rotator Cuff Pathology

A cause-and-effect relationship exists between rotator cuff inflammation and rotator cuff impingement syndrome. Impingement of the rotator cuff muscles occurs when there is decreased space through which the rotator cuff muscles pass. This impingement, in its initial stages, often results in the inflammation of the rotator cuff. Likewise, inflammation of the rotator cuff muscles results in the enlargement of the tendons, decreasing the subacromial space and increasing the likelihood of impingement of the musculature.

This sequence of events creates a closed cycle in which one condition exacerbates the other. When allowed to proceed unchecked, the ultimate outcome is a shoulder with greatly diminished function. To athletes participating in overhead sports, impingement syndrome and/or rotator cuff pathology are often career threatening.

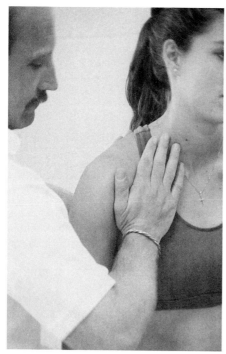

Figure 11–40. Acromioclavicular compression test. Compressing the clavicle and scapula causes the clavicle to ride over or under the acromion process if the coracoclavicular ligaments are lax.

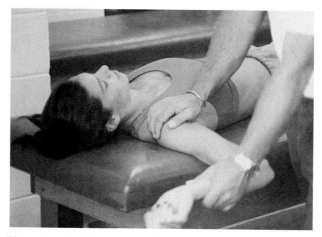

Figure 11–42. Relocation test for anterior glenohumeral instability. This test is performed in the same manner as the apprehension test, but the athlete is lying supine. During the movement the examiner applies pressure to prevent the humerus from moving anteriorly on the glenoid fossa.

Rotator Cuff Impingement Syndrome

Caused by a decrease in space below the coracoacromial arch, the structures that lie beneath this area are impinged between the acromion process and the humeral head (Fig. 11–46). Passing through this area are the rotator cuff tendons (primarily the supraspinatus tendon), the long head of the biceps brachii, the subacromial bursa, the GH joint capsule, and the head of the humerus. The most common cause of impingement is anatomical variation in the coracoacromial arch that produces a mechanical wear on the rotator cuff, subacromial bursa, and the long head of the biceps tendon.[26]

A relationship between poor scapular biomechan-

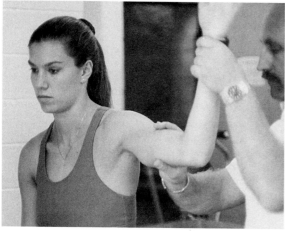

Figure 11–41. Apprehension test for anterior glenohumeral instability. With the shoulder abducted to 90°, externally rotating the humerus causes the humeral head to glide anteriorly. The athlete attempts to stop this movement if the fear of a dislocation exists.

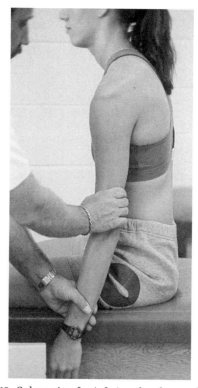

Figure 11–43. Sulcus sign for inferior glenohumeral instability. This test is performed in a manner similar to the traction test, but the examiner is looking for a depression between the acromioclavicular joint and the humeral head, indicating inferior displacement of the humerus. A modification of this test is to stabilize the scapula by placing a hand in the athlete's axilla.

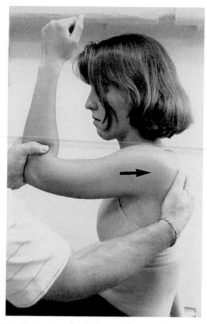

Figure 11–44. Posterior glenohumeral apprehension test for instability. The examiner attempts to displace the humeral head posteriorly on the glenoid fossa.

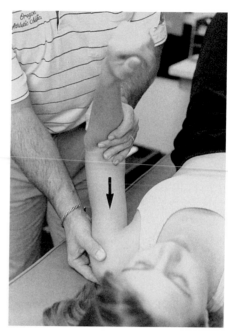

Figure 11–45. Tests for posterior glenohumeral instability in the plane of the scapula.

ics and impingement syndromes has been suggested.[27,28] In this case, the scapula does not rotate appropriately to allow the superior GH structures to pass beneath the coracoacromial arch. The chief complaint associated with rotator cuff impingement is pain during overhead movements and an associated painful arc (Table 11–10).

Test for Rotator Cuff Impingement

Most commonly, impingement occurs from the supraspinatus tendon's being trapped between the humeral head and the acromion process. Therefore, most impingement tests attempt to duplicate this mechanism. Signs of impingement may be manifest during midrange of active or passive range of motion (painful arc) and at the extreme end-point of humeral elevation.

Shoulder Impingement Test

This test is used to determine the impingement of the supraspinatus or long head of the biceps tendon between the humeral head and the acromion process and/or the coracoacromial arch (Fig. 11–47).

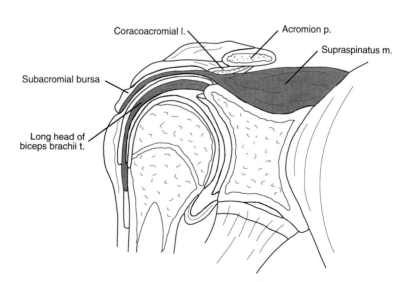

Figure 11–46. Structures involved in shoulder impingement syndrome. If the humeral head does not depress during abduction, the long head of the biceps brachii, the subacromial bursa, and the supraspinatus tendon are impinged between the acromion process and the head of the humerus.

Coracoacromial l.

Acromion p.

Supraspinatus m.

Subacromial bursa

Long head of biceps brachii t.

Shoulder Impingement Test (Fig. 11–47)

Position of athlete	Sitting or standing. The shoulder, elbow, and wrist are in the anatomical position.
Position of examiner	Standing lateral or forward of the involved side. The athlete's shoulder is stabilized on the posterior aspect. The examiner's other hand grips the athlete's arm at the elbow joint.
Evaluative procedure	With the elbow extended, the glenohumeral joint is passively moved through forward flexion.
Positive test results	Pain with motion, especially near the end of the range of motion.
Implications	Pathology is present in the rotator cuff group (especially the supraspinatus) or the long head of the biceps brachii tendon. The motion of the test impinges these structures between the greater tuberosity and the inferior side of the acromion process and acromioclavicular joint.

Modification of the Shoulder Impingement Test

This modification of the shoulder impingement test positions the greater tuberosity to more readily compress the structures passing beneath the coracoacromial arch (Fig. 11–48).

Modification of the Shoulder Impingement Test (Fig. 11–48)

Position of athlete	Sitting or standing. The shoulder, elbow, and wrist are in the anatomical position.
Position of examiner	Standing lateral or forward of the involved side. The athlete's shoulder is stabilized on the posterior aspect. The examiner's other hand grips the athlete's arm at the elbow joint.
Evaluative procedure	1. With the elbow flexed, the glenohumeral joint is forward flexed to 90°. At this point the humerus is passively internally rotated. 2. The shoulder is abducted to 90° and the glenohumeral joint is passively internally rotated.
Positive test results	Pain with motion, especially near the end of the range of motion.
Implications	Pathology is present in the rotator cuff group (especially the supraspinatus) or the long head of the biceps brachii tendon. The motion of the test impinges these structures between the greater tuberosity and the inferior side of the acromion process.

Rotator Cuff Tendinitis

Athletes suffering from rotator cuff tendinitis typically describe a slow onset of the symptoms. In the early stages the athlete complains of pain following activity deep within the shoulder in the subacromial area. The symptoms then progress to pain during activity and, finally, to constant pain with most activities of daily living. Factors contributing to the onset of rotator cuff pathology are a decreased muscle balance between the internal and external rotators, capsular laxity, and impingement syndromes.

The shoulder is predisposed to rotator cuff tendinitis by the relatively poor vascularization of the tendons, a fact that also hinders the healing process.

The supraspinatus muscle is perhaps the most susceptible of the rotator cuff group to inflammatory conditions. In addition to its poor blood supply, pressure is placed on this tendon by the humeral head, "wringing" it dry of blood and other vital fluids.

The relative severity of rotator cuff pathology is largely based on the presence of tearing within the tendons (Table 11–11). Tears to the tendons may result from a single traumatic force or, more commonly, especially in older athletes, from the accumu-lation of microtrauma (overuse injuries). **Partial-thickness tears** are short, longitudinal lesions in the tendon, initially involving only the superficial fibers. When partial-thickness tears go

Table 11–10. Evaluative Findings of Rotator Cuff Impingement

Examination Segment	Clinical Findings	
History	Onset Location of pain: Mechanism:	Insidious. Beneath, and lateral to, the acromion process. Repetitive overhead motion impinging the rotator cuff muscles (especially the supraspinatus) and long head of the biceps tendon among the humeral head, acromion, and coracoacromial arch.
Inspection	The shoulder may be postured for comfort.	
Palpation	Tenderness exists beneath the acromion process, over the greater and lesser tuberosities, and over the bicipital groove.	
Functional tests	Active, passive, and resisted movements of glenohumeral internal and external rotation and flexion result in pain and/or weakness. Abduction in the range of 70° to 120° results in pain. Activities of daily living and athletic events requiring overhead movement result in pain.	
Ligamentous tests	A complete ligamentous and capsular screen should be conducted to rule out glenohumeral and acromioclavicular laxity.	
Neurological tests	Not applicable.	
Special tests	Shoulder impingement test and its modification.	
Comments	Impingement may result secondary to glenohumeral instability. The inflammatory response caused by rotator cuff impingement, if untreated, leads to rotator cuff tendinitis, long head of the biceps brachii tendinitis, subacromial bursitis, or rotator cuff tears.	

untreated, a **full-thickness tear** may develop (full-thickness tears may also develop secondary to a single traumatic force). Severe dysfunction of the supraspinatus or infraspinatus can lead to atrophy that is visible during inspection of the scapula.

The posterior rotator cuff muscles, the infraspinatus and teres minor, play an important function in the throwing motion. In addition to externally rotating the humerus during the cocking phase of the throw, these muscles eccentrically contract to decrease the velocity of the arm during the follow-through phase. The eccentric contraction can lead to microtearing or inflammation of these muscles, eventually giving way to larger tears.

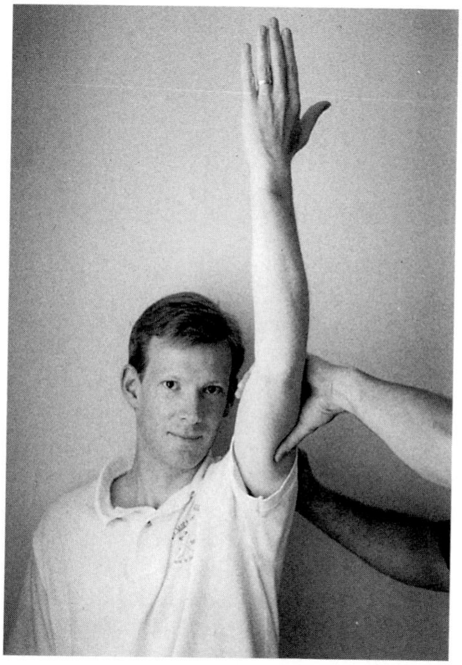

Drop Arm Test

This test uses the eccentric force of gravity to detect lesions in the supraspinatus muscle. During the controlled motion from full abduction to adduction, athletes suffering from tears in the rotator cuff tendons are unable to control the rate of fall once the humerus reaches the position of 90-degrees abduction. Another approach is to have the athlete attempt to hold the shoulder in 90-degrees abduction while the examiner applies a downward tap (Fig. 11–49). The result of the drop arm test may manifest itself during the examination of active abduction and adduction (see top of page 360).

Empty Can Test for Supraspinatus Pathology

This test isolates pathology of the supraspinatus tendon by increasing its tension while simultaneously placing mechanical pressure on it. The empty can test earned its name through its resemblance to the position of the hand and arm when draining a beverage can (Fig. 11–50) (see middle of page 360).

Figure 11–47. Shoulder impingement syndrome test.

Drop Arm Test (Fig. 11–49)

Position of athlete	Standing or sitting. The arm is fully abducted with the elbow straight.
Position of examiner	Standing lateral to, or behind, the involved extremity.
Evaluative procedure	The athlete slowly lowers the arm to the side.
Positive test results	The arm falls uncontrollably from a position of 90° to the side.
Implications	The inability to control adduction of the glenohumeral joint is indicative of lesions to the rotator cuff, especially the supraspinatus.
Modification	If the athlete is able to control adduction through the entire range of motion, a derivative of the drop arm test may be implemented: • The athlete holds the humerus in 90° abduction. • The examiner applies gentle pressure on the distal forearm. • A positive test result causes the arm to fall against the side of the body, indicating lesions to the rotator cuff.

Empty Can Test (Fig. 11–50)

Position of athlete	Sitting. The glenohumeral joint is abducted to 90° while the elbow is extended and the palm faces upward.
Position of examiner	Standing facing the athlete. One hand is placed on the superior portion of the midforearm to resist the motion of abduction.
Evaluative procedure	The evaluator resists abduction (applies a downward pressure) while the athlete internally rotates the glenohumeral joint and horizontally flexes the shoulder to 30°. (The ending position is similar to the position used when draining a can.)
Positive test results	Weakness or pain accompanying the movement.
Implications	The supraspinatus tendon (1) is being impinged between the humeral head and the coracoacromial arch, (2) is inflamed, or (3) contains a lesion.

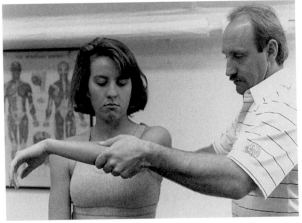

Figure 11–48. Modification of the shoulder impingement test.

Biceps Tendon Pathology

As stated by Norkin and Levangie, the relevance of the long head of the biceps tendon to the GH joint "may have more to do with dysfunction than with function. That is, its contribution to normal glenohumeral motion has less impact than its contribution to shoulder problems."[29] Otherwise stated, the long head of the biceps tendon provides very little force in moving the GH joint. During overhead movements, the tendon must slide within its sheath, located in the bicipital groove. When the tendon is inflamed, these movements produce pain and decrease the GH joint's functional ability.

Biceps tendinitis may result from rotator cuff dysfunction, from overuse of the biceps brachii muscle,

Table 11–11. Evaluative Findings of Rotator Cuff Tears

Examination Segment	Clinical Findings	
History	Onset Location of pain: Mechanism:	Acute or insidious. Deep within the shoulder beneath the acromion process. Acute: Dynamic overloading of the muscle of bony impingement. Insidious: Muscle imbalance, impingement, capsular laxity and/or drying and fraying of the muscle.
Inspection	In chronic cases, inspection of the scapula may indicate atrophy of the supraspinatus.	
Palpation	There is tenderness in the subacromial and proximal deltoid region.	
Functional tests	Isolation of the supraspinatus muscle results in pain. Pain exists during overhead motions. Pain may be present with resisted range of motion tests, especially abduction, internal rotation, and external rotation.	
Ligamentous tests	Tests to rule out glenohumeral and acromioclavicular laxity and impingement.	
Neurological tests	Not applicable.	
Special tests	Drop arm test; empty can test.	
Comments	The impingement sign is positive. Rotator cuff tendinitis often follows rotator cuff impingement syndrome.	

or from impingement. The transverse ligament, which holds the tendon in the bicipital groove, may become stretched or torn as the result of sudden forceful extension or external rotation of the shoulder accompanied by elbow flexion, causing the rapid increase of tension within the tendon.

Yergason's Test

This test may reproduce subluxation of the long head of the biceps tendon out of its groove or may elicit pain along the tendon as a result of tendini-tis. The athlete flexes the elbow and supinates the forearm against resistance while the examiner moves the humerus into external rotation (Fig. 11–51). Damage to the transverse ligament may result in the tendon's displacing from its groove or, in the case of tendinitis, may result in pain along the head of the biceps tendon.

Speed's Test

Speed's test is used to confirm the presence of inflammation in the long head of the biceps ten-

Yergason's Test (Fig. 11–51)

Position of athlete	Seated or standing. Glenohumeral joint is in the anatomical position. The elbow is flexed to 90°. The forearm is supinated 90° so that the lateral border of the radius faces upward.
Position of examiner	Positioned lateral to the athlete on the involved side. The olecranon is stabilized inferiorly and maintained close to the thorax. The forearm is stabilized proximal to the wrist.
Evaluative procedure	The athlete flexes the forearm against resistance while the examiner concurrently moves the glenohumeral joint into external rotation.
Positive tests	Pain and/or snapping in the bicipital groove.
Implications	Primary: Snapping or popping in the bicipital groove indicates a tear or laxity of the transverse humeral ligament. This pathology prevents the ligament from securing the long head of the tendon in its groove. Secondary: Pain with no associated popping in the bicipital groove may be indicative of bicipital tendinitis.

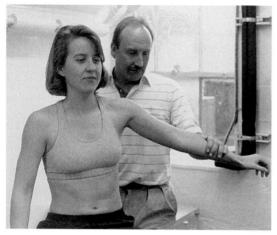

Figure 11–49. Drop arm test. This test is performed by passively abducting the shoulder of the athlete, who then lowers the arm to the side. In the presence of a rotator cuff tear, the arm falls from a position of 90°. As shown, the test may be modified by the examiner's applying pressure on the arm as it is held at 90°.

don (Fig. 11–52). Unlike Yergason's test, this technique does not replicate the subluxation of the tendon and may be used to differentiate bicipital tendinitis from a subluxating tendon (see middle of this page).

Subacromial Bursitis

Chronic rotator cuff impingement or rotator cuff tears, if untreated, ultimately lead to inflammation of the subacromial bursa. It is difficult to differentiate between these two maladies. Subacromial bursitis causes positive results from impingement tests and tests for supraspinatus tendinitis.

Thoracic Outlet Syndrome

Thoracic outlet syndrome is caused by pressure on the medial cord of the brachial plexus, the subclavian artery, and/or the subclavian vein (collectively known as the neurovascular bundle). Its etiol-

Speed's Test (Fig. 11–52)

Position of athlete	Sitting, standing, or prone. The glenohumeral joint is in the anatomical position. The elbow is extended and the forearm supinated.
Position of examiner	Standing lateral to and in front of the involved limb. The fingers of one hand are positioned over the bicipital groove. The forearm is stabilized proximal to the wrist.
Evaluative procedure	The clinician resists flexion of the glenohumeral joint while palpating tenderness over the bicipital groove.
Positive test results	Pain along the long head of the biceps brachii tendon, especially in the bicipital groove.
Implications	Pain associated only with resisted glenohumeral flexion is indicative of advanced tendinitis of the long head of the biceps tendon, whereas pain that is elicited only by palpating over the bicipital groove indicates that the tendon inflammation is in its earlier stages.

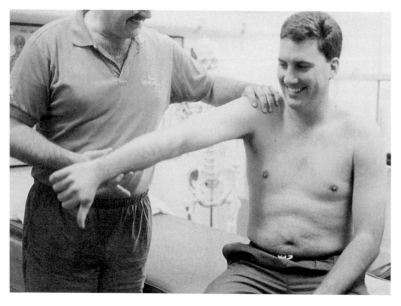

Figure 11–50. Empty can test for supraspinatus involvement.

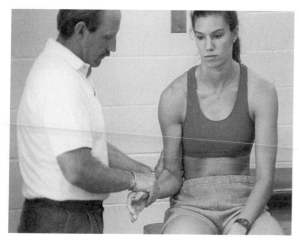

Figure 11–51. Yergason's test for pathology of the long head of the biceps tendon.

ogy may be linked to the presence of a cervical rib or pressure placed on the neurovascular bundle as it is impinged between the clavicle and the first thoracic rib secondary to tightness of the pectoralis minor or the scalenus anticus muscle.

Present in a small percentage of the population, the cervical rib is a congenital outgrowth of the seventh cervical vertebra. This structure places pressure on the neurovascular bundle, especially when the shoulder girdle is pulled inferiorly. The presence of a cervical rib does not necessarily predispose an athlete to thoracic outlet syndrome. Of all individuals possessing cervical ribs, fewer than 10

percent display the clinical signs and symptoms of thoracic outlet syndrome.[30]

The neurovascular bundle passes between the clavicle and the first thoracic rib and is therefore susceptible to pressure on its anterior surface. Poor posture, drooping shoulders, prolonged pressure on the upper surfaces of the first rib, or acute trauma may lead to the onset of thoracic outlet syndrome.

The signs and symptoms of thoracic outlet syndrome may be neurological or vascular in nature (Table 11–12). Neurological symptoms tend to be found along the distribution of the medial cord of the brachial plexus (C8 and T1) because of its proximity to the first thoracic rib. Clinical symptoms are generally manifest along the distribution of the ulnar nerve; decreased function along the median nerve may also be noted.

Vascular signs and symptoms reflect the specific structure being obstructed. Occlusion of the subclavian artery presents signs and symptoms typical of decreased blood flow. Blockage of the subclavian vein is characterized by edema in the distal upper extremity and, if untreated, may result in thrombophlebitis.

Positive test results for thoracic outlet syndromes are not necessarily definitive of any underlying pathology. Athletes who test positive for thoracic outlet syndrome should be referred to a physician for further evaluation.

Adson's Test

The underlying principle in any test for thoracic outlet syndrome is the pressure placed on the neurovascular bundle. Adson's test attempts to depress the shoulder girdle and place the medial cord of the brachial plexus, the subclavian artery, and the subclavian vein on stretch while simultaneously placing pressure on the bundle from the anterior scalene muscle (Fig. 11–53) (see top of page 364).

Allen Test

The Allen test is similar to Adson's test but is used to identify pressure caused by the pectoralis minor's being placed on the neurovascular bundle (Fig. 11–54) (see middle of page 364).

Military Brace Position for Costoclavicular Involvement

This test evaluates costoclavicular obstruction of the neurovascular bundle (Fig. 11–55) (see bottom of page 364).

Scapular Injuries

Because of its relatively flat contour and its protection from trauma by the overlying musculature and protective equipment, the scapula is rarely injured. Blows to the posterior surface overlying the

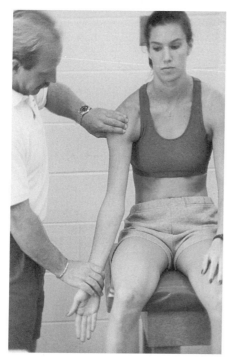

Figure 11–52. Speed's test for tendinitis of the long head of the biceps brachii muscle.

Adson's Test (Fig. 11–53)

Position of athlete	Sitting. The shoulder is abducted to 30°. The elbow is extended and the thumb is pointing upward. The head is looking toward the involved side.
Position of examiner	Standing behind the athlete. One hand is positioned so that the radial pulse is felt.
Evaluative procedure	While still maintaining a feel for the radial pulse, the examiner externally rotates and extends the shoulder while the athlete extends the neck. The athlete is then instructed to inhale deeply and hold the breath.
Positive test results	The radial pulse disappears or markedly diminishes.
Implications	The subclavian artery is being occluded between the anterior and middle scalene muscles.
Comment	This test often produces false-positive results.

Allen Test (Fig. 11–54)

Position of athlete	Sitting. The shoulder is abducted to 30°. The elbow is extended and the thumb is pointing upward. The head is looking forward.
Position of examiner	Standing behind the athlete. One hand is positioned so that the radial pulse is felt.
Evaluative procedure	The elbow is flexed to 90° while the clinician abducts the glenohumeral joint to 90°. The shoulder is then horizontally extended and externally rotated. The athlete then looks toward the opposite shoulder.
Positive test results	The radial pulse disappears.
Implications	The pectoralis minor muscle is compressing the neurovascular bundle.
Comment	This test often produces false-positive results.

Military Brace Position (Fig. 11–55)

Position of athlete	Standing. The shoulders are in a relaxed posture. The head is looking forward.
Position of examiner	Standing behind the athlete. One hand is positioned to locate the radial pulse on the involved extremity.
Evaluative procedure	The athlete retracts the shoulders as if coming to military attention. The arm is extended and abducted to 30°. The neck and head are hyperextended.
Positive test results	The radial pulse disappears.
Implications	The subclavian artery is being blocked by the costoclavicular structures of the shoulder.

Table 11–12. Evaluative Findings
of Thoracic Outlet Syndrome

Neurological onset:
- Numbness
- Pain
- Paresthesia
Note: These symptoms normally occur over the ulnar
  nerve distribution
Arterial onset:
- Coldness of the skin
- *Pallor*
- Cyanosis in the fingers
- Muscular weakness
Venous onset:
- Muscular and joint stiffness
- Edema
- Venous engorgement
- Thrombophlebitis

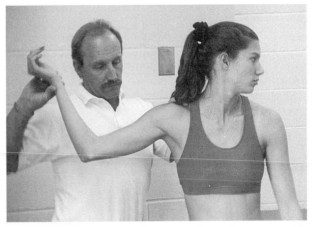

Figure 11–54. Allen test for thoracic outlet syndrome caused by the pectoralis minor muscle.

scapula during athletic competition generally result in damage to the skin and muscles rather than to the bone itself.

Although rare, reports of scapular fractures in football have been reported.[31,32] Incidence of scapular fractures is higher among players at high-impact positions wearing relatively small shoulder pads. Fractures may occur to the body of the scapula, but most often in the glenoid fossa, glenoid neck, or coracoid process secondary to a GH dislocation.

Fractures of the scapula may present with many of the signs and symptoms of rotator cuff inflammation through decreased strength during abduction and external rotation. Any athlete suffering from a GH dislocation should also have a radiographic evaluation to rule out a secondary fracture to the glenoid or coracoid process.

Humeral Injuries

Although not frequent, humeral fractures do occur in athletics, especially in collision sports. This condition is marked by extreme pain and dysfunction. In many cases a disruption in the continuity of the humeral shaft is observed. Although the vast majority of humeral fractures occur as the result of a high-impact force, spontaneous fractures occurring during pitching have also been reported.[33] Fractures in the region of the surgical neck can threaten the radial nerve.

A common finding of glenohumeral dislocation is that of a **Hill-Sachs lesion**. The lesion is a small ar-

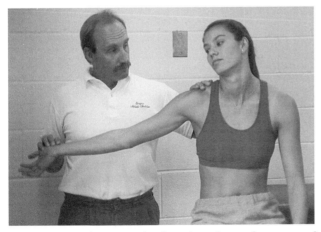

Figure 11–53. Adson's test for thoracic outlet syndrome caused by the anterior scalene muscle.

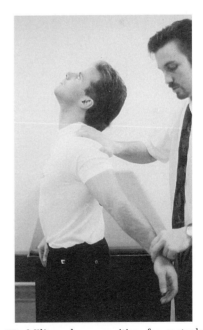

Figure 11–55. Military brace position for costoclavicular obstruction of the neurovascular bundle.

Pallor: Lack of color in the skin.

ticular cartilage defect on the humeral head caused by the impact of the humeral head on the glenoid fossa as the humerus dislocates. The lesion is typically found along the posterior aspect of the humeral head following an anterior dislocation. Lesions found on the anterior portion of the humeral head following a posterior dislocation are termed reverse Hill-Sachs lesions.

The Hill-Sachs lesion itself is used as a diagnostic tool in determining the severity of the dislocation. In those athletes reporting that the shoulder dislocated but spontaneously relocated, the lesion may be present on x-ray examination. The lesion itself is rarely symptomatic but may lead to early degeneration of the glenohumeral joint.

An untreated hematoma within the biceps brachii muscle can result in myositis ossificans ("blocker's exostosis") (see Fig. 2–2). This condition is marked by decreased range of motion during elbow flexion and extension and, in chronic cases, the calcified mass may be palpable.

ON-FIELD EVALUATION OF SHOULDER INJURIES

The most important findings to be ruled out during the immediate evaluation of injuries to the shoulder complex are fractures and dislocations. In many cases the presence of these conditions may be confirmed through visual inspection or palpation of the area. When a humeral fracture or glenohumeral joint dislocation is suspected, the presence of a distal pulse must be determined. The absence of this pulse warrants the immediate transportation of the athlete to a hospital.

Pain radiating through the shoulder and into the arm may indicate damage to one or more cervical nerve roots. A complete evaluation of the cervical and/or thoracic spine should be performed first when the mechanism of injury or description of the symptoms implicates possible cervical spine trauma. It is important not to make any unnecessary movements of the athlete until the possibility of spinal injury has been eliminated. Trauma to the spleen or myocardial dysfunction may also refer pain into the shoulder.

The on-field evaluation of shoulder injuries is complicated by the presence of shoulder pads in sports such as football, ice hockey, lacrosse, and motorcross racing. The examiner must become familiar with how to work around these pads and, if necessary, how to remove them without further aggravating the athlete's injury

Palpation Under the Shoulder Pads

Shoulder pads are characterized by the presence of at least one cantilever arching over the acromion process and the deltoid muscle group (Fig. 11–56). The space provided by the cantilever provides enough room for the clinician to reach under the shirt and palpate the humeral head, the AC joint, and the distal clavicle. By unfastening the strap that passes beneath the axilla and loosening the sternal fasteners, more room may be provided. It is also possible to palpate the proximal structures of the shoulder girdle by entering the shoulder pads from the neck opening.

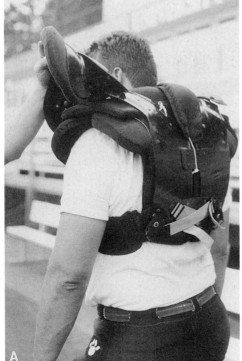
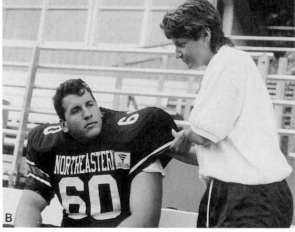

Figure 11–56. (*A*) The cantilever of football shoulder pads. (*B*) By reaching under the cantilever, the humeral head, acromioclavicular joint, and distal clavicle can be palpated.

Because the clinician is palpating these structures without actually being able to see them, care must be used when applying pressure. The initial palpation should be gentle, following the contours of the shoulder girdle while checking for gross deformity.

Removal of Shoulder Pads

Certain injuries such as AC or SC joint sprains, GH dislocations, or clavicular fractures require the removal of the shoulder pads to further evaluate the condition, to begin treatment of the area, or to transport the athlete. This must be done with as little movement of the injured extremity as possible to prevent further insult to the injured structures.

If the athlete's jersey is loose-fitting, the examiner first removes the uninjured arm. Once this is complete, the examiner slides the shirt up and over the head, then drops it down over the injured arm. In many cases it is easier to remove the shirt and shoulder pads as a single unit (Fig. 11–57). If the shirt is extraordinarily tight-fitting or a practice jersey, or in the case of a medical emergency, it may be cut off the athlete. Athletic trainers may deem that the problems

associated with delay in safely and quickly removing the shirt outweigh the drawbacks of cutting it off.[34]

INITIAL MANAGEMENT OF ON-FIELD INJURIES

The following is suggested protocol for the initial management of major injuries to the shoulder girdle and upper arm. In emergency situations or when proper splinting materials are not available, the athlete's jersey may be used as a sling or the hand can be tucked into the belt of the pants (Fig. 11–58).

Fractures of the Clavicle

When fractures of the clavicle are suspected, the shoulder should be immobilized to prevent movement of the fractured segments and the athlete transported to a physician for a definitive diagnosis. Although a rare occurrence, secondary damage to nerves and blood vessels have resulted from clavicular fractures.[35]

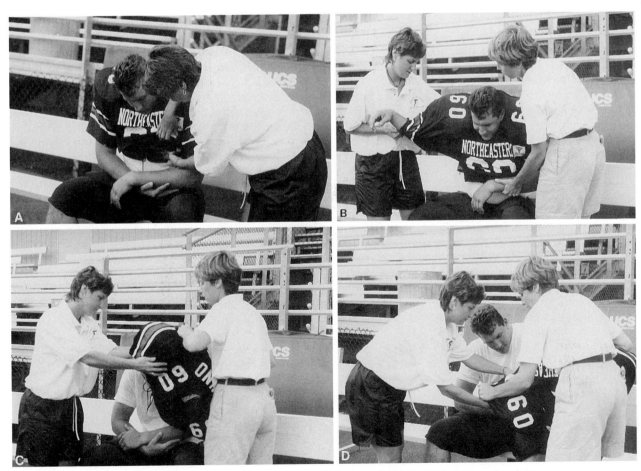

Figure 11–57. Removing shoulder pads (the athlete's left arm is injured). (*A*) Unsnap the chest straps. (*B*) Pull the shirt off the uninjured arm. (*C*) Lift the shoulder pads and shirt over the athlete's head. (*D*) Slide the shoulder pads from around the injured arm.

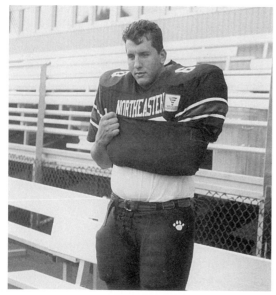

Figure 11–58. A temporary sling can be made by pulling the shirt up and over the involved arm.

The shoulder may be immobilized through the use of a sling or triangular bandage. A sling and swath approach may be more comfortable for the athlete by taking the weight of the arm off the involved clavicle.

Acromioclavicular Joint Injuries

Athletes displaying the signs and symptoms of an AC joint sprain should be immobilized in a position that lessens the displacement between the clavicle and the acromial process. Initially this may be achieved through the use of a foam pad with a hard shell held in place over the acromial process by a

spica wrap, and a sling supporting the weight of the arm (Fig. 11–59).

Physicians most commonly choose to treat all but the most severe AC dislocations nonsurgically.[10,17,36] Comparative follow-up studies of surgical and nonsurgical management of AC dislocations indicate that shoulders treated nonsurgically display little residual decrease in range of motion or in strength deficits.[10]

Athletes suffering from AC joint contusions, in addition to the standard modality protocol, should have the joint protected with additional padding during activity. Such protection may be obtained through the use of a foam doughnut pad with a hard shell held in place by an elastic spica wrap or elastic tape.

Glenohumeral Dislocations

Because of the possibility of a dislocated humeral head causing additional trauma to the blood and nerve supply to the arm, it is important to monitor the athlete's radial pulse, check for circulation in the fingertips, and perform a sensory screen of the involved arm. Absence of a pulse indicates a medical emergency.

To transport the athlete, the arm should be fixed in the position it has assumed through the use of a moldable splint (metal or vacuum) or toweling placed between the humerus and torso. A sling or elastic wrap may be used to support the weight of the arm. It is important to keep the wrist and hand exposed so that the radial pulse may be rechecked. The athlete should be transported supine on a stretcher or spineboard.

Because of the threat of causing additional trauma to the glenohumeral structures, on-field reductions of GH dislocations should *not* be performed by any-

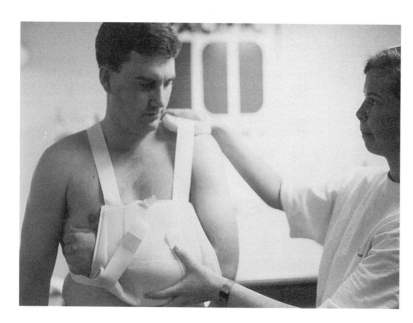

Figure 11–59. Management of an acromioclavicular joint sprain. A commercially available device (shown) or a sling and swath can be used to immobilize the shoulder and apply pressure to the acromioclavicular joint.

one other than a physician. Forced reduction of the humeral head may damage the glenoid fossa, the coracoid process, or the neurovascular structures in the area. The athlete should be immediately transported to a physician once the shoulder has been immobilized.

Humeral Fractures

Fractures of the humeral shaft may be marked by gross deformity and extreme pain. However, fractures of the humeral head may occur secondary to glenohumeral dislocations and therefore go initially unnoticed because of the attention placed on the joint.

Fractures of the humeral shaft should be splinted in the position they are found, using a moldable aluminum splint or a vacuum splint. The wrist and fingers should remain exposed so that the radial pulse, circulation to the fingers, and sensation of the fingers can be monitored. The athlete should be transported supine or on a stretcher, and immediate physician referral is indicated.

REFERENCES

1. Perry, J: Normal upper extremity kinesiology. Phys Ther 58:265, 1978.
2. Culham, E, and Peat, M: Functional anatomy of the shoulder complex. Journal of Orthopedic and Sports Physical Therapy 18:342, 1993.
3. Norkin, CC, and Levangie, PK: The shoulder complex. In Norkin, CC, and Levangie, PK: Joint Structure and Function: A Comprehensive Analysis, ed 2. FA Davis, Philadelphia, 1992, p 219.
3a. Rothstein, JM, Roy, SH, and Wolf, SL: Rehabilitation Specialist's Handbook. FA Davis, Philadelphia, 1991.
4. Norkin, CC, and Levangie, PK: The shoulder complex. In Norkin, CC, and Levangie, PK: Joint Structure and Function. A Comprehensive Analysis, ed 2. FA Davis, Philadelphia, 1992, p 220.
5. Kessler, RM, and Hertling, D: The shoulder and shoulder girdle. In Hertling, D, and Kessler, RM: Management of Common Musculoskeletal Disorders. Physical Therapy Principles and Procedures, ed 2. JB Lippincott, Philadelphia, 1990, p 171.
5a. Kendall, FP, and McCreary, EK: Muscles: Testing and Function, ed 3. Williams & Wilkins, Baltimore, 1983.
5b. Daniels, L, and Worthingham, C: Muscle Testing: Techniques of Manual Examination, ed 5. WB Saunders, Philadelphia, 1986.
6. Doody, SG, and Waterland, JC: Shoulder movements during abduction in the scapular plane. Arch Phys Med Rehabil 51:595, 1970.
7. Hollinshead, WH, and Jenkins, DB: The shoulder. In Hollings-head, WH, and Jenkins, DB: Functional Anatomy of the Limbs and Back, ed 5. WB Saunders, Philadelphia, 1981.
8. Boublik, M, and Hawkins, RJ: Clinical examination of the shoulder complex. Journal of Orthopedic and Sports Physical Therapy 18:379, 1993.
9. Norkin, CC, and Levangie, PK: The shoulder complex. In Norkin, CC, and Levangie, PK: Joint Structure and Function: A Comprehensive Analysis, ed 2. FA Davis, Philadelphia, 1992, p 223.
10. Tibone, J, Sellers, R, and Tonino, P: Strength testing after third degree acromioclavicular dislocations. Am J Sports Med 20:328, 1992.
11. Chandler, TJ, et al: Shoulder strength, power, and endurance in college tennis players. Am J Sports Med 20:445, 1992.
12. Wilk, KE, et al: The strength characteristics of internal and external rotator muscles in professional baseball pitchers. Am J Sports Med 21:61, 1993.
13. Reynolds, RS, and Hirschman, LD: An examination of the concentric and eccentric strength of the shoulder rotators (abstr). Athletic Training: Journal of the National Athletic Trainers Association 26:154, 1991.
14. Speer, KP: Anatomy and pathomechanics of shoulder instability. Operative Techniques in Sports Medicine 1:252, 1993.
15. Prime, HT, Doig, SG, and Hooper, JC: Retrosternal dislocation of the clavicle: A case report. Am J Sports Med 19:92, 1991.
16. Bach, BR, VanFleet, TA, and Novak, PJ: Acromioclavicular injuries: Controversies in treatment. The Physician and Sports Medicine 20:87, 1992.
17. Bach, BR, and Novack, PJ: Chronic acromioclavicular joint pain: An overlooked problem. The Physician and Sports Medicine 21:63, 1993.
18. Gartsman, GM: Arthroscopic resection of the acromioclavicular joint. Am J Sports Med 21:71, 1993.
19. Gartsman, GM, et al: Arthroscopic acromioclavicular joint resection: An anatomical study. Am J Sports Med 19:2, 1991.
20. Terry, GC, et al: The stabilizing function of passive shoulder restraints. Am J Sports Med 19:26, 1991.
21. Jobe, FW, et al: Anterior capsulolabral reconstruction of the shoulder in athletes in overhand sports. Am J Sports Med 19:428, 1991.
22. Tsia, L, et al: Shoulder function in patients with unoperated anterior shoulder instability. Am J Sports Med 19:469, 1991.
23. Hurley, JA, et al: Posterior shoulder instability: Surgical versus conservative results with evaluation of glenoid version. Am J Sports Med 20:396, 1992.
24. Greenan, TJ, et al: Posttraumatic changes in the posterior glenoid and labrum in a handball player. Am J Sports Med 21:153, 1993.
25. Warner, JJP, et al: Static capsuloligamentous restraints to superior-inferior translation of the glenohumeral joint. Am J Sports Med 20:675, 1992.
26. Burns, TP, and Turba, JE: Arthroscopic treatment of shoulder impingement in athletes. Am J Sports Med 20:13, 1992.
27. Kamkar, A, Irrgang, JJ, and Whitney, SL: Nonoperative management of secondary shoulder impingement syndrome. Am J Sports Med 17:212, 1993.
28. Shankwiler, JA, and Burkhead, WZ: Diagnosis, evaluation, and conservative treatment of impingement syndrome. Operative Techniques in Sports Medicine 1:89, 1994.
29. Norkin, CC, and Levangie, PK: The shoulder complex. In Norkin, CC, and Levangie, PK: Joint Structure and Function: A Comprehensive Analysis, ed 2. FA Davis, Philadelphia, 1992, p 228.
30. Baker, CL, and Liu, SH: Neurovascular injuries to the shoulder. Journal of Orthopedic and Sports Physical Therapy 18:360, 1993.
31. Culpepper, MI, and Roberts, JM: Case report: Fracture of the scapula in a professional football player. Athletic Training: Journal of the National Athletic Trainers Association 20:35, 1985.
32. Cain, TE, and Hamilton, WP: Scapular fractures in professional football players. Am J Sports Med 20:363, 1992.
33. Branch, T, et al: Spontaneous fractures of the humerus during pitching: A series of 12 cases. Am J Sports Med 20:468, 1992.
34. McCarthy, M: Personal communication, July 1994.
35. Bartosh, RA, Dugdale, TW, and Nelson, R: Isolated musculocutaneous nerve injury complicating closed fracture of the clavicle: A case report. Am J Sports Med 20:356, 1992.
36. Martel, JR: Clavicular nonunion: Complications with the use of mersilene tape. Am J Sports Med 20:360, 1992.
37. Tibone, J, Sellers, R, and Tonio, P: Strength testing after third degree acromioclavicular dislocations. Am J Sports Med 20:328, 1992.

12

The Elbow and Forearm

Serving as the link between the powerful movements of the shoulder and the *fine motor control* of the hand, the elbow is often overlooked as an area of potentially disabling injury. Even minor injuries to the elbow can severely hamper the athlete's ability to perform the most rudimentary of athletic skills.

Fractures or other trauma involving the forearm or elbow can result in impairment of the neurovascular structures supplying the wrist, hand, and fingers. Because of this the examination of the elbow and forearm is often expanded to include the distal structures of the hand.

CLINICAL ANATOMY

Three bones—the humerus, the radius, and the ulna—form the elbow joint, with the radius and ulna continuing on to form the bony structure of the forearm. The distal end of the humerus flares to form the medial and lateral epicondyles. The larger of these epicondyles, the **medial epicondyle**, is demarcated on its distal anteromedial border by the **trochlea**. Covered by articular cartilage, this structure serves as the axis for rotation of the ulna on the humerus. Separated from the trochlea by the trochlear groove, the **capitulum** forms the lateral humeral articulating surface on the distal border of the **lateral epicondyle**. Unlike the trochlea, the dome-shaped capitulum does not extend to the posterior aspect of the humerus. Located immediately above the capitulum, the **radial fossa** is an indentation in the lateral epicondyle that accepts the radial head during elbow flexion (Fig. 12–1). The distal end of the humerus is anteriorly rotated 30 degrees relative to the humeral shaft.[1]

The medial border of the forearm is formed by the **ulna**. Its proximal anatomy is structured to allow articulation with both the humerus and radius. The **semilunar notch**, an indentation lined with articular cartilage, fits snugly around the trochlea. The proximal border is formed by the **olecranon process**, a projection that fits into the humeral **olecranon fossa** during complete extension of the elbow. The distal border of the semilunar notch is formed by the **coronoid process**, which is received by the coronoid fossa during elbow flexion. Medial and slightly distal to the coronoid process, the **radial notch** is an indentation that accepts the radial head (Fig. 12–2).

The lateral bone of the elbow and forearm is the **radius**. Its proximal articulating surface is disk-shaped and concave to allow gliding and rotation on the capitulum. The border of the proximal radius is also covered with articular cartilage to allow it to rotate on the ulna. Distal to the proximal radial head is the **bicipital tuberosity** (radial tuberosity), the insertion site for the biceps brachii. The **radial shaft** is triangular and broadens medially and laterally at its distal end to form the **radial head.**

Articulations and Ligamentous Anatomy

In order to function properly, the elbow relies on the integrity of four individual articulations: the humeroulnar joint, the humeroradial joint, the proximal radioulnar joint, and the distal radioulnar joint. The motion of forearm flexion and extension occurs at the humeroulnar and humeroradial joint, whereas the motion of forearm *supination* and *pronation* occurs at the humeroradial, superior radioulnar, and inferior radioulnar joints.

Humeroulnar and Humeroradial Joints

A modified hinge joint, the humeroulnar articulation allows for 1 degree of freedom of movement: flexion and extension. The design of this joint may allow up to 5 degrees of internal rotation of the ulna on the humerus, but this motion is generally considered to be an accessory one.

Fine motor control: Specific control of the muscles allowing for completion of small, delicate tasks.
Supination (forearm): Movement at the radioulnar joints allowing for the palm to turn upward, as if holding a bowl of soup.
Pronation (forearm): Movement at the radioulnar joints allowing for the palm to be turned downward.

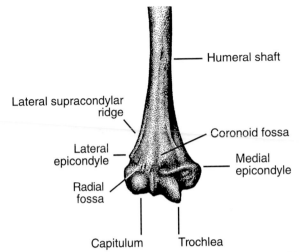

Figure 12-1. Bony anatomy of the distal humerus. The trochlea articulates with the ulna; the capitulum, with the radius.

Also a modified hinge joint, the humeroradial joint permits 2 degrees of freedom of movement: (1) flexion and extension as the radial head glides around the capitulum and (2) internal and external rotation of the radius on the capitulum during the movements of pronation and supination.

Proximal and Distal Radioulnar Joints

The **proximal radioulnar joint** is formed by the convex medial rim of the radial head and the con-

cave radial notch of the ulna; the **distal radioulnar joint** is formed by an articular disk between the radius and ulna. The radioulnar joint has 1 degree of freedom of movement, pronation and supination, and its alignment is maintained by an interosseous membrane spanning the inner (facing) borders of these two bones, classifying it as a syndesmotic joint. During supination, motion at the superior joint occurs as the radius rotates and crosses over the ulna. At the inferior joint the disk and ulnar notch of the radius sweeps across the ulna. The reverse occurs during pronation.

Ligamentous Support

Support of the medial elbow against valgus forces is obtained from the **ulnar collateral ligament (UCL)**, which is divisible into three unique sections (Fig. 12-3). The **anterior oblique band** originates from the inferior surface of the medial epicondyle and passes anterior to the axis of rotation to insert on the medial aspect of the coronoid process. Unlike the other elbow ligaments, the anterior oblique band is easily distinguishable from the joint capsule. Taut throughout the elbow's range of motion, this band is the primary restraint against valgus force. The **transverse oblique band**, originating from the medial epicondyle and inserting on the coronoid process, provides little, if any, support to the medial elbow.[1] Inserting on the olecranon process, the **posterior oblique band** is taut in flexion beyond 60 degrees.

Lateral support of the elbow is derived from the radial collateral, lateral ulnar collateral, and the accessory lateral collateral ligaments (Fig. 12-4). The most important lateral stabilizing structure is the **lateral ulnar collateral ligament (LUCL)**. Arising from the middle of the lateral epicondyle and in-

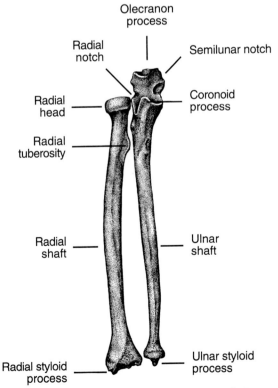

Figure 12-2. Bony anatomy of the radius and ulna.

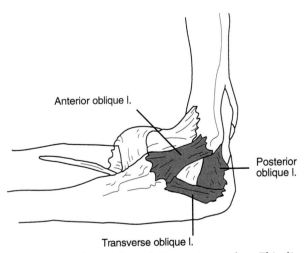

Figure 12-3. Ulnar collateral ligament complex. This ligament is formed by the anterior oblique ligament, the posterior oblique ligament, the transverse oblique ligament, and the lateral ulnar collateral ligament, which is visible on the lateral view.

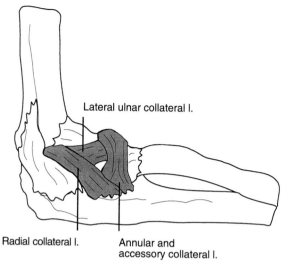

Figure 12-4. Lateral ligaments of the elbow. This group is formed by the radial collateral ligament, the lateral ulnar collateral ligament, and the annular ligament. The lateral ulnar collateral ligament is a part of the ulnar collateral ligament complex. The annular ligament is responsible for maintaining the relationship between the proximal radius and ulna.

serting on the tubercle of the ulna, the LUCL provides lateral support of the ulna that is independent of the other lateral ligaments and is considered to be a component of the ulnar collateral ligament complex. Disruption of this ligament results in a rotatory-type instability of the elbow joint.

The **radial collateral ligament (RCL)** is a thickened area in the lateral joint capsule spanning the distance between the lateral epicondyle and the annular ligament. In addition to resisting varus stresses, the RCL is important in maintaining the close relationship between the humeral and radial articulating surfaces.

Encircling the radial head, the **annular ligament** is a fibro-osseous structure that permits internal and external rotation of the radius on the ulna. Both ends of the annular ligament attach to the coronoid process and form four-fifths of a circle, with the remaining one-fifth being formed by the radial notch. This articulation receives additional support from the attachment of the RCL and the fibrous attachment of the supinator muscle. The distal end of the annular ligament narrows to conform to the shape of the radial head, preventing the radius from migrating distally.

During extreme supination the anterior fibers of the annular ligament become taut; during hyperpronation the posterior fibers are taut. When a varus stress is applied to the elbow, the **accessory lateral collateral ligament (ALCL)** assists the annular ligament and the RCL in preventing the separation of the radius from the ulna.

Interosseous Membrane

A dense band of fibrous connective tissue, the fibers of the interosseous membrane run obliquely

from the radius to the ulna and span the distance between the proximal and distal radioulnar joints (Fig. 12-5). This fibrous arrangement serves as a stabilizer against axial forces applied to the wrist, transmitting force from the radius to the ulna, which then transmits the force to the humerus. A gap is present near its distal end to allow small blood vessels to pass to the posterior aspect of the forearm. The interosseous membrane also serves as the origin for many of the muscles acting on the wrist and hand.

Muscular Anatomy

The muscles inserting on the proximal radius and ulna act to flex or extend the elbow and pronate or supinate the forearm. Many of the prime movers of the wrist and hand originate from the humeral epicondyles. The actions, origins, insertions, and innervation of the muscles producing elbow and forearm motion are presented in Table 12-1. Chapter 13 discusses the forearm muscles acting on the wrist and hand.

Elbow Flexor/Supinator Group

The **biceps brachii, brachialis,** and **brachioradialis** are the prime flexors of the elbow. The relative position of the forearm (pronated or supinated) determines which of the muscles provides the primary contribution to the movement. When the forearm is supinated the biceps brachii is the prime flexor; when the forearm is pronated the brachialis is the primary contributor to flexion. When the forearm is

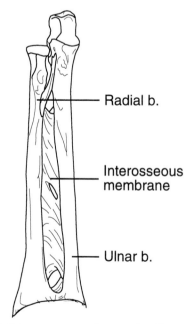

Figure 12-5. Interosseous membrane. The fibrous arrangement of this structure transmits force absorbed by the radius at the wrist to the ulna.

Table 12–1. Muscles Acting on the Elbow and Forearm

Muscle	Action	Origin	Insertion	Nerve	Root
Anconeus	Elbow extension Stabilizes ulna during pronation and supination	• Posterior surface of the lateral epicondyle	• Lateral border of the olecranon process	Radial	C7, C8
Biceps brachii	Elbow flexion Forearm supination Shoulder flexion	• Long head: Supraglenoid tuberosity of scapula • Short head: Coracoid process of scapula	• Radial tuberosity	Musculo-cutaneous	C5, C6
Brachialis	Elbow flexion	• Distal one-half of anterior humerus	• Coronoid process of ulna • Ulnar tuberosity	Musculo-cutaneous	C5, C6
Brachioradialis	Elbow flexion Forearm pronation Forearm supination	• Supracondylar ridge of humerus	• Styloid process of radius	Radial	C5, C6
Extensor carpi radialis brevis	Wrist extension Ulnar deviation	• Lateral epicondyle via the common extensor tendon • Radial collateral ligament	• Base of the 3rd metatarsal	Radial	C6, C7
Extensor carpi radialis longus	Elbow flexion Wrist extension Ulnar deviation	• Supracondylar ridge	• Radial side of the 2nd metacarpal	Radial	C6, C7
Extensor carpi ulnaris	Wrist extension Ulnar deviation	• Lateral epicondyle via the common extensor tendon	• Ulnar side of the base of the 5th metacarpal	Deep radial	C6, C7, C8
Extensor digitorum	Wrist extension MCP extension IP extension	• Lateral epicondyle via the common extensor tendon	• Into the dorsal surface of the proximal base of the middle and distal phalanges of each of the four fingers	Deep radial	C6, C7, C8
Flexor carpi radialis	Elbow flexion Forearm pronation Wrist flexion Radial deviation	• Medial epicondyle via the common flexor tendon	• Bases of the 2nd and 3rd metacarpal bones	Median	C6, C7
Flexor carpi ulnaris	Elbow flexion Wrist flexion Ulnar deviation	Humeral head: • Medial epicondyle via the common flexor tendon Ulnar head: • Medial border of the olecranon • Proximal two-thirds of the posterior ulna	• Pisiform • Hamate • 5th metacarpal	Ulnar	C8, T1
Flexor digitorum profundus	DIP flexion PIP flexion Wrist flexion	• Anteromedial proximal three-fourths of ulna and associated interosseous membrane	• Bases of the medial 4 phalanges	Palmar interosseous	C8, T1

continued

Table 12–1. Muscles Acting on the Elbow and Forearm (*Continued*)

Muscle	Action	Origin	Insertion	Nerve	Root
Flexor digitorum superficialis	PIP flexion MCP flexion Wrist flexion	Humeral head: • Medial epicondyle via the common flexor tendon • Ulnar collateral ligament Ulnar head: • Coronoid process Radial head: • Oblique line of radius	• Middle sides of the 4 phalanges	Median	C7, C8, T1
Palmaris longus	Wrist flexion Elbow flexion	• Medial epicondyle via the common flexor tendon	• Flexor retinaculum • Palmar aponeurosis	Median	C6, C7
Pronator quadratus	Forearm pronation	• Anterior surface of the distal one-fourth of ulna	• Lateral portion of the distal one-fourth of the radius	Palmar interosseous	C8, T1
Pronator teres	Forearm pronation Elbow flexion	Humeral head: • Proximal to the medial epicondyle of humerus Ulnar head: • Coronoid process	• Middle one-third of the lateral radius	Median	C6, C7
Supinator	Forearm supination	• Lateral epicondyle • Radial collateral ligament • Annular ligament • Supinator crest of ulna	• Proximal one-third of radius	Deep radial	C6, C7, C8
Triceps brachii	Elbow extension Shoulder adduction	Long head: • Infraglenoid tuberosity of scapula Lateral head: • Posterolateral surface of the proximal one-half of the humeral shaft Medial head: • Posteromedial surface of the humerus	• Olecranon process of ulna	Radial	C7, C8

Muscle actions, origins, and insertions adapted from Kendall and McCreary[1a]; innervations adapted from Daniels and Worthingham.[1b]

in its neutral position (radial side upward) the brachioradialis is the primary flexor. The **supinator** is assisted by the biceps brachii and brachioradialis during forceful supination. The brachioradialis also serves to pronate the forearm from the supinated position. The anterolateral bulk of the forearm muscles is formed by the extensor carpi radialis longus, extensor carpi radialis brevis, and the extensor digitorum muscles (Fig. 12–6).

Elbow Extensor/Pronator Group

Those muscles acting to extend the elbow, the **triceps brachii** and **anconeus**, do not influence pronation or supination of the forearm, although the anconeus does stabilize the ulna during these movements (Fig. 12–7). A twin set of muscles, the **pronator teres**, located proximally on the forearm, and the distal **pronator quadratus**, are

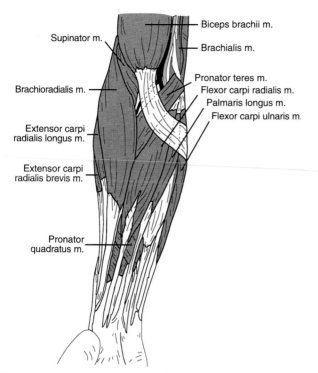

Figure 12-6. Anterior muscles of the forearm. These muscles serve primarily to flex the elbow, wrist, and fingers.

the primary forearm pronators. The remaining medial bulk is formed by the flexor carpi radialis longus, palmaris longus, and flexor carpi ulnaris muscles. These muscles are described in Chapter 13.

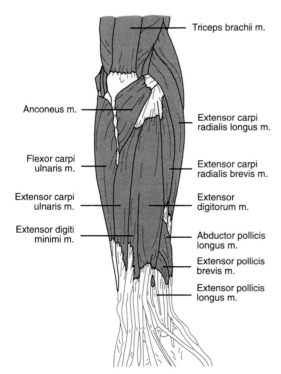

Figure 12-7. Posterior muscles of the forearm. These muscles serve to extend the elbow, wrist, and fingers.

Nerves

Three primary nerves cross the elbow: the median nerve, ulnar nerve, and radial nerve. Their relatively superficial course across the elbow and in the distal portion of the forearm predispose them to acute, traumatic injury. Figure 12-8 presents the sensory distribution of these nerves in the hand.

Median Nerve

Crossing the anterior elbow in the same path as the brachial artery, the median nerve courses deep within the forearm muscles to follow the flexor digitorum superficialis down the middle of the anterior forearm. As it approaches the wrist, the median nerve becomes superficial once again as it passes between the flexor digitorum superficialis and flexor carpi radialis tendons (beneath the palmaris longus) to pass within the carpal tunnel and enter the hand. With the exception of the flexor carpi ulnaris and the medial portion of the flexor digitorum profundus, the median nerve supplies all of the wrist flexor muscles and the pronator teres and pronator quadratus.

Ulnar Nerve

The ulnar nerve enters the elbow by traveling around the posterior portion of the medial epicondyle. After superficially crossing the joint line it courses deep to follow the ulnar artery to the middle of the forearm. At this point it moves lateral to the flexor carpi ulnaris tendon and crosses the wrist joint superficial to the flexor retinaculum. The ulnar nerve innervates the flexor carpi ulnaris muscle and the medial portion of the flexor digitorum profundus.

Radial Nerve

Crossing the lateral aspect of the elbow's joint line between the brachioradialis and brachialis muscles, the radial nerve soon diverges into two branches. The **superficial branch** is the direct continuation of the radial nerve and provides sensation to the dorsum of the wrist, hand, and thumb (see Fig. 12-8). The **deep branch** provides entirely muscular innervation, including the extensor carpi radialis brevis, the supinator, and the extensor digitorum muscle. Therefore, it is possible to sever the deep branch of the radial nerve and not experience any sensory loss.

Bursae

Several bursae are found in the elbow region, but few have clinical significance. Commonly injured in athletics is the **subcutaneous olecranon bursa** that

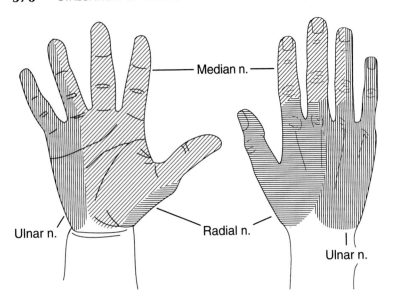

Figure 12–8. The median, ulnar, and radial nerve sensory distribution in the hand. Note that texts differ on the exact delineation between the cutaneous areas serviced by the individual nerves.

is located between the olecranon and the skin. This bursa is usually injured following a direct blow to the olecranon. The other significant bursa is the **subtendinous olecranon bursa**. This structure is located between the tendon of triceps brachii and the olecranon and may become inflamed secondary to repetitive stresses applied to the joint.

CLINICAL EVALUATION OF THE ELBOW AND FOREARM

The elbow may be directly traumatized by valgus or varus forces, forced hyperextension, or direct blows to the olecranon process or the epicondyles. More commonly, however, the elbow is injured secondary to overuse from the inherently unnatural motion of throwing. The stresses placed on the elbow are increased when improper technique is used or the athlete is compensating for shoulder pain by altering elbow motion. An overview of the evaluation of elbow and forearm injuries is presented in Table 12–2.

History

The onset and location of the athlete's symptoms are among the most important facts surrounding elbow trauma. Determining the cause-and-effect relationship between the mechanism and onset of injury and the athlete's symptoms is helpful in the successful treatment of the athlete's condition.

The elbow may be the site of referred pain from the cervical spine, shoulder, or hand. The examiner must be thorough in ruling out sources of pain other than the elbow itself. The clinician should derive the following information from the history-taking process in an attempt to ascertain the mechanism leading to the injury, the structures involved in the injury, and the nature of the pain.

- **Location of the symptoms:** The examiner should begin the examination by localizing the area of pain, the type of pain, and any dysfunction noted by the athlete, remembering the possibility of these symptoms being referred by trauma that is proximal or distal to the elbow (Table 12–3). Referred pain usually presents itself through symptoms localized within the distribution of a specific nerve or nerve root.

- **Onset of the symptoms:** Elbow pain may have an acute or chronic onset. The athlete with traumatic injury is usually capable of noting the specific onset of their pain. Chronic conditions of the elbow may initially produce minor symptoms related to activity but these symptoms can rapidly progress to constant pain.

- **Mechanism of injury:** The elbow is well protected at the side of the body and is not subjected to an overburden of harmful stress. The elbow can be acutely injured as the athlete generates a high amount of stress while throwing or while lifting weights. The elbow can also be acutely injured if the hand is planted on the playing surface and forces are transmitted across the joint.

Most elbow injuries tend to be caused by repetitive low-load stresses. Throwing a ball or using a racquet can cause stresses that are capable of resulting in tendinitis or neuritis in the elbow. Adolescent athletes are vulnerable to repetitive stress-type injuries at open growth plates as stresses are transmitted across these areas. If the athlete is a pitcher, the level of activity, including the number of innings pitched and the total number of pitches, assists in determining the potential of overuse.

Table 12–2. Evaluation of the Elbow and Forearm

History	Inspection	Palpation	Functional Tests	Ligamentous Tests	Neurological Tests	Special Tests
Location of the pain	Anterior Structures	Anterior Structures	Active Range of Motion	Valgus stress test	Radial nerve	Elbow sprains
Onset of the symptoms	Carrying angle	Biceps brachii	Flexion	Varus stress test	Medial nerve	Ulnar collateral ligament
Mechanism of injury	Cubital fossa	Cubital fossa	Extension		Ulnar nerve	Posterolateral rotatory instability test
Technique	Swelling	Medial Structures	Pronation			Radial collateral ligament
Associated sounds	Medial Structures	Medial epicondyle	Supination			Epicondylitis
Associated sensations	Flexor muscle mass	Ulna	Passive Range of Motion			Lateral epicondylitis tennis elbow test
Previous history	Lateral Structures	Ulnar collateral ligament	Flexion			Medial epicondylitis
General medical health	Alignment	Wrist flexor group	Extension			Nerve trauma
	Cubital recurvatum	Lateral Structures	Pronation			Tinel's sign
	Extensor muscle mass	Lateral epicondyle	Supination			Forearm compartment syndrome
	Posterior Structures	Radial head	Resisted Range of Motion			
	Bony alignment	Capitulum	Flexion			
	Olecranon process and bursa	Radial collateral ligament	Extension			
		Annular ligament	Pronation			
		Brachioradialis	Supination			
		Wrist extensors				
		Posterior Structures				
		Olecranon process				
		Olecranon fossa				
		Olecranon bursa				
		Ulnar nerve				
		Triceps brachii				

Table 12–3. Possible Trauma Based on the Location of Pain

	Location of Pain			
	Lateral	**Anterior**	**Medial**	**Posterior**
Soft tissue	Annular ligament sprain Radial collateral ligament sprain Radiocapitular chondromalacia Lateral epicondylitis (tennis elbow) Radial nerve trauma	Biceps brachii tendinitis Median nerve trauma Soft tissue sprain (hyperextension)	Ulnar collateral ligament sprain Medial epicondylitis Ulnar nerve trauma	Olecranon bursitis Triceps brachii tendinitis
Bony	Avulsion of the common extensor tendon Lateral epicondyle fracture Ulnar fracture	Osteochondral fracture	Avulsion of the common flexor tendon Medial epicondyle fracture Radius fracture	Fracture of the olecranon process

• **Technique:** Overuse injuries should lead the examiner to suspect improper technique or poor biomechanics at the athlete's elbow. The athlete should be questioned regarding changes in technique or increases in the intensity or duration of play. Questions raised during the history-taking process regarding the athlete's biomechanics may necessitate that the examiner work with the athlete and coach in further evaluating technique and making corrections as needed.

• **Associated sound and sensations:** An elbow that chronically locks, clicks, or pops during movement may have loose bodies within the joint. The presence of these structures may be confirmed through palpation or diagnostic imaging.

• **Previous history:** Many times the athlete reports symptoms similar to those of previous elbow pain. Pain that is associated with seasonal activity may be related to poor conditioning at the season's onset.

Athletes suspected of having referred pain from the cervical spine should be asked about a history of previous trauma or dysfunction in this area.

• **General medical health:** The athlete should be questioned regarding other medical conditions. Certain vascular problems, neurological involvement, or diseases may predispose the elbow to inflammatory or degenerative injuries or illnesses.

Inspection

The upper arm, elbow, and forearm should be inspected for the presence of contusions, ecchymosis, scars, and swelling. These conditions can place pressure on the radial, median, and ulnar nerves, radiating symptoms into the forearm and hand.

Inspection of the Anterior Structures

• **Carrying angle:** The angle formed by the long axis of the humerus and ulna, the carrying angle, ranges from 10 to 15 degrees of valgus in men and is slightly greater in women. Normally this angle is reduced or entirely eliminated during flexion.[1] The examiner should note the presence of an increased carrying angle, cubitus valgus, or a decreased angle, cubitus varus (Fig. 12–9). Baseball pitchers may exhibit cubitus valgus in the throwing arm, an adaptation to repeated valgus loading during the throwing motion.[2] Other deviations of this angle may reflect a fracture of one or more bones or their epiphyseal plates.

• **Cubital fossa:** The cubital fossa is a triangular area demarcated by the brachioradialis muscle laterally and the pronator teres medially. The proximal border is formed by an imaginary line connecting the medial and lateral epicondyle. Swelling can place pressure on the neurovascular structures passing though the fossa (Fig. 12–10).

• **Swelling:** Observing from the anterior aspect, the examiner can compare the joints bilaterally. Gross swelling often leads to deformity on the lateral and/or medial sides of the elbow and should lead the examiner to suspect a severe injury such as ligamentous rupture, acute tendinitis, or an avulsion fracture.

Inspection of the Medial Structures

• **Flexor muscle mass:** The wrist flexor muscle mass is observable along the medial aspect of the elbow and forearm. The mass widens approximately 2 to 3 inches below the elbow. Loss of girth along the medial forearm can occur secondary to prolonged immobilization or from disuse associated with long-term tendinitis.

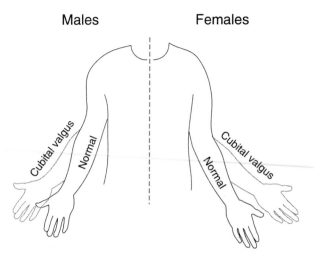

Males   Females

Figure 12–9. Angular relationships at the elbow. On average, women have an increased angle between the midline of the forearm and the humerus (the "carrying angle") relative to men. Longtime participation in overhand throwing sports increases this angle.

Inspection of the Lateral Structures

• **Alignment of the wrist and forearm:** The wrist should be centered on the forearm. Compression of the radial nerve as it crosses the elbow joint can inhibit innervation of the wrist extensors, resulting in **drop wrist syndrome.**[3]

• **Cubital recurvatum:** The alignment of the forearm and humerus when the elbow is fully extended should be noted. This is normally a straight line, but extension beyond 0 degrees (cubital recurvatum) is common, especially in female athletes (Fig. 12–11).

• **Extensor muscle mass:** The wrist extensor muscle mass is observable along the lateral aspect of

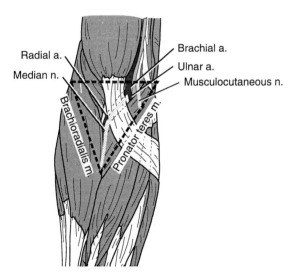

Figure 12–10. Cubital fossa. Passing through this area are the brachial artery and its two subdivisions (the radial and ulnar arteries), the median nerve, and the musculocutaneous nerve.

the elbow and forearm. The mass widens approximately 1 to 2 inches below the elbow. Loss of girth along the lateral forearm can occur secondary to prolonged immobilization or disuse following long-term tendinitis.

Inspection of the Posterior Structures

• **Bony alignment:** When the elbow is flexed to 90 degrees, the medial epicondyle, lateral epicondyle, and olecranon process form an isosceles triangle. When the elbow is extended, these structures should lie within a straight line. Deviation from this alignment may reflect bony pathology.

• **Olecranon process and bursa:** Flexion of the elbow makes the bony contour of the olecranon process visible. Acute injury or overuse conditions may cause the olecranon bursa to rupture, swell, or inflame, masking the outline of the olecranon (Fig. 12–12).

Palpation

Many of the structures of the upper extremity insert or originate at the elbow, making careful, precise palpation a must for the examiner. Tenderness elicited with palpation must be correlated with other subjective and physical findings. Some areas, like the humeral condyles, may be tender in the uninjured elbow.

Palpation of the Anterior Bony Structures

The muscle mass over the anterior portion of the elbow precludes the bony palpation of these structures.

Palpation of the Anterior Musculature and Related Soft Tissue

• **Biceps brachii:** The muscle belly of the biceps brachii is palpated along the anterior aspect of the humerus. The muscle should be palpated along its length until its tendon inserts into the radius. The distal biceps brachii tendon can be ruptured with a forceful eccentric contraction, resulting in obvious deformity of the muscle (Fig. 12–13).

• **Cubital fossa:** Passing within the cubital fossa, the brachial artery and median nerve can be palpated medial to the biceps brachii tendon. The musculocutaneous nerve also passes through this area but it cannot be palpated as it runs underneath the pronator teres muscle (see Fig. 12–10).

Palpation of the Medial Bony Structures

• **Medial epicondyle:** The medial epicondyle is prominent along the distal aspect of the humerus as it flares away from the shaft of the bone. The

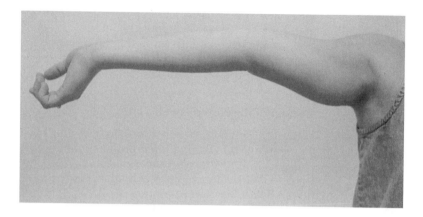

Figure 12–11. Cubital recurvatum. A normal hyperextension of the elbow.

common wrist flexor tendon attaches at the epicondyle; palpation of the epicondyle elicits exquisite tenderness in the presence of medial epicondylitis.

- **Ulna:** The base of the ulna can be located distal to the elbow's medial joint space. The shaft is prominent throughout its length, especially along its medial and posterior (dorsal) surfaces. The anterior aspect of the shaft can be palpated along the distal two-thirds of its length as it arises from beneath the mass of the wrist flexors to its point of articulation with the wrist.

Palpation of the Medial Musculature and Related Soft Tissue

- **Ulnar collateral ligament:** For better identification of the UCL, the elbow should be flexed between 20 and 30 degrees. The anterior oblique ligament can be directly palpated as it crosses the angle formed by the humerus and ulna.

- **Wrist flexor group:** Near their origin on the medial epicondyle, the bellies of the wrist flexors cannot be distinguished from one another. Hoppenfeld[4] describes a technique to approximate the individual wrist flexors and the pronator teres (Fig. 12–14). Their individual tendons become identifiable as they near the wrist.

Palpation of the Lateral Bony Structures

- **Lateral epicondyle:** Smaller than the medial epicondyle, the lateral epicondyle is prominent as it projects from the distal end of the humerus. This structure should be palpated for tenderness caused by inflammation of the common origin of the wrist extensors or the epicondyle itself.

- **Radial head:** The examiner should move slightly distal from the lateral joint line to locate the base of the radius. This structure is palpable underneath the posterior aspect of the wrist extensor muscles and becomes more identifiable as it rolls beneath the examiner's finger as the forearm is pronated and supinated. During flexion and extension of the elbow the radial head moves with the forearm.

- **Capitulum:** The examiner moves proximally from the radial head, across the joint line, to find the rounded capitulum. While passively pronat-

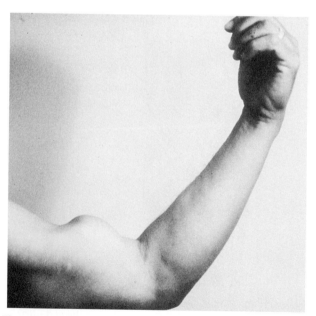

Figure 12–13. Rupture of the biceps brachii muscle. The athlete is still able to actively flex the elbow, but supination strength is markedly decreased.

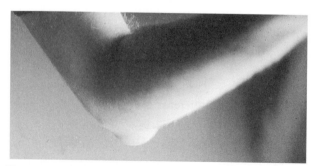

Figure 12–12. Inflammation of the subcutaneous olecranon bursa. This structure is often traumatized by a direct blow to the olecranon process.

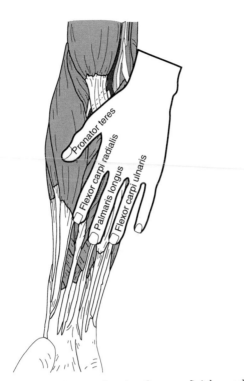

Figure 12–14. Method of approximating the superficial muscles of the flexor forearm. (Adapted from Hoppenfeld,[4] p 44.)

ing and supinating the forearm with the elbow bent to various degrees of flexion, the capitulum and radial head are palpated for the presence of crepitus indicating radiocapitular chondromalacia.[5]

Palpation of the Lateral Musculature and Related Soft Tissue

- **Radial collateral ligament:** The RCL is located between the radial head and the capitulum. Although the RCL is not normally identifiable, its length should be palpated for signs of tenderness.

- **Annular ligament:** This structure cannot be identified during palpation, but the area overlying the radial head should be palpated for the presence of tenderness, crepitus, or swelling.

- **Brachioradialis:** The most anterior of the elbow flexor muscles, the brachioradialis is made prominent by the athlete's resisting elbow flexion while the forearm is held in the neutral position (Fig. 12–15).

- **Wrist extensors:** Resisting wrist extension makes the extensor carpi radialis longus and brevis muscles become prominent. With the forearm pronated, the wrist extensors can be palpated distal to the lateral epicondyle. The superficial muscle is the extensor carpi radialis longus; the inferior, the extensor carpi radialis brevis.

Palpation of the Posterior Bony Structures

- **Olecranon process:** The ulna's olecranon process is the prominent rounded bone on the posterior aspect of the elbow. This structure should be palpated for tenderness or mobility relative to the length of the ulna. A forced hyperextension of the elbow may cause a fracture.

- **Olecranon fossa:** With the athlete's elbow partially flexed and the triceps muscle relaxed, the examiner can palpate the olecranon fossa.

Palpation of the Posterior Musculature and Related Soft Tissue

- **Olecranon bursa:** The olecranon's superficial bursa is not palpable unless it is inflamed. Inflammation of this structure can result in a large amount of swelling and tenderness.

- **Ulnar nerve:** With the elbow in full extension, the examiner palpates the sulcus formed by the medial epicondyle and the medial border of the olecranon process for the ulnar nerve, identifiable as a thin, cordlike structure. The examiner must determine if this nerve can be displaced from the sulcus by gently moving it medially and laterally. Inflammation of the nerve may result in Tinel's sign—burning, pain, or paresthesia along the medial border of the forearm and little finger—during palpation.

- **Triceps brachii:** Slightly flexing the elbow makes the fibers of the triceps tendon brachii stand out from their attachment on the olecranon. The posterolateral portion of this muscle is formed by the lateral head of the triceps and the posteromedial portion by the long head. The medial head runs deep to the long head but becomes palpable over the medial aspect of the distal humerus. The length of the triceps brachii should be palpated for tenderness or deformity.

Functional Testing

The motions at the elbow joint are limited to flexion/extension and pronation/supination. If epicondylitis or trauma to the ulnar, median, or radial nerve is suspected, range of motion testing of the wrist and fingers should be incorporated.

Active Range of Motion (Fig. 12–16)

- **Flexion and extension:** The vast majority of the elbow's range of motion is composed of flexion, ranging between 145 to 155 degrees from the neutral position and occurring in the sagittal plane around a coronal axis. Extension is usually limited at 0 degrees by the olecranon process, but hyperextension is common (see Fig. 12–11).

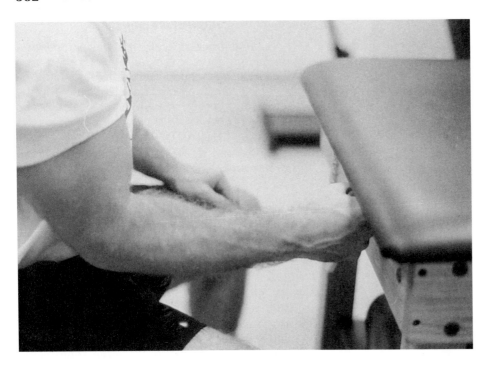

Figure 12–15. Making the brachioradialis more prominent. An isometric contraction with the forearm in the neutral position and the elbow flexed to 90° causes the brachioradialis to become prominent.

• **Pronation and supination**: The neutral position for forearm pronation and supination is the thumb and radius pointing upward. The total range of motion is 170 to 180 degrees, with approximately 90 degrees of motion in each direction. This movement occurs in the transverse plane around the longitudinal axis when the subject is in the anatomical position.

Passive Range of Motion (Fig. 12–17)

• **Flexion and extension**: To passively move the forearm, the elbow is positioned in extension with the forearm supinated and the shoulder joint stabilized to prevent compensatory motion. Soft tissue approximation between the bulk of the bi-

ceps brachii muscle and the muscles of the anterior forearm limit elbow flexion. Extension is limited by the bony contact between the olecranon process and the olecranon fossa of the humerus.

• **Pronation and supination**: The examiner should position the shoulder in the neutral position and flex the elbow to 90 degrees. The forearm should be supported so that the radius and thumb are pointing upward and the elbow is supported against the torso to prevent shoulder motion. During pronation the end-feel may be hard as the radius and ulna contact each other or firm secondary to stretching of distal radioulnar ligaments and the interosseous membrane. Supination normally meets with a firm end-feel caused by the stretching of the distal radioulnar ligament and the interosseous membrane.

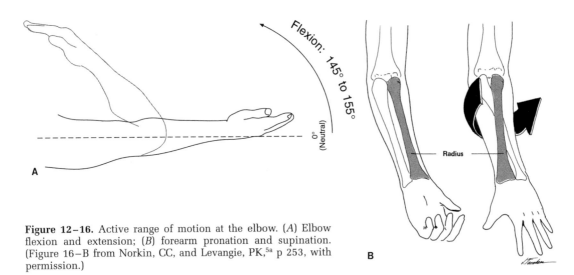

Figure 12–16. Active range of motion at the elbow. (*A*) Elbow flexion and extension; (*B*) forearm pronation and supination. (Figure 16–B from Norkin, CC, and Levangie, PK,[5a] p 253, with permission.)

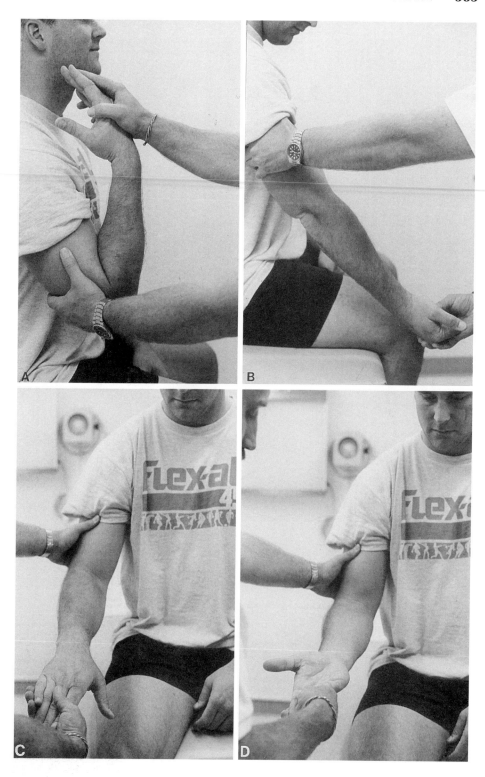

Figure 12–17. Passive range of motion for (A and B) flexion and extension and (C and D) pronation and supination.

Resisted Range of Motion (Fig. 12–18)

- **Flexion and extension**: With the athlete sitting or standing, the examiner positions the shoulder in the neutral position. To better isolate the biceps brachii, the forearm is supinated; for the brachioradialis, the forearm is placed in the neutral position; and for the brachialis the forearm is pronated. The examiner stabilizes the anterior humerus, being careful not to compress the involved muscles. Resistance is applied over the distal forearm.

- **Pronation and supination**: With the athlete sitting, the examiner places the shoulder in the neutral position and the lateral radial border pointing

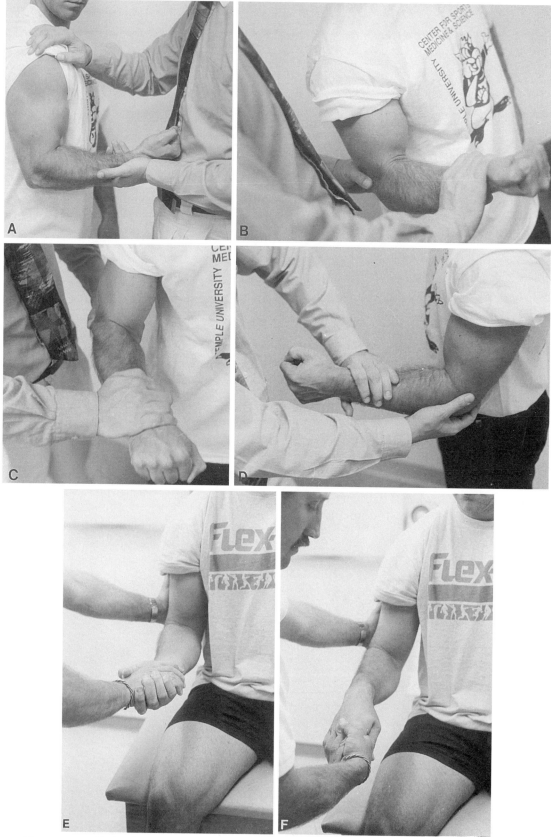

Figure 12–18. Resisted range of motion for (*A*) elbow extension and flexion isolating the (*B*) biceps brachii, (*C*) brachialis, and (*D*) the brachioradialis. (*E* and *F*) Resisted forearm supination and pronation.

upward. Stabilization occurs over the elbow to ensure that shoulder abduction or adduction does not assist in the movement. Resistance may be provided with a hand-shake grip or may be applied to the palmar surface of the forearm during pronation and on the dorsal surface during supination.

Even injured athletes are capable of overpowering the clinician during this test. An alternative method of resisting pronation and supination is through the use of a 1-inch diameter dowel. The athlete grasps the middle of the dowel as if holding a baseball bat. The examiner then applies resistance to both ends of the dowel as the athlete pronates and supinates the forearm.

Ligamentous Testing

Single plane instability of the elbow joint can be tested only in the frontal plane when the joint is not fully extended. Valgus and varus stress testing of the fully extended elbow is meaningless because the olecranon process is securely locked within its humeral fossa.

Test for Medial Ligament Instability

The anterior oblique portion of the UCL is the primary restraint of the medial elbow against valgus stress. Trauma to this structure displays valgus laxity throughout the range of motion, and injury to the other medial ligaments is unlikely without first damaging the anterior oblique portion of the UCL (Fig. 12–19).

Valgus Stress Test (Fig.12–19)

Position of athlete	Standing or sitting. The athlete's elbow is flexed to 25°.
Position of examiner	Standing lateral to the joint being tested. One hand supports the lateral elbow with the fingers reaching behind the joint to palpate the medial joint line. The opposite hand grasps the distal forearm.
Evaluative procedure	A valgus force is applied to the joint. The procedure is repeated with the elbow in various degrees of flexion.
Positive test results	Increased laxity compared with the opposite side, or pain.
Implications	Sprain of the ulnar collateral ligament, especially the anterior oblique portion. Laxity beyond 60° of flexion also implicates involvement of the posterior oblique fibers.

Test for Lateral Ligament Instability

Straight plane varus instability of the elbow occurs when the RCL is damaged. Involvement of the annular ligament, ALCL, or LUCL increases the instability by allowing the radial head to separate from the ulna. The integrity of these structures is determined through varus stress tests (Fig. 12–20).

Varus Stress Test (Fig. 12–20)

Position of athlete	Standing or sitting. The elbow is flexed to 15°.
Position of examiner	Standing medial to the joint being tested. One hand supports the medial elbow with the fingers reaching behind the joint to palpate the lateral joint line. The opposite hand grasps the distal forearm.
Evaluative procedure	A varus force is applied to the elbow. This process is repeated with the joint in various degrees of flexion.
Positive test results	Increased laxity compared with the opposite side, or the athlete describes pain.
Implications	Moderate laxity reflects trauma to the radial collateral ligament. Gross laxity may also indicate damage to the annular or accessory lateral collateral ligament, causing the radius to displace from the ulna.

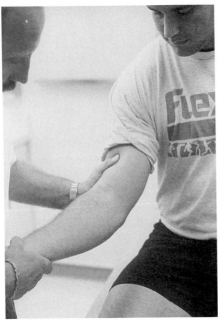

Figure 12–19. Valgus stress testing of the ulnar collateral ligament complex.

Neurological Testing

The innervation of the brachial plexus continues from the shoulder into the elbow, forearm, and hand. Nerve impingement occurring in the cervical or shoulder region results in disruption of the sensory and/or motor function in the elbow and forearm. Likewise, nerve trauma in the elbow refers its symptoms into the wrist, hand, and fingers. (see Neurological Screen on page 387).

Pathologies and Related Special Tests

This section discusses the evaluation of acute and chronic elbow injuries. The number of special tests for the elbow is relatively limited compared with the other joints described in this text. The conclusion of specific injuries is based on the correlation between the athlete's history of injury and examination findings.

Elbow Sprains

Because the elbow is stabilized by the locking of the olecranon process in its fossa when the joint is extended, strain is placed on the ligaments when the elbow is flexed. A valgus or varus blow delivered to a flexed elbow is dissipated by one of the collateral ligaments. As with knee injuries, the trauma to involved structures becomes more complex when a rotational component is added to the stress. When a valgus or varus force is placed on an extended elbow, the olecranon process should be evaluated for injury as well as the collateral ligament.

Ulnar Collateral Ligament

The ulnar collateral ligament is stressed secondary to a valgus loading of the humeroulnar joint. Acutely, this stress results from a force delivered to the lateral elbow. Valgus loading of the UCL also normally occurs during normal athletic movements but is especially great during the overhand pitching motion. The force load generated during this motion is so great that the UCL cannot tolerate the tension on its own and must rely on the triceps brachii, the wrist flexor-pronator muscles, and the anconeus to provide dynamic stabilization of this joint.[6]

The athlete complains of pain on the medial aspect of the elbow that is intensified with motion. Depending on the severity of the injury, swelling may be present on the anterior, medial, and posterior borders of the joint. The anterior oblique section is traumatized in most UCL sprains and its length from the medial epicondyle to the coronoid process is tender. If the elbow is flexed past 60 degrees, the posterior oblique band may be painful as well. Range of motion testing may reveal pain secondary to stretching of the ligaments or from joint instability. Valgus stress testing demonstrates laxity at various degrees of flexion (Table 12–4). Because of the relationship of the ulnar nerve to the medial elbow, a neurological examination of the forearm, wrist, hand, and fingers may also be required.

Tears of the lateral ulnar collateral ligament permit a transient rotatory subluxation of the humero-

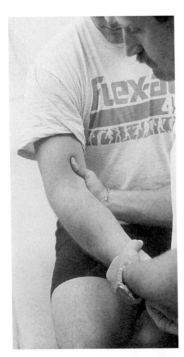

Figure 12–20. Varus stress testing of the radial collateral ligament.

Neurological Screen

Nerve Root Level	Sensory Testing	Motor Testing	Reflex Testing
C6	Musculocutaneous n.	Musculocutaneous n. (C5 & C6)	Brachioradialis
C7	Radial n.	Radial n.	Triceps brachii
C8	Ulnar n. (mixed)	Radial n.	None
T1	Med. brachial cutaneous n.	Med. brachial cutaneous n.	None

ulnar joint and an associated subluxation of the radiohumeral joint.[7] This results in the radius and ulna acting as a single unit as they rock away from the articulating surfaces of the humerus. Clinically, this condition can be evaluated through the posterolateral rotatory-instability test.

Posterolateral Rotatory-Instability Test of the Elbow
This evaluative technique is used to determine the presence of humeroulnar and humeroradial subluxa-

tion that occurs during elbow flexion (Fig. 12–21).[8] A positive test result causes visible and palpable reduction of these joints (see top of page 388).

Radial Collateral Ligament

Injury to the RCL complex is relatively rare, especially compared with its medial counterpart. This is largely based on the fact that in most positions the body shields the elbow from varus forces. Additionally, the stresses placed on the elbow joint during

Posterolateral Rotatory-Instability Test (Fig. 12–21)

Position of athlete	Lying supine. The elbow is extended and the forearm is pronated.
Position of examiner	Standing at the side of the athlete. One hand grasps the distal forearm while the other palpates the radiohumeral and ulnohumeral joints by cupping the elbow medially.
Evaluative procedure	The examiner flexes and supinates the forearm and administers an axial load on the forearm while applying a valgus force on the elbow.
Positive test results	Palpable and visible reduction of the humeroulnar and humeroradial joints.
Implications	Tear of the lateral ulnar collateral ligament of the elbow.

Table 12–4. Evaluative Findings of an Ulnar Collateral Ligament Sprain

Examination Segment	Clinical Findings
History	Onset: Acute or insidious. Location of pain: Medial aspect of elbow. Mechanism: Acute: Valgus stress placed on the ulnar collateral ligament. Insidious: Repeated valgus loading of the medial elbow (e.g., the overhand pitching motion).
Inspection	Swelling may be present in the anterior, medial, and posterior aspects of the elbow.
Palpation	Palpation of the medial elbow, from the medial epicondyle to the coronoid process, may elicit tenderness and crepitus.
Functional tests	AROM: This is limited owing to stretching of the ligaments or joint instability. PROM: Pain is elicited by stretching of the ligaments. RROM: Strength is decreased secondary to pain and joint instability.
Ligamentous tests	Valgus stress testing of the elbow in various degrees of flexion (e.g., 25°, 45°, 60°, 90°).
Neurological tests	Sensory and motor testing of the ulnar nerve distribution.
Special tests	Posterolateral rotatory instability test of the elbow.

throwing and racquet sports are absorbed by the UCL and the wrist extensor muscles.

Varus forces placed on the lateral elbow ligaments can result in trauma to the RCL and, possibly, the annular ligament. Trauma to this ligament or its component parts (see Fig. 12–4) not only results in varus laxity, but also may disrupt the articulation between the radial head and the capitulum. The signs and symptoms of RCL sprains are similar to those of UCL trauma but may be compounded by pain, laxity, or weakness during pronation and supination.

Epicondylitis

Both the lateral and medial epicondyles serve as the origin for many of the muscles acting on the wrist and fingers. The relatively small area in which these muscles attach to the epicondyles results in a large amount of force being applied to a small area. The most common ailment afflicting the epicondyles is inflammation of the periosteum and the as-

sociated muscles. Prolonged stress loads may result in stress or avulsion fractures.

Lateral Epicondylitis

Inflammation of the lateral epicondyle irritates the common attachment of the wrist extensor group leading to inflammation of these structures. Although any or all of these muscles' functions may be inhibited, the extensor carpi radialis brevis is the most predisposed. Repeated, forceful contractions of the wrist extensor muscles result in the accumulation of degenerative forces at their attachment site. The relatively small area of attachment for these muscles causes a great force load to be applied to the bone as these muscles contract.

Lateral epicondylitis is prevalent in racquet sports, affecting more than half of all regular tennis players,[9] leading to its colloquial name, "**tennis elbow.**" Most common in individuals over 40 years old, the chief complaint is pain over the lateral epicondyle and decreased grip strength. In racquet sports the

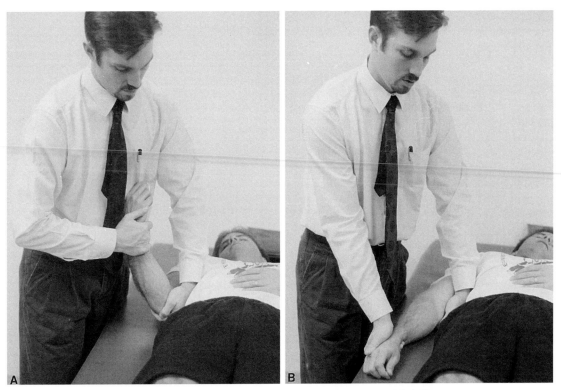

Figure 12–21. Test for posterolateral rotatory instability of the elbow.

symptoms are increased during backhand strokes. Inspection of the painful area may reveal swelling, and palpation of the area is painful to the athlete. Active wrist extension results in pain that is worsened when this motion is resisted. Pain elicited during passive stretching of the extensor muscles and resisted finger extension has also been demon-strated to be a reliable indicator of this condition.[10] The **tennis elbow test** is sensitive to even mild cases of lateral epicondylitis (Table 12–5).

Tennis Elbow Test

Pain associated with lateral epicondylitis may be reproduced during palpation of involved structures

Test for Tennis Elbow (Fig. 12–22)

Position of athlete	Seated with the tested elbow flexed to 90°, the forearm pronated, and the fingers flexed.
Position of examiner	Standing lateral to the athlete. One hand is positioned over the dorsal aspect of the wrist and hand.
Evaluative procedure	The examiner resists wrist extension while palpating the lateral epicondyle and common attachment of the wrist extensors.
Positive tests	Pain in the lateral epicondyle.
Implications	Lateral epicondylitis (tennis elbow).

and during resisted wrist extension. The tennis elbow test combines these two facets of the evaluation into a single step (Fig. 12–22).

Medial Epicondylitis

Activities involving the swift, powerful snapping of the wrist and pronation of the forearm load the medial epicondyle. As with its lateral counterpart, medial epicondylitis involves point tenderness at the site of the muscle's attachment. The length of the pronator teres muscle may be tender as well (Table 12–6). In young baseball pitchers, the tension build-up in the medial epicondyle may result in the common tendon being avulsed from its attachment site, "**little leaguer's elbow**" (Fig. 12–23).

Table 12–5. Evaluative Findings of Lateral Epicondylitis

Examination Segment	Clinical Findings
History	Onset: Insidious. Location of pain: Lateral epicondyle and proximal portion of the common tendons of the wrist extensors. Mechanism: Overuse syndrome involving repeated, forceful wrist extension.
Inspection	Swelling may be present over the lateral epicondyle.
Palpation	Pain and possible crepitus over the lateral epicondyle and proximal portion of the common wrist extensor tendon.
Functional tests	AROM: There is pain with combined wrist extension and elbow flexion. PROM: Pain occurs during passive wrist flexion when the elbow is extended. RROM: Pain occurs with resisted wrist extension and with resisted finger extension when the elbow is extended.
Ligamentous tests	Not applicable.
Neurological tests	Not applicable.
Special tests	Tennis elbow test.
Comments	In racquet sports, pain is worsened with the backhand stroke and may be related to improper size of the handle or a too tightly strung racquet.

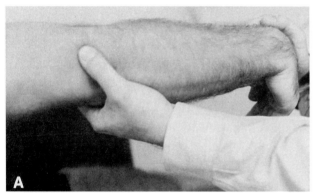

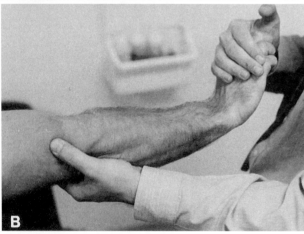

Figure 12–22. Tests for tennis elbow. (*A*) Lateral epicondyle is palpated while the wrist is passively flexed. (*B*) Lateral epicondyle is palpated while the examiner resists wrist extension.

Nerve Trauma

The superficial location of the ulnar nerve and the tunnels through which the radial and median nerves pass can result in traumatic or insidious impediment of their functions. Inhibition of these nerves in the area of the elbow radiates their symptoms distally and result in dysfunction in the wrist, hand, and fingers characterized by paresthesia, decreased grip strength, and the inability to actively extend the wrist.

As the **ulnar nerve** crosses the medial aspect of the elbow's joint line, it is relatively superficial, predisposing it to concussive forces. If the nerve's supporting structures are unstable, the nerve may chronically subluxate as the forearm is flexed, resulting in a progressive inflammation. A decrease in the cross-sectional size of the cubital tunnel can compress the ulnar nerve.[11]

Impairment of the ulnar nerve manifests its symptoms through decreased sensory and motor function in the hand and fingers. Acute trauma of the ulnar nerve causes a burning sensation in the little finger and ring finger and decreased function of their flexor muscles and the flexor carpi ulnaris. Chronic neurological deficit to these muscles causes the hand to radially deviate during flexion and inhibits the ability to make a fist because of a lack of flexion in the fourth and fifth DIP joints, characterized by a ***clawhand*** position.

The **radial nerve** is most often injured by deep lacerations of the elbow or secondary to fractures of the radius. The deep branch of the radial nerve is dedicated to motor function of the thumb's extensors and

Clawhand: Hand positioning characterized by hyperextension of the proximal phalanges and flexion of the middle and distal phalanges resulting from trauma to the median and ulnar nerves.

Table 12–6. Evaluative Findings of Medial Epicondylitis

Examination Segment	Clinical Findings
History	Onset: Insidious. Location of pain: Medial epicondyle and the proximal portion of the adjacent wrist flexor and pronator muscles. Mechanism: Repeated, forceful flexion and/or pronation of the wrist.
Inspection	The area over the medial epicondyle is swollen.
Palpation	Point tenderness and crepitus are found over the medial epicondyle. The proximal portion of the wrist flexor group, especially the pronator teres, is tender.
Functional tests	AROM: Pain occurs during wrist flexion; wrist extension may result in pain secondary to stretching the involved muscles. PROM: Pain occurs during wrist extension. RROM: Strength is decreased and pain occurs during wrist flexion.
Ligamentous tests	Not applicable.
Neurological tests	Neurological check of the ulnar nerve distribution.
Special tests	None.
Comments	Prolonged epicondylitis can result in calcification of the involved structures.

flexors of the metacarpophalangeal (MCP) joints; there is no sensory loss associated with trauma to this nerve segment. If the superficial branch is lacerated there is sensory loss on the posterior forearm and hand. Inflammation or irritation of the ulnar and radial nerves as they cross the elbow joint can be detected through Tinel's sign (Fig. 12–24).

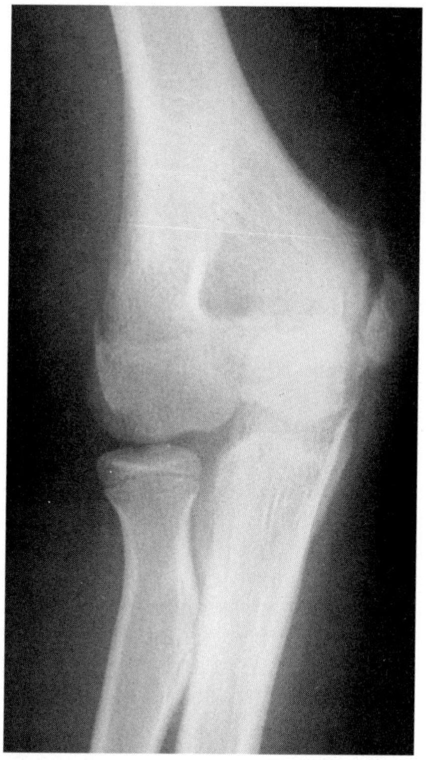

Entrapment of the radial nerve, **radial tunnel syndrome (RTS)**, clinically resembles lateral epicondylitis. Radial tunnel syndrome differs from epicondylitis in that the symptoms of RTS persist for more than 6 months with tenderness over the radial tunnel, and the symptoms are reproduced with resisted supination and during resisted extension of the middle finger.[12]

The **median nerve** is typically injured or compressed on the distal portion of the forearm. However, pressure in the cubital fossa can compress the nerve as it crosses the joint line. The most common clinical manifestation of median nerve trauma, **carpal tunnel syndrome,** is discussed in the following chapter.

Figure 12–23. Avulsion of the origin of the wrist flexor muscles, "little leaguer's elbow." This condition can mimic medial epicondylitis.

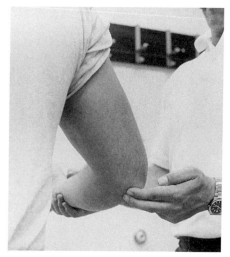

Figure 12–24. Tinel's sign for radial neuropathy. In the presence of neuropathy, tapping on the ulnar (shown) or radial nerve results in a burning sensation in the hand.

Forearm Compartment Syndrome

Similar to the compartmental syndromes discussed in the lower leg, the forearm, being a compartmentalized structure, carries the risk of inflamed tissues compromising circulation to the hand. Although this condition is rare in athletics, it may be initiated by hypertrophic muscles, hemorrhage, or fractures. In its early stages, forearm compartment syndrome is marked by the athlete's complaint of pressure in the forearm, sensory disruption in the hand and fingers, decreased muscular strength, and pain during passive elongation of the involved muscles. As the condition becomes more chronic or increases in severity, a decrease or absence of the radial and/or ulnar pulse is noted.

ON-FIELD EVALUATION OF ELBOW AND FOREARM INJURIES

In most instances, acute injuries of the elbow do not require an on-field evaluation and subsequent management of the condition. The exceptions to this are elbow dislocations and fractures of the forearm. In these cases the athlete remains down on the playing surface.

Inspection

The primary tool in the evaluation of these conditions is inspection of the injured area. Elbow dislocation and forearm fractures both tend to result in gross deformity, but radial and/or ulnar fractures are inherently more noticeable.

- **Alignment of forearm and wrist:** The length of the radius and ulna is observed for any gross deformity and the relationship between the forearm and wrist noted. A complete fracture of either of the long bones alters the wrist's position relative to the forearm.

- **Posterior triangle of the elbow:** The alignment of the medial epicondyle, lateral epicondyle, and the olecranon process is noted. These structures should form an isosceles triangle; any deviation of this relationship is indicative of a dislocation. In the event of a posterior dislocation the olecranon process becomes overly prominent.

If either of these condition exist, the evaluation should be immediately terminated and the athlete referred to a physician following appropriate immobilization.

History

Once the possibility of a fracture or dislocation has been ruled out the examiner should establish the circumstances surrounding the injury:

- **Position of the arm:** When the hand is supporting the body weight, the arm is in a closed kinetic chain. Blows to the forearm, elbow, or humerus must be absorbed by the elbow's supportive structures.

- **Type of force involved:** The nature of the force delivered to the elbow should be ascertained. Landing on the palm of the hand delivers a longitudinal force up the radius that is transferred to the ulna by the interosseous membrane. A force to the lateral side of the elbow places stress on the UCL, and a medial force stresses the RCL. A force from the posterior aspect of the elbow results in hyperextension of the joint and places shear forces on the olecranon process. A blunt force places compressive forces on the tissues beneath the location of the impact.

Palpation

Palpation should be performed to confirm the suspicion of injury established during the history-taking process while also ruling out any other gross trauma.

- **Alignment of the elbow:** The medial epicondyle, lateral epicondyle, and olecranon are palpated for tenderness, crepitus, and improper alignment.

- **Collateral ligaments:** The RCL and UCL should be palpated along their lengths so as to identify any pain or crepitus along these structures. Crepitus at the ligament's origin or insertion can indicate an avulsion.

- **Radius and ulna:** The length of the radius and ulna are palpated for tenderness, deformity, or false joints indicative of a fracture.

Functional Tests

Before deciding whether to splint the arm or not, the athlete's willingness and ability to move the elbow should be established:

- **Active range of motion:** The athlete should first be asked to wiggle the fingers, move the wrist through flexion/extension and radial/ulnar deviation, and then through forearm pronation/supination and elbow flexion/extension. The inability to perform any one of these steps or significant pain with these motions warrants the immobilization of the elbow, forearm, and wrist before the athlete is removed from the field.

- **Passive range of motion:** After the athlete has displayed the ability to actively and willingly move the elbow, the examiner should passively move the joint through its ranges of motion. Osteochondral fractures cause a premature endpoint in the range of motion. Fractures of the olecranon process cause pain at the terminal range of extension.

• **Resistive range of motion:** Although this portion of the examination can be delayed until the athlete is removed to the sideline, the examiner may wish to establish a baseline strength for future comparison. Nerve root compression may result in a short-term loss of strength that rapidly returns to normal.

Neurological Screen

The immediate evaluation of elbow injuries may necessitate the neurological assessment of the forearm and hand. The reader should refer to the Neurological Testing section of this chapter and see Figure 12–8.

ON-FIELD MANAGEMENT OF ELBOW AND FOREARM INJURIES

The most significant injuries facing the athletic trainer during the on-field evaluation are dislocations of the elbow joint and fractures of the forearm (Fig. 12–25). These conditions must be carefully managed to prevent further trauma to the involved structures and to protect the neurovascular network to the hand.

Dislocations of the Elbow

The forces needed to dislocate the elbow are very high. Injuries of this magnitude cause extreme pain and perhaps *hysteria* in the athlete. The elbow must be immobilized in the position in which it is found, yet allowing for the distal pulse to be monitored. The athlete must be immediately transported for physician intervention.

Forearm Fractures

Fractures of the radius and/or ulna may compromise the neurovascular supply to the wrist and hand. Because of this, the presence of the distal pulses should be constantly monitored following the injury. At that time, the elbow, forearm, and wrist must be immobilized to minimize movement of the fractured bones. The athlete must be immediately transported once the area has been stabilized and the athlete treated for shock.

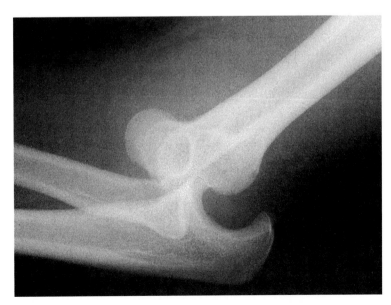

Figure 12–25. Posterior dislocation of the elbow. This condition results in obvious deformity of the joint. Note that the humeroulnar and humeroradial joints are involved.

Hysteria: An increased or heightened state of panic.

REFERENCES

1. Stroyan, M, and Wilk, KE: The functional anatomy of the elbow complex. Journal of Orthopedic and Sports Physical Therapy 17:279, 1993.
1a. Kendall, FP, and McCreary, EK: Muscles: Testing and Function, ed 3. Williams & Wilkins, Baltimore, 1983.
1b. Daniels, L, and Worthingham, C: Muscle Testing: Techniques of Manual Examination, ed 5. WB Saunders, Philadelphia, 1986.
2. King, JW, Brelsford, HJ, and Tullos, HS: Analysis of the pitching arm of the professional baseball pitcher. Clin Orthop 67:116, 1969.
3. Doughty, MP: Drop wrist: Complications following a comminuted fracture of the radius. Orthotic glove designed to permit participation. Athletic Training: Journal of the National Athletic Trainers Association 22:221, 1987.
4. Hoppenfeld, S: Physical examination of the elbow. In Hoppenfeld, S: Physical Examination of the Spine and Extremities. Appleton-Century-Crofts, New York, 1976, p 44.
5. Andrews, JR, et al: Physical examination of the thrower's elbow. Journal of Orthopedic and Sports Physical Therapy 17:269, 1993.
5a. Norkin, CC, and Levangie, PK: Joint Structure and Function: A Comprehensive Analysis, ed 2. FA Davis, Philadelphia, 1992.
6. Werner, SL, et al: Biomechanics of the elbow during baseball pitching. Journal of Orthopedic and Sports Physical Therapy 17:274, 1993.
7. Nestor, BJ, O'Driscoll, SW, and Morrey, BF: Ligamentous reconstruction for posterolateral rotatory instability of the elbow. J Bone Joint Surg Am 74:1235, 1992.
8. O'Driscoll, SW, Bell, DF, and Morrey, BF: Posterolateral rotatory instability of the elbow. J Bone Joint Surg Am 73:440, 1991.
8a. Fleisig, S, Dillman, CJ, and Andrews, JR: Biomechanics of the shoulder during throwing. In Andrews, JR, and Wilk, KE (eds): The Athlete's Shoulder. Churchill Livingstone, New York, 1994.
8b. Souza, TA: The shoulder in throwing sports. In Souza, TA (ed): Sports Injuries of the Shoulder. Churchill Livingstone, New York, 1994.
9. Sterling, JC, et al: Tennis elbow: A brief review of treatment. Athletic Training: Journal of the National Athletic Trainers Association, 23:316, 1988.
10. Haker, E: Lateral epicondylalgia: Diagnosis, treatment, and evaluation. Critical Reviews in Physical and Rehabilitation Medicine 5:129, 1993.
11. Barker, C: Evaluation, treatment, and rehabilitation involving a submuscular transposition of the ulnar nerve at the elbow. Athletic Training: Journal of the National Athletic Trainers Association 23:10, 1988.
12. Lutz, FR: Radial tunnel syndrome: An etiology of chronic lateral elbow pain. Journal of Orthopedic and Sports Physical Therapy 14:14, 1991.

13

The Wrist, Hand, and Fingers

In many types of athletic competition the wrist, hand, and fingers are the body areas most exposed to injury. The need to have unrestricted use of these body parts limits the amount of protective equipment that can be reasonably used by most athletes. The physical ramification of injury to this area stems from the gross and fine motor movements required not only for competition, but also for the activities of daily living.

The functional disability of these injuries is largely dependent on the athlete's sport, position, and the dominance of the injured hand. In football, a hand injury that has little consequence to a lineman could be disabling to a quarterback or wide receiver. In a sport such as basketball, injuries to the non-shooting hand have less consequence than those involving the shooting hand. The necessity for a thorough understanding of the anatomical relationship between the tendons, bones, and nerves and the possible ramifications of their injury cannot be understated.

CLINICAL ANATOMY

The distal portions of the radius and ulna, 8 carpal bones, 5 metacarpals, and 14 phalanges, form the skeleton of the wrist, hand, and fingers (Fig. 13–1). The **distal radius** broadens to form a small **ulnar notch** on its medial surface to accept the ulnar head, while the **radial styloid process** projects off its anterolateral border. The **ulnar head** is more circular, with the **ulnar styloid process** arising from its medial surface.

Having unusual shapes and irregular surfaces, the **carpal bones** are aligned in two rows (Fig. 13–2). From lateral to medial, the **proximal row** consists of the scaphoid (navicular), lunate, triquetrum, and the pisiform; the **distal row** is formed by the trapezium, trapezoid, capitate, and hamate. The pisiform "floats" on the triquetrum, acting as a sesamoid bone for the flexor carpi ulnaris, modifying its angle of pull. The scaphoid is the most commonly fractured of the carpals and the lunate is the most commonly dislocated.

Much of the length of the hand is formed by the **metacarpals (MCs),** numbered from I (thumb) to V (little finger). Shaped similarly to long bones, the proximal articulating surfaces are concave to accept the carpals, and the distal surfaces are convex to accept the proximal phalanx of each of the fingers. Each finger has a **proximal, middle,** and **distal phalanx** except the thumb, which has only a proximal and distal phalanx.

Two small sesamoid bones are located over the distal end of the first metacarpal. These mobile bones improve the mechanical line of pull of the muscles acting on the thumb (see Fig. 13–2).

Articulations and Ligamentous Support

The motion produced by the wrist, hand, and fingers occurs through the interaction of many joints, which form numerous force couples with their associated muscles. An overview of the interactions involving specific joints is described in this section.

Distal Radioulnar Joint

This articulation is formed by the ulnar head and the ulnar notch of the radius and allows 1 degree of freedom of movement: pronation/supination. This motion is produced by the radius gliding around the ulnar, but the ulna does display slight anterior and medial movement during supination and posterior and lateral movement during pronation. The distal radioulnar joint functions concurrently with the proximal radioulnar joint to produce forearm supination and pronation. Restriction of motion at either of these joints limits pronation and supination along the entire forearm.

Radiocarpal Joint

The radiocarpal articulation is an ellipsoid joint that provides 2 degrees of freedom of movement: flexion/extension and radial/ulnar deviation. The joint is formed by the distal end of the radius articulating with the scaphoid and lunate, and the trian-

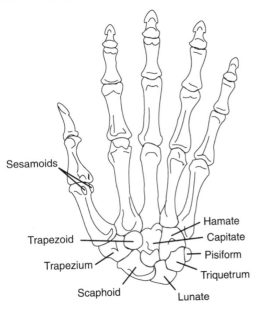

Figure 13–1. Carpal bones of the hand.

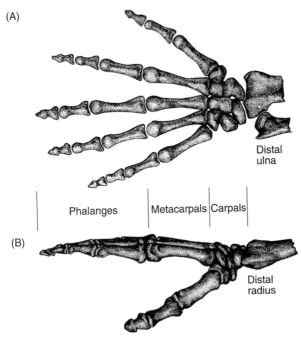

Figure 13–2. Bones of the wrist and hand, formed by the radius and ulna, 8 carpal bones, 5 metacarpals, and 14 phalanges.

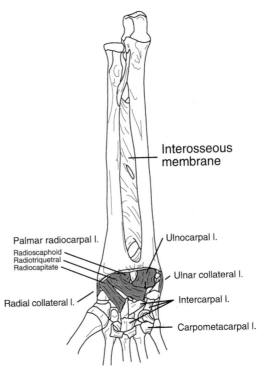

Figure 13–3. Palmar (volar) ligaments of the wrist and hand.

gular fibrocartilaginous disk articulating with the lunate and triquetrum. The ulna is buffered from the proximal row of carpals by the disk and therefore does not directly articulate with the carpals.

The joint is covered by an articular capsule reinforced by ligamentous thickenings (Fig. 13–3). The **radial collateral ligament (RCL)**, originating off the styloid process and inserting on the scaphoid and trapezium, limits **ulnar deviation** and becomes taut when the wrist is at the extreme ranges of flexion and extension. The **ulnar collateral ligament (UCL)** arises from the ulna's styloid process and attaches on the medial aspect of the triquetrum **dorsally** and the pisiform palmarly. This ligament checks radial deviation and becomes taut at the end-ranges of flexion and extension.

The most important ligament for controlling motion and wrist stability is the **palmar (volar) radiocarpal ligament.**[1] This structure originates from the anterior surface of the distal radius and courses obliquely and medially to split into three individual segments, each named for the bone to which it attaches: the **radiocapitate ligament**, the **radiotriquetral ligament**, and the **radioscaphoid ligament**. As a unit, these ligaments maintain the alignment of the associated joint structures and limit hyperextension of the wrist and hand. Medially, the small **palmar (volar) ulnocarpal ligament** originates from the distal ulna, blends in with the UCL, and attaches to the lunate and triquetrum.

The **dorsal radiocarpal ligament** is the only major ligament on the dorsal surface of the wrist (Fig. 13–4). Arising from the posterior surface of the distal radius and styloid process, this ligament attaches to the lunate and triquetrum to limit wrist flexion.

Ulnar deviation: Movement of the hand toward the ulnar side of the forearm.
Dorsal: Referring to the posterior aspect of the hand and forearm relative to the anatomical position.

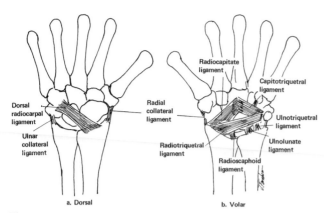

Figure 13-4. Dorsal ligaments of the wrist and hand. (From Norkin, CC, and Levangie, PK,[1] p 267, with permission.)

Intercarpal Joints

Each carpal bone is fixated to its contiguous carpal in the same row by small palmar, dorsal, and interosseous ligaments. This ligamentous arrangement allows for very little gliding movement between the bones adjacent to one another within a row.

Midcarpal Joints

The proximal and distal carpal rows are separated by a single joint cavity with small fibrous projections connecting the rows. This structure allows limited movements of flexion/extension, radial/ulnar deviation, and glide.

Carpometacarpal Joints

The first three metacarpals articulate with a single carpal: MC I, with the trapezium; MC II, trapezoid; and MC III, capitate. The fourth and fifth metacarpals articulate with the hamate to form one of the **carpometacarpal (CMC) joints** (see Fig. 13-2). The first CMC joint, that of the thumb, has a synovial cavity separate from the lateral four joints. Classified as a saddle joint, the first CMC joint is capable of 2 degrees of freedom of movement: flexion/extension and abduction/adduction. An accessory rotational component occurs concurrently with these motions, allowing for **opposition**, a combined movement that allows the thumb to touch each of the four fingers (the return motion from opposition is **reposition**).

The CMC joints II through IV are *plane synovial joints* having 1 degree of freedom of movement, flexion/extension, whereas the fifth CMC joint has 2 degrees of movement, flexion/extension and abduction/adduction. Several small ligaments support these joints and allow progressively more motion with each medial joint. The second and third CMC joints are practically immobile; the fourth and fifth

have greater mobility, allowing the hand to strongly grip small objects.

Metacarpophalangeal Joints

Condyloid joints capable of 2 degrees of freedom of movement, flexion/extension and abduction/adduction, the five metacarpophalangeal (MCP) articulations represent the union between the concave articular surface of the proximal phalanx of each finger and the convex articular surface of the associated metacarpal (MC). While the thumb is capable of abducting and adducting at any point in the range of motion, the maximum amount of this movement in the lateral four fingers is possible only when they are fully extended.

Support against valgus and varus forces is provided by pairs of collateral ligaments running obliquely from the dorsal aspect of the side of the metacarpal to the palmar aspect of the phalanx. As the fingers are flexed these ligaments tighten, limiting the amount of abduction and adduction available to the joint.

The palmar aspect of the MCP joints is reinforced by a thick fibrocartilaginous **palmar (volar) ligament**. The dorsal aspects of the lateral four MCP joints are reinforced by the expanse of the extensor hood. Reinforcement is also provided by the deep transverse metacarpal ligament. These strong bands limit abduction/adduction and reinforce the palmar ligaments.

Muscular Anatomy

The muscles of the wrist and hand must function under a broad spectrum of circumstances and demands. The same muscles that are used to strongly grip a bat are also called on to perform the most delicate of motor skills. Those muscles acting on the wrist, including the long muscles of the fingers, are described in Table 13-1. The intrinsic muscles of the hand are presented in Table 13-2.

The natural, relaxed position of the hand and fingers is one of slight flexion. This positioning is caused by the relative shortness of the finger flexors. This concept can be demonstrated by noting how the fingers flex as the wrist is passively extended.

Extensor Muscles

Located on the posterolateral portion of the forearm, the wrist's extensor muscles are divided into two groups, both innervated by the radial nerve. The reader should refer to Figures 12-6 and 12-7 for the location of these muscles relative to the forearm and Figures 13-5 and 13-6 for their insertion on the wrist and hand.

Plane synovial joint: A synovial joint formed by the gliding between two or more bones.

Table 13–1. Muscles Acting on the Wrist and Hand

Muscle	Action	Origin	Insertion	Nerve	Root
Abductor pollicis longus	1st CMC joint abduction 1st CMC joint extension Assists in radial deviation of the wrist	• Posterior surface of the distal ulna • Posterior surface of the distal radius • Adjoining interosseous membrane	• Radial side of the base of the 1st metacarpal	Deep radial	C6, C7
Extensor carpi radialis brevis	Wrist extension Wrist radial deviation	• Lateral epicondyle via the common extensor tendon • Radial collateral ligament	• Base of the 3rd metatarsal	Radial	C6, C7
Extensor carpi radialis longus	Elbow flexion Wrist extension Wrist radial deviation	• Supracondylar ridge	• Radial side of the 2nd metacarpal	Radial	C6, C7
Extensor carpi ulnaris	Wrist extension Wrist ulnar deviation	• Lateral epicondyle via the common extensor tendon	• Ulnar side of the base of the 5th metacarpal	Deep radial	C6, C7, C8
Extensor digitorum	Wrist extension MCP extension IP extension	• Lateral epicondyle via the common extensor tendon	• Into the dorsal surface of the proximal base of the middle and distal phalanges of each of the four fingers	Deep radial	C6, C7, C8
Extensor pollicis brevis	1st MCP joint extension 1st CMC joint extension 1st CMC joint abduction Assists in wrist radial deviation	• Posterior surface of the distal radius • Adjoining interosseous membrane	• Dorsal surface of the base of the proximal phalanx of the thumb	Deep radial	C6, C7
Extensor pollicis longus	1st IP joint extension 1st MCP joint extension 1st CMC joint extension Assists in wrist extension Assists in wrist radial deviation	• Posterior surface of the middle one-third of the ulna • Adjoining interosseous membrane	• Dorsal surface of the base of the distal phalanx of the thumb	Deep radial	C6, C7, C8
Flexor carpi radialis	Elbow flexion Forearm pronation Wrist flexion Wrist radial deviation	• Medial epicondyle via the common flexor tendon	• Bases of the 2nd and 3rd metacarpal bones	Median	C6, C7
Flexor carpi ulnaris	Elbow flexion Wrist flexion Wrist ulnar deviation	Humeral head • Medial epicondyle via the common flexor tendon Ulnar head • Medial border of the olecranon • Proximal two-thirds of the posterior ulna	• Pisiform • Hamate • 5th metacarpal	Ulnar	C8, T1

Table 13–1. Muscles Acting on the Wrist and Hand (*Continued*)

Muscle	Action	Origin	Insertion	Nerve	Root
Flexor digitorum profundus	DIP flexion PIP flexion Wrist flexion	• Anteromedial proximal three-fourths of ulna and associated interosseous membrane	• Bases of the medial 4 phalanges	Palmar interosseous	C8, T1
Flexor digitorum superficialis	PIP flexion MCP flexion Wrist flexion	Humeral head • Medial epicondyle via the common flexor tendon • Ulnar collateral ligament Ulnar head • Coronoid process Radial head • Oblique line of radius	• Middle sides of the 4 phalanges	Median	C7, C8, T1
Flexor pollicis longus	1st IP joint flexion 1st MCP joint flexion Assists in wrist flexion	• Anterior surface of the radius • Adjoining interosseous membrane • Coronoid process of ulna	• Palmar surface of the base of the distal phalanx of the thumb	Palmar interosseous	C8, T1
Palmaris longus	Wrist flexion Elbow flexion	• Medial epicondyle via the common flexor tendon	• Flexor retinaculum • Palmar aponeurosis	Median	C6, C7

Muscle actions, origins, and insertions adapted from Kendall and McCreary[1a]; innervations adapted from Daniels and Worthingham.[1b]

The superficial muscles **extensor carpi radialis longus and brevis** and **extensor carpi ulnaris** are the primary wrist extensors. The **extensor digitorum** is the primary extensor of the lateral four fingers' interphalangeal (IP) joints and serves to assist in wrist extension. The **brachioradialis** is also located in the superficial compartment, but it does not directly influence wrist movement.

The deep compartment contains the thumb's extensors, the **extensor pollicis longus** and the **extensor pollicis brevis**, and its primary abductor, the **abductor pollicis longus**. The long extensor of the second finger, the **extensor indicus**, is also located in this compartment. The remaining deep muscle, the **supinator**, is capable of supinating the forearm at all angles of elbow flexion, whereas the biceps brachii is most efficient when the elbow is at 90 degrees.

The extensor muscles are secured to the posterior portion of distal radius and ulna by the **extensor retinaculum**. This strong, transverse band increases the efficiency of the muscles' pull and prevents bowstringing when the wrist is extended.

Flexor Muscles

The anteromedial forearm is divided into compartments. The superficial compartment houses the wrist's flexor muscles, the **flexor carpi radialis, palmaris longus**, and **flexor carpi ulnaris**. The **flexor digitorum superficialis**, responsible for flexion of the four proximal interphalangeal (PIP) joints, and the **pronator teres** are also located in this compartment. The location of these muscles is presented in Figure 12–6 and their insertion on the wrist and hand in Figure 13–6. The deep compartment is formed by the **flexor digitorum profundus**, flexing both the PIP and distal interphalangeal (DIP) joints; the **flexor pollicis longus**; and the **pronator quadratus**.

The flexor muscles are supplied by the median nerve, with the exception of the flexor carpi ulnaris and the fourth and fifth portions of the flexor digitorum profundus, which are supplied by the ulnar nerve.

Palmar Muscles

The hand's intrinsic muscles are grouped into thenar, central, hypothenar, and adductor interosseous compartments. The thenar eminence is the mass found over the thumb's palmar surface and is formed by the **abductor pollicis brevis, flexor pollicis brevis**, and **opponens pollicis** muscles, and the tendon of **flexor pollicis longus** (Fig. 13–7). On the ulnar aspect, the fleshy mound at the base of the lit-

Table 13–2. Intrinsic Muscles of the Hand

Muscle	Action	Origin	Insertion	Nerve	Root
Abductor digiti minimi	Abduction of the 5th finger Assists in opposition	• Tendon of flexor carpi ulnaris • Pisiform	By two slips into the 5th finger • Ulnar side of the base of the proximal phalanx • Ulnar border of the extensor expansion	Ulnar	C8, T1
Abductor pollicis brevis	1st CMC joint abduction 1st MCP joint abduction Assists in opposition	• Flexor retinaculum • Trapezium • Scaphoid	• Radial surface of the base of the proximal phalanx of the thumb • Via a slip into the extensor expansion	Median	C6, C7
Adductor pollicis	1st CMC joint adduction 1st MCP joint adduction 1st MCP joint flexion Assists in opposition	• Capitate bone • Bases of 2nd and 3rd metacarpals • Palmar surface of 3rd metacarpal	• Ulnar surface of the base of the proximal phalanx of the thumb • Via a slip into the extensor expansion	Deep palmar branch	C8, T1
Dorsal interossei	Abduction of the 3rd, 4th, and 5th fingers Assist in MCP flexion Assist in extension of the IP joints	Thumb • Ulnar border of 1st metacarpal • Radial border of 2nd metacarpal 2nd, 3rd, & 4th fingers • Adjacent sides of metacarpals	Thumb • Radial border of the 2nd finger 2nd • Radial side of the 3rd finger 3rd • Ulnar side of 3rd finger 4th • Ulnar side of 4th finger	Deep palmar branch	C8, T1
Flexor digiti minimi	5th MCP joint flexion Assists in opposition	• Hook of the hamate bone • Flexor retinaculum	• Ulnar border of the proximal phalanx of the 5th finger	Ulnar	C8, T1
Flexor pollicis brevis	1st MCP joint flexion 1st CMC joint flexion Assists in opposition	• Flexor retinaculum • Trapezoid • Capitate	• Radial surface of the base of the proximal phalanx • Via a slip into the extensor expansion	Median Deep palmar branch	C6, C7 C8, T1
Lumbricales	Flexion of the 2nd through 5th MCP joints Extension of the PIP and DIP joints	1st & 2nd • Radial surface of flexor profundus tendons 3rd • Adjacent sides of flexor profundus tendons of 3rd and 4th fingers 4th • Adjacent sides of flexor profundus tendons of the 4th and 5th fingers	• Radial border of the extensor tendons of the respective digits	1st & 2nd Median 3rd & 4th Deep palmar branch	C6, C7 C8, T1

Table 13–2. Intrinsic Muscles of the Hand (*Continued*)

Muscle	Action	Origin	Insertion	Nerve	Root
Opponens digiti minimi	Opposition of the 5th finger	• Hook of the hamate bone • Flexor retinaculum	• Ulnar border of the length of the 5th metacarpal	Ulnar	C8, T1
Opponens pollicis	Thumb opposition	• Flexor retinaculum • Trapezium	• Length of the 1st metacarpal	Median	C6, C7
Palmar interossei	Adducts 1st, 2nd, 4th, and 5th fingers Assists in flexion of the MCP joints	Thumb • Ulnar border of the 1st metacarpal 2nd • Ulnar border of the 2nd metacarpal 3rd • Radial border of the 4th metacarpal 4th • Radial border of the 5th metacarpal	Thumb • Ulnar border of thumb 2nd • Ulnar side of 2nd finger 3rd • Radial side of ring finger • Radial side of little finger	Deep palmar branch	C8, T1

tle finger, the hypothenar eminence, contains the **abductor digiti minimi** and the **opponens digiti minimi** muscles.

Passing through the central compartment are the tendons of **flexor digitorum superficialis** and **flexor digitorum profundus**. Four **lumbrical** muscles originate off the radial side of each slip of the flexor digitorum profundus tendon. Crossing the MCP joint on the palmar side, the lumbrical continues around the phalanx to insert into the extensor hood. Because of their attachment on the extensor hood, the lumbricals serve to flex the MCP

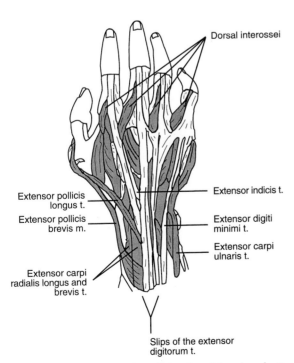

Figure 13–5. Intrinsic muscles of the dorsal hand and attachments of the long finger extensors.

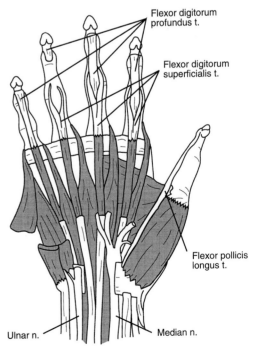

Figure 13–6. Intrinsic palmar muscles and long finger flexors. Note the location of the ulnar and median nerves.

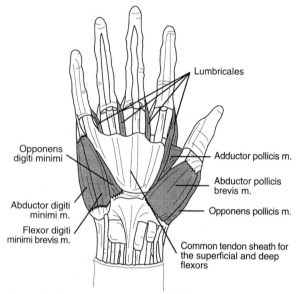

Figure 13–7. Intrinsic muscles of the thumb and little finger.

joints and extend the PIP and DIP joints. The entire central compartment is covered by the **palmar aponeurosis** (volar plate).

The adductor interosseous compartment fills the void between metacarpals. The webspace between the thumb and index finger is filled by **adductor pollicis muscle.** Three spaces between the remaining metacarpals are filled by four palmar and four dorsal **interosseous muscles.** Referenced from the third MC, the palmar interossei adduct the fingers and the dorsal interossei abduct them.

The Carpal Tunnel

Many of the anterior muscles acting on the wrist and fingers cross the radiocarpal joint through the carpal tunnel (Fig. 13–8). A fibro-osseous structure, the tunnel's floor is formed by the proximal carpal bones and its roof by the transverse carpal

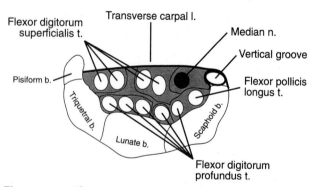

Figure 13–8. The carpal tunnel. Inflammation of the tendons passing through the carpal tunnel increases the volume within this fixed space. If the volume continues to increase, the median nerve is compressed, resulting in neurologic symptoms in the hand.

ligament. Ten structures pass through the tunnel: the median nerve, the flexor pollicis longus tendon, the four slips of the flexor digitorum superficialis, and the flexor digitorum profundus tendons. Inflammation of these structures compresses the median nerve and results in paresthesia in the second, third, and fourth fingers and decreased grip strength.

CLINICAL EVALUATION OF INJURIES TO THE WRIST, HAND, AND FINGERS

In order to preserve function and prevent permanent deformity, injuries to the wrist, hand, and fingers must be readily recognized and treated. The evaluation of this area is somewhat eased by the relatively subcutaneous location of most of the structures, but this makes these structures vulnerable to otherwise minor forces and/or trauma (Table 13–3).

An evaluation of the elbow, shoulder, and cervical spine may also be indicated when the history, mechanism, or symptoms suggest involvement of these structures. Impairment of the nerves in these areas may manifest their symptoms through decreased sensation and strength in the hand.

History

The conditions leading to the onset of the athlete's complaints are a valuable resource in determining the structures and pathology involved. The history-taking process should be structured so that the location of the symptoms, the mechanism of injury, and the duration of the symptoms are clearly identified.

- **Location of pain:** Because the structures of the wrist and hand are so close to one another, enough detail should be gained during the history-taking process to localize the symptoms as specifically as possible. Trauma to the cervical spine, shoulder, elbow, and forearm can radiate symptoms into the wrist and hand. Injury to the median, ulnar, and radial nerves can radiate symptoms into their specific distributions in the hand (see Fig. 12–8).

- **Mechanism of injury:** The majority of injuries to the wrist and hand are caused by a single traumatic force. In the case of acute trauma, the mechanism of injury must be ascertained as closely as possible so that the injured structure(s) can be localized. Athletes describing an injury of insidious onset should be asked which activities increase or decrease the symptoms.

- **Relevant sounds or sensations:** Fractures and dislocations may have an associated popping sound and the athlete may describe a snapping sensation.

Table 13–3. Evaluation of the Wrist and Hand

History	Inspection	Palpation	Functional Tests	Ligamentous Tests	Neurological Tests	Special Tests
Location of pain	General	Anteromedial	Wrist	Valgus stress	Radial nerve	Wrist Pathology
Mechanism of injury	Posture of the	Structures	Active range of	testing—	Median nerve	Wrist sprains
Relevant sounds	hand	Ulnar head	motion	radiocarpal	Ulnar nerve	Triangular
Relevant sensation	Gross deformity	Ulnar collateral	Flexion	joint		fibrocartilage
Duration of symptoms	Palmar creases	ligament	Extension	Varus stress		injury
Description of	Areas of cuts or	Triquetrum	Radial deviation	testing—		Carpal tunnel
symptoms	scars	Pisiform	Ulnar deviation	radiocarpal		syndrome
Previous history		Hamate	Passive range of	joint		Phalen's test
General medical health	Wrist and Hand	Wrist flexor group	motion	Glide testing of		
	Continuity of the	Flexor carpi ulnaris	Flexion	the wrist		Hand Pathology
	distal radius	Flexor digitorum	Extension			Scaphoid fractures
	and ulna	profundus	Radial deviation			Perilunate and
	Continuity of the	Palmaris longus	Ulnar deviation			lunate dislocations
	carpals	Flexor carpi radialis	Resisted range of			
	Alignment of the	Carpal tunnel	motion	Valgus stress		Finger Pathology
	knuckles		Flexion	testing—IP		Collateral ligament
	Ganglion cyst	Posterolateral	Extension	joints		injuries
		Structures	Radial deviation	Varus stress		Boutonnière
	Thumb and	Lateral epicondyle	Ulnar deviation	testing—IP		deformity
	Fingers	Radial shaft		joints		Finger fractures
	Alignment of	Distal radius and	Thumb—CMC	Ulnar collateral		Mallet finger
	fingernails	styloid process	Active range of	ligament—		Jersey finger
	Boutonnière	Radial collateral	motion	thumb		
	deformity	ligament	Flexion			Thumb Pathology
	Mallet finger	Scaphoid	Extension			deQuervain's
	Jersey finger	Wrist extensor group	Abduction			syndrome
		Extensor carpi	Adduction			Finkelstein's test
		radialis longus	Opposition			Thumb sprains
		Extensor carpi	Passive range of			MCP joint
		ulnaris	motion			dislocation
		Extensor carpi	Flexion			Thumb fractures
		radialis brevis	Extension			
		Extensor digitorum	Abduction			

continued

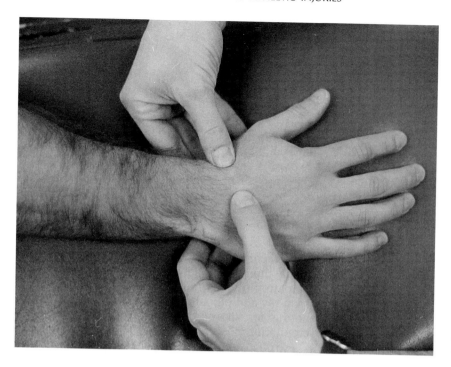

Figure 13–16. Palpation of the lunate. The examiner's left thumb (on the patient's ulnar side) indicates the location of the lunate.

and index finger and is more easily identified if the athlete actively abducts the thumb.

- **Central compartment:** Lying between the thenar and hypothenar compartments, the palmar aponeurosis is the most superficial structure within the central compartment. Palpation along the metacarpals may reveal the fingers' flexor tendons.
- **Hypothenar compartment:** The hypothenar mass is palpated along the ulnar border of the

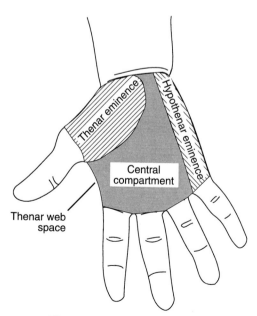

Figure 13–17. Zones of the hand.

palm. The musculature within this area cannot be specifically identified.

Functional Tests

The thumb is discussed as an individual unit as it pertains to the CMC joint. Its MCP and IP joints are described in the finger range of motion section. A summary of the end-feels obtained from passive range of motion testing for the wrist, hand, fingers, and thumb is presented in Table 13–4. The reader should refer to Table 13–1 and Table 13–2 for the innervations of these muscles. An encapsulated version of the muscles influencing each motion is presented in Table 13–5.

Wrist Range of Motion Testing

The motions of pronation and supination are described in Chapter 12.

- Active range of motion
  - **Flexion and extension:** A total of 155 to 175 degrees of motion occurs in the sagittal plane around a coronal axis. Flexion accounts for 80 to 90 degrees and extension ranges from 75 to 85 degrees. The fingers should be relaxed to ensure the maximum amount of motion (Fig. 13–18A).
  - **Radial and ulnar deviation:** Approximately 55 degrees of motion are permitted though the range of radial and ulnar deviation. This motion occurs in the frontal plane around an anteroposterior axis. From the neutral position,

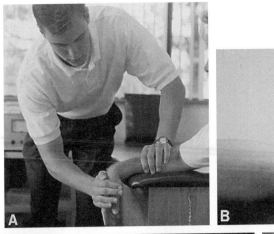

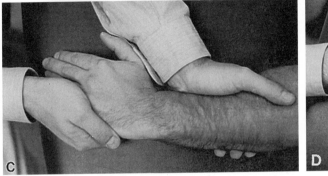

Figure 13–19. Passive range of motion of the wrist: (*A*) ... ulnar deviation.

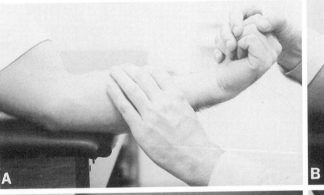

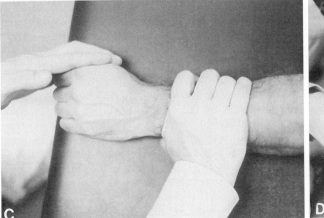

Figure 13–20. Resisted range of motion at the wrist: (*A*) ... ulnar deviation.

Table 13–4. Normal End-Feels Obtained During Passive Range of Motion Testing

Area	Motion	End-Feel	Tissues
Wrist	Flexion	Firm	Dorsal radiocarpal ligament and joint capsule
	Extension	Firm	Palmar radiocarpal ligament and joint capsule
	Radial deviation	Hard	Scaphoid striking styloid process of radius
Thumb (CMC)	Flexion	Soft	Approximation of thenar eminence and the palm
	Extension	Firm	Anterior joint capsule, flexor pollicis brevis, opponens pollicis, first dorsal interossei
	Abduction	Firm	Stretching of the webspace
	Adduction	Soft	Approximation of thenar eminence and palm
	Opposition	Firm	Thumb and 5th finger touching
Fingers and thumb (MCP)	Flexion	Hard	Proximal phalanx contacts the metacarpal
	Extension	Firm	Tension in the volar plate
	Abduction	Firm	Stretching of the collateral ligaments and webspace
	Adduction	Firm	Stretching of the collateral ligaments and webspace
Fingers (PIP)	Flexion	Hard	Proximal and middle phalanges contact
	Extension	Firm	Stretching of the volar plate
Fingers (DIP) and thumb (IP)	Flexion	Firm	Tension in dorsal joint capsule and collateral ligaments
	Extension	Firm	Stretching of palmar joint capsule and volar plate

Adapted from Norkin and White.[1d]

35 degrees of ulnar deviation and 20 degrees of radial deviation are permitted by the joint structure (Fig. 13–18B).

- Passive range of motion
  - **Flexion and extension:** The athlete is positioned so that the wrist is over the edge of the table with the hand facing downward. The forearm is stabilized to prevent pronation/supination during the motion. The normal end-feel for extension is firm owing to stretching of the palmar radiocarpal ligament and palmar joint capsule. During flexion, a firm end-feel arises from the soft tissue stretch of the dorsal radiocarpal ligament and joint capsule (Fig. 13–19A).
  - **Radial and ulnar deviation:** The wrist and forearm are positioned in the same manner as for passive flexion and extension. The normal end-feel for radial deviation is hard as the scaphoid contacts the styloid process of the radius. During ulnar deviation a firm end-feel occurs as the radial collateral ligament is stretched (Fig. 13–19B).
- Resisted range of motion
  - **Flexion and extension:** During flexion, resistance is provided to the palmar surface of the hand with the forearm supinated and stabilization occurs over the posterior portion of the distal forearm. When resisting extension, the opposite positioning is assumed: resistance is

applied to the dorsal aspect of the hand and stabilization occurs over the anterior portion of the distal forearm (Fig. 13–20A).
  - **Radial and ulnar deviation:** *Radial* and ulnar *deviation* is most easily performed with the fingers flexed. Stabilization is provided by grasping the distal aspect of the forearm. Resistance to radial deviation is provided on the thumb side of the hand and on the opposite border during ulnar deviation (Fig. 13–20B).

Thumb Range of Motion Testing—

Carpometacarpal Joint

- Active range of motion
  - **Flexion and extension:** Thumb flexion and extension occurs in the frontal plane around an anteroposterior axis. The majority of this motion, 60 to 70 degrees, is flexion (Fig. 13–21A). Only a trace amount of true CMC extension is permitted.
  - **Abduction and adduction:** In the anatomical position, this motion occurs in the sagittal plane around a coronal axis. Abduction, best exemplified by the position the thumb assumes when holding a beverage can, accounts for the total motion of 70 to 80 degrees (Fig. 13–21B). True adduction is limited by the phalanx striking the second MC.

Radial deviation: Movement of the hand toward the radial (thumb) side.

Table 13–5. Actions of the Muscles of the Wrist, Hand, and Fingers

Wrist Flexion	Wrist Extension
Flexor carpi radialis	Extensor carpi radialis brevis
Flexor carpi ulnaris	Extensor carpi radialis longus
Flexor digitorum profundus	Extensor carpi ulnaris
Flexor digitorum superficialis	Extensor digitorum
Flexor pollicis longus	Extensor pollicis longus
Palmaris longus	
Wrist Ulnar Deviation	*Wrist Radial Deviation*
Extensor carpi ulnaris	Abductor pollicis longus
Flexor carpi ulnaris	Extensor carpi radialis brevis
	Extensor carpi radialis longus
	Extensor pollicis brevis
	Extensor pollicis longus
	Flexor carpi radialis
Finger MCP Flexion	*Finger MCP Extension*
Dorsal interossei	Extensor digitorum
Flexor digitorum profundus	
Flexor digitorum superficialis	
Flexor digiti minimi (5th finger)	
Lumbricales	
Palmar interossei	
Finger PIP Flexion	*Finger PIP Extension*
Flexor digitorum profundus	Dorsal interossei
Flexor digitorum superficialis	Extensor digitorum
	Lumbricales
Finger DIP Flexion	*Finger DIP Extension*
Flexor digitorum profundus	Dorsal interossei
	Extensor digitorum
	Lumbricales
Finger Adduction	*Finger Abduction*
Palmar interossei	Abductor digiti minimi (5th finger)
	Dorsal interossei
Thumb Flexion	*Thumb Extension*
Flexor pollicis brevis	Abductor pollicis longus
Flexor pollicis longus	Extensor pollicis brevis
	Extensor pollicis longus
Thumb IP Flexion	*Thumb IP Extension*
Flexor pollicis longus	Extensor pollicis brevis
	Extensor pollicis longus
Thumb Adduction	*Thumb Abduction*
Adductor pollicis brevis	Abductor pollicis brevis
	Abductor pollicis longus
	Extensor pollicis brevis

○ **Opposition:** Opposition is the combined motion of flexion, adduction, and rotation of the first phalanges and is demonstrated by touching the thumb to the little finger (see Fig. 13–13). Because of these combined move-

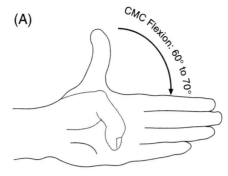

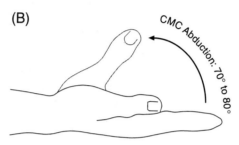

Figure 13–21. Active range of motion of the first carpometacarpal joint: (*A*) flexion; (*B*) abduction.

Figure
sion. (B
the wri

the forearm is fully supinated and the wrist is in 0 degrees of flexion and extension. The examiner brings the athlete's thumb and fifth finger toward each other. Normally, the two fingers should touch each other.

- Resisted range of motion
  ○ **Flexion and extension:** During both motions stabilization is provided to the first MC. Flexion is resisted on the palmar aspect of the first phalanx, and resistance is applied to the dorsal aspect during extension (Fig. 13–23A).
  ○ **Abduction and adduction:** The wrist and lateral four metacarpals are stabilized as resistance is given on the lateral border of the proximal phalanx when the thumb is abducted. During adduction, the resistance is applied to the medial border of the proximal phalanx (Fig. 13–23B).
  ○ **Opposition:** The athlete touches and holds the tips of the thumb and little finger together. The examiner then attempts to spread the fingers and compares the results with those found on the opposite side (Fig. 13–23C).

Finger Range of Motion Testing

- Active range of motion
  ○ **Flexion and extension of the metacarpopha-**

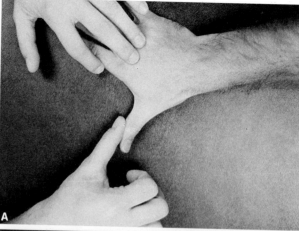

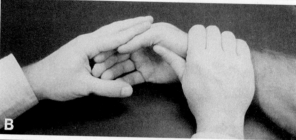

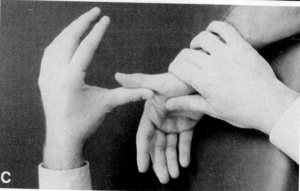

Figure 13–22. Passive range of motion of the first carpometacarpal joint: (*A*) abduction; (*B*) flexion; (*C*) extension.

langeal joints: Flexion and extension of the MCP and IP joints occur in the sagittal plane around a coronal axis. A maximum of 105 to 135 degrees of motion is allowed at the MCP joint, with 20 to 30 degrees occurring during extension from the neutral position and the remaining 85 to 105 degrees accounted for during flexion (Fig. 13–24A).
○ **Abduction and adduction of the metacarpophalangeal joints:** Twenty to 25 degrees of motion are allowed during abduction and the return motion of adduction. The movement occurs in the frontal plane around an anteroposterior axis (Fig. 13–24B).
○ **Flexion and extension of the interphalangeal joints:** Flexion and extension of the interphalangeal joints range from 80 to 90 degrees at the

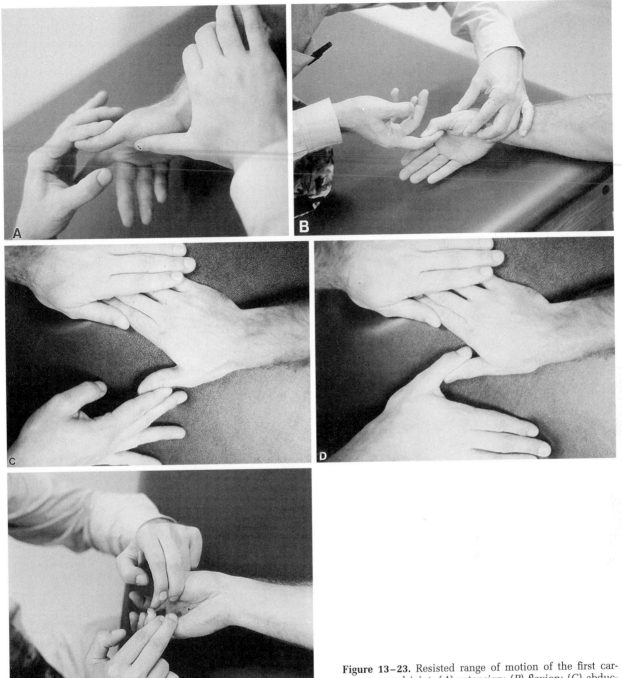

Figure 13–23. Resisted range of motion of the first carpometacarpal joint: (*A*) extension; (*B*) flexion; (*C*) abduction; (*D*) adduction; (*E*) opposition.

thumb, 110 to 120 degrees at the PIP, and 80 to 90 degrees at the DIP joints of the fingers (Fig. 13–24C and D).

• Passive range of motion

   ◦ **Flexion and extension of the metacarpophalangeal joints:** While stabilizing the metacarpal, the examiner grasps the proximal phalanx of the finger being tested. The fingers are resting in their natural amount of flexion. During flexion, a hard end-feel is to be expected as

the proximal phalanx contacts the metacarpal. Tightening of the volar plate leads to a firm end-feel during extension of the MCP joint (Fig. 13–25A).

   ◦ **Abduction and adduction of the metacarpophalangeal joints:** The athlete's arm should be positioned so that the palm is resting flat against the table with the metacarpals stabilized to prevent wrist motion. The examiner grasps the finger over the PIP joint. For both ab-

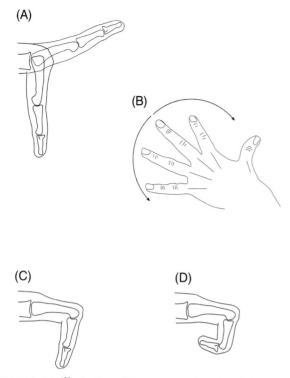

Figure 13–24. Illustration of finger range of motion: (*A*) metacarpophalangeal flexion and extension; (*B*) metacarpophalangeal abduction; (*C*) flexion of the proximal interphalangeal joint; (*D*) flexion of the proximal and distal interphalangeal joints.

duction and adduction a firm end-feel is normal because of tension in the collateral ligaments of the MCP joint and a stretching of the webspace.

○ **Flexion and extension of the interphalangeal joints:** The phalanx proximal to the joint being tested is stabilized, while force is applied to the phalanx of the distal bone. The normal end-feel for the PIP joint is hard during flexion as the two phalanges contact each other, although a soft end-feel can occur by soft tissue approximation (Fig. 13–25B). During extension, the stretching of the palmar joint capsule and the volar plate gives a firm end-feel (Fig. 13–25C). The DIP joints and the thumb's IP joint have a firm end-feel during flexion from tension in the dorsal joint capsule and the collateral ligaments. During extension, a firm end-feel is caused by stretching of the palmar joint capsule and the volar plate.

• Resisted range of motion
  ○ **Flexion and extension of the metacarpophalangeal joints:** Flexion and extension of the fingers' MCP joints are typically tested as a unit. For each motion the hand is stabilized across the metacarpals with care not to compress or impinge them. During flexion, resistance is de-

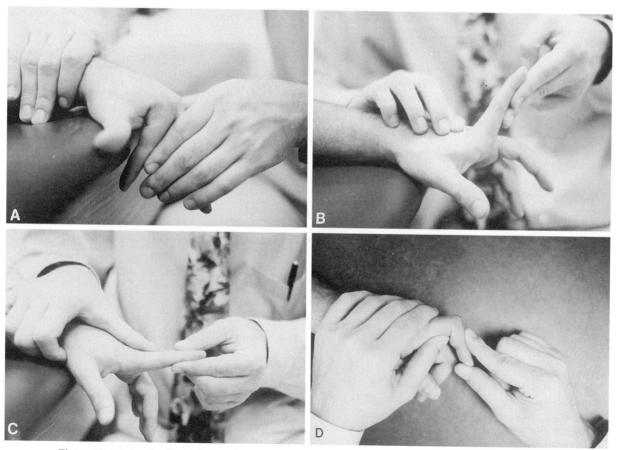

Figure 13–25. Passive finger range of motion: (*A*) flexion and (*B*) extension of the metacarpophalangeal joint; (*C*) extension of the proximal interphalangeal joint; (*D*) flexion of the distal interphalangeal joint.

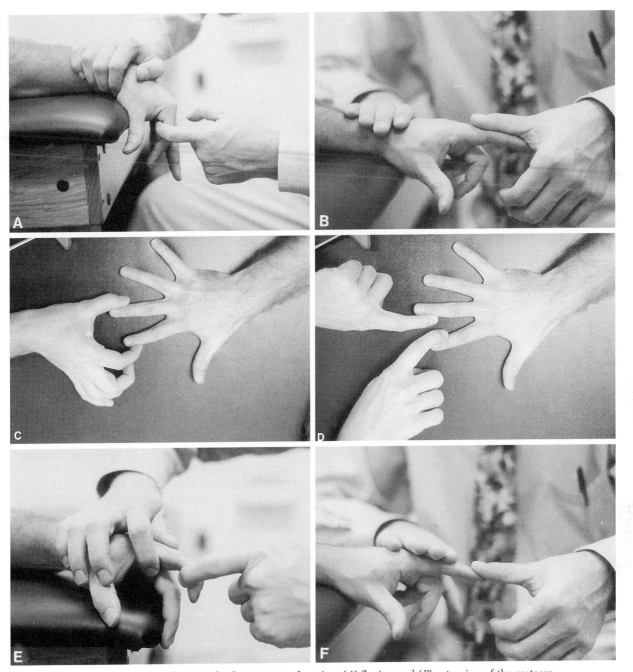

Figure 13–26. Resisted testing for finger range of motion: (*A*) flexion and (*B*) extension of the metacar-pophalangeal joint; (*C*) adduction and (*D*) abduction of the metacarpophalangeal joints; (*E*) resisted flex-ion of the proximal interphalangeal joint and (*F*) extension of the distal interphalangeal joint.

livered across the palmar aspect of the proxi-mal phalanges. During extension, resistance is applied to the dorsal aspect of the proximal phalanges (Fig. 13–26A).

○ **Abduction and adduction of the metacar-pophalangeal joints:** Resisted abduction is tested by having the athlete first spread the fin-gers. Pressure is then applied to the distal pha-langes of the two fingers being tested, squeez-ing them together. Adduction is tested by having the athlete tightly squeeze the fingers

together. The examiner then attempts to sepa-rate them (Fig. 13–26B).

○ **Flexion and extension of the interphalangeal joints:** To resistively test the interphalangeal joints, the examiner stabilizes the phalanx proximal to the joint.

Resistance is provided on the palmar surface of the phalanx distal to the joint being tested during flexion and the dorsal surface when test-ing extension. These joints are typically tested individually (Fig. 13–26C).

Grip Dynamometry

A manual dynamometer can be used to quantitatively measure an athlete's grip strength (Fig. 13–27). These results can then be used to objectively measure bilateral strength deficits, identify, and document progress through the rehabilitation program.

Grip Dynamometry (Fig. 13–27)

Position of athlete	Holding the grip dynamometer with the elbow flexed to 90° and the radioulnar joint in its neutral position.
Position of examiner	Standing in front of the athlete, viewing the dynamometer's gauge.
Evaluative procedure	The dynamometer is set at one of five specified settings (1, 1.5, 2, 2.5, and 3 inches). The athlete squeezes the dynamometer's handle with maximum force at every setting, with adequate recovery time allowed between bouts. The values are recorded and the test is repeated on the opposite hand.
Positive test results	Injured nondominant hand: More than 10% bilateral strength deficit when compared with the dominant hand. Injured dominant hand: More than 5% bilateral strength deficit when compared with the nondominant hand.
Implications	A decreased grip strength.
Comment	Because of the wide range of variation in grip strength, the outcome of each of these tests is most meaningful when compared against a baseline measure.

Ligamentous and Capsular Testing

Although injury to the ligamentous tissues surrounding the wrist and hand is common, there are no specific tests to check the integrity of the specific ligaments. The ligaments of the wrist are stressed with overpressure during the evaluation of passive range of motion (Table 13–6).

Tests for Collateral Support of the Wrist Ligaments

The UCL provides lateral support against valgus forces (radial deviation) and the RCL checks varus forces (ulnar deviation). These two ligaments also function cooperatively to limit wrist flexion and extension. Their integrity may be partially established through valgus and varus stress testing (Fig. 13–28) and by assessing glide between the proximal carpal row and the radius (Fig. 13–29). One should note that these tests not only check the integrity of the collateral ligaments but also may elicit signs of trauma to the triangular fibrocartilage.

Valgus and Varus Stress Testing of the Radiocarpal Joint (Fig. 13–28)

Position of athlete	Sitting. The elbow is flexed to 90°, the forearm is pronated, and the fingers assume the relaxed position of flexion.
Position of examiner	Standing lateral to the wrist being tested. One hand grips the distal forearm and the other grasps the hand across the metacarpals.
Evaluative procedure	UCL: A valgus stress is applied, radially deviating the wrist. RCL: A varus stress is applied, ulnarly deviating the wrist.
Positive test results	Pain or laxity as compared with the same ligament on the opposite wrist.
Implications	Stretching or tearing of the ulnar collateral or radial collateral ligament.
Comment	Pain may be elicited in the presence of trauma to the triangular fibrocartilage or the palmar or dorsal radiocarpal or ulnocarpal ligaments.

Glide Testing of the Wrist (Fig. 13–29)

Position of athlete	Sitting. The elbow is flexed to 90°, the forearm is pronated, and the fingers assume the relaxed position of flexion.
Position of examiner	Standing lateral to the wrist being tested. One hand grips the distal forearm and the other grasps the hand across the metacarpals.
Evaluative procedure	A shear force is applied to the wrist by gliding the distal segment in a radial and ulnar direction and then in a superior and inferior direction.
Positive test results	Pain or significant glide when compared with the opposite side.
Implications	Tear or stretching of the collateral ligaments or trauma to the triangular fibrocartilage.
Comment	This motion stresses both collateral ligaments; the determination of which ligament is involved is based on the location of pain.

Tests for Collateral Support of the Interphalangeal Joints

The integrity of the 14 IP joints' collateral ligaments can be determined through valgus and varus stress testing. Although these tests will demonstrate laxity in cases of a complete rupture of the ligament, pain may also be used as a measure of the relative severity of the injury (Fig. 13–30).

Valgus and Varus Stress Testing of the Interphalangeal Joints (Fig. 13–30)

Position of athlete	Sitting or standing.
Position of examiner	Standing in front of the athlete, stabilizing the phalanx proximal to the joint being tested.
Evaluative procedure	The examiner grasps the phalanx distal to the joint being tested and applies a valgus stress to the joint. A varus stress is then applied to the joint.
Positive test results	Increased gapping, compared with the same motion on the same finger of the opposite hand.
Implications	Collateral ligament sprain.
Comment	Except in the case of a complete disruption of the ligament, the degree of injury to the ligament cannot be established.

Test for Support of the Collateral Ligaments

The only MCP joint that is routinely stress tested is the thumb's ulnar collateral ligament (Fig. 13–31). Because of the alignment of the fingers, the only other MCP collateral ligaments that are frequently injured are the ulnar collateral ligament of the MCP joint of the index finger and the radial collateral ligament of the little finger.

Ulnar Collateral Ligament of the Thumb (Fig. 13–31)

Position of athlete	Seated.
Position of examiner	Standing in front of the athlete. The examiner stabilizes the first metacarpal with one hand and its proximal phalanx with the other.
Evaluative procedure	While stabilizing the first metacarpal with the thumb slightly abducted and extended, the examiner adducts the thumb, applying stress to the ulnar collateral ligament. The test is repeated with the joint in varying degrees of flexion.
Positive test results	The ulnar side of the first metacarpophalangeal joint gaps farther than the uninjured side and/or the athlete describes pain.
Implications	Stretching or tearing of the ulnar collateral ligament.

Neurological Testing

Most commonly, nerves of the hand, wrist, and fingers are affected by pathology proximal to the forearm, although trauma in this region can lead to localized symptoms. The distributions of the specific nerves of the upper arm are presented in Chapter 9 (see Neurological Screen on page 421).

Pathologies and Related Special Tests

The majority of injuries to the wrist, hand, and fingers are traumatic in their onset. Despite the constant use of these areas, overuse injuries are relatively rare in athletics. Any injury to this area involves the possible ramification of significant disability in both athletic competition and the activities of daily living. Although similar in nature, trauma to the thumb and trauma to the fingers are discussed in separate sections because of the potential differences in the functional outcomes.

Wrist Pathology

Trauma to the wrist can affect the distal portion of the radius and ulna; the collateral, volar, and dorsal ligaments; the triangular fibrocartilage; or neurovascular structures. The mechanisms of injury for most of these conditions are very similar, calling for careful inspection, palpation, and functional testing of the involved structures.

Wrist Sprains

Because wrist sprains are caused by many of the same mechanisms as for other pathologies of the wrist and hand, the conclusion of a wrist sprain is often based on the exclusion of other injuries.[2] The possibilities of carpal fractures, triangular fibrocartilage tears, and carpal tunnel syndrome must first be

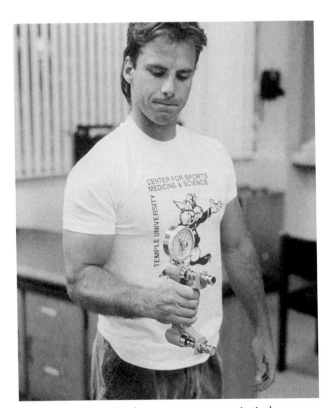

Figure 13–27. Use of a dynamometer to quantitatively measure grip strength.

Table 13–6. Ligaments Stressed During Wrist Passive Range of Motion

Passive Movement	Ligaments Stressed	
	Primary	**Secondary**
Extension	Palmar ulnocarpal	Radial collateral
	Palmar radiocarpal	Ulnar collateral
Flexion	Dorsal radiocarpal	Radial collateral
		Ulnar collateral
Radial deviation	Ulnar collateral	
Ulnar deviation	Radial collateral	

Neurological Screen

Nerve Root Level	Sensory Testing	Motor Testing	Reflex Testing
C6	Musculocutaneous n.	Musculocutaneous n.(C5 & C6)	Brachioradialis
C7	Radial n.	Median and Ulnar n.	Triceps brachii
C8	Ulnar n. (mixed)	Radial n.	None
T1	Med. brachial cutaneous n.	Med. brachial cutaneous n.	None

eliminated before making the determination of a wrist sprain. Sprains of the distal radioulnar ligaments can lead to a dislocation of the distal ends of these two bones, especially in the presence of an associated fracture.[3]

Active range of motion is limited in all directions secondary to pain, with the restriction occurring equally during flexion and extension. Pain occurs during passive range of motion or during valgus and varus stress testing as the involved ligaments are stretched with overpressure, although pain may be duplicated by the ligaments' being pinched between two bones (Table 13−7). There are no additional specific tests to confirm the presence of wrist ligament sprains.

Triangular Fibrocartilage Injury

Trauma to the triangular fibrocartilage and its closely associated UCL can result in permanent disability of the wrist if left unrecognized and untreated.[4] Forced hyperextension results in pain along the ulnar side of the wrist and is accompanied by decreased wrist motion secondary to pain. During palpation, close attention should be devoted

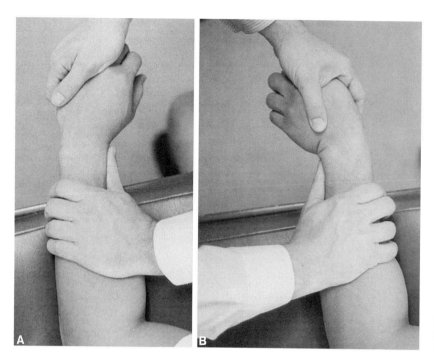

Figure 13–28. (*A*) Valgus and (*B*) varus stress testing of the radiocarpal joint (relative to the anatomical position).

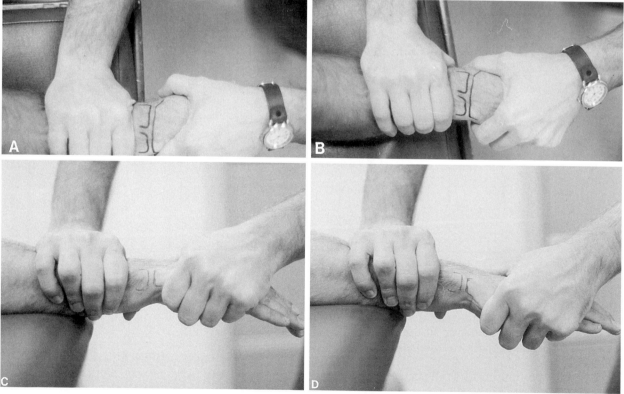

Figure 13–29. Testing of radiocarpal glide: (*A*) radial glide; (*B*) ulnar glide; (*C*) superior glide; (*D*) inferior glide.

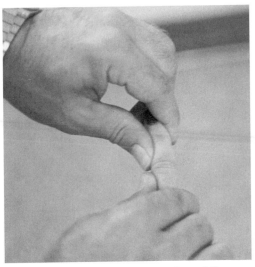

Figure 13–30. Stress testing the ulnar collateral ligament of the proximal interphalangeal joint. This test should be repeated for the radial collateral ligament.

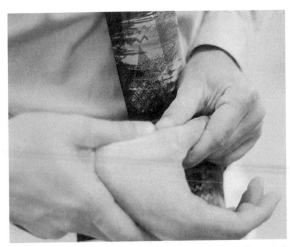

Figure 13–31. Stress testing the thumb's ulnar collateral ligament of the metacarpophalangeal joint.

to the ulnar styloid process, as it can be avulsed by the UCL (Table 13–8). Any suspicion of injury to the triangular fibrocartilage should warrant referral to a physician for further evaluation.

Carpal Tunnel Syndrome

Carpal tunnel syndrome (CTS) refers to the signs and symptoms caused by the compression of the median nerve as it passes through the carpal tunnel (see Fig. 13–8). The most frequently cited cause of CTS is fibrosis of the synovium of the flexor tendons secondary to tenosynovitis of the flexor tendons.[5,6] Although this is not a common athletic injury, CTS may occur with repetitive microtrauma, with acute trauma to the carpal tunnel, or as the result of progressive degeneration of the carpal tun-

Table 13–7. Evaluative Findings of Wrist Sprains

Examination Segment	Clinical Findings
History	Onset: Acute. Location of pain: Pain emanates from the palmar and dorsal aspects of the wrist near the joint line. Mechanism: Tensile forces are placed on the ligaments as the joint is forced past its normal range of motion.
Inspection	Swelling is localized to the joint line.
Palpation	Tenderness, which is over the involved tissues, tends to be more diffuse than with other wrist injuries such as scaphoid fractures or tears of the triangular fibrocartilage.
Functional tests	AROM: This is limited as the sprained tissues are placed on stretch. Motion in the opposite direction may also be limited as the capsule and ligamentous tissues become pinched as the movement is performed. PROM: This is limited as the sprained tissues are placed on stretch. RROM: Isometric testing in a neutral position may not elicit pain. Providing resistance through the range of motion exhibits weakness secondary to pain.
Ligamentous tests	None; ligamentous integrity is determined by overpressure during passive range of motion testing.
Neurological tests	Not applicable.
Special tests	None.
Comments	The diagnosis of a wrist sprain is made after the possibility of carpal fractures, triangular cartilage tears, and other traumatic injury has been ruled out.

Table 13-8. Evaluative Findings of Injury to the Triangular Fibrocartilage

Examination Segment	Clinical Findings		
History	Onset:		Acute. The athlete may not present the injury to the examiner until some time after its onset, thinking that the symptoms may subside on their own.
	Location of pain:		Distal to the ulna along the medial one-half of the wrist. The UCL of the wrist may also be tender.
	Mechanism:		Forced hyperextension of the wrist, compressing the triangular fibrocartilage.
Inspection	Diffuse swelling around the wrist is possible, although acutely no swelling may be visible..		
Palpation	Point tenderness distal to the ulna along the medial one-half of the wrist's joint line. The UCL may also display tenderness.		
Functional tests	AROM: Motion is limited, especially into extension. PROM: Motion is limited, especially into extension. RROM: Isometric testing may be normal. Resistance through the range of motion is limited, especially as the wrist is brought into extension.		
Ligamentous tests	Stressing the ulnar collateral ligament elicits pain, although laxity may not be present.		
Neurological tests	Not applicable.		
Special tests	None.		
Comments	Triangular fibrocartilage tears may be easily confused with a sprain of the wrist's ulnar collateral ligament. Persistence of symptoms should alert the examiner to injury beyond a simple wrist sprain. Athletes suspected of suffering from triangular fibrocartilage tears should be referred to a physician for further evaluation.		

nel's structures. The resulting symptoms of CTS can have a drastic deleterious effect on the athlete's performance.

The athlete experiences paresthesia and pain along the median nerve distribution (thumb, index, middle, and lateral half of the ring finger), with the symptoms often occurring at night because of impeded venous return.[7] Inspection of the hand may reveal atrophy of the thenar muscles, and grip strength is often decreased.[8] Bilateral manual muscle testing of the abductor pollicis brevis reveals weakness on the involved side[9] (Table 13-9). A positive Tinel's sign is elicited over the carpal tunnel (Fig. 13-32) and results of Phalen's test are positive.

Phalen's Test

Phalen's test is used to put pressure on the median nerve by placing overpressure on the wrist during flexion. In the recommended procedure, the clinician manually applies this pressure to avoid the possible compression of the thoracic outlet duplicating the symptoms associated with the traditional methods of detecting carpal tunnel syndrome. (Fig. 13-33).

Phalen's Test (Fig. 13-33)

Position of athlete	Seated.
Position of examiner	Standing in front of the athlete.
Evaluative procedure	The examiner applies overpressure during passive wrist flexion and holds the position for 1 minute. This procedure is then repeated for the opposite extremity.
Positive test results	Tingling in the distribution of the median nerve distal to the carpal tunnel.
Implications	Median nerve compression.
Modification	The traditional version of this test, in which the athlete maximally flexes the wrists by pushing the dorsal aspects of the hands together, is not recommended because the athlete may shrug the shoulders, causing compression of the median branch of the brachial plexus as it passes through the thoracic outlet.

Table 13–9. Evaluative Findings of Carpal Tunnel Syndrome

Examination Segment	Clinical Findings
History	Onset: Insidious. Location of pain: Paresthesia and/or pain in the hand, wrist, and fingers. The symptoms may radiate up the length of the arm. Mechanism: Repetitive wrist movement involving flexion and extension.
Inspection	Palmar aspect of the wrist may appear to be thickened.
Palpation	Palpation directly over the palmar aspect of the wrist may be tender.
Functional tests	AROM: The wrist motion may be slightly limited owing to stiffness, although active range of motion may be normal. PROM: Median nerve symptoms may increase as the wrist is fully extended or fully flexed. RROM: Strength of the abductor pollicis brevis is decreased.
Ligamentous tests	Not applicable.
Neurological tests	May exhibit decreased sensation along the median nerve distribution of the hand (palmar aspect of the thumb, fingers II and III, and the lateral aspect of IV).
Special tests	Tinel's sign; Phalen's test.
Comments	This condition is typically found in the person who performs repetitive wrist and hand movements such as typing and may become more pronounced in a student-athlete population with the increase in computer use in academic work.

Wrist Fractures

Fractures of the distal radius and/or ulna frequently occur secondary to the athlete's landing on an outstretched arm. The term "Colles' fracture" is often used to describe any fracture of the distal radius. However, a true Colles' fracture is a nonarticular fracture of the radius approximately 1.5 inches proximal to the radiocarpal joint, where the distal radius is displaced dorsally.[10] On an x-ray film view, the wrist appears as an upside-down fork (Fig. 13–34). The terms "Smith's fracture" and "reverse Colles' fracture" are used to describe a fracture in which the distal radius is displaced palmarly.[11] Fractures of the wrist involve the immediate loss of function and possible deformity (Table 13–10).

Hand Pathology

The majority of injuries to the hand—to the carpals and metacarpals—are traumatic in nature. The carpals are most commonly injured following hyperflexion or hyperextension of the wrist and the metacarpals following axial loading of the bone. Both groups of bones are also susceptible to crushing forces.

Scaphoid Fractures

The majority of all carpal fractures involve the scaphoid because of its function as a bony block limiting wrist extension.[12] Receiving its blood supply from the distal end, a fracture compromises nutrition to the proximal portion, causing a high incidence of **nonunion fractures** and malunion fractures secondary to avascular **necrosis** (Fig. 13–35).[13] Unresolved fractures or chronically impaired circulation to the scaphoid can result in **Preiser's disease**.

The chief complaint is of a constant ache in the area of the anatomical snuff box that is worsened with palpation on its palmar and dorsal aspects (see Fig. 13–14). Pain occurs with active and resisted wrist extension near the end of the range of motion where the scaphoid contacts the radius. Exquisite pain is produced with overpressure during passive flexion and extension, and the athlete may have a decreased grip strength on the involved side. Compression of the first metacarpal toward the scaphoid may also produce pain.

Any athlete with pain in the area of the anatomical snuff box following a hyperextension mechanism should be treated as having a fracture of the scaphoid (Table 13–11). The wrist should be immo-

---

Nonunion fracture: A fracture that fails to spontaneously heal within the normal time frame for the involved bone.

Necrosis: The death of one or more cells.

Preiser's disease: Osteoporosis of the scaphoid, resulting from a fracture or repeated trauma.

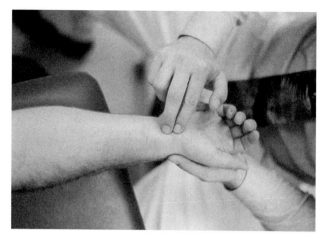

Figure 13-32. Tinel's test performed over the median nerve. In the presence of carpal tunnel syndrome, this test results in pain and paresthesia radiating into the middle finger.

bilized and the athlete referred to a physician. Fracture lines are not always visible on the initial x-ray examination and follow-up radiographs may be ordered as indicated.[14]

Perilunate and Lunate Dislocations

Forced hyperextension of the wrist and hand can disassociate the lunate from the rest of the carpals, resulting in its displacement either dorsally or palmarly. As the limits of the wrist and hand extension are exceeded, the scaphoid strikes the radius, rupturing the volar ligaments connecting the scaphoid to the lunate. As the force continues, the distal carpal row is stripped away from the lunate, result-

ing in the lunate's resting dorsally relative to the other carpals, a **perilunate dislocation**. Further extension leads to rupture of the dorsal ligaments, relocating the carpals and rotating the lunate. The lunate then rests volarly relative to the carpals, a **lunate dislocation**. Each of these types of dislocations may spontaneously reduce themselves.

The athlete's chief complaint is pain along the lateral border of the wrist and hand, limiting range of motion. A bulge may be visible on the palmar or dorsal aspect of the hand (Table 13-12). The displacement of the lunate or swelling can cause paresthesia in the middle finger.[15] A fracture of the scaphoid should be suspected with any lunate dislocation because of the similarity in their mechanisms of injury. Athletes with these injuries can present with no significant physical findings other than pain, so these injuries must be diagnosed through radiographs. Repeated trauma to the lunate can result in *Kienböck's disease*.

Metacarpal Fracture

The metacarpals are typically fractured secondary to a compressive force, such as punching with a closed fist, along the bone's shaft. In football the incidence of metacarpals involved in fractures is evenly divided among the five digits. In basketball most fractures involve the fourth and fifth metacarpals.[16] It is common for the athlete to hear the bone snapping as it fractures and describe immediate pain along one or more metacarpals. Gross deformity at the fracture site may be observed as one end of the bone rides over the other end, or the fracture site may be obscured by localized swelling along the dorsum of the hand (Fig. 13-36). Palpa-

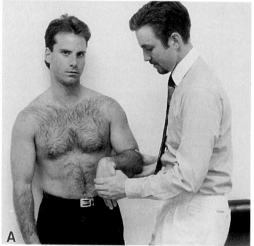
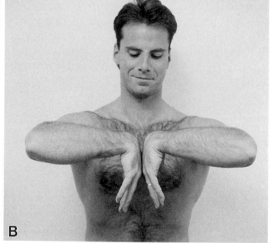

Figure 13-33. Phalen's test for carpal tunnel syndrome. (*A*) Method advocated in the text. (*B*) Traditional method.

Kienböck's disease: Osteochondritis or slow degeneration of the lunate bone.

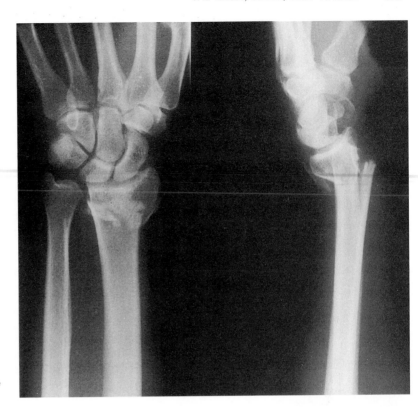

Figure 13–34. X ray of a Colles' fracture. Note the distal displacement of the radius.

Table 13–10. Evaluative Findings of Wrist Fractures

Examination Segment	Clinical Findings	
History	Onset:	Acute.
	Location of pain:	Distal forearm, proximal wrist. The athlete may describe hearing and feeling a cracking sensation.
	Mechanism:	A hyperextension mechanism, possibly combined with a rotatory component, placing tensile, compressive, or shear forces on the radius and/or ulna (e.g., landing on an outstretched arm).
Inspection	Gross deformity of the long bones may be present. The onset of swelling occurs rapidly.	
Palpation	Discontinuity of the long bones may be felt and the area is tender to the touch. The examiner should locate the radial and ulnar pulses to ensure an adequate blood supply to the hand and fingers. The bony palpation phase may be omitted if gross deformity is present.	
Functional tests	In the event of obvious gross deformity of the long bones, range of motion testing should not be conducted.	
Ligamentous tests	Not applicable.	
Neurological tests	Not applicable.	
Special tests	Not applicable.	
Comments	Suspected fractures should be appropriately splinted and the athlete immediately referred to a physician.	

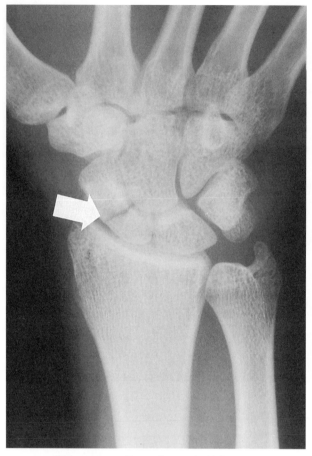

Figure 13-35. X ray of a scaphoid fracture.

tion reveals local tenderness over the fracture site. The actual bony fragments and/or crepitus may be palpated and the presence of a false joint established. The presence of a nondisplaced fracture may be confirmed through the long bone compression test (Fig. 13-37). The range of motion of the involved finger, and possibly of the hand, is limited by pain and the athlete is unable to make a fist (Table 13-13).

Fractures of the fifth metacarpal are termed **"boxer's fractures"** because of their common incidence following an improperly thrown punch. This type of fracture is characterized by a depressed fifth knuckle that, on radiography, reveals an overlapping of the bone.

Finger Pathology

The unprotected exposure to trauma makes finger injuries prevalent in athletics. Frequently these injuries go unreported or there is a significant lapse between the onset of the injury and its report. Often gross deformity is associated with these conditions, especially with joint dislocations. However, the athlete may reduce these malalignments out of instinct.

Collateral Ligament Injuries

Trauma to the collateral ligaments can range from simple sprains to complete dislocations caused from a unilateral stress being applied to an ex-

Table 13-11. Evaluative Findings of Scaphoid Fractures

Examination Segment	Clinical Findings
History	Onset: Acute. Location of pain: Proximal portion of the lateral wrist in the anatomical snuff box. Mechanism: Crushing mechanism caused by a forceful hyperextension of the wrist.
Inspection	Swelling may be localized in the anatomical snuff box.
Palpation	Palpation of the scaphoid as it sits in the anatomical snuff box elicits pain and tenderness, although crepitus may not be present. Pain may also be produced during palpation of the scaphoid's palmar aspect. Compression of the first metacarpal toward the scaphoid may elicit pain.
Functional tests	AROM: Pain is produced at the terminal range of motion, especially during extension. Radial deviation increases pain as the scaphoid is impinged between the radius, lunate, and trapezium. PROM: Overpressure produces exquisite pain during extension. Pressure during flexion may also produce pain. Radial deviation increases pain. RROM: The athlete's grip strength may be reduced.
Ligamentous tests	Not applicable.
Neurological tests	Not applicable.
Special tests	Not applicable.
Comments	Athletes describing pain in the anatomical snuff box following a mechanism involving forced hyperextension of the wrist should be managed as if they have a scaphoid fracture until it is ruled out by a physician. Scaphoid fractures may not appear on standard radiographs until several weeks after the injury but may be recognized on a bone scan within 72 hours after injury.

Table 13–12. Evaluative Findings of a Perilunate or Lunate Dislocation

Examination Segment	Clinical Findings
History	Onset: Acute. Location of pain: Lateral wrist and hand. Paresthesia along the median nerve distribution. Mechanism: Forced hyperextension of the wrist and hand.
Inspection	A bulge caused by the displacement of the lunate may be seen on the palmar or dorsal aspect of the hand.
Palpation	The lunate can be prominent during palpation, especially when it is displaced dorsally. Point tenderness and crepitus are present over the lunate.
Functional tests	Range of motion in all planes is limited secondary to pain.
Ligamentous tests	Not applicable.
Neurological tests	The sensory distribution of the median nerve should be evaluated for paresthesia.
Special tests	None.
Comments	An associated scaphoid fracture should be suspected with both perilunate and lunate dislocations.

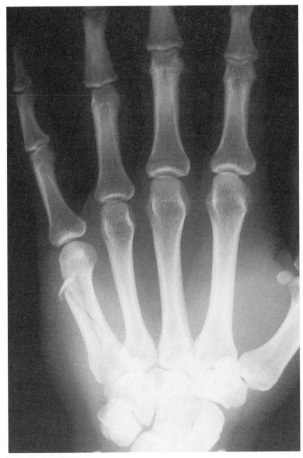

Figure 13–36. X ray of a metacarpal fracture, the so-called "boxer's fracture."

tended finger. The athlete experiences pain at the affected joint and may report self-reducing the joint after a dislocation. Active motion and passive motion are limited secondary to pain and swelling. With the exception of a complete disruption of the ligament, valgus and varus stress testing do not accurately distinguish the severity of the injury.

Boutonnière Deformity

A rupture of the central extensor tendon causes it to slip dorsally on each side of the PIP joint, changing its line of pull on this joint from that of an ex-

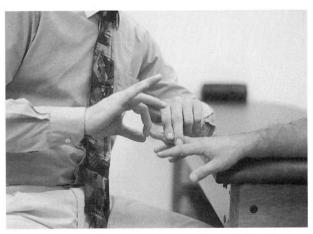

Figure 13–37. Long bone compression test for phalanx fracture. The examiner flicks the tip of the finger. Pain arising from a phalanx is a positive result.

Table 13–13. Evaluative Findings of Metacarpal Fractures

Examination Segment	Clinical Findings
History	Onset: Acute. Location of pain: Along the shaft of one or more metacarpals. Mechanism: Longitudinal compression of the bone (direct contact), a crushing force (being stepped on), or a shear force (hyperextension of the finger).
Inspection	Gross deformity of the bone may be visible. There is localized swelling over the involved metacarpal(s), and knuckle(s), which may spread to the entire dorsum of the hand. Fractures of the 5th, and possibly 4th, metacarpals may result in a depression or shortening of the knuckles (boxer's fracture). The fingernail may be abnormally rotated when the athlete makes a fist.
Palpation	Exquisite tenderness is present over the fracture site. Bony fragments or crepitus may be present. A false joint may be displayed. NOTE: Palpation should not be performed if a fracture is clearly evident during inspection.
Functional tests	AROM: This is limited owing to pain. In some instances the athlete is unable to make a fist. PROM: This is limited owing to pain. RROM: This is limited owing to pain.
Ligamentous tests	Not applicable.
Neurological tests	Not applicable.
Special tests	Long bone compression test.
Comments	If a fracture is evident during inspection, the evaluation should be immediately terminated, the hand appropriately splinted, and the athlete immediately referred to a physician.

tensor to one of a flexor. The resulting position of the finger is extension of the DIP joint and flexion of the PIP joint, a boutonnière deformity (Fig. 13–38 and see Fig. 13–11A). The athlete describes a longitudinal force on the finger, such as being struck with a ball. Pain occurs on the dorsal aspect of the PIP joint and the boutonnière deformity is visible. In acute cases, the athlete is unable to extend the PIP joint, but the examiner can passively return the joint to its normal position. However, in chronic cases, a mechanical block is formed against even passive extension of the joint.

An injury to the volar plate can cause a flexion deformity of the PIP joint that resembles a boutonnière deformity, a **pseudo-boutonnière deformity** (Fig. 13–39). Hyperextension of the finger causes the volar plate to split along the finger's long axis and slide dorsally past the joint's axis. The PIP joint cannot be extended either actively or passively.

Finger Fractures

Fractures of the **distal phalanx** are the most common fractures of the hand and occur most frequently in the thumb and middle finger. One reason for this high incidence of injury is the attachments of the flexor and extensor tendons. Avulsions of these tendons result in the inability to completely flex or extend the distal phalanx. The distal phalanx is also vulnerable to crushing mechanism (e.g., being stepped on) and longitudinal compression and rotation (e.g., a blow to the tip of the finger). The **middle phalanx** is the least frequently fractured phalanx and tends to fracture at the distal portion of the shaft. Injuries to the **proximal phalanx** usually have concurrent tendon and skin trauma. A direct blow to the finger often results in a transverse or comminuted fracture; a twisting or rotational force causes a spiral fracture (Fig. 13–40).

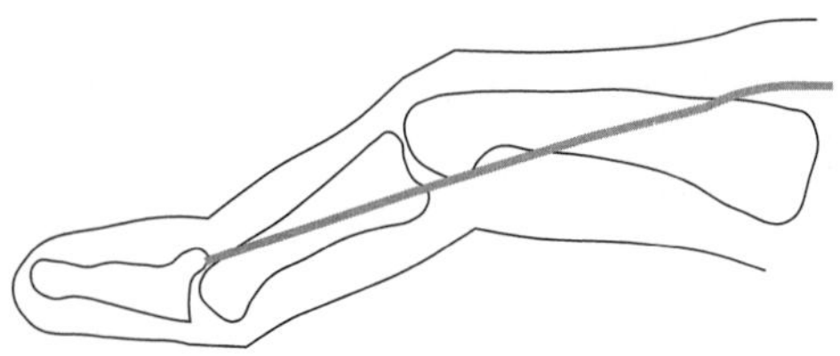

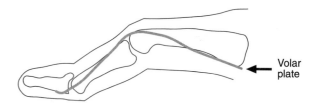

Volar plate

Figure 13–38. Illustration of the structures involved in a boutonnière deformity. The central extensor tendon slips dorsally past the proximal interphalangeal joint.

Figure 13–39. Illustration of a pseudoboutonnière deformity. The volar plate slips dorsally past the proximal interphalangeal joint.

The signs and symptoms of phalanx fractures are similar to those of metacarpal fractures (see Table 13–13). The athlete may describe hearing a snap at the time of injury, especially when the proximal or middle phalanges are injured. Pain is centered over the fracture site and gross deformity may be present in the finger's alignment. Soft tissue swelling and hematoma formation increase the amount of pain associated with the fracture and impair the ability to palpate the injured area. Active range of motion is limited by pain or bony derangement. During finger flexion, a spiral or oblique fracture causes the portion of the finger distal to the fracture site to rotate so that the fingernails are not in line with each other.

Complications of Finger Fractures

Mallet finger occurs when an avulsion or stretching of an extensor tendon results in the inability to fully extend the distal phalanx (Fig. 13–41 and see Fig. 13–11B). This occurs when the DIP is forced into flexion, such as when the fingertip is struck with a ball. In addition to being unable to actively extend the finger, the athlete reports pain in the distal phalanx, which rests at approximately 25 to 35 degrees of flexion. Active

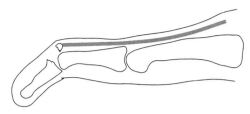

Figure 13–41. Illustration of a mallet finger. The extensor tendon is avulsed from its attachment on the distal phalanx.

flexion is still present and the phalanx can be passively moved into extension.

An avulsion of the flexor digitorum profundus tendon, **jersey finger**, results in the athlete's being unable to flex the DIP joint (Fig. 13–42 and see Fig. 13–11C). This commonly occurs as the athlete grasps another athlete's jersey, forcing the finger into extension as the finger is attempting to flex and hold onto the opponent. The jersey finger injury is described as being one of three types.[17]

First-degree: The bony attachment is left intact and the ruptured tendon retracts to the PIP joint.
Second-degree: A portion of the bony attachment is avulsed and the tendon retracts to the palm.
Third-degree: A fragment of bone is avulsed with the tendon's insertion and retracts to the PIP joint.

On casual inspection and functional testing the involved finger appears to be normal. The finger is painful, but little swelling or disfiguration is noted. The fingers appear to flex and extend normally, with an increase in pain noted during flexion. The tell-tale sign occurs when the examiner stabilizes the PIP joint in extension and requests that the athlete flex the DIP joint, but the athlete is unable to do so.

Thumb Pathology

The thumb is involved in most aspects of athletics and the position it assumes when gripping, catching, or in the "ready position" exposes it to po-

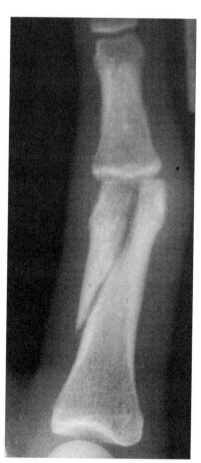

Figure 13–40. X ray of a phalanx fracture. Note that this is a spiral fracture involving the articular surface.

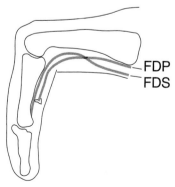

Figure 13–42. Illustration of "jersey finger." The distal interphalangeal joint cannot be flexed secondary to an avulsion of the flexor digitorum profundus tendon (FDP = flexor digitorum profundus; FDS = flexor digitorum superficialis).

tentially injurious forces in all planes. Unlike the other digits, the thumb is also susceptible to overuse conditions.

deQuervain's Syndrome

deQuervain's syndrome is a tenosynovitis of the extensor pollicis brevis and abductor pollicis longus tendons, which are encased by a fibrous sheath having a common synovial lining. Repetitive stress results in the compartment's becoming inflamed, and prolonged inflammation causes a thickening and narrowing of the tendon's sheath. A history of this condition reveals a mechanism of repetitive motions usually involving radial deviation.[18] The athlete has pain at the radial styloid process and dorsum of the thumb, which radiates proximally into the forearm. Swelling may be lo-cated over the styloid process and thenar eminence. Radial and ulnar deviation of the wrist results in pain as do flexion and abduction of the thumb (Table 13–14). Although not conclusive, **Finkelstein's test** may be used to support or refute the presence of deQuervain's syndrome.

Finkelstein's Test

Finkelstein's test involves the athlete's actively flexing and abducting the thumb by making a fist around the thumb and then ulnarly deviating the wrist (Fig. 13–43).[19] This motion passively stretches the extensor pollicis brevis and abductor pollicis longus muscles. Results of this test are often positive in otherwise normal wrists, so the results must be correlated with other evaluative findings.

Finkelstein's Test (Fig. 13–43)

Position of athlete	Seated or standing.
Position of examiner	Standing in front of the athlete.
Evaluative procedure	The athlete flexes and adducts the thumb, tucking the thumb under the fingers by making a fist. The athlete ulnarly deviates the wrist.
Positive test results	Increased pain in the area of the radial styloid process.
Implications	deQuervain's syndrome (tenosynovitis of the extensor pollicis brevis and abductor pollicis longus tendons).
Comments	Results of this test are often positive in otherwise healthy wrists, so the results must be correlated with other findings of the evaluation.

Table 13–14. Evaluative Findings of deQuervain's Syndrome

Examination Segment	Clinical Findings	
History	Onset:	Insidious.
	Location of pain:	Over the radial styloid process and thenar eminence, radiating into the forearm. Complaints of pain are increased during radial and ulnar deviation.
	Mechanism:	Repetitive stress often involving radial deviation.
Inspection	There is swelling over the styloid process and in the involved tendons.	
Palpation	Pain is felt over the styloid process, thenar eminence, and the length of the extensor pollicis brevis and abductor pollicis longus muscles.	
Functional tests	AROM: Wrist: Pain occurs with radial and ulnar deviation. Thumb: Pain occurs with flexion and adduction. PROM: Wrist: Pain occurs with ulnar deviation. Thumb: Pain occurs with flexion and adduction. RROM: Wrist: Pain occurs with radial deviation. Thumb: Pain occurs with extension and abduction.	
Ligamentous tests	Not applicable.	
Neurological tests	Not applicable.	
Special tests	Finkelstein's test.	
Comments	The definitive diagnosis of deQuervain's syndrome is made by a physician.	

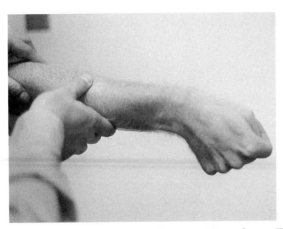

Figure 13–43. Finkelstein's test for deQuervain's syndrome. This test results in a duplication of the symptoms. Note that many false positive results are elicited by this test.

Thumb Sprains

The ulnar collateral ligament of the MCP joint is injured 10 times more often than its radial counterpart.[20] This structure may be acutely sprained by hyperabduction and/or hyperextension of the MCP joint, or it may be traumatized secondary to a repetitive stress. In the case of acute trauma, an associated avulsion fracture may occur around the MC joint. The term "gamekeeper's thumb" was coined to describe the stretching of this ligament suffered by individuals whose duty it was to snap the neck of small game that had just been captured during hunting. Regardless of the onset of this injury, it is important to recognize it because of the potential impairment of thumb opposition.

The athlete's chief complaint is pain along the ulnar aspect of the joint, which hinders the ability to forcefully pinch or grasp smaller objects. Swelling tends to be localized in the adductor compartment and thenar eminence. During palpation, tenderness is elicited over the UCL, with special attention paid to its proximal and distal attachments, noting for signs of an avulsion. Pain is produced and a strength deficit noted during opposition of the thumb and index finger (Table 13–15). Stress testing of the UCL demonstrates an increase in the amount of gapping present as compared with the uninjured hand. Stress testing should be carried out with the thumb extended as well as flexed.[21]

Metacarpophalangeal Joint Dislocation

Dislocation of the MCP joint is most common in the thumb and occurs when the volar plate is avulsed from the head of the first metacarpal.[22] The mechanism of injury is extension and abduction, and a fracture of the proximal phalanx or first metacarpal may occur concurrently. The involved joint has obvious deformity and is unable to demonstrate active motion because of pain.

Thumb Fractures

Fractures of the first metacarpal are similar to the description given for metacarpal fractures of the hand. Fractures of the first metacarpal that extend into the articular surface are termed **Benett's fractures** (Fig. 13–44). Because of the thumb's potential loss of function secondary to instability at the CMC joint, this type of fracture often requires the need for an internal or external fixation of the bony fracture.

Table 13–15. Evaluative Findings of an Ulnar Collateral Ligament Sprain of the Thumb

Examination Segment	Clinical Findings
History	Onset: Acute or chronic. Location of pain: Along the ulnar aspect of the first metacarpophalangeal joint. Mechanism: Acute: Hyperextension and/or hyperabduction of the first metacarpophalangeal joint. Chronic: Repetitive flexion and/or adduction of the joint.
Inspection	Swelling is localized in the adductor compartment and thenar eminence.
Palpation	Pain is felt along the ulnar border of the joint. The examiner should note for the presence of bony fragments indicating an avulsion of the ligament.
Functional tests	AROM: Pain occurs during extension, adduction, and opposition of the thumb. PROM: Pain occurs during thumb extension and adduction. RROM: Weakness is experienced during flexion and abduction. Pinch strength is decreased.
Ligamentous tests	Test for ulnar collateral ligament instability.
Neurological tests	Not applicable.
Special tests	None.
Comments	Significant UCL sprains should be referred to a physician for further evaluation to rule out an avulsion fracture.

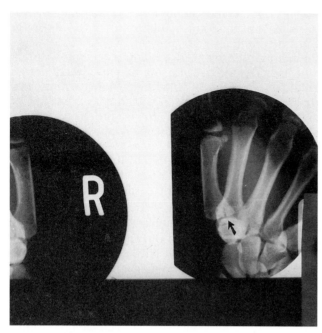

Figure 13–44. X ray of a Bennett's fracture.

ON-FIELD MANAGEMENT OF WRIST, HAND, AND FINGER INJURIES

Most often, athletes with a wrist, hand, or finger injury leave the field on their own, cradling and protecting the injured extremity. The examiner must carry out a complete inspection of the injured area, a task that is somewhat eased by the relatively superficial nature of the structures. With the exception of trauma to the carpal bones, deformity is usually obvious and may involve open or closed fractures and/or dislocation of the fingers.

Typically the injured hand and wrist are not covered by equipment. In certain sports such as football, ice hockey, and lacrosse the athlete may wear a glove. In these cases the glove is most easily, and with the least amount of pain, removed by the athlete.

Wrist Fractures and Dislocations

Fractures of the radius and/or ulna as well as dislocations of the radiocarpal joint must be immobilized in the position in which they are found, using a vacuum-type splint (Fig. 13–45). Before splinting the area, the radial and ulnar arterial pulses should be evaluated. As with any fracture, the joint itself or the joint above and below the fracture site should be immobilized.

Suspected fractures or dislocations of the carpal bones can be carefully supported and the athlete moved off the field to be further evaluated. If a fracture is suspected, the wrist should be immobilized as previously described.

Interphalangeal Joint Dislocation

Dislocation of an IP joint results in obvious deformity (Fig. 13–45). In some instances the athlete instinctively reduces the dislocation by applying traction to the finger. However, the on-field reduction of these dislocations is discouraged because of the possibility of an underlying fracture or an avulsed piece of bone or ligament becoming lodged within the joint space. The palmar aspect of the injured finger should be splinted in the position in which it was found, an ice pack applied to the dorsal side, and the athlete referred to a physician.

Hand and Finger Fractures

When fractures of the hand are suspected, the hand should be splinted so that the wrist and fingers are also immobilized, but the fingernails should remain uncovered so that their vascularity can be checked. Finger fractures should be splinted in the position in which they are found using an aluminum splint that also immobilizes the MCP joint, although a standard tongue depressor is often sufficient. Table 13–16 describes the splinting position for other common finger injuries.

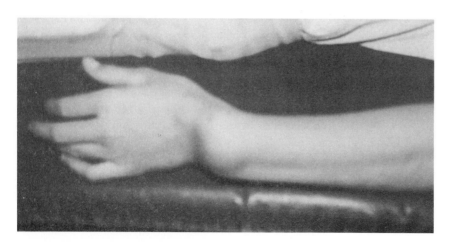

Figure 13–45. Wrist dislocation. Note that the radius and ulna are displaced posteriorly to the hand (relative to the anatomical position).

Table 13–16. Splinting of Common Finger Injuries

Deformity	Splinting Position
Jersey finger	Distal interphalangeal joint in flexion
Mallet finger	Distal interphalangeal joint in extension
Boutonnière deformity	Proximal and distal interphalangeal joints in extension

Lacerations

Because of the relatively superficial location of the tendons and nerves in the wrist, hand, and fingers, they are vulnerable to damage from even shallow lacerations. As with any cut, the possibility of infection exists. Any laceration involving the fascia below the cutaneous level should be referred to a physician to rule out the possibility of trauma to these structures and the possible need for suturing.

REFERENCES

1. Norkin, CC, and Levangie, PK: The wrist and hand complex. In Norkin, CC, and Levangie, PK: Joint Structure and Function: A Comprehensive Analysis, ed 2. FA Davis, Philadelphia, 1992, p 267.
1a. Kendall, FP, and McCreary, EK: Muscles: Testing and Function, ed 3. Williams & Wilkins, Baltimore, 1983.
1b. Daniels, L, and Worthingham, C: Muscle Testing: Techniques of Manual Examination, ed 5. WB Saunders, Philadelphia, 1986.
1c. Stanley, BG, and Tribuzi, SM: Concepts in Hand Rehabilitation. FA Davis, Philadelphia, 1992.
1d. Norkin, CC, and White, DJ: Measurement of Joint Motions: A Guide to Goniometry, ed 2. FA Davis, Philadelphia, 1995.
2. Frykman, GK, and Nelson, EF: Fractures and traumatic conditions of the wrist. In Hunter, J, et al: Rehabilitation of the Hand: Surgery and Therapy, ed 3. CV Mosby, St Louis, 1990, p 267.
3. Trousdale, RT, et al: Radio-ulnar dissociation. A review of twenty cases. J Bone Joint Surg Am 74:1486, 1992.
4. Palmer, AK, and Werner, FW: The triangular fibrocartilage complex of the wrist—anatomy and function. J Hand Surg [Am] 6:153, 1981.
5. Phalen, GS: The carpal tunnel syndrome: Seventeen years' experience in diagnosis and treatment of 654 hands. J Bone Joint Surg Am 48:211, 1966.
6. Phalen, GS: The carpal tunnel syndrome: Clinical evaluation of 598 hands. Clin Orthop 83:29, 1972.
7. Inglis, AE, Straub, LR, and Williams, CS: Median nerve neuropathy at the wrist. Clin Orthop 83:48, 1972.
8. Bechtol, C: Grip test: The use of a dynamometer with adjustable handle spacings. J Bone Joint Surg Am 36:L820, 1954.
9. Zimmerman, GR: Carpal tunnel syndrome. Journal of Athletic Training 29:22, 1994.
10. Colles, A: On the fracture of the carpal extremity of the radius. Edinb Med Surg J 10:182, 1814.
11. Thoms, FB: Reduction of Smith's fractures. J Bone Joint Surg Br 39:463, 1959.
12. Cave, EF: The carpus with reference to the fractured navicular bone. Arch Surg 40:54, 1940.
13. Taleisnick, J, and Kelly, PJ: The extraosseous and intraosseous blood supply to the scaphoid bone. J Bone Joint Surg Am 48:1126, 1966.
14. Dobyns, JH, and Linsheid, RL: Fractures and dislocations in the wrist. In Rockwood, CA, and Green, DP (eds): Fractures in Adults, ed 2. JB Lippincott, Philadelphia, 1984, p 411.
15. Campbell, RD, Lance, EM, and Yeoh, CB: Lunate and perilunate dislocations. J Bone Joint Surg Br 46:55, 1964.
16. Rettig, RC, et al: Metacarpal fractures in the athlete. Am J Sports Med 17:567, 1989.
17. Leddy, JP, and Packer, JW: Avulsion of the profundus tendon insertion in athletes. J Hand Surg [Am] 2:66, 1977.
18. Lipscomb, PR: Stenosing tenosynovitis at the radial styloid process. Ann Surg 134:110, 1951.
19. Finklestein, H: Stenosing tendovaginitis at the radial styloid process. J Bone Joint Surg Am 12:509, 1930.
20. Lane, LB: Acute grade III ulnar collateral ligament ruptures: A new surgical and rehabilitation protocol. Am J Sports Med 19:234, 1991.
21. McCue, FC, Mayer, V, and Moran, DJ: Gamekeeper's thumb: Ulnar collateral ligament rupture. Journal of Musculoskeletal Medicine 5:53, 1988.
22. Rettig, AC: Hand injuries in football players: Soft-tissue trauma. The Physician and Sportsmedicine 19:97, 1991.

14

The Eye

Resulting from a direct blow, an impalement, or a chemical invasion, trauma to the eye requires an accurate assessment so that proper management and further evaluation by an *ophthalmologist* can be initiated. Failure to recognize trauma to the eye and/or improper management can result in permanent dysfunction, including blindness.

Racquet sports, in which the ball can reach speeds up to 140 mph, boxing, and golf are most often associated with catastrophic injury to the eye, but traumatic injury to the eye can occur in all sports, with basketball being the most common.[1] Ninety percent of all eye injuries can be prevented through the use of approved protective eye wear.

CLINICAL ANATOMY

The eye sits encased within the conical bony **orbit**, surrounding all but the anterior aspect of the eye. In addition to protecting and stabilizing the eye, the orbit also serves as an attachment site for some of the extrinsic muscles acting on the eye. The **orbital margin** (periorbital region) comprises the **frontal bone**, forming the supraorbital margin; the **zygomatic bone** and a portion of the frontal bone, forming the lateral margin; and the zygomatic bone and **maxillary bone**, forming the infraorbital margin (Fig. 14-1).

The anterior portion of the orbit's roof is formed by the frontal bone, with a portion of the **sphenoid bone** forming its posterior aspect. Medially the orbit is formed by the very thin **ethmoid bone**, and the floor, by the maxillary, zygomatic, and **palatine bones**. Laterally the orbit is the thickest, composed of the zygomatic bone and the sphenoid bone. The **superior orbital fissure**, an opening between the lesser and greater wings of the sphenoid bone, is located between the lateral wall and the roof. This fissure allows the cranial nerves, arteries, and veins to communicate with the eye. The orbit's posterior aspect is marked by the **optic canal**, the foramen through which the optic nerve passes to reach the brain.

The Eye

The mass of the eye is a fibrous, fluid-filled structure collectively referred to as the **globe**. Its white layering, the **sclera**, encompasses the posterior five-sixths of the globe and becomes continuous with the sheath of the optic nerve as the nerve continues posteriorly and merges with the brain's fibrous lining. The dark central aperture of the eye, the **pupil**, is surrounded by pigmented contractile tissue, the **iris** (Fig. 14-2). The **conjunctiva** is a thin mucous membrane covering the sclera and lines the inside of the eyelids. Anteriorly, the conjunctiva is continuous with the transparent **cornea**. The cornea is the main structure involved in bending light rays entering the eye.

Suspended by ligaments arising from the **ciliary body**, the **lens** is a clear elastic structure located behind the iris that serves to sharpen and focus visual rays on the globe's posterior surface, the **retina**. The innermost surface (the surface facing the center of the globe) of the retina contains nervous tissues having an outward layer of darkly pigmented vascular tissue, the **choroid**. Light rays strike the nervous tissues, stimulating the **rods** and **cones**, photoreceptors located on the globe's posterior surface. Each receptor passes its stimulus through a complex network of nerves until the impulses are collected and transmitted to the brain via the **optic nerve**. Rods and cones are absent at the optic nerve, thus causing a blind spot in the field of vision (Fig. 14-3).

Eyelids act as shutters to protect the eye from accidental direct contact by reflexively closing when an object comes close to the exposed globe and by preventing airborne dust and dirt from entering the eye. The conjunctiva of the globe is continuous with the inner surfaces of the eyelids, secreting a fluid that moistens and lubricates the anterior portion of the eye.

Ophthalmologist: A medical doctor specializing in injury, diseases, and abnormalities of the eye.

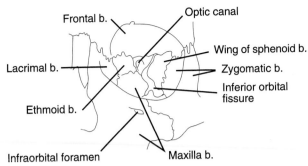

Figure 14–1. Bony anatomy of the orbit and orbital rim (periorbital region).

Muscular Anatomy

Six muscles control the movement of the globe (Fig. 14–4). The inferior, medial, lateral, and superior **rectus muscles** rotate the globe toward the contracting muscle (e.g., the inferior rectus rotates the eye downward). The two **obliques**, the inferior and superior, move the eye diagonally relative to the muscle's orientation (e.g., the inferior oblique directs the eye upward and laterally) (Table 14–1).

Visual Acuity

The quality of an individual's vision is most commonly determined through the use of **Snellen's chart** (Fig. 14–5). This method determines the athlete's ability to clearly see letters based on a normalized scale. An athlete having 20/20 vision (**emmetropia**) is able to read the letters on the 20-ft line of an eye chart when standing 20 ft from the chart, indicating that the light rays come into focus precisely on the retina. **Myopia**, nearsightedness, occurs when the light rays come into focus in front of the retina, making only those objects very close to the eyes distinguishable. **Hypermetropia** (hyperopia), farsightedness, results when the light rays come into focus at a point behind the retina. Athletes who demonstrate significant diminished visual acuity may require further assessment to enhance performance and ensure safe participation.

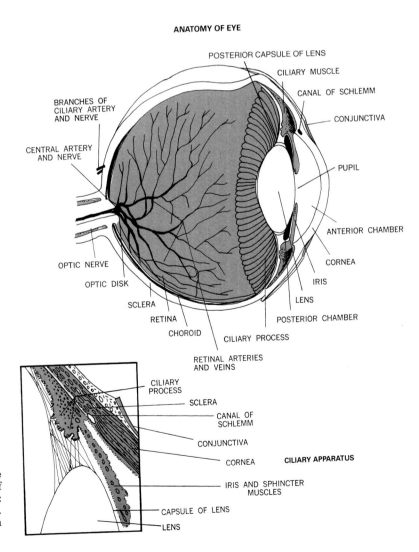

Figure 14–2. Cross-sectional view of the anatomy of the eye with an enlargement of the ciliary apparatus. (From Thomas, CL [ed]: Taber's Cyclopedic Medical Dictionary, ed 17. FA Davis, Philadelphia, 1993, p 698, with permission.)

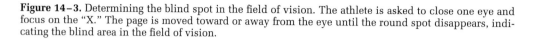

Figure 14–3. Determining the blind spot in the field of vision. The athlete is asked to close one eye and focus on the "X." The page is moved toward or away from the eye until the round spot disappears, indicating the blind area in the field of vision.

CLINICAL EVALUATION OF EYE INJURIES

Blunt trauma to the eye can result in injury to the globe and its related structures, laceration of the periorbital skin, or a fracture of the bony orbit. Infections, diseases, allergies, and brain trauma can also lead to dysfunction of the eye. Because of the eye's delicate nature, all maladies involving the eye should be handled with the utmost care and urgency (Table 14–2). The supplies necessary for the evaluation and management of eye injuries are presented in Table 14–3.[2]

History

A complete history is most useful in determining the nature and extent of the athlete's eye injury. With the exception of dysfunction occurring secondary to infection, disease, or allergy, all eye injuries have an acute onset.

Location and description of the symptoms: The athlete may complain of **photophobia**. Complaints of scratchiness or "something in the eye" may be caused not only by a foreign body but also by a displaced contact lens or a **corneal abrasion**. Itching of the eye is usually associated with edema of the conjunctiva (chemosis) caused by an allergy. Disruption of

the normal visual field may also be described. These findings are discussed in the Functional Testing section of this chapter.

Injury mechanism: The size and elastic properties of the object striking the eye are key determinants of the subsequent injury. Hard objects that are larger than the orbital rim transmit forces directly to the eye's bony margin. Elastic objects or objects smaller than the orbital margin deliver forces directly to the eye. Elastic objects are of particular concern as the expansive force may be of a magnitude sufficient to rupture the globe.

Size Relative to the Orbit	Elastic Property	Resulting Pathology
Larger	Hard	Orbital fracture, periorbital contusion
Larger	Elastic	Blow-out fracture, ruptured globe, corneal abrasion, traumatic iritis
Smaller	Hard	Ruptured globe, corneal abrasion, corneal laceration, traumatic iritis
Smaller	Elastic	Ruptured globe, blow-out fracture, corneal abrasion, traumatic iritis

Injury may also be caused by chemicals or other foreign substances entering the eye. In athletics, the common substances that may be encountered in addition to dirt and sand are lime (or other field marking agents), chlorine, or fertilizers and pesticides used for maintaining grass fields. If a foreign substance enters the eye, a sample of it should be transported to the hospital with the athlete.

Prior visual assessment: The athlete's medical record should be used to ascertain prior visual acuity, the need for corrective lenses (glasses or contact lenses), and any relevant history of previous eye injuries.

Inspection

Because all but the most anterior portion of the eye is hidden from view, trauma to its external structures, the eyelid and the eyebrow, may mask underlying pathology. The presence of the findings

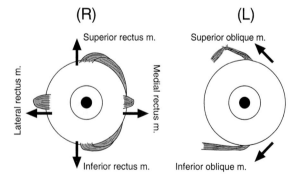

Figure 14–4. Extrinsic muscles of the eye. The right eye is used to present the rectus muscles, which move the globe in the cardinal planes. The left eye describes the oblique muscles, which abduct and adduct the globe.

Photophobia: The eye's intolerance to light.

Table 14-1. Extrinsic Eye Muscles

Muscle	Action	Origin	Insertion	Nerve	Root
Inferior rectus	Rotates globe downward	From a tendinous ring on the posterior aspect of the orbit	Middle of the inferior aspect of the anterior globe	Oculomotor	CN III
Superior rectus	Rotates globe upward	From a tendinous ring on the posterior aspect of the orbit	Middle of the superior aspect of the anterior globe	Oculomotor	CN III
Medial rectus	Rotates globe medially	From a tendinous ring on the posterior aspect of the orbit	Middle of the medial aspect of the anterior globe	Oculumotor	CN III
Lateral rectus	Rotates globe laterally	From a tendinous ring on the posterior aspect of the orbit	Middle of the lateral aspect of the anterior globe	Abducens	CN VI
Inferior oblique	Rotates globe superiorly and medially	From the floor of the anterior orbit, maxillary bone	Middle of the inferior aspect of the anterior globe, posterior to the inferior rectus	Oculomotor	CN III
Superior oblique	Rotates globe inferiorly and laterally	From a tendinous ring on the posterior aspect of the orbit	Middle of the superior aspect of the anterior globe, posterior to the superior rectus	Trochlear	CN IV

CN = cranial nerve.

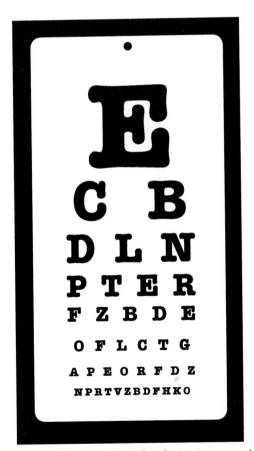

Figure 14–5. Snellen-type chart. This device is commonly used to determine an individual's visual acuity.

listed in Table 14–4 indicates the need for immediate referral for further assessment by an ophthalmologist, as do any questions regarding the nature or extent of injury to the eye.

The Periorbital Area

• **Discoloration:** A simple **orbital hematoma** (or black eye) is common with blunt injuries and may have no consequence other than its abnormal appearance. However, external trauma to the eyelid, orbit, or conjunctiva may alter their function and indicate trauma to the eye itself.[3]

• **Gross deformity:** Gross bony deformity of the orbit is rare and its presence indicates a significant condition requiring immediate medical intervention. The loose skin surrounding the eye and eyelid is easily swollen after an injury and the swelling is often less significant than it appears. Lacerations are common secondary to direct trauma and should be managed using the appropriate universal precautions.

The Globe

• **General appearance:** The examiner observes the appearance of the globe as it sits within the orbit relative to the uninvolved eye. Orbital frac-

Table 14–2. Evaluation of the Eye

History	Inspection	Palpation	Functional Tests	Ligamentous Tests	Neurological Tests	Special Tests
Location of the symptoms	Periorbital Area	Orbital margin	Vision assessment	Not applicable	Cranial nerve check	Orbital fracture
Description of the symptoms	Discoloration	Related areas	Pupil reaction to light		Numbness of lateral	Corneal abrasion
Injury mechanism	Gross deformity	Soft tissue	Eye motility		nose and cheek	Fluorescein strips
Prior visual assessment					Pupillary response	Cobalt-blue light
Eyewear worn	Globe					Corneal laceration
	General					Iritis
	appearance					Detached retina
	Eyelids					Ruptured globe
	Cornea					Conjunctivitis
	Conjunctiva					Foreign bodies
	Sclera					
	Iris					
	Pupil shape and					
	size					

Table 14–3. Supplies Needed for the Evaluation and Management of Eye Injuries

Evaluation Supplies	Management Supplies
Snellen's chart or similar	Eye shield
Penlight	Eye patch
Cobalt-blue light	Tape
Small mirror	Plunger for removing hard
Fluorescein strips	contact lenses
Antibiotic eyedrops	Sterile irrigation solution
Anesthetic eyedrops	Sterile cotton swabs
Telephone number of	Contact lens case
ophthalmologist	Steri-Strips or butterfly
Telephone number of	bandages
hospital and poison	
control center	

tures can cause the globe to be displaced inferiorly or posteriorly (enophthalmos) or to bulge anteriorly (exophthalmos) within the orbit.[4]

- **Eyelids:** The examiner inspects the eyelid for signs of acute injury, such as swelling, ecchymosis, and/or lacerations, which may obscure serious underlying pathology of the globe (Fig. 14–6). An infection of a ***ciliary gland*** or ***sebaceous gland***, a stye, is caused by bacteria and results in general lid edema, focal tenderness, and redness of the involved lid.

- **Cornea:** Normally crystal clear, any discoloration of the cornea indicates trauma warranting the immediate termination of the evaluation and subsequent referral to an ophthalmologist. Increased intraocular pressure may result in corneal cloudiness. **Hyphema**, the collection of blood within the anterior chamber of the eye, is caused by the rupture of a blood vessel supplying the iris (Fig. 14–7).

- **Conjunctiva:** The normal appearance of the conjunctiva is transparent as it covers the white sclera anteriorly. To view the inferior portion of the conjunctiva, the examiner gently pulls down on the athlete's eyelid as the athlete looks upward. To view the upper conjunctiva, the examiner gently lifts the upper eyelid while the athlete looks downward. If a foreign body is suspected, the upper conjunctiva is viewed by gently everting the upper eyelid with a cotton-tipped applicator (Fig. 14–8).

- **Sclera:** Leakage of the superficial blood vessels, ***subconjunctival hematoma***, is a common benign condition but is of concern because of its potential to conceal underlying pathology (Fig. 14–9).[5] The appearance of a black object on the sclera should be viewed with concern, as it may actually be the inner tissue of the eye bulging outward through a wound.

Table 14–4. Findings Sufficient to Immediately Refer the Athlete to an Ophthalmologist

History	Inspection	Palpation	Functional Tests	Neurological Tests
Loss of all or part of the visual field	Foreign body protruding into the eye	Crepitus of the orbital rim	Restricted eye movement	Numbness over the lateral nose and cheek
Persistent blurred vision	Laceration involving the margin of the eyelid		Double vision occurring with eye movement	Pupillary reaction abnormality
Diplopia	Deep laceration of the lid			
Photophobia	Inability to open the eyelid because of swelling			
Throbbing or penetrating pain around the eye	Protrusion of the globe (or other obvious displacement)			
Mechanism for a ruptured globe	*Injected* conjunctiva with a small pupil			
	Loss of corneal clarity			
	Hyphema			
	Pupillary distortion			
	Unilateral pupillary dilation or constriction			

Ciliary gland: A form of sweat gland on the eyelid.
Sebaceous gland: Oil-secreting gland of the skin.
Injected: Congested with blood or other fluids forced into an area.
Subconjunctival hematoma: Leakage of the superficial blood vessels beneath the sclera.

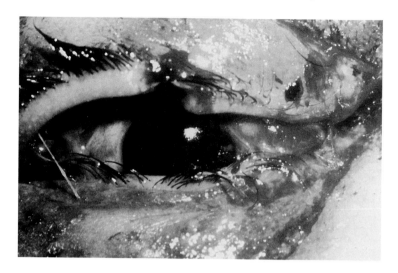

Figure 14–6. Laceration of the eyelid. This injury may also conceal underlying eye trauma.

• **Iris:** Marked conjunctival injection adjacent to the cornea indicates the presence of inflammation, iritis.

• **Pupil shape and size:** The pupils are normally equal in size and shape, although *anisocoria* may be congenital or associated with brain trauma. Any irregularity in the pupil's shape is an ominous sign of a serious injury. An elliptical or "teardrop" pupil is of serious concern because of the possibility of a **corneal laceration** or **ruptured globe** (Fig. 14–10).

Palpation

Assessment of eye injuries should never include palpation nor probing of the globe itself. Superficial bony structures and the soft tissue about the eye may be safely palpated for signs of an injury.

Bony Palpation

• **Orbital margin:** The examiner palpates the circumference of the orbital rim for signs of tenderness or crepitus indicating the presence of an orbital fracture. The bony prominence of the orbit may become obscured secondary to swelling (Fig. 14–11).

• **Related areas:** Injuries caused by blunt trauma should also include a general palpation of the frontal, nasal, and zygomatic bones to rule out concurrent injury.

Soft Tissue Palpation

The eyelid and skin surrounding the eye may be palpated, but injury to these areas is usually apparent during inspection.

Functional Tests

During the preparticipation physical examination the athlete's visual acuity, required corrective devices (glasses and/or contact lenses), and history of previous eye injury should be deter-

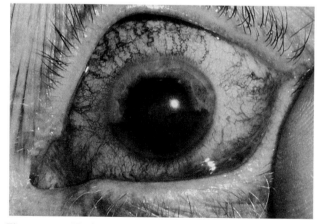

Figure 14–7. Hyphema, a collection of blood within the anterior chamber of the eye.

Anisocoria: Unequal pupil sizes; may be a benign congenital condition or may occur secondary to brain trauma.

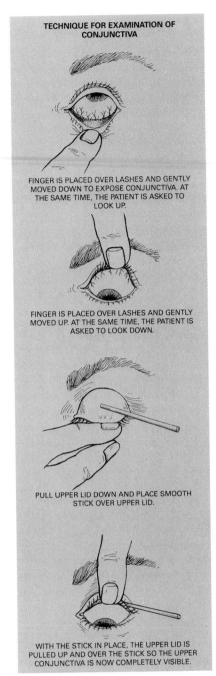

TECHNIQUE FOR EXAMINATION OF CONJUNCTIVA

FINGER IS PLACED OVER LASHES AND GENTLY MOVED DOWN TO EXPOSE CONJUNCTIVA. AT THE SAME TIME, THE PATIENT IS ASKED TO LOOK UP.

FINGER IS PLACED OVER LASHES AND GENTLY MOVED UP. AT THE SAME TIME, THE PATIENT IS ASKED TO LOOK DOWN.

PULL UPPER LID DOWN AND PLACE SMOOTH STICK OVER UPPER LID.

WITH THE STICK IN PLACE, THE UPPER LID IS PULLED UP AND OVER THE STICK SO THE UPPER CONJUNCTIVA IS NOW COMPLETELY VISIBLE.

Figure 14–8. Inspection of the upper surface of the eye. The upper eyelid is inverted around a cotton-tipped applicator to expose the upper portion of the sclera and conjunctiva. (From Thomas, CL [ed]: Taber's Cyclopedic Medical Dictionary, ed 17. FA Davis, Philadelphia, 1993, p 699, with permission.)

mined and included as a part of the medical record. Any congenital pupillary changes, nystagmus, or other deformity should also be noted to compare with any subsequent examination findings.

> **Vision assessment:** Vision can be assessed through the use of Snellen's chart (see Fig. 14–5), a near-vision card, or even a newspaper or game program. Vision assessment should be performed monocularly (one eye) and binocularly (both eyes). Athletes who require the use of glasses or contact lenses should be wearing these at the time of the vision assessment. Athletes should be able to read the 20/20 line on Snellen's chart or be able to read standard newspaper print held 16 inches from the eye.[6] If the athlete is unable to read the chart, fingers may be held up at different distances. Athletes who do not display 20/20 vision or describe diplopia following an injury should be referred for evaluation by an ophthalmologist.
>
> Blurred vision that clears upon blinking the eye indicates the formation of mucus or other debris floating in the surface of the eye and is not considered to be a significant finding.[2] Loss of portions of the visual field, typically described as a shade or curtain being pulled over the eye, can indicate a detached retina. Double vision can indicate an orbital fracture, brain trauma, damage to the optic or cranial nerves, or injury to the eye's extrinsic muscles.
>
> **Pupil reaction to light:** Pupillary dysfunction is also associated with significant head trauma and may include dilation, diminished reactivity to light, or asymmetry (see top of page 444).
>
> **Eye motility:** The eyes' ability to perform a complete sweep of the range of motion in a smooth, symmetrical manner through the eye's field of gaze is a key finding of the examination (Fig. 14–12). Asymmetrical motion or movement that results in double vision is considered to be a significant finding (see middle of page 444).

Neurological Tests

The muscles of the eye are controlled sympathetically or parasympathetically by cranial nerves III, IV, and VI. A discussion of these nerves and their direct influence on the eyes is found in Chapter 16. Numbness in the cheek and lateral nose corresponds to the distribution of the infraorbital nerve and is indicative of an orbital floor fracture.

Pathologies and Related Special Tests

Injury to the globe almost always results in some degree of visual impairment, with or without outward signs of trauma. Periorbital injuries usually have no associated visual change. The potential of an associated head trauma during the assessment of eye injuries should be considered.

Pupillary Reaction Test

Position of athlete	Sitting.
Position of examiner	Standing in front of the athlete.
Evaluative procedure	A card, or the athlete's hand, is held in front of the eye not being tested. A penlight is used to shine light into the athlete's pupil for 1 sec and then removed. The examiner observes for the pupil constricting when the light is applied and dilating when the light is removed. This process is repeated for the opposite eye.
Positive test results	A pupil that is unresponsive to light or reacts sluggishly compared with the opposite eye.
Implications	A mechanical or neurological deficit of the iris.

Test for Eye Motility

Position of athlete	Seated.
Position of examiner	Standing in front of the athlete, hold a finger approximately 2 ft from the athlete's nose.
Evaluative procedure	The athlete focuses on the examiner's finger. The examiner moves the finger upward, downward, left, and right relative to the starting point. The athlete follows this motion using only the eye and is allowed to fix the gaze at the terminal end of each movement. The finger is then moved through the diagonal fields of gaze.
Positive test results	Asymmetrical tracking of the eyes or double vision produced at the end of the range of motion.
Implications	Decreased motility of the eyes.

Orbital Fracture

A blow to the eye received by an object that is larger than the orbit itself may result in a fracture of the frontal, zygomatic, or maxillary bones of the orbital rim. A deformable or irregularly shaped object, such as a ball or an elbow, can also deliver force to the globe with a magnitude sufficient to cause the

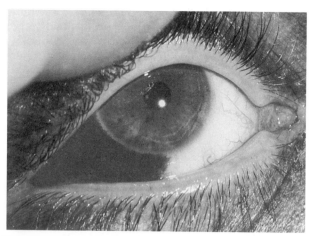

Figure 14–9. Subconjunctival hemorrhage. This condition by itself is usually benign but may conceal underlying pathology.

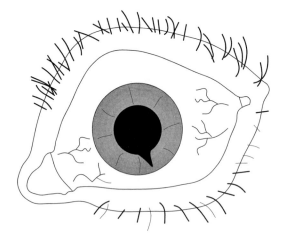

Figure 14–10. Teardrop pupil. This condition, or any other deviation in the normally round shape of the pupil, indicates serious underlying pathology such as a corneal laceration or ruptured globe.

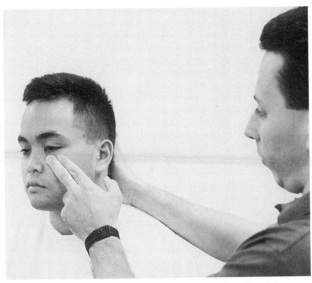

Figure 14–11. Palpation of the infraorbital rim. Only a physician should palpate the globe itself.

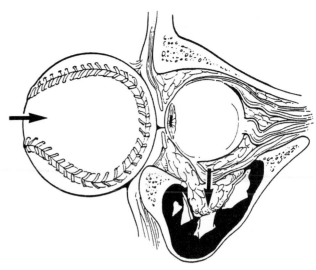

Figure 14–13. Mechanism for an orbital floor "blow-out" fracture. The object striking the eye causes the globe to expand downward, rupturing the relatively thin floor. (From Matthews,[8] with permission.)

orbital floor or medial wall to rupture (Fig. 14–13). With this injury, termed a **blow-out fracture**, the athlete may have signs of diplopia when attempting to look upward and outward, a sunken or retracted globe, and numbness in the infraorbital area, although all of these symptoms may not be present.[7] Pieces of the maxillary portion of the orbital floor may entrap the inferior rectus muscle, mechanically limiting the athlete's ability to look upward (Fig. 14–14). The globe may seen sunken into the orbit or may bulge outward.[8]

Fractures of the medial wall of the orbit may initially be asymptomatic and go undiagnosed until the athlete blows his or her nose, at which time air escapes the nasal passage, enters the orbit, and exits from under the eyelids. A floor fracture or its subsequent swelling may cause infraorbital nerve entrapment, resulting in numbness of the lateral nose and cheek.

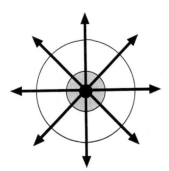

Figure 14–12. Field of gaze for the eye. An inspection of eye motility should involve these directions, noting equality of movement between the eyes.

Any deformity of the orbit, caused by bony fractures, entrapment of a muscle, or edema can disorient the eye's alignment and result in diplopia. The athlete may also describe periods of nausea and vomiting. Fractures of the orbital rim may produce focal tenderness and crepitus during palpation, although these symptoms are not always associated with a blow-out fracture (Table 14–5).

Corneal Abrasion

Scratching of the cornea may be caused by an external force directly striking the eye or by a foreign object such as sand or dirt being caught between the cornea and the eyelid. Contact lenses may also create a corneal abrasion. Subsequent blinking of the eyelids results in pain and the sensation of a foreign body on the eye, which may or may not still be present.

The eye sympathetically tears in an attempt to wash any invading particles from the eye. The athlete may describe a sharp, stabbing pain caused by exposed corneal nerves. If the abrasion involves the central visual axis, the athlete's vision may be blurred (Table 14–6). Under normal conditions the abrasion is not visible to the unaided eye and the definitive diagnosis is made through the use of fluorescein strips and a cobalt-blue light. The fluorescein strips serve as a dye that is absorbed only by the cells that are exposed after a corneal laceration (Fig. 14–15). When a cobalt-blue light is shined on the area, the abrasion becomes obvious.

Fluorescein Strip Test

Position of athlete	Seated or prone.
Position of examiner	Standing in front of or beside the athlete.
Evaluative procedure	The fluorescein strip is soaked with sterile saline solution. The wet fluorescein strip is touched lightly to the conjunctiva of the lower lid for a few seconds. The athlete then blinks the eye to spread the solution. Care must be taken to avoid placing the strip directly on the cornea. In a darkened room, the cobalt-blue light is used to illuminate the eye.
Positive test results	When viewed with the cobalt-blue light, corneal abrasions appear as a bright yellow-green pattern on the eye.
Implications	A corneal abrasion.

Corneal Laceration

Direct trauma from a sharp object to the eye can result in partial-thickness or full-thickness tears of the conjunctiva.[9] Partial-thickness tears are similar in their signs and symptoms to corneal abrasions (see Table 14–6), but with these lacerations the actual trauma to the cornea may be visible. Full-thickness tears are readily apparent either by the disruption in the normal translucent appearance of the cornea, a shallow anterior chamber, or the obvious opening of the laceration and subsequent spilling of its contents. Last, an irregularly shaped (elliptical or teardrop) pupil is suggestive of a corneal laceration.

Iritis

Minor blunt trauma to the eye can activate an inflammatory reaction within the anterior chamber, resulting in the "red eye" appearance associated with iritis. Although the inflammation of the iris itself may occur without pain, the athlete may describe the sensation of pressure within the globe and experience marked sensitivity to light. On inspection, the involved pupil is constricted relative to the opposite side, although in certain cases it appears dilated or normal.[10] The inflammatory cells within the anterior chamber may cause blurred vision. Assessment of pupillary reaction, determined through the use of a penlight, reveals a pupil that reacts sluggishly when compared with that of the uninjured eye (Table 14–7).

Detached Retina

A jarring force to the head can result in an interruption in the communication of the retina and the choroid. Although this mechanism can be delivered to the head, the jarring motion associated with sneezing may also be sufficient. The actual detachment of the retina is caused by the vitreous humor's seeping between the retina and the choroid, interrupting the nervous input being relayed to the optic nerve.

The athlete complains of flashes of light, halos, or blind spots within the normal field of vision. Retinal detachment can be diagnosed only by an ophthalmologist and normally requires surgical correction.

Ruptured Globe

The most catastrophic injury to the eye is a ruptured globe. Severe blunt trauma delivered to the globe itself (i.e., little or no force being dissipated by the orbital rim) can result in a rupture of the sclera, causing it to subsequently spill its contents. Commonly, these tears occur behind the insertion of the eye's extrinsic muscles (where the sclera is the thinnest) and therefore may not be visible, although black specks on the sclera are indicative of the contents of the eye spilling outward.

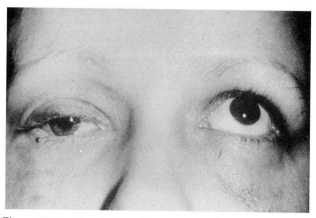

Figure 14–14. Restriction of eye motion following a blow-out fracture of the orbital floor. The athlete's right eye is unable to gaze upward, indicating an entrapment of the inferior rectus muscle.

Table 14–5. Evaluative Findings of an Orbital Fracture

Examination Segment	Clinical Findings
History	Onset: Acute. Location of pain: Orbital margin and possibly within the eye and orbit. Mechanism: A direct blow to the periorbital area or the globe itself. A blow-out fracture results when a blow increases the amount of pressure within the orbit, causing the orbital floor or medial wall to fracture.
Inspection	Ecchymosis and swelling may be present in the periorbital area. The eye may appear sunken posteriorly into the socket (enophthalmos) or may bulge outward (exophthalmos). A laceration of the periorbital area or eyelid may be associated with trauma.
Palpation	There may be tenderness in the periorbital area, although a blow-out fracture may produce no tenderness.
Functional tests	Vision: Diplopia, especially on end-gaze, may be described by the athlete. This is caused by an alteration in the shape of the orbit or may be secondary to the bony impingement of the eye's intrinsic musculature or to edema. Blurred vision may also be described. ROM: Although not a prerequisite symptom, blow-out fractures may result in the affected eye's inability to look upward or outward.
Ligamentous tests	Not applicable.
Neurological tests	Sensory testing of the cheek and lateral nose for infraorbital nerve involvement.
Special tests	CT scan, MRI, or x ray may be used to view the orbit.
Comments	Athletes suspected of suffering from an orbital fracture should be referred to an ophthalmologist for further evaluation. Athletes suspected of suffering a blow-out fracture should be instructed to refrain from blowing the nose.

Table 14–6. Evaluative Findings of a Corneal Abrasion

Examination Segment	Clinical Findings
History	Onset: Acute. Location of pain: Over the cornea and surrounding the conjunctiva, normally reported as "something in my eye." The pain may be intense. Mechanism: Direct contact to the cornea or a foreign object (e.g., sand) between the cornea and the eyelid, causing an abrasion.
Inspection	The eyes may water. Conjunctival redness is present. A small foreign object may be present. The actual abrasion is not visible under normal conditions.
Palpation	Not applicable.
Functional tests	Possible sensitivity to light. Vision may be blurred secondary to increased watering of the eye or to scratching of the central cornea.
Ligamentous tests	Not applicable.
Neurological tests	Not applicable.
Special tests	The presence of a corneal abrasion is definitively diagnosed through fluorescein strips and a cobalt-blue light.
Comments	Athletes suspected of having a corneal abrasion should be immediately referred to a physician, with the eye patched.

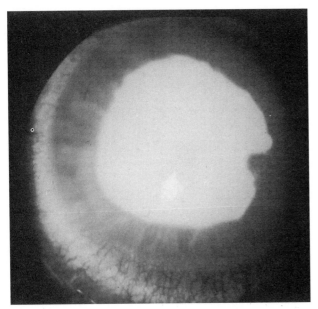

Figure 14–15. Corneal abrasion viewed with the use of fluorescein strips and a cobalt-blue light to highlight the abraded area.

Athletes suffering from a ruptured globe have pain and total or partial loss of vision. On inspection the globe may appear disoriented in the orbit and the anterior chamber may seem unusually deep. The conjunctiva has marked edema (chemosis), and the pupil may be elliptical or teardrop-shaped. Hyphema or a dark, coffee grain–like substance may be viewed within the anterior chamber as well (Table 14–8). However, many ruptured globes are relatively asymptomatic.

Athletes suspected of suffering from a ruptured globe should have an eyeshield placed over the eye and be immediately transported to the hospital. No type of eye drops should be administered and, because of the possibility of the need for immediate surgery, the athlete should be instructed not to eat or drink.

Conjunctivitis

Conjunctivitis, or "pinkeye," is the result of a viral or bacterial infection of the conjunctiva. The athlete usually first experiences the symptoms of conjunctivitis upon waking in the morning, at which time the eyelids may stick together and the eye burns and itches. The involved eye is red and swollen. The nature of the discharge usually dictates the etiology; that is, a watery discharge indicates a viral infection, whereas a yellow or green discharge indicates a bacterial infection. The affected eye may also be sensitive to light (Table 14–9). Note that this condition may develop secondary to improper cleaning and care of contact lenses.

Athletes with conjunctivitis, a highly contagious condition, should be instructed not to touch the affected eye to avoid spreading the contamination to the uninvolved eye. Likewise, athletes diagnosed with this condition should be barred from contact sports or from entering a swimming pool to prevent transmission of the disease to other athletes. Bacterial conjunctivitis is easily treated with antibacterial eyedrops. Therefore, athletes suspected of suffering from conjunctivitis should be immediately referred to a physician.

Table 14–7. Evaluative Findings of Traumatic Iritis

Examination Segment	Clinical Findings
History	Onset: Acute. Location of pain: Photophobia. Mechanism: A traumatic force to the eye that elicits an inflammatory cycle.
Inspection	The conjunctiva adjacent to the cornea is injected. The involved pupil may be constricted but on occasion may be dilated or normal.
Palpation	Not applicable.
Functional tests	The pupil is sluggishly reactive to light. Photophobia is usually described.
Ligamentous tests	Not applicable.
Neurological tests	Pupillary reaction.
Special tests	Not applicable.
Comments	Blunt trauma can result in a tearing of the iris sphincter, leading to permanent pupillary deformity.

Table 14–8. Evaluative Findings of a Ruptured Globe

Examination Segment	Clinical Findings
History	Onset: Acute. Location of pain: Throughout the eye. Mechanism: Severe blunt trauma to the globe.
Inspection	The globe may be obviously deformed. The anterior chamber may appear deepened. Hyphema or a black, grainy substance may be visible within the anterior chamber. The pupil may be elliptical or teardrop-shaped. The contents of the globe may bulge outward through the sclera, appearing as a black "foreign object" on the eye.
Palpation	Not applicable.
Functional tests	Vision is lost or markedly decreased in the affected eye.
Ligamentous tests	Not applicable.
Neurological tests	Not applicable.
Special tests	Not applicable.
Comments	Athletes suspected of having a ruptured globe should immediately be transported to the hospital, with a shield covering the eye. Patches should not be used, as direct pressure on the globe is to be avoided. No food or fluids should be permitted, as immediate surgery may be required.

Table 14–9. Evaluative Findings of Conjunctivitis

Examination Segment	Clinical Findings
History	Onset: Acute. Symptoms normally appear when the athlete awakes in the morning. Location of pain: Itchy, burning sensation in the affected eye. Photophobia may also be described. Mechanism: Viral or bacterial infection. This condition may result from improper cleaning and care of contact lenses.
Inspection	The involved eye appears red. Lid swelling may be present. Conjunctivitis is usually accompanied by a discharge. If a discharge is present, the color should be noted.
Palpation	Palpation is performed using latex gloves to prevent the infection from spreading to the examiner. The eyelids feel fluid-filled and boggy.
Functional tests	The athlete may complain of the eyelids sticking together. Vision may be hindered in the affected eye secondary to the inability to open the eye, swelling, and discharge.
Ligamentous tests	Not applicable.
Neurological tests	Not applicable.
Special tests	None.
Comments	Viral conjunctivitis is highly contagious and will likely spread to the other eye. Athletes suffering from this condition should refrain from contact with other athletes or from entering a swimming pool. Athletes suspected of suffering from conjunctivitis should be referred to a physician for further evaluation. The athlete must refrain from wearing contact lenses.

Foreign Bodies

A foreign body in the eye is a troublesome but usually benign condition that clears once the object has been removed from the eye; on occasion, however, a foreign object can lead to corneal abrasions. Additionally, foreign bodies are not to be confused with the impalement of the eye by an object.

An attempt should be made to locate the material causing the discomfort, as described in the Inspection section of this chapter. Once the particle has been located, it may be flushed out of the eye using a saline solution or water. A moistened cotton applicator or the corner of a gauze pad may also be used to blot the contaminant from the eye. Dry cotton should not be used on the eye as the fibers will stick to it and may induce a corneal abrasion. Athletes should be instructed to refrain from the instinct of rubbing the eye, as this may worsen the problem. Discomfort may be reduced by having the athlete hold the upper eyelid outward, allowing the eye to tear, possibly washing the particle from the eye.

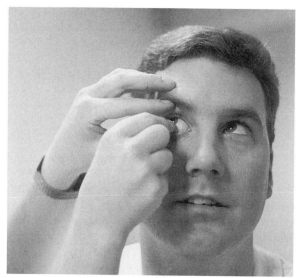

Figure 14–16. Removing a soft contact lens. Care must be taken not to insult the cornea or conjunctiva during this procedure.

ON-FIELD MANAGEMENT OF EYE INJURIES

The correct initial management of eye injuries greatly increases the chances of the long-term viability of the eye. Likewise, improper management can worsen the severity of the injury and increase the likelihood of permanent disability.

Removal of Contact Lenses

Trauma to the eye when swelling is imminent, such as with a periorbital contusion, requires that contact lenses be removed as soon as possible after the injury. Ideally, this is best performed by the athlete. However, certain circumstances may require assistance, because either the athlete is unable to do so or he or she cannot find the contact lens on the eye.

Hard contact lenses may be removed through the use of a plungerlike device or may be manually manipulated from the eye in the following manner:

• The athlete opens the eyes as wide as possible.

• The examiner pulls the outer margin of the eyelids laterally.

• While holding a hand under the eye to catch the lens, the athlete blinks, forcing the lens out of the eye.

Soft contact lenses should never be plucked directly from the eye, especially when they are resting on the cornea, as this may result in serious trauma to the eye. The following procedure is recommended for the removal of soft contact lenses (Fig. 14–16):

• The athlete is asked to look upward. This motion lifts a portion of the lens off the cornea.

• A finger is placed against the raised portion of the contact lens.

• The lens is manipulated inferiorly and laterally, to where it can be pinched between the fingers and safely removed from the eye.

• If the contact lens is torn, it is important to remove all pieces from the eye.

Orbital Fractures

Fractures to the orbital rim that are asymptomatic (other than pain) may require no extraordinary treatment other than ice packs loosely applied to the periorbital area, avoiding direct pressure on the globe. Fractures that cause pain during eye movement should be shielded with a plastic or metal guard, again avoiding direct pressure on the globe (Fig. 14–17). Because the eyes move in unison, the athlete should be instructed to gaze straight ahead with the uninvolved eye, thus limiting voluntary eye movement.

Penetrating Eye Injuries

Corneal lacerations and ruptured globes should be managed through the use of an eye shield, as described in the previous section. No attempt should be made to remove an object that is impaling the eye, and direct pressure on the globe should be avoided. If the object is protruding some distance outside of the eye, a foam, plastic, or paper cup may be used to cover and protect the eye. In this case both eyes should be covered to minimize movement.

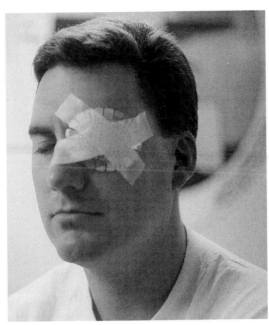

Figure 14-17. Protecting the eye with a metal shield. Because the eyes move in unison, it is recommended that the person close the uninvolved eye or stare straight ahead.

Chemical Burns

Following a chemical burn the eye should be thoroughly irrigated with large amounts of saline solution or water. The eye should then be patched and the athlete, along with a sample of the invading substance, immediately transported to a hospital.

REFERENCES

1. Zagelbaum, B: Sports-related eye trauma: Managing common injuries. The Physician and Sportsmedicine 21:25, 1993.
2. Whyte, DJ: Eye injuries. Athletic Training: Journal of the National Athletic Trainers Association 22:207, 1987.
3. Sandusky, JC: Field evaluation of eye injuries. Athletic Training: Journal of the National Athletic Trainers Association 16:254, 1981.
4. Halling, AH: The importance of clinical signs and symptoms in the evaluation of facial fractures. Athletic Training: Journal of the National Athletic Trainers Association 17:102, 1982.
5. Jeffers, JB: Considerations of anatomy, physiology, and pathology of sports related ocular injuries. Athletic Training: Journal of the National Athletic Trainers Association 20:195, 1985.
6. Erie, JC: Eye injuries. Prevention, evaluation, and treatment. The Physician and Sportsmedicine 19:108, 1991.
7. Forrest, LA, Schuller, DE, and Strauss, RH: Management of orbital blow-out fractures. Case reports and discussion. Am J Sports Med 17:217, 1989.
8. Matthews, B: Maxillofacial trauma from athletic endeavors. Athletic Training: Journal of the National Athletic Trainers Association 25:132, 1990.
9. Belin, MW: Foreign bodies and penetrating injuries to the eye. In Catalano, RA (ed): Ocular Emergencies. WB Saunders, Philadelphia, 1992, p 203.
10. Bruckner, AJ: Diagnosis and management of injuries to the eye and orbit. In Torg, JS: Athletic Injuries to the Head, Neck, and Face, ed 2. Mosby-Year Book, St Louis, 1991, p 659.

15

The Face and Related Structures

Even when athletes use appropriate equipment and padding, portions of the face, nose, mouth, and ears are vulnerable to injury. Rules requiring the use of facemasks and mouthguards have reduced the number and severity of injuries to the maxillofacial area. For maximum protection, these devices must be properly fitted and athletes should be encouraged to use mouthguards during both practices and games, even in sports in which their use is not mandated.

Injuries to the facial structures are significant because of their relationship to neurological function, the potential of permanent physical deformity and disability, and, in the case of throat injuries, the threat to life itself by compromising the airway. A quick, accurate evaluation of injury to these areas is necessary to determine severity and to immediately initiate appropriate treatment and management, lessening the probability of any long-term consequences.

CLINICAL ANATOMY

The face is formed by the **frontal, maxillary, nasal,** and **zygomatic bones** (Fig. 15–1). Composing a large portion of the anterior face, the maxilla forms a portion of the inferior orbits of the eye, the nasal cavity, and the oral cavity. The superior row of teeth is fixed within the **alveolar process** along the maxilla's inferior border. The **zygoma** is fused to the maxilla anteriorly and the **temporal bones** posteriorly, forming the prominent **zygomatic arch** beneath the eyes. Providing the cheek with its surface structure, disruption of the zygomatic arch can have a drastic effect on the face's physical appearance. The zygoma also serves an important role in ocular function by forming a portion of the lateral and inferior rim of the eye's orbit.

Anteriorly, the body of the **mandible** forms the chin. Diverging laterally from the point of the chin, the **ramus** of the mandible begins at the angle of the jaw and continues its course posteriorly and superiorly. The convex **mandibular condylar processes** sit at the end of the ramus, forming the inferior aspect of the **temporomandibular joint (TMJ)**. Anterior to the mandibular condylar process is the site of attachment of the temporalis muscle, the **coronoid process**. Injury to the mandible can potentially involve the alveolar process and thus affect the *occlusion* of the teeth.

Temporomandibular Joint Anatomy

With the exception of the TMJ, joints between the maxillofacial bones are solid. Pathology to the TMJ, a synovial articulation between the mandibular condylar process and the temporal bone, can result in *malocclusion* and has been implicated as the cause of headaches, cervical musculature strain, and overall muscle weakness. Correction of the occlusion with specially formed mouthpieces has been suggested to solve these problems.

Movement at the TMJ is necessary for communication and the *mastication* of food. The superior temporal articulation, from anterior to posterior, consists of the **articular tubercle, articular eminence, glenoid fossa,** and **posterior glenoid spine** (Fig. 15–2). The actual articulating area for the mandibular condylar process is the convex articular eminence. The anterosuperior portion of the mandibular condylar process and the articular eminence are covered with the thickest area of fibrocartilaginous tissue in the joint, enabling these surfaces to withstand the stresses associated with joint movement.

Occlusion: The process of closing or being closed.
Malocclusion: A deviation in the normal alignment of two opposable tissues (e.g., the mandible and maxilla).
Mastication: The chewing of food.

452

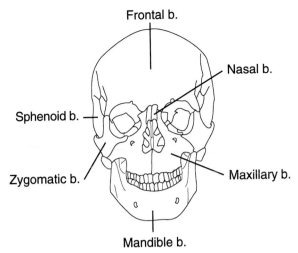

Figure 15-1. Bony anatomy of the face.

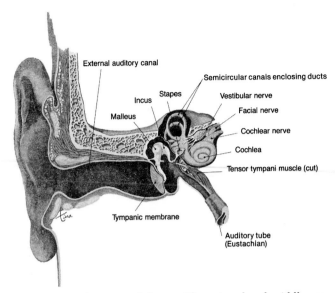

Figure 15-3. Anatomy of the ear. The external and middle ear are separated by the tympanic membrane. The middle and inner ear are divided by the oval window. (From Rothstein, JM, Roy, SH, and Wolf, SL,[1b] p 440, with permission.)

An articular disk is located between the two bones and the entire joint is encased by a synovial joint capsule. The disk is concave on both its superior and inferior surfaces, allowing a smooth articulation between two convex bones. The disk has sturdy attachments to the mandible, attaching anteriorly and posteriorly to the capsule and surrounding tissues. Medially and laterally there are no attachments to the joint capsule so that the disk has freedom of movement in the anteroposterior direction as the mouth opens and closes.[1]

The Ear

The ear comprises three sections: the external ear, the middle ear, and the inner ear (Fig. 15-3). The design of the ear permits it to focus and change acoustical energy into an electrical signal that can be interpreted by the brain. The ear also functions to maintain balance during athletic competition and daily activities.

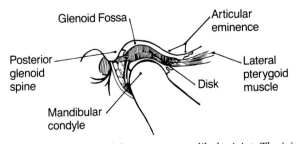

Figure 15-2. Anatomy of the temporomandibular joint. The joint structure allows the mandibular condyle to glide forward as the mouth is opened. Trauma to the disk results in a locking or catching as the mouth is opened and closed. (From Norkin, CC, and Levangie, PK,[1a] p 195, with permission.)

The External Ear

The shape of the external ear is maintained by an accumulation of cartilaginous tissue, the **auricle** (pinna). The shape of the external ear functions as a funnel, collecting and focusing sound waves into the **external auditory meatus** to be passed on to the middle ear. Although the auricle is sturdy enough to maintain the shape of the ear, the cartilage is capable of being deformed and quickly returning to its original shape, a mechanism that efficiently disperses many of the forces to which the external ear is exposed.

The Middle Ear

The outer barrier of the middle ear is the **tympanic membrane**, or eardrum. Functioning like a microphone picking up sound, sound waves strike the tympanic membrane, causing it to oscillate. Three small bones, the **auditory ossicles**, are aligned in a chain formed by the **malleus, incus,** and **stapes** that transmits the vibrations of the tympanic membrane to the **oval window** of the inner ear.

The middle ear is connected to the nasal passages by the **eustachian tube**. This structure regulates the amount of pressure within the middle ear.

The Inner Ear

Within the inner ear, the mechanical vibrations caused by sound waves are encoded into electrical impulses to be interpreted as sound by the brain.

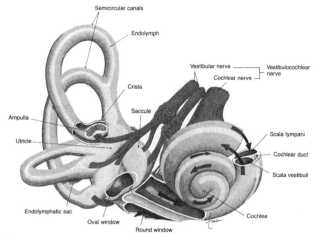

Figure 15–4. Inner ear. Here mechanical sound waves are converted into nervous impulses that are sent along to the brain for processing. (From Rothstein, JM, Roy, SH, and Wolf, SL,[1b] p 441, with permission.)

The structures of the inner ear, the **cochlea** and the **semicircular canals**, sit within a bony, fluid-filled labyrinth formed within the temporal bone (Fig. 15–4). Acoustic signals are passed along the cochlea, a bony structure that moves up and down in response to these signals. This movement is detected by fine hair cells and subsequently translated into electrical impulses by the **vestibulocochlear nerve**.

The semicircular canals are fluid-filled. As the head is tilted from an upright position, the fluid in the canals is moved. The feedback from this movement is provided to the brain, assisting in maintaining balance and an upright posture of the head and body.

The Nose

The paired, wafer-thin **nasal bones** arise off the facial bones to meet with extensions of the **frontal bones** and **maxillary bones**, forming the **nasal bridge**. The **nasal septum**, formed on its posterior half by the **vomer bone** and the perpendicular plate of the **ethmoid bone**, meets with the **nasal cartilage** anteriorly to separate the nasal passage into two halves. The floor of the nasal cavity is formed by the **hard palate** anteriorly and the **soft palate** posteriorly (Fig. 15–5).

The external nasal openings, the **nostrils**, allow air to flow into the nasal passages, through the inferior, middle, and superior **choanae**, and into the **pharynx** to be transmitted to the lungs via the **trachea**. The nasal passages are lined with **mucosal cells** that warm and humidify cool, dry air prior to inspiration into the lungs. These cells also produce mucus that, along with the nasal hairs, traps foreign particles, preventing them from being passed along to the lungs.

The Throat

Because the **larynx** is the most superficial and prominent structure of the throat, it is the area most susceptible to traumatic injury. Covered superiorly by the prominent **thyroid cartilage** (Adam's apple) and inferiorly by the **cricoid cartilage**, the larynx is well protected from all but the most severe blows. Inferior to the cricoid cartilage, the **trachea**'s semicircular cartilage serves as its protective covering until it descends behind the sternum (Fig. 15–6).

The **hyoid bone** is located in the anterior neck between the mandible and the larynx and functions as the tongue's attachment site. This U-shaped bone is

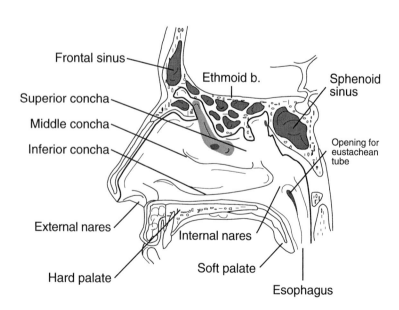

Figure 15–5. Cross section of the nasal passage.

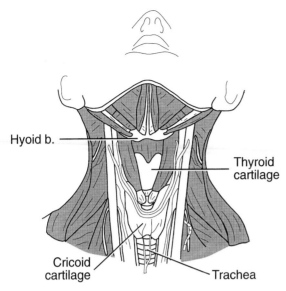

Figure 15-6. Anatomy of the upper trachea. The larynx lies behind the thyroid and cricoid cartilages.

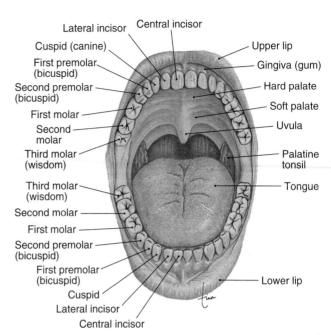

Figure 15-7. Oral cavity. (From Rothstein, JM, Roy, SH, and Wolf, SL,[1b] p 834, with permission.)

suspended by ligaments arising from the temporal bones and has the distinction of being the only bone in the body that does not articulate with another bone. The hyoid consists of a central body with two pairs of laterally and posteriorly projecting structures, the greater and lesser **cornua**.

The Lips

Formed by connective tissue and a thin covering of skin, the lips contain a small layer of transparent cells over a network of vascular capillaries. The rest of the oral cavity is covered by a membrane that produces the protective mucus throughout the digestive system (see Chap. 10). The mouth is divided into the **oral vestibule**, from the lips to the teeth, and the **oral cavity**, everything past the teeth, leading to the trachea.

The tongue is a skeletal muscle covered by mucous membrane (Fig. 15-7). Its surface is covered with **papillae** and **taste buds**. The papillae are small, rough projections on the surface of the tongue that assist in the movement of food during chewing. The taste buds allow us to appreciate the flavor of whatever we are ingesting. The tongue is connected on its underside to the floor of the oral cavity by the **lingual frenulum**. This small piece of mucous membrane can be injured during trauma to the tongue or mouth.

The Teeth

There are 32 permanent teeth, divided equally into upper and lower rows. Each row is formed by four different types of teeth, each serving a different function (see Fig. 15-7 and Table 15-1). Individu-

ally, each tooth has three major anatomical areas: the **root**, the **neck**, and the **crown**. The roots are anchored to the alveolar process by **cementum** and small **periodontal ligaments**. The alveolar process and root are covered to the base of the tooth's neck by the **gums**.

Each tooth is formed by **dentin**, a hard, calcified substance covered by an even harder substance, **enamel**. The tooth's core is formed by the **pulp chamber**, housing a strong connective tissue (**pulp**), nerves, and blood vessels (Fig. 15-8). The nerves and blood vessels enter from the underlying bone through the apical foramen and course through the root canal up into the pulp cavity.

Muscular Anatomy

For the purposes of this chapter, the maxillofacial muscles are classified as being either the muscles of mastication or muscles of expression. Injury to these muscles occurs secondary to lacerations, dislocations, fractures, or cranial nerve involvement. Additional facial muscles acting on the eye and eyelids are discussed in Chapter 14.

Table 15-1. Classification and Function of the Teeth per Row

Type	Number	Function
Incisors	4	Cutting
Canines (cuspids)	2	Tearing
Premolars (bicuspids)	4	Crushing and grinding
Molars	6	Crushing and grinding

STRUCTURE OF TOOTH

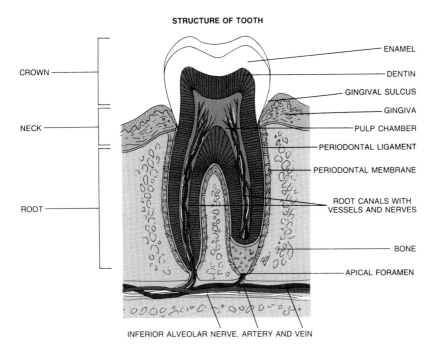

CROWN

NECK

ROOT

ENAMEL

DENTIN

GINGIVAL SULCUS

GINGIVA

PULP CHAMBER

PERIODONTAL LIGAMENT

PERIODONTAL MEMBRANE

ROOT CANALS WITH
VESSELS AND NERVES

BONE

APICAL FORAMEN

INFERIOR ALVEOLAR NERVE, ARTERY AND VEIN

Figure 15–8. Cross-sectional anatomy of a tooth. (From Thomas, CL [ed]: Taber's Cyclopedic Medical Dictionary, ed 17, Beth Anne Willert, MS, medical illustrator. FA Davis, Philadelphia, 1993, p 2010, with permission.

Muscles of Mastication

The primary muscle for flexing the jaw (closing the mouth) is the **masseter**, spanning the distance between the mandibular angle and the inferior portion of the zygomatic arch. The mouth is opened by the contraction of the **digastric, mylohyoid, medial pterygoid,** and **lateral pterygoid** muscles.

Muscles of Expression

The muscles of expression, those that move the lips, cheeks, nose, eyebrows, and forehead, have little clinical significance. The lack of symmetrical movement or hypertonicity of the facial muscles indicates pressure being placed on one or more cranial nerves (see Chapter 16).

EVALUATION OF FACIAL INJURIES

The evaluation of a specific segment of the face need not encompass all aspects of otherwise unrelated structures. However, a secondary screen of these areas should be conducted to rule out any concurrent injury. An outline of the evaluation of these structures is presented in Table 15–2.

With the exception of TMJ dysfunction, athletic-related injury to these areas almost always has an acute onset. Systemic illness or local disease, found in this area includes *sinusitis*, upper respiratory infections, and *dental caries*.

History

The history phase of the examination of athletic-related injury to facial structures is most likely to be concise, owing to the acute trauma involved. Obvious deformity to the structure is often found. Despite the presence of an obvious injury to a particular structure, trauma to adjacent areas must also be ruled out. Injuries to the larynx may impede the athlete's ability to speak.

The Ear

- **Location of the pain:** Direct blows to the external ear commonly result in pain in the affected area. Complaints of pressure within the middle or inner ear indicate an infection or a tympanic membrane rupture. Athletes with otitis externa, infection of the external auditory meatus, present with intense, chronic pain accompanied by itching.

- **Onset:** In contrast to symptoms of ear infections, the onset of symptoms of most injuries is acute. The progressive worsening of symptoms is indicative of an infection or other disease state.

- **Activity and injury mechanism:** Most athletic-related ear injuries stem from a blunt trauma to the auricle and are especially prevalent in those sports in which headgear is not mandated. An athlete may suffer a rupture of the

---

Sinusitis: Inflammation of the nasal sinus.
Dental caries: A destructive disease of the teeth; cavities.

Table 15–2. Evaluation of Injuries to the Face and Related Structures

History	Inspection	Palpation	Functional Tests	Ligamentous Tests	Neurological Tests	Special Tests
Location of the pain Onset Activity Injury mechanism Other symptoms	Ear 　Auricle 　Tympanic membrane 　Periauricular area Nose 　Alignment 　Epistaxis 　Septum and mucosa Eyes and Face 　The throat 　Respiration 　Thyroid cartilage 　Cricoid cartilage Face and Jaw 　Bleeding 　Ecchymosis 　Symmetry 　Muscle tone Oral Cavity 　Lips 　Teeth 　Tongue 　Lingual frenulum 　Gums	Ear 　Periauricular area 　External ear Nose 　Nasal bone 　Nasal cartilage Throat 　Hyoid bone 　Cartilages Face 　Zygoma 　Maxilla 　Forehead Jaw 　Mandible 　Temporomandibular joint Teeth	Ear 　Hearing 　Balance Nose 　Smell TMJ involvement	Not applicable	Ear 　Hearing 　Balance Nose 　Smell	Ear Pathology 　Auricular hematoma 　Tympanic membrane rupture 　Otitis externa 　Otitis media Nasal Pathology Throat Injury Facial Fractures 　Mandibular fractures 　Tongue blade test 　Zygoma fractures 　Maxillary fractures 　LeFort's fractures Dental Injuries 　Tooth fracture 　Tooth luxation Temporomandibular Joint

tympanic membrane secondary to a slapping blow to the ear that results in sufficient pressure on the middle ear to cause the membrane to rupture, an injury that is predisposed to infection of the middle ear. A physical puncture of the tympanic membrane may occur from an object entering the external auditory meatus. Infections to the middle ear are usually preceded by upper respiratory infections, resulting in inflamed mucous membranes blocking the eustachian tubes.

- **Other symptoms:** Because the inner ear plays a key role in the maintenance of equilibrium, the athlete may describe *tinnitus* and/or dizziness. With infection, pressure changes within the middle or inner ear cause the ear to feel congested. This condition may be aggravated by pressure changes associated with airplane travel.

The Nose

- **Location of the pain:** Athletic-related nasal trauma almost always involves direct trauma. Pain is centered over the nose itself but may also radiate throughout the eyes, face, and forehead.
- **Onset:** The onset of injury is often, if not always, acute. The insidious onset of nasal symptoms should lead the examiner to suspect the presence of a disease or illness.
- **Activity and injury mechanism:** The mechanism of injury is a direct blow to the nasal bone and/or nasal cartilage. Spontaneous *epistaxis* may occur as the result of competing in a hot, dry environment.
- **Symptoms:** Besides obvious pain, the athlete usually reports bleeding. The athlete should be evaluated for a possible concussion, as the forces needed to fracture a nose are also sufficient to cause closed head trauma (see Chapter 16).
- **Previous history:** The athlete should be questioned regarding a history of past nasal trauma. A prior nasal fracture can result in deformity that can be mistaken for an acute injury.

The Throat

- **Location of the pain:** Acute throat trauma manifests itself with pain in the anterior portion of the neck. Pain arising from illness (e.g., sore throat) is described as being deep within the neck.

- **Onset:** Throat injuries typically have an acute onset.
- **Activity and injury mechanism:** Usually the athlete is struck with an object such as a bat, ball, or an opponent's elbow.
- **Symptoms:** A blow that crushes the larynx may result in the athlete's inability to speak. Respiratory distress can occur secondary to an obstruction of the airway.

Maxillofacial Injury

- **Location of the pain:** The athlete usually pinpoints the pain to an exact site. Dental injuries can almost always be pinpointed by the athlete to one or more teeth.
- **Onset:** Maxillofacial injuries are almost always acute and the direct result of trauma. The exceptions are nonathletic dental problems (e.g., dental caries).
- **Activity and injury mechanism:** The typical mechanism of injury is blunt trauma from an object or competitor. Balls, various forms of sticks and bats, and opponents all pose potential risks for inflicting maxillofacial injuries. Lacerating trauma to the lips or tongue can be self-inflicted as the athlete accidentally bites these areas.
- **Other symptoms:** The facial bones are a large component of the orbit of the eye cavity. Secondary to facial trauma, the athlete may complain of difficulty with eye movements and vision (see Chapter 14). An athlete may not immediately report seemingly minor injuries to the TMJ but may later notice pain or clicking at the TMJ while chewing or difficulty chewing because of malocclusion.

Inspection

Close inspection of the facial structures is vital to the accurate evaluation and management of injuries to this area. Gross inspection of the injured area is often inadequate to determine the presence of underlying pathology. The primary inspection includes a check for obvious lacerations to the face and mouth, as these injuries are usually found concurrently with other trauma. Because trauma to the face and mouth involves the respiratory system, the athlete's airway must be immediately assessed. In cases of injury to the mouth, the oral cavity should be inspected for blockage by a mouthguard, piece of tooth, or other material that could become lodged in

---

Tinnitus: Ringing in the ears.
Epistaxis: A nosebleed.

the airway and great care taken to remove any loose objects to avoid blockage.

The Ear

- **The auricle:** The examiner observes the outer ear for signs of a contusion or laceration. High-velocity impact of the auricle, as occurs when hit with a baseball, may cause a piece of the outer ear to be avulsed (Fig. 15–9). Formation of a hematoma within the auricle can result in the characteristic cauliflower ear (Fig. 15–10). Otitis externa will be evident as the external ear, including the external auditory meatus, is reddened and inflamed.

- **The tympanic membrane:** The eardrum is visualized through the use of an otoscope (Fig. 15–11). The membrane itself should appear shiny, translucent, and smooth without any perforations. Suspected disruption of the tympanic membrane or fluid within the auditory canal should immediately be referred for further medical evaluation. Infection of the middle ear causes the membrane to appear distended secondary to the collection of fluids, pus, and other debris. These substances may also occlude the membrane.

- **Periauricular area:** The examiner carefully inspects the area surrounding the ear for signs of a basilar skull fracture, characterized by ecchymosis around the mastoid process and known as **Battle's sign**.

The Nose

- **Alignment:** The nose is inspected for proper alignment. Normally, the nose is symmetrical

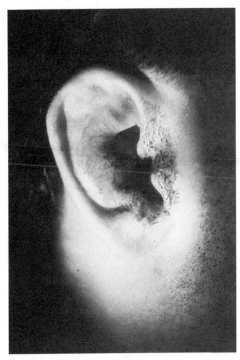

Figure 15–10. Auricular hematoma, or "cauliflower ear." This condition is shown in its acute stage. If the hematoma is allowed to develop, the underlying cartilage is destroyed, resulting in permanent deformity of the external ear. Hearing acuity is affected secondary to the decreased ability to funnel sound waves into the middle ear.

on each side of the sagittal plane. Asymmetry may be present owing to a fracture or swelling. Any question regarding the presence of a deformity can be resolved by asking the athlete to view his or her nose in a mirror to see if it looks "normal."

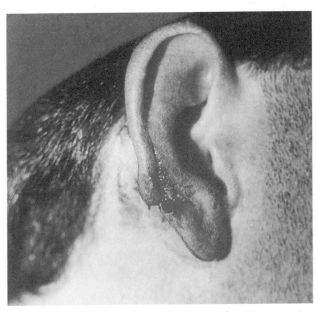

Figure 15–9. Laceration of the external ear. This injury requires suturing to prevent permanent deformity of the ear.

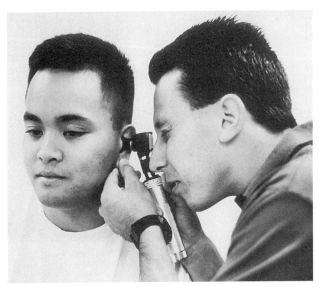

Figure 15–11. Viewing the tympanic membrane through the use of an otoscope. The otoscope must be used with care and only after proper training. Improper use of the otoscope can puncture the tympanic membrane.

- **Epistaxis:** Bleeding from the nasal passage is common following trauma to the nasal bones and is usually the result of mucosal laceration.[2,3] Laceration of the skin covering the nose is also common in these injuries and may or may not have an associated fracture.

- **Septum and mucosa:** The nasal septum and its mucosal lining can be viewed using an otoscope or penlight (Fig. 15–12). On inspection the septum should be symmetrical and straight; asymmetry or angulation of the nasal passage indicates a deviated septum.[4] Bony fragments may also be seen within the nasal passage.

- **Eyes and face:** The area beneath the eyes should be inspected for the presence of ecchymosis. Following a nasal fracture, blood follows the contour of the bone to rest beneath the eyes, a clinical sign termed "**raccoon eyes**" (Fig. 15–13).

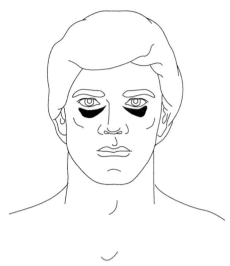

Figure 15–13. "Raccoon eyes." Following a nasal fracture, blood lost because of hemorrhage follows the contour of the face and pools beneath the eyes. This condition can also result from a skull fracture.

The Throat

- **Respiration:** Even relatively minor blows to the throat can be sufficient to disrupt breathing. The athlete's breathing pattern should be observed for signs of respiratory distress. Any difficulty in breathing should be considered a medical emergency.

- **Thyroid and cricoid cartilage:** These cartilages should be inspected for deformity. Swelling may appear rapidly and obliterate the borders of the thyroid cartilage. Any deformity in this structure should be treated as a medical emergency because of the potential jeopardy to the airway.[5]

The Face and Jaw

- **Bleeding:** Facial lacerations are often accompanied by profuse bleeding. Although controlling bleeding takes precedence, the possibility of underlying trauma should not be overlooked (see On-Field Management of Facial Lacerations).

- **Ecchymosis:** The presence of periorbital ecchymosis may be the result of fracture to the nasal bones, maxilla, or zygoma. Ecchymosis below the alveolar process and at the angle of the mandible is common after mandibular fracture.

- **Symmetry:** Inspection of the uninjured face usually reveals symmetry between the right and left halves. With facial pathology such as zygomatic fracture or TMJ injury, this symmetry may be lost secondary to bony deformity or swelling. Inspection of the face should also include inspecting the athlete's eye movements for equality. If the maxilla or zygoma is fractured the movement of the eyes may be asymmetrical.

- **Muscle tone:** As the athlete responds to the examiner's questions, the examiner should observe the movements of the mouth, eyebrows, and forehead symmetry. A unilateral paralysis of the facial muscles, **Bell's palsy**, is the result of traumatic or organic inhibition of the facial nerves.

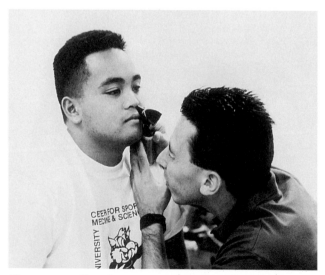

Figure 15–12. Use of an otoscope to view the nasal septum.

Bell's palsy: Inhibition of the facial nerve secondary to trauma or disease, resulting in flaccidity of the facial muscles. In individuals suffering from Bell's palsy the face on the involved side appears elongated.

The Oral Cavity

- **Lips:** Any laceration protruding onto the lips should be referred to a physician for further evaluation. These injuries have a high potential for infection and scarring.
- **Teeth:** Although many types of tooth fractures are readily apparent during gross inspection, chipped teeth and fractures involving the root are more subtle. Both the inner and outer sides of the tooth's surfaces should be inspected for chipped crowns. The use of a penlight and dental mirror assists in this process (Fig. 15–14).
- **Tongue:** The dorsal and ventral surfaces of the tongue should be inspected for lacerations.
- **Lingual frenulum:** As the athlete lifts the tongue, the examiner observes for the integrity of the lingual frenulum (Fig. 15–15). This structure can become lacerated secondary to teeth fractures.
- **Gums:** The examiner inspects the inner and outer border of the gums for lacerations, an abscess, or *gingivitis*.

Palpation

The relatively subcutaneous location of the facial bones and mandible eases the palpation of these structures. Although the internal structures of the ears, nose, and throat cannot be palpated, the overlying and surrounding areas should be examined for tenderness and concurrent injury.

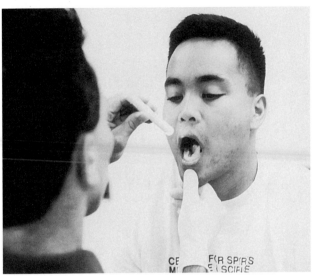

Figure 15–15. Inspection of the lingual frenulum. The athlete is asked to lift the tongue to the roof of the mouth.

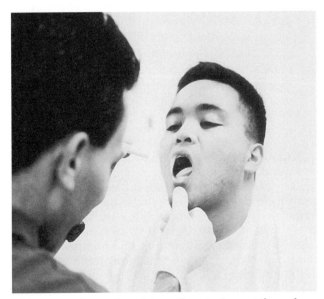

Figure 15–14. Inspection of the oral cavity. Inspect the oral cavity to rule out tooth fractures and to locate the source of bleeding.

The Ear

- **Periauricular area:** To rule out the presence of a fracture, the examiner palpates the temporal bone surrounding the external ear and its mastoid process.
- **External ear:** The auricle is palpated to determine tenderness and swelling. In cases of repeated trauma to the external ear, as commonly occurs in wrestlers, hard nodules may be felt within the auricle. Pain associated with a middle or inner ear infection is increased by tugging on the earlobe.

The Nose

- **Nasal bone:** The examiner begins palpating the nasal bone at the point that the zygomatic and maxillary bones merge beneath the eye (Fig. 15–16). Applying light, yet firm, pressure, the examiner continues palpation medially to the base of the nasal bone and up to the bridge of the nose, noting painful areas and/or crepitus. From the upper boundaries of the nasal bone, the examiner proceeds upward and laterally to palpate the frontal bone above the nose and eyes.
- **Nasal cartilage:** From the bridge of the nose, palpation continues distal to the nasal cartilage at the tip of the nose. Normally, this structure should align with the center of the bridge.

Gingivitis: Inflammation of the gums.

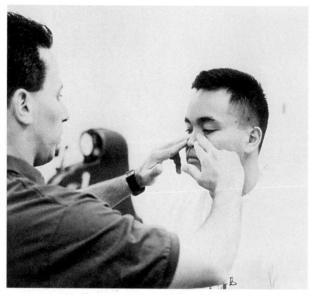

Figure 15–16. Palpation of the nose. Palpation of the nose is begun along the zygomatic arch, working toward the nasal bone.

The Throat

- **Hyoid bone:** The hyoid bone is palpable approximately one finger's breadth superior to the thyroid cartilage. The integrity of the hyoid bone can be determined by gently grasping it between the thumb and index fingers. The bone should glide downward as the athlete swallows.
- **Cartilages:** The examiner begins palpation of the cartilages at the sternal notch. Palpation continues upward to find the series of depressions and hardened bands of the tracheal cartilage and then moving farther up to find the cricoid cartilage and the thick body of the thyroid cartilage.

The Face

- **Zygoma:** Palpation of the face begins at the junction between the temporal and zygomatic bones, just anterior to the auditory canals and above the TMJ. The examiner palpates anteriorly and medially along the zygomatic arches as they pass beneath the eyes and merge with the maxillary bones bilaterally.
- **Maxilla:** From the crest of the zygomatic arch, the examiner palpates upward along the maxillary bones. The fused joint where the maxillary and nasal bones join is marked by a sudden slope. Palpation continues to the crest of the nasal bones. The remainder of the maxillary bone is palpated by moving inferiorly from the nose and outward along the upper margin of the teeth.
- **Forehead:** After returning to the starting position above the TMJ, the examiner palpates su-

periorly along the lateral portion of the orbits. The lateral edge of the eyebrow is used to approximate the junction between the zygomatic and frontal bones. If indicated by the athlete's description of the location of pain, the forehead and periorbital area should be palpated for tenderness and/or crepitus.

The Jaw

- **Mandible:** Palpation of the chin is begun at the mental protuberance (cleft of the chin). The examiner progresses posteriorly, palpating the lateral and posterior portion of the mandible as well as the lower alveolar processes. The mandibular ramus and the lateral border of the angle of the mandible become obscured by the masseter muscle.
- **Temporomandibular joint:** Open the athlete's jaw to move the coronoid process from under the zygomatic arch. Although this structure is often not directly palpable, the area can be palpated for underlying tenderness.

  Placing the tips of the index and middle fingers over the athlete's TMJ, the examiner notes the presence of any clicking or crepitus as the athlete opens and closes the mouth (Fig. 15–17). These conditions are pathological and indicate a disruption of the joint's normal biomechanics. As the mouth is fully opened, a small depression should be felt within the joint as the mandibular head and neck slide forward. Inflammation and swelling can fill this area.

  The posterior aspect of the TMJ is palpated by placing the fifth finger in the opening of the external auditory meatus (Fig. 15–18). The bilateral movement of the TMJ should be smooth and equal as the athlete opens and closes the mouth. Any discrepancy in this motion is indicative of TMJ dysfunction, a TMJ dislocation, or a mandibular fracture.

The Teeth

Palpation of the teeth after an oral injury should be undertaken with caution. Gentle pressure is sufficient to check the integrity of the tooth's attachment to the alveolar processes (Fig. 15–19). An alternative is to have the athlete use the tongue to apply this pressure. Any suspicion of a loosened tooth warrants consultation with a dentist. The procedure for the management of a lost tooth is covered in the on-field management of these injuries.

Functional Tests

The functional tests for the ear, nose, and throat provide limited information about the athlete's pathology. They do, however, provide valuable in-

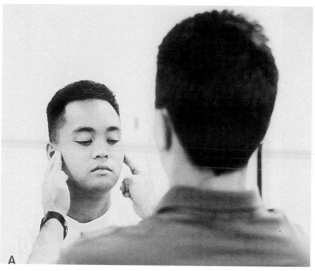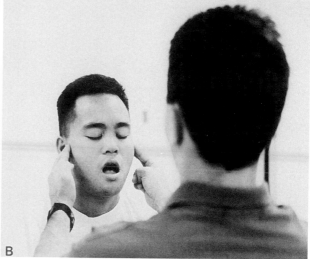

Figure 15–17. Palpation of the external temporomandibular joint. The temporomandibular joint is palpated while the athlete opens and closes the mouth. Asymmetry of movement and clicking or locking of the joint are noted.

formation concerning hearing, balance, smell, and swallowing function.

The Ear

- **Hearing:** Transitory hearing loss is to be expected immediately following a blow to the ear. The failure of a return to normal hearing within 1 hour after injury is significant and warrants referral of the athlete for further medical evaluation.
- **Balance:** The athlete should be questioned regarding balance and dizziness, each of which may occur secondary to either ear or brain trauma. Discussion of assessment of an athlete's sense of balance appears in Chapter 16.

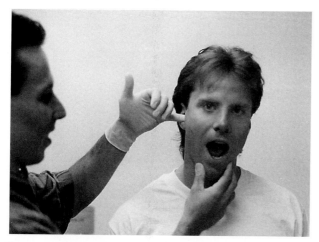

Figure 15–18. Palpation of the internal temporomandibular joint. Using rubber gloves, the examiner lightly places a finger in the outermost portion of the auditory canal to further palpate the mechanics of the temporomandibular joint as the athlete opens and closes the mouth

The Nose

- **Smell:** The athlete's olfactory senses may be obscured by epistaxis but should return once the bleeding has subsided. The loss of olfactory function is more commonly attributed to brain trauma than to trauma directly to the nose itself.

TMJ Involvement

Functional testing for TMJ pathology involves having the athlete slowly open and close the mouth. The clinician should select a point, such as the junction between the two middle lower incisors, to use as a reference as the athlete opens and closes the mouth (Fig. 15–20).[6] The jaw should move smoothly and evenly with no interruption. Following injury to the TMJ, mandible, or maxilla, opening and closing the jaw may demonstrate a side-to-side deviation and the athlete's bite may be maloccluded.

Lateral excursion of the jaw can also be evaluated for distance and quality using the same reference point for the lower jaw and comparing it to the point between the incisors of the upper jaw. The athlete is asked to move the jaw to the right and then to the left. The distance that the lower reference point moves relative to the upper reference point is measured with a ruler and compared bilaterally. The movement should be equal and should be completed in a smooth and pain-free manner.

Neurological Testing

Loss of the associated special senses (hearing and smell) can indicate the presence of closed head trauma that has disrupted one or more cranial

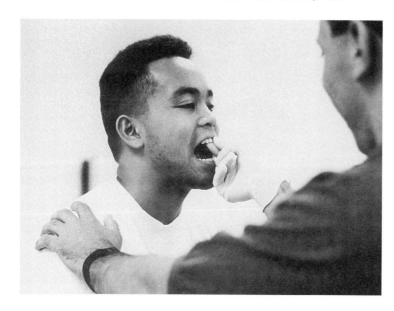

Figure 15–19. Palpation of the teeth. Because of the possibility of exposure to bloodborne pathogens, rubber gloves must be worn during this process.

nerves. The evaluation of these conditions is described in Chapter 17.

Pathologies and Related Special Tests

Pathology to the ear, nose, and throat is relatively uncommon in athletics, largely as a result of the use of protective mouthguards and headgear. Also, rules have been implemented to decrease the possibility of injury by prohibiting blows to the face and head. Although limited in number, injuries to this area can involve major trauma and have potential long-term complications of impaired hearing, smell, and speech. Laryngeal injury can be life-threatening secondary to obstruction of the airway.

Ear Pathology

Most athletic-related ear injuries are the result of a single traumatic force or may be caused by invading organisms and diseases. This trauma may be visible to the unaided eye or it may not be visible to untrained personnel, requiring the decision to refer the athlete to a physician based on the complaints reported.

Auricular Hematoma

Repeated episodes of blunt trauma or shearing forces to the external ear can result in an auricular hematoma,[7] also termed a "cauliflower ear." Swelling within the skin of the outer ear develops within hours of the injury. Pooling of blood between the skin and the cartilage separates the two, depriving the cartilage of its source of nutrition. With time the hematoma can scar, causing a deformed appearance to the external ear (see Fig. 15–10).

The athlete's chief complaint is pain in the external and middle ear, accompanied by ecchymosis and swelling of the auricle. The external ear should be inspected for open wounds and drainage from

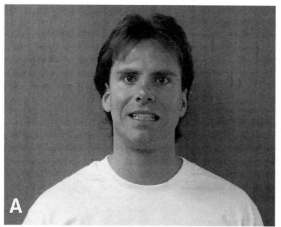
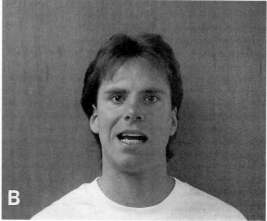

Figure 15–20. Observation for malocclusion of the teeth. (*A*) Normally, the mandible travels in a straight line. (*B*) Trauma to the temporomandibular joint or a fracture of the mandible causes the jaw to track laterally and results in a malalignment of the teeth.

Table 15–3. Evaluative Findings of an Auricular Hematoma ("Cauliflower Ear")

Examination Segment	Clinical Findings	
History	Onset:	Acute or chronic.
	Location of pain:	The external ear.
	Mechanism:	A single or repeated trauma to the external ear, resulting in a subcutaneous hematoma.
Inspection	The external and possibly the middle ear appears violently red. Swelling secondary to a hematoma may be visible.	
Palpation	Palpation of an acute injury produces pain and confirms the presence of a hematoma. Palpation of a chronic injury may reveal hardened nodules within the ear.	
Functional tests	The athlete's hearing and balance should be checked.	
Ligamentous tests	Not applicable.	
Neurological tests	Impairment of cranial nerve VIII.	
Special tests	Hearing and balance.	
Comments	Suspected auricular hematomas should be immediately referred to a physician.	

the middle ear. Palpation reveals increased tenderness and, initially, the "boggy" feel of swelling. Untreated cases with scarring feel hardened on palpation and appear smooth (Table 15–3). In cases of injury to the external ear, the examiner should carefully assess the inner ear with an otoscope (see tympanic membrane).[8]

In cases caused by a blow to the head, brain trauma must also be ruled out. A concurrent basilar skull fracture may result in ecchymosis at the mastoid process (Battle's sign). An athlete suspected of having a concurrent skull fracture should be immediately referred to a physician for a definitive diagnosis.

Often, the physician elects to drain the blood from within the hematoma, decreasing the amount of separation between the skin and the cartilage. Following this procedure, or as a method of initial management of this condition, the ear may be casted with pieces of plaster casting material or gauze and **flexible collodion**.[9–11]

Tympanic Membrane Rupture

The mechanism of injury for a tympanic membrane rupture is usually a sudden change of air pressure on the tympanic membrane caused by blunt trauma or by a decreased ability to regulate inner ear pressure secondary to an infection. The membrane may also be ruptured through direct trauma, such as the athlete's sticking a sharp object in the ear. The signs and symptoms of tympanic membrane ruptures are presented in Table 15–4.

To view the tympanic membrane, the examiner should use an otoscope with a speculum that fits snugly within the ear canal without being painful. The speculum need be placed only slightly into the ear canal to view the structures. Insertion into the external auditory meatus is eased by gently tugging down on the earlobe to better align the canal.

Reddish-brown **cerumen** may be seen as the speculum enters the ear canal. Any fluids in the canal are unusual and minimally indicate a rupture to the tympanic membrane. In a worst-case scenario, this is caused by a skull fracture. Disruption of the tympanic membrane warrants the referral of the athlete for further examination by a physician.

Otitis Externa

Otitis externa, an infection of the external auditory meatus, is usually caused by inadequate drying of the ear canal and has been termed "swimmer's ear" because of its prevalence in water activities.[12] The dark, damp environment encourages the growth of bacteria or fungus, resulting in the inflammation of the external auditory meatus. The athlete's chief complaint is one of constant pain, possibly accompanied by itching, in the ear. The area is red and a discharge from the middle ear may be present. Tugging on the earlobe usually increases pain.

Otitis Media

Upper respiratory infections can cause an inflammation of the ear's mucous membranes, block-

---

Flexible collodion: A mixture of ether, alcohol, cellulose, and camphor, which dries to form a firm, protective layer.

Cerumen: A reddish-brown wax formed in the auditory meatus.

Table 15–4. Evaluative Findings of a Tympanic Membrane Rupture

Examination Segment	Clinical Findings
History	Onset: Acute. Location of pain: Pain in the middle ear, radiating inward and outward. The pain is often excruciating. Mechanism: A mechanical pressure that causes the tympanic membrane to burst (a slap to the ear or a blocked sneeze) or a mechanical intrusion through the membrane (e.g., cleaning the ears with a ballpoint pen).
Inspection	Inspection of the ear with the unaided eye normally produces no remarkable findings. Inspection with an otoscope reveals redness and the perforation may be visible.
Palpation	Not applicable.
Functional tests	There is a marked hearing loss in the involved ear. Valsalva's maneuver may result in the audible escape of air from within the inner ear.
Ligamentous tests	Not applicable.
Neurological tests	Not applicable. (In this case hearing reduction is the result of a mechanical deficit.)
Special tests	Hearing.
Comments	The resulting pain and inflammatory response may result in transient dizziness. The ear must be kept dry and the athlete referred to a physician.

ing the eustachian tubes and increasing the pressure within the inner ear. In addition to having a history of upper respiratory problems, the athlete complains of blockage, pressure, and pain within the inner ear. Inspection with an otoscope reveals fluid build-up and an opaque and possibly bulging tympanic membrane. Athletes suffering from otitis media may describe hearing loss in the affected ear.

Nasal Injuries

The most commonly fractured bones of the face and skull, the nasal bones are fractured by a direct blow to the nose.[13] Bleeding typically occurs immediately following the trauma but is usually easily controlled (see On-Field Management of Nasal Injuries). Athletes competing in contact or collision sports often have a history of prior nasal fractures. However, deformity of the nose should not automatically be assumed to be pre-existing.

The athlete's chief complaint, other than bleeding, is pain on and around the nose. On inspection, the nose may be visibly deformed, but the lack of a deformity does not conclusively rule out a nasal fracture. Swelling in and around the nose may obscure minor deformities and make palpation difficult. With time, ecchymosis develops and settles under the inferior aspect of the athlete's eyes ("raccoon eyes"). Palpation reveals tenderness at the fracture site and the surrounding areas. Crepitus may be identifiable at the fracture site as well (Table 15–5).

Repeated nasal trauma can result in necrosis of the nasal cartilage. As the cartilage dies, the bridge of the nose begins to collapse, resulting in a **saddle nose deformity** when the athlete is viewed in profile (Fig. 15–21).

The internal nose should be inspected for the presence of a **deviated septum** through the use of an otoscope or penlight. The athlete should attempt to breathe through one nostril while holding the opposite one closed. The nostril should close during inhalation and breathing should be unobstructed. The exhalation should be easy and unencumbered. If a nasal fracture and/or deviated septum is suspected, the athlete should be referred to a physician.

Throat Injury

Trauma to this area often results in respiratory distress and the inability to speak, both leading to agitation on the part of the athlete. The insulting blow to the anterior throat, if it includes the *carotid sinus*,[14] can result in the athlete's losing consciousness. Pain is increased as the athlete attempts to swallow or take deep, gasping breaths of air. Bruising over and around the larynx is com-

---

Carotid sinus: An area near the common carotid artery that, when stimulated, results in vasodilation and a lowering of the heart rate. When this occurs suddenly, unconsciousness may result.

Table 15–5. Evaluative Findings of Nasal Fractures

Examination Segment	Clinical Findings
History	Onset: Acute. Location of pain: The bridge of the nose and nasal cartilage; may radiate into the frontal and zygomatic bones. Mechanism: A direct blow to the nose.
Inspection	The nose may be visibly deformed. Bleeding normally accompanies nasal fractures. Ecchymosis may accumulate beneath one or both eyes ("raccoon eyes"). The internal nose should be inspected using an otoscope or penlight for the presence of a deviated septum.
Palpation	Palpation of the traumatized area elicits pain. Crepitus may be felt over the fracture site.
Functional tests	The sense of smell and breathing through the nose may be obstructed by bleeding and/or a deviated septum.
Ligamentous tests	Not applicable.
Neurological tests	Not applicable.
Special tests	None.
Comments	Athletes who have sustained a nasal fracture should also be screened for injury to the eyes or head.

mon and the usual palpable definition of the larynx is lost because of deformity and/or swelling. The inside of the mouth should be examined with the use of a penlight for the presence of bloody sputum, indicating an injury to the inside of the throat. Palpation may reveal a displaced cartilage and extreme tenderness or crepitus (Table 15–6). No attempt should be made to correct any deviations because of the possibility of worsening the condition.[15] Immediate referral to a physician is

indicated because airway compromise may develop as swelling continues.

Facial Fractures

Protective facial equipment, such as a football helmet's facemask or a catcher's mask, is useful in deflecting many otherwise injurious forces. However, most equipment leaves at least a portion of the face exposed to potential injury.

Mandibular Fractures

Mandibular fractures are the second most common type of facial fracture, ranking behind nasal fractures, and are the result of a high-velocity impact to the jaw.[16] The chief complaint of a mandibular fracture is pain in the jaw that is increased by opening and closing the mouth. Difficulty with or discrepancies in jaw movement may also be noted by the athlete (Fig. 15–22). Crepitus may be felt during palpation of the fracture site. Mandibular fractures almost always result in a malocclusion of the jaw and teeth, a fact that should direct the clinician to refer the athlete for physician evaluation (Table 15–7). The **tongue blade test** may be used to reinforce the suspicion of a mandibular fracture.

Tongue Blade Test

The tongue blade test is used to determine the presence of mandibular fracture by measuring the athlete's ability to maintain a firm bite (Fig. 15–23).[17]

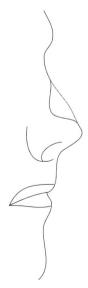

Figure 15–21. Saddle-nose deformity. Repeated trauma or other condition causing necrosis of the nasal cartilage can result in deformity of the nose.

Tongue Blade Test (Fig. 15–23)

Position of athlete	Seated.
Position of examiner	Standing in front of the athlete. The clinician places a tongue blade in the athlete's mouth.
Evaluative procedure	As the athlete attempts to hold the tongue blade in place, the examiner rotates (twists) the blade.
Positive test results	The athlete is unable to maintain a firm bite and/or pain is elicited.
Implications	Possible mandibular fracture.

Zygoma Fractures

Blows to the cheek and inferior periorbital area can result in a fracture of the zygomatic arch. Pain is described at the site of injury, and attempted eye movements may increase the pain or be performed with difficulty. Subconjunctival hematoma and periorbital swelling may be noted. Increased pain is elicited with palpation along the zygomatic arch and the lateral rim of the eye socket. Occasionally a step-off deformity is noted as the examiner palpates over the fracture site.[16]

Maxillary Fractures

Isolated fractures of the maxillae tend to occur concurrently with nasal fractures. The athlete describes pain through the midportion of the face. De-formity found on inspection is rare, but ecchymosis and swelling along the alveolar processes are common. Crepitus may be elicited at the fracture site.

LeFort's Fractures

The LeFort system is used to classify midface fractures. Because these fractures are normally the result of extremely high-impact forces (e.g., automobile accidents), their incidence in athletics is unusual. Figure 15–24 presents the LeFort classification system and identifies the bony segments involved. This type of fracture is so extensive that when the upper teeth are pulled forward the fractured segment and the associated portion of the face are also displaced forward, roughly resembling the anterior drawer test in the knee. Sinus fluid may also be observed running from the nose.

Table 15–6. Evaluative Findings of Throat Trauma

Examination Segment	Clinical Findings
History	Onset: Acute. Location of pain: Anterior neck, possibly radiating into the chest secondary to an obstructed airway. Mechanism: A crushing force to the anterior neck.
Inspection	Bruising or other signs of trauma are present over the anterior throat. Swelling and/or deformity may be present. The mouth and throat may show bloody sputum. The athlete may be coughing in an attempt to clear the airway.
Palpation	Palpation produces tenderness. Crepitus is present. Displacement of the cartilage or fracture of the hyoid bone may be felt.
Functional tests	The athlete has difficulty breathing. There is an inability to speak (or difficulty speaking).
Ligamentous tests	Not applicable.
Neurological tests	Not applicable.
Special tests	Not applicable.
Comments	Immediate referral to a physician is indicated. Ice packs may be applied to control the swelling, but care must be taken not to compress the traumatized tissues. The athlete's vital signs should continue to be monitored.

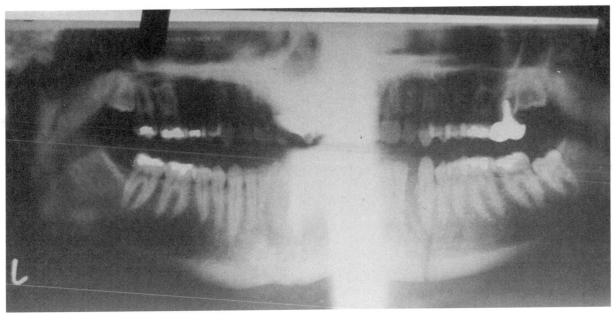

Figure 15-22. X-ray view of a mandibular fracture.

Dental Injuries

Oral injury rates have been determined for both female and male intercollegiate athletes.[18,19] In female athletes the injury rate ranges from 1.5 percent in softball to 7.5 percent in basketball, with soccer, field hockey, and lacrosse having high rates also. The rates for field hockey and lacrosse are surprisingly high considering approximately 90 percent of the participants wear mouthguards. The highest oral injury rates for male athletes occur in basketball, at 10 percent, followed by ice hockey, lacrosse, football, soccer, baseball, and volleyball, totaling 16 percent. The examiner must carefully evaluate oral injuries to ensure that their management is undertaken promptly and that physical deformity and disability are limited.

The preparticipation physical examination questionnaire should ascertain the presence of dental appliances such as crowns, caps, or porcelain implants. This dental work must be evaluated for loosening, fracture, or luxation along with the natural dental structures. The numeric system used by dentists in referencing the teeth is presented in Figure

Table 15-7. Evaluative Findings of a Mandibular Fracture

Examination Segment	Clinical Findings	
History	Onset:	Acute.
	Location of pain:	Ramus or mental protuberance of mandible.
	Mechanism:	Direct blow to the mandible on its anterior or lateral aspects.
Inspection	Swelling and/or gross deformity may be seen over the fracture site. Malocclusion of the teeth may be noted.	
Palpation	Tenderness, crepitus, or bony deformity is present over the fracture site.	
Functional tests	Pain is experienced when opening and closing the mouth, or this motion is prohibited secondary to pain. The mandible may track laterally.	
Ligamentous tests	The structures of the temporomandibular joint may be affected. However, the integrity of these structures should not be checked in the presence of a known fracture.	
Neurological tests	Cranial nerves V and/or VII may be traumatized by the fracture (see Chapter 16).	
Special tests	Tongue blade test.	
Comments	Mandibular fractures may also be accompanied by a temporomandibular joint dislocation. Athletes suspected of suffering a mandibular fracture or dislocation should be referred to a physician for further evaluation and treatment.	

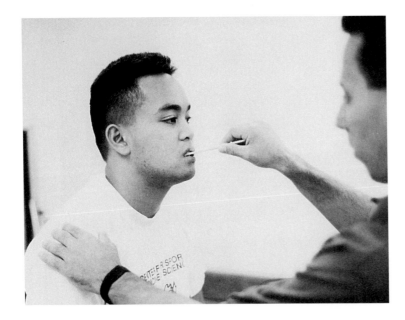

Figure 15–23. Tongue blade test for temporomandibular strength. The examiner twists the tongue blade as the athlete bites down.

15–25. With all dental injuries, the examiner must establish the presence of a suitable airway, rule out the presence of head injury, and evaluate concurrent lacerations.

Tooth Fracture

Tooth fractures range from a simple chip of the crown to a full avulsion of the crown from its roots and are classified on a scale of I to IV (Fig. 15–26). Class I injuries, chip fractures, may be subtly noticed by the athlete during eating, drinking, talking, or other activity in which the tongue is scraped across the teeth; these injuries may be self-evalu-

ated by the athlete's looking in a mirror. Class II fractures and above are more easily recognized secondary to pain, sensitivity to extreme temperatures of food or drink, or obvious deformity. The degree of sensitivity depends on the extent of the fracture. Fractures into the enamel are usually minor irritations, whereas fractures into the dentin and those as deep as the pulp cavity are painful and sensitive to hot and cold temperatures.

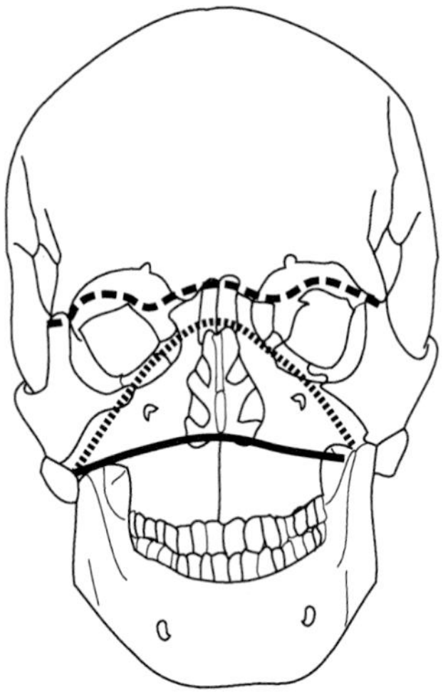

Le Fort I ————
Le Fort II ••••••••••
Le Fort III ‐ ‐ ‐ ‐ ‐ ‐

Figure 15–24. Classification of LeFort's fractures. Type I fractures involve only the maxillary bone; type II extend up into the nasal bone; type III cross the zygomatic bones and the orbit.

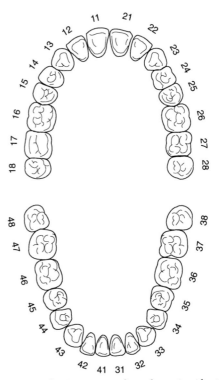

Figure 15–25. Numbering system for referencing the teeth. The upper right teeth are numbered by 10s, the upper left by 20s, the lower left by 30s, and the lower right by 40s.

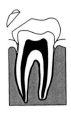
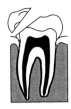
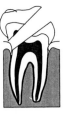
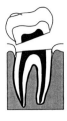

Figure 15–26. Classification scheme for tooth fractures.

Class I   Class II   Class III   Class IV

Tooth Luxation

Luxations of the teeth range from a tooth's being avulsed from the socket to its being driven into the bone (Fig. 15–27). A subtle tooth dislocation, one that is loosened in its socket, is not always visibly recognized. The athlete may discover it while chewing or applying pressure on it with the tongue. An **intruded tooth** is marked by its depression into the alveolar process relative to the contiguous teeth and to its match on the opposite side. An **extruded tooth** is partially withdrawn from the bone and may be tilted anteriorly or posteriorly, or twisted. A **tooth avulsion** is marked by the intact tooth's being displaced from the alveolar process.

Another cause of a luxated tooth is the fracture of its root (Fig. 15–28). A fracture of the cervical third of the tooth may be repaired or permanently secured through the use of dental hardware, whereas fractures to the middle third typically result in the loss of the tooth. The best prognosis occurs when the fracture occurs in the apical third (root) because the tooth is not greatly displaced in its socket.

The teeth can be evaluated for loosening through gentle palpation. If uncertainty exists as to whether a tooth has been partially dislodged, the athlete may be given a mirror to conduct a self-assessment. A tooth that is loose should be left in place so that it can be properly managed by a dentist.

In the event of an avulsed tooth, the athlete is keenly aware of the injury. Other types of tooth luxations result in pain, bleeding from the socket, and temperature hypersensitivity. Once recognized, the condition must be properly managed to maximize the potential of saving the tooth. Management of the luxated tooth is found in the On-Field Management of Injuries section of this chapter.

Temporomandibular Joint

Injury to the TMJ can include sprains, cartilage tears, subluxations, or dislocations. The determination of the specific pathology is less important than the need to identify the fact that TMJ dysfunction exists.

In athletics the TMJ is usually injured when the athlete is hit either on the point of the chin or across the jaw. The initial complaint is jaw pain and possibly clicking at the joint. On inspection the mouth of the athlete may open and close in an asymmetrical fashion, causing the lower jaw to deviate in one direction. Palpation should be carefully performed to rule out a mandibular fracture. Palpation of the TMJ reveals localized tenderness and possibly crepitus or clicking at the joint (Table 15–8).

Dislocations often result in an observable displacement of the mandible, although subtle dislocations that spontaneously reduce may be less evident (Fig. 15–29). The mechanism for this injury is a blow of sufficient force to move the mandible laterally, such as being punched. The rotation of the mandible causes the joint opposite the direction of displacement to anteriorly dislocate. As

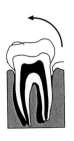
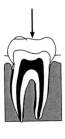
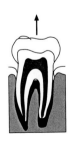
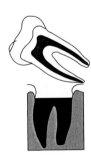

Figure 15–27. Classification scheme for tooth luxations.

Partial displacement   Intrusion   Extrusion   Total avulsion described during the inspection portion of this chapter, the upper and lower teeth suffer a malalignment, and movement of the jaw may be significantly impaired.

Blows to the point of the mandible, driving the bone toward the skull, may result in a fracture along the mandibular ramus or, on rare occasion, the temporal bone. Similar to TMJ dislocations, mandibular fractures result in malocclusion of the teeth, crepitus and deformity over the fracture site, and the inability to normally open and close the mouth.

Measuring TMJ Range of Motion

The ability of the athlete to fully open the mouth should be evaluated, as full range of motion is usually limited with TMJ injury. The ability to open the mouth is evaluated by seeing how many of the athlete's knuckles can be placed in the fully opened mouth. The use of this test allows for the size variation in athletes because the size of their mouth opening is relative to the size of their knuckles.[6] The athlete should be able to place two knuckles within the mouth (Fig. 15–30).

Determination of TMJ Motion (Fig. 15–30)

Position of athlete	Seated or standing.
Position of examiner	In front of the athlete.
Evaluative procedure	The athlete attempts to place as many flexed knuckles as possible between the upper and lower teeth.
Positive test results	The athlete is unable to place a minimum of two knuckles within the mouth.
Implications	Decreased tempomandibular joint range of motion.

ON-FIELD MANAGEMENT OF MAXILLOFACIAL INJURIES

Athletes who have sustained an injury to the maxillofacial area usually remain on the playing surface because of both pain and fear. Owing to the proximity of the maxillofacial area to the airway, the presence of an unencumbered airway must be established. It is not unusual for the athlete to sustain a laceration and a concurrent injury to the maxillofacial structures. After establishing the presence of an airway, the responder must control bleeding before proceeding with a complete evaluation. As with all open wounds, the examiner must abide by the universal precautions for bloodborne pathogens.

Lacerations

By far the most common injury to this area of the body is lacerations. Even when pathology to other structures is present, a laceration is a common concurrent finding. Only cases of airway obstruction have a higher priority in injury management than the control of bleeding.

Lacerations can potentially mask underlying injuries. After the bleeding is controlled, the area around the laceration should be palpated for tenderness. The examiner must be careful to delineate between tenderness from the insulting blow that caused the injury and any actual fractures that may have occurred.

The presence of any foreign particles or objects within the laceration must be determined prior to any subsequent treatment. An imbedded object should be left in place. The surrounding area can be cleaned and dressed until the object can be removed and the wound further managed by a physician.

Next, the extent of the wound must be determined. As a general rule, any facial laceration should be referred for evaluation by a physician for possible suturing to limit the extent and visibility of any scars; this should occur within the 24 hours following the injury, but the sooner the better.[16] If the bleeding can be controlled and the wound closed and dressed with a sterile bandage, the athlete may return to competition. The bandage covering the wound must be sufficient to protect other competitors from contact with the athlete's blood.

In the case of lacerations of the throat, the athlete should be assessed for difficulty with breathing and should be transported by trained personnel who can aid the athlete en route to the hospital. If the laceration avulses a piece of the ear, nose, or tongue, the

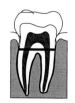 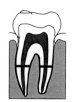 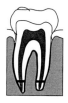

Cervical third   Middle third   Apical third

Figure 15–28. Classification scheme for root fractures.

Table 15–8. Evaluative Findings of Temporomandibular Joint Dysfunction

Examination Segment	Clinical Findings	
History	Onset:	Acute, insidious, or chronic.
	Location of pain:	Area of the temporomandibular joint; possible clicking or locking of the joint.
	Mechanism:	Trauma to the mandibular or progressive joint degeneration.
Inspection	Inspection of the joint may be unremarkable. Swelling may be located over the joint. Malocclusion of the jaw may be noted.	
Palpation	Tenderness exists over the joint surfaces. Palpation of the external and internal structures may reveal clicking as the athlete opens and closes the mouth.	
Functional tests	The athlete's jaw should be observed for true inferior and superior movement as the mouth is opened or closed. Any lateral deviation in the motion indicates joint pathology.	
Ligamentous tests	Not applicable.	
Neurological tests	Not applicable, although TMJ dysfunction has been implicated in causing headaches, decreased strength, and other symptoms.	
Special tests	None.	
Comments	Athletes suffering from persistent TMJ pain should be referred to a physician for further evaluation.	

avulsed tissue should be cleaned with sterile water, wrapped in sterile gauze, put on ice, and transported with the athlete to the medical facility for possible reimplantation. Microsurgical techniques may be able to salvage these parts, giving the athlete a better cosmetic repair and normal function.

Laryngeal Injuries

Laryngeal injuries present a difficult decision for the examiner because of their potential to become life-threatening. Early signs of potentially catastrophic injury include progressive swelling (indicating bleeding), crepitation (indicating the presence of subcutaneous air), audible **stridor** (indicating a narrowing of the airway), and blood exiting the oral cavity.[20]

The decision must be made to move the athlete to the sideline prior to transport or to transport the athlete directly from the field. In cases in which the athlete has trouble breathing, it is prudent to stabilize the athlete and transport him or her to a hospital using emergency medical personnel capable of managing an obstructed airway. The athlete may first be moved to the sideline if no signs of breathing difficulty are noted. Ice may be applied to the anterior throat, but care must be taken not to compress the underlying structures. The pressure applied could be enough to displace the injured area, causing obstruction of the airway.

Facial Fractures

The forces required to fracture the facial bones (zygoma, frontal, maxillary, and mandible) are usually of considerable magnitude. The athlete is not only "down" from the injury, but it is also common

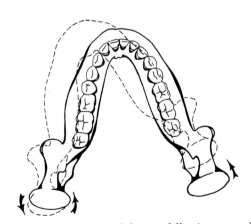

Figure 15–29. Malocclusion of the jaw following a mandibular dislocation. Correlate this illustration with Figure 15–20B. (From Perry, JF, Rohe, DA, and Garcia, AO,[20a] with permission.)

Stridor: A harsh, high-pitched sound resembling blowing wind, experienced during respiration.

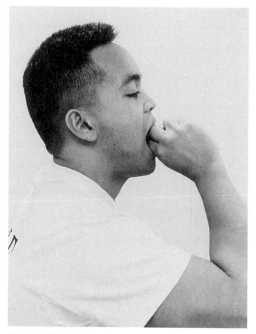

Figure 15–30. Method for determining temporomandibular joint range of motion. An athlete should be able to open the mouth wide enough to accept two knuckles.

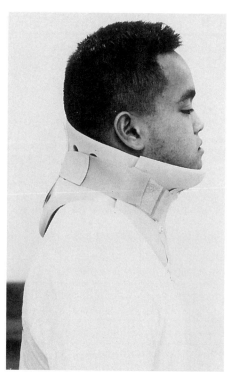

Figure 15–31. Use of a Philadelphia collar for immobilizing a suspected mandibular fracture. Applying too much pressure to the fracture site should be avoided.

to be stunned or rendered unconscious by head injury from the incident. In this case the head injury takes precedence and the examiner should follow the evaluation and on-field management of the head injury (see Chapter 16).

In cases in which the athlete has not sustained a head injury, the responder must calm the athlete. Facial fractures are usually stable and remain so, providing that the athlete is carefully moved. Athletes with suspected facial fractures can be removed to the sideline for further evaluation and treatment. If the athlete has an obvious fracture, movement of the athlete's head and neck should be restricted. As long as it does not increase the athlete's discomfort, a Philadelphia collar can be used to stabilize the jaw and prevent unwanted motion while the athlete is transported to a medical facility (Fig. 15–31).

Temporomandibular Injuries

The temporomandibular joint may be injured along with the mandible from a blow to the jaw. If a fracture of the mandible is unlikely, the athlete can be carefully assisted to the sideline for a full assessment of the TMJ. Injuries that produce malocclusion warrant the removal of the athlete from participation immediately and referral to a physician or dentist. If the TMJ is dislocated the athlete can be immobilized with a Philadelphia collar as long as it does not create further pain. This athlete should also be referred immediately for treatment.

Nasal Fractures

Nasal fractures are almost always accompanied by epistaxis, which must be controlled before further evaluation or management of the injury. Although squeezing the nostrils and tilting the head forward is an adequate form of management for nasal bleeding, this method may be prohibited secondary to pain arising from the fracture. The nose may be packed with rolled gauze or a tampon that has been cut into quarters. (These should be precut and kept in the athletic trainer's medical kit.)

The nose, nasal cartilage, and adjacent maxillary, zygomatic, and frontal bones should be palpated for tenderness and/or crepitus. If the nose is obviously deformed, the athlete should be discouraged from viewing the injury in a mirror or feeling the deformity, as doing so may increase his or her anxiety or cause the onset of shock. Suspected nasal fractures may be packed with a small bag of ice to assist in controlling pain and limiting the amount of bleeding until the athlete is seen by a physician.

Dental Injuries

An athlete suffering tooth trauma usually reports to the sidelines for evaluation. As continued participation can result in a complete tooth avulsion, athletes suffering from any form of tooth injury, other

Table 15–9. Emergency Management of Teeth Injuries

- Before reimplanting an avulsed tooth, it must be rinsed off with a pH-balanced preserving solution or sterile saline solution. The tooth may be held in its socket by the athlete's biting on gauze. The clinician should make sure the tooth is reimplanted in its proper orientation.
- If the tooth is not reimplanted immediately, it should be stored in a secure biocompatible storage environment such as an Emergency Tooth Preserving System or in fresh whole milk in a plastic container with a tightly fitting top.
- No attempt should be made to clean, sterilize, or scrape the tooth in any way other than as noted above.
- The athlete and the tooth should be transported to a dentist as quickly as possible.

than a class I fracture, should be removed from competition and evaluated by a dentist (see Fig. 15–26).

A fractured tooth is usually not of immediate danger to the athlete unless the remaining portion is loose. If no loosening has occurred, the athlete can return to activity as long as a mouthpiece is used and the injury followed up with a dentist as soon as possible. The athlete should expect extreme discomfort, especially if the fracture penetrates the pulp cavity.

Every reasonable attempt should be made to find a tooth that has been luxated. With proper care as recommended by the American Dental Association[21] and the American Association of **Endodontics**,[22] it is estimated that 90 percent of all avulsed teeth can be reimplanted for the life of the athlete.[23] The primary problem leading to failure of the tooth to survive involves the death of the periodontal ligament attached to the avulsed tooth. All treatment should focus on the survival of this ligament.[24–26] To improve the tooth's chances of survival the emergency procedures found in Table 15–9 should be followed.[23] The team dentist should be consulted prior to the start of the season so that the protocol for these conditions can be established and followed.

REFERENCES

1. Bourbon, BM: Anatomy and biomechanics of the TMJ. In Krauss, SL: TMJ Disorders: Management of the Craniomandibular Complex. Churchill-Livingstone, New York, 1988.
1a. Norkin, CC, and Levangie, PK: Joint Structure and Function: A Comprehensive Analysis, ed 2. FA Davis, Philadelphia, 1992.
1b. Rothstein, JM, Roy, SH, and Wolf, SL: The Rehabilitation Specialist's Handbook. FA Davis, Philadelphia, 1991.
2. Jordan, L: Acute nasal and septal injuries. The Eye, Ear, Nose, and Throat Monthly 53:51, 1974.
2a. Perry, JF, Rohe, DA, and Garcia, AO: The Kinesiology Workbook, ed 2. FA Davis, Philadelphia, 1996.
3. Olsen, K, Carpenter, R, and Kern, E: Nasal septal injury in children. Arch Otolaryngol Head Neck Surg 106:317, 1980.
4. Sitler, M: Nasal septal injuries. Athletic Training: Journal of the National Athletic Trainers Association 21:10, 1986.
5. Bechman, SM: Laryngeal fracture in a high school football player. Journal of Athletic Training 28:217, 1993.
6. Friedman, MH, and Weisberg, J: The temporomandibular joint. In Gould, JA, and Davies, GJ (eds): Orthopaedic and Sports Physical Therapy. CV Mosby, St Louis, 1985, p 581.
7. Savage, R, Bevinino, J, and Mustafa, E: Treatment of acute otohematoma with compression sutures. Ann Emerg Med 10:641, 1981.
8. Fincher, AL: Use of the otoscope in the evaluation of common injuries and illnesses of the ear. Journal of Athletic Training 29:52, 1994.
9. Keating, TM, and Mason, J: A simple splint for wrestler's ear. Journal of Athletic Training 27:273, 1992.
10. Odom, CJ, and McCandless, R: Contour casting for cauliflower ear. Athletic Training: Journal of the National Athletic Trainers Association 17:114, 1982.
11. Grosse, SJ, and Lynch, JM: Treating auricular hematoma. Success with a swimmer's nose clip. The Physician and Sportsmedicine 19:98, 1991.
12. Schelkun, PH: Swimmer's ear. Getting patients back in the water. The Physician and Sportsmedicine 19:85, 1991.
13. Schendel, SA: Sports-related nasal injuries. The Physician and Sportsmedicine 18:59, 1990.
14. Storey, MD, Schatz, CF, and Brown, KW: Anterior neck trauma. The Physician and Sportsmedicine 17:85, 1989.
15. Schuller, DE, and Schleuning, AJ: DeWeese and Saunders' Otolaryngology—Head and Neck Surgery, ed 8. CV Mosby, St Louis, 1994, p 123.
16. Matthews, B: Maxillofacial trauma from athletic endeavors. Athletic Training: Journal of the National Athletic Trainers Association 25:132, 1990.
17. Halling, AH: The importance of clinical signs and symptoms in the evaluation of facial fractures. Athletic Training: Journal of the National Athletic Trainers Association 17:102, 1982.
18. Morrow, RM, and Bonci, T: A survey of oral injuries in female college and university athletes. Athletic Training: Journal of the National Athletic Trainers Association 24:236, 1989.
19. Morrow, RM, et al: Report of a survey of oral injuries in male college and university athletes. Athletic Training: Journal of the National Athletic Trainers Association 26:338, 1991.
20. Fabian, RL: Sports injury to the larynx and trachea. The Physician and Sportsmedicine 17:111, 1989.
20a. Perry JF, Rohe, DA, and Garcia, AO: The Kinesiology Workbook, ed 2. FA Davis, Philadelphia, 1996.
21. Ad Hoc Committee on Treatment of the Avulsed Tooth. American Association of Endodontists: Recommended guidelines for the treatment of the avulsed tooth. Journal of Endodontics 9:571, 1983.
22. Accepted Dental Therapeutics. American Dental Association, 1984, Chicago, p 72.
23. Krasner, P: The athletic trainer's role in saving avulsed teeth. Athletic Training: Journal of the National Athletic Trainers Association 24:139, 1989.
24. Andreasen, JO: Periodontal healing after reimplantation of traumatically avulsed human teeth. Assessment by mobility testing and radiography. Acta Odontol Scand 33:325, 1975.
25. Andreasen, JO, and Kristersson, L: The effect of limited drying or removal of the periodontal ligament. Periodontal healing after reimplantation of mature permanent incisors in monkeys. Acta Odontol Scand 39:1, 1981.
26. Andreasen, JO: Relationship between cell damage in the periodontal ligament after reimplantation and subsequent development of root resorption. A time-related study in monkeys. Acta Odontol Scand 39:15, 1981.

Endodontics: The field of dentistry specializing in the management of injuries and diseases affecting the pulp of a tooth.

16

Head and Neck Injuries

The greatest fear of virtually every coach, parent, fan, and medical staff is that of an athlete's suffering a catastrophic head or neck injury as a result of participation in sports. Fortunately, the overall rate of injury to these body areas is very low; when it does occur, however, the outcome can be fatal.

Those sports in which blows to the head are commonplace—football, baseball, and ice hockey—have rules mandating the use of protective headgear. A properly fitting mouthpiece is beneficial in preventing brain injury caused by a blow to the chin, and its use should be recommended in all contact and collision sports. The use of helmets has greatly reduced the number and severity of head injuries in football, but various styles and brands have differing degrees of effectiveness.[1-3] Ironically, the football helmet has been implicated in increasing the number of injuries to the cervical spine.

Regular inspection of equipment is imperative to ensure that it is properly maintained and continues to provide adequate protection for the athlete. Also, it is mandatory that athletes be knowledgeable about the risks associated with participation in sports and be instructed in the proper techniques necessary to avoid serious head and neck injury.

This chapter is dedicated to the immediate and follow-up evaluation and management of head and neck injuries. A well-organized procedure for the emergency management of head and neck trauma is crucial to this process and must be rehearsed regularly with the medical staff to ensure appropriate care. Chapter 10 describes the cervical spine's anatomy, evaluation of insidious cervical spine conditions, and injury to the brachial plexus.

CLINICAL ANATOMY

The brain is almost totally encased in bone with the exception of a small opening on the skull's base, through which the brain stem and spinal cord pass. The skull (or cranium) is formed by paired **parietal** and **temporal** bones laterally, the **frontal** bone, and the posteriorly projecting **occipital** bone (Fig. 16–1). In adults, these bones are rigidly fused by **cranial sutures**, making the skull a single structure. However, the sutures of infants and children are more pliable, as they are constantly remodeled during growth.

The design of the skull allows for maximum protection of the brain. The density of the bone serves to decrease the amount of physical shock transmitted inwardly. The rounded shape of the skull also has protective qualities. When an object strikes a rounded object, it tends to be quickly deflected. Consider, for example, two scenarios: dropping a brick on a tabletop and dropping a brick on a basketball. When the brick hits the tabletop, it stays there, transmitting its force into the table. When a brick is dropped onto a basketball, however, although some of the force is transmitted into the ball, the remaining force is removed as the brick deflects. Last, the skin covering the skull greatly increases the cranium's ability to protect the brain by absorbing and redirecting forces from the skull. The skin greatly increases the skull's strength, increasing its breaking force from 40 lb per square inch to 425 to 490 lb per square inch.[4]

The Brain

Because the brain is the most complex and least understood mechanism on the planet, its anatomy and function are presented in this chapter only superficially, as they relate to athletic injuries. Table 16–1 presents an encapsulated description of the major brain areas and their primary functions.

The Cerebrum

The largest section of the brain, the cerebrum is formed by two **hemispheres** separated by the **longitudinal fissure**. Each hemisphere is divided into **frontal**, **parietal**, **temporal**, and **occipital** lobes, which are separated by sulci and fissures and are named for the overlying cranial bones (Fig. 16–2).

The cerebrum is responsible for controlling the body's primary **motor** functions, in terms of both gross muscle contraction and coordination of the muscle contractions in a specific sequence. **Sensory** information such as temperature, touch, pain, pressure, and proprioception is processed in this region of the brain, along with the **special senses**, visual, auditory, olfactory, and taste. **Cognition**, including

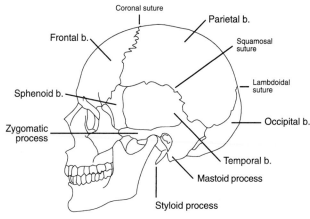

Figure 16–1. Lateral view of the bones of the skull.

spatial relationships, behavior, memory, and association, also occurs in the cerebrum.

With a few exceptions, the cerebrum communicates contralaterally with the rest of the body. The right hemisphere controls the motor actions and interprets much of the sensory input of the body's left side, and vice versa. Clinically, motor impairment of the body's left side may reflect trauma to the brain's right hemisphere.

The Cerebellum

Designed to allow the quick processing of both incoming and outgoing information, the cerebellum

provides the functions necessary to maintain **balance** and **coordination**. Visual, tactile, auditory, and proprioceptive information from the cerebrum is routed to the cerebellum for immediate processing. The outgoing information is relayed to the muscles via the cerebrum in order to properly orchestrate the necessary movements.

Fluid, synergistic motions, whether performing a back flip in gymnastics or lifting a cup of coffee, are initiated and controlled by the cerebellum. Facilitative impulses are relayed from the cerebellum to the contracting muscles, while an inhibitory stimulus is sent to the antagonistic muscles. Individuals who have suffered trauma to the cerebellum are recognizable by their uncoordinated, segmental, robotlike movements.

The Diencephalon

Formed by the **thalamus, hypothalamus,** and **epithalamus,** the diencephalon acts as a processing center for conscious and unconscious brain input. In its gatekeeper role, sensory information ascending the spinal cord is monitored by the thalamus, routing the specific types of information to the appropriate area of the brain. In addition to regulating some of the body's hormones, the hypothalamus is the center of the body's autonomic nervous system, regulating *sympathetic* and *parasympathetic nerve* activity. Body temperature, water balance, gastrointestinal activity, hunger, and certain emotions are controlled by the hypothalamus.

The Brain Stem

Formed by the **medulla oblongata** (medulla) and the **pons,** the brain stem serves to relay information to and from the central nervous system and to control many of the body's involuntary systems. Literally translating as "bridge," the **pons** serves to link the cerebellum to the brain stem and spinal cord, connecting the upper and lower portions of the central nervous system. Additionally, receptors in the pons regulate the respiratory rate.

The medulla serves as the interface between the spinal cord and the rest of the brain. Involuntary functions of heart rate, respiration, blood vessel diameter (vasodilation and vasoconstriction), coughing, and vomiting are regulated by the **medullary centers.**

The Meninges

The brain and spinal cord are buffered from the hard bony surfaces of the cranium and spinal col-

Table 16–1. Brain Function by Area

Area	Function
Cerebrum	Provides motor function.
	Processes sensory information (touch, pain, temperature, and so on).
	Processes the special senses (vision, hearing, smell, taste).
	Provides cognition.
	Provides memory.
Cerebellum	Maintains balance and coordination.
	Provides for smooth, synergistic muscle control.
Diencephalon	Routes afferent information to the appropriate cerebral areas.
	Regulates body temperature.
	Maintains the necessary water balance.
	Controls emotions (anger and fear).
Brain stem	Regulates the respiratory rate.
	Regulates the heart rate.
	Controls the amount of peripheral blood flow.

Sympathetic nervous system: The part of the central nervous system supplying the involuntary muscles.
Parasympathetic nervous system: A series of specific effects controlled by the brain regulating smooth muscle contractions, slowing the heart rate, and constricting the pupil.

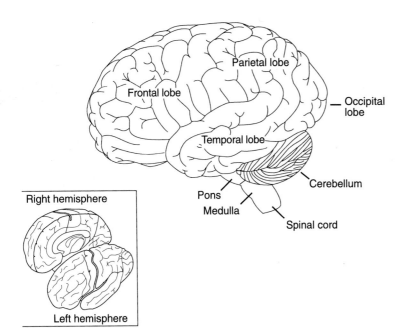

Figure 16–2. Regions of the brain, with insert showing the cerebral hemispheres.

umn by three membranes, the meninges. The progressive densities of the meninges support and protect the brain and spinal cord. Arterial and venous blood supplies are provided through these structures, as are the production and introduction of the cerebrospinal fluid (CSF).

The Dura Mater

Literally translating as "hard mother," the dura mater is the outermost meningeal covering, also serving as the periosteum for the skull's inner layer. The **falx cerebri** is a fold in the dura mater in the longitudinal fissure between the two cerebral hemispheres. The void between the two cerebellar hemispheres is filled by another fold of the dura mater, the **falx cerebelli**.

Arteries in the dura mater, the **meningeal arteries**, primarily supply blood to the cranial bones. Blood supply to the dura mater is provided by fine branches from the meningeal arteries. At various points around the brain the dura mater forms two layers. The space between these layers forms the **venous sinuses**, which serve as a drainage conduit to route used blood into the internal jugular veins in the neck.

The Arachnoid Mater

The name "arachnoid" is gained from this structure's resemblance to a cobweb ("arachne" is the Greek word for spider). Like a cobweb, the fibers forming the arachnoid are thin, yet relatively resilient to trauma. The arachnoid mater is separated from the dura mater by the very narrow **subdural space**. Beneath the arachnoid is a wider separation, the **subarachnoid space**, containing the CSF.

The Pia Mater

The internal meningeal membrane, the pia mater, envelops the brain, forming its outer "skin." This delicate membrane derives its name from the Latin word for tender; therefore, the pia mater is the "tender mother." The pia mater follows the brain's contour, riding into its fissures and sulci.

Cerebrospinal Fluid

Originating from the **choroid plexuses** deep within the brain and secreted by cells surrounding the cerebrum's blood vessels, CSF slowly circulates around the brain and spinal cord within the subarachnoid space. From the lateral ventricles, CSF is forced into the third and fourth ventricles by a pressure gradient. Once in the fourth ventricle, a small proportion of the CSF enters the central canal of the spinal cord. The remaining fluid flows down the spinal cord on its posterior surface and returns to the brain on the anterior portion of the subarachnoid space.

Because of the presence of the subarachnoid space and its watery content, the central nervous system (CNS) floats within the body. This arrangement serves as another buffer against force being transmitted to the CNS. This may be illustrated by the following. Using two Mason jars, one is filled completely with water and left the other empty. A raw egg is placed in each jar and the lid replaced. When the jar that has no water in it is shaken, the egg breaks. When the jar filled with water is shaken, the egg does not break. Although beneficial in dissipating the high-velocity impacts associated with collision sports, this protective configuration is most useful in buffering more repetitious forces, such as those seen when running.

Blood Circulation in the Head

When the body is at rest, the brain demands 20 percent of the body's oxygen uptake. For each degree (centigrade) the body's core temperature increases, the brain's need for oxygen increases by 7 percent. Blood supply to the brain is provided by the two **vertebral arteries** and the two **common carotid arteries**. Each common carotid artery diverges to form an **internal carotid** artery and an **external carotid** artery. The external carotid arteries continue upward to supply blood to the head and neck, with the exception of the brain. The internal

carotid arteries move toward the center of the cranium to assist in supplying the brain with blood.

The two internal carotid arteries and the two vertebral arteries converge to form a collateral circulation network, the **circle of Willis** (Fig. 16–3). If one of the cranial arteries is obstructed, the design of the circle of Willis permits at least a partial supply of blood to the affected area.

EVALUATION OF HEAD AND NECK INJURIES

The ability of the athletic trainer to identify and properly manage serious head and neck injury may affect whether an athlete lives, dies, or becomes permanently disabled. Although some signs and

VASCULAR ANATOMY OF BRAIN

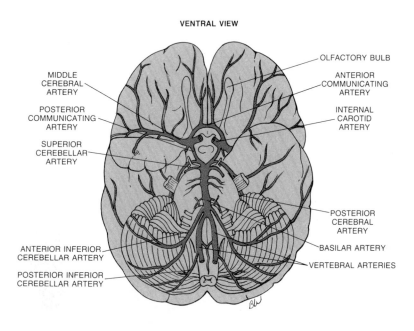

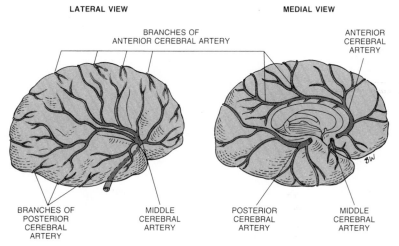

Figure 16–3. Blood supply to the brain. The Circle of Willis provides collateral circulation to the brain's regions. (From Thomas, CL [ed]: Taber's Cyclopedic Medical Dictionary, ed 17, Beth Anne Willert, MS, medical illustrator. FA Davis, Philadelphia, 1993, p 262, with permission.)

symptoms of brain trauma are blatantly obvious, such as unconsciousness, some potentially catastrophic head injuries initially have few, if any, outward signs or symptoms. This section describes the signs and symptoms of brain and spine trauma. The following section describes the on-field management of these conditions. Many of these evaluative procedures are performed on the field.

Catastrophic injury is almost always followed by litigation.[5] For this reason, the athletic trainer must thoroughly document the events leading up to the injury, how the injury is managed on the field, and the athlete's disposition at the time of transport to the hospital. Additional information should describe any unusual circumstances surrounding the injury and copies of any waivers the athlete may have signed prior to competing in the sport.

Evaluation Scenarios

Before discussing how to evaluate and manage head and neck injuries, the possible scenarios under which an evaluation may have to be performed must be considered. The best-case scenario is one in which the athlete is conscious and responsive to stimuli. The worst-case scenario is that of a prone, unconscious athlete who is devoid of an airway, breathing, or circulation (ABC). In this case the decisions made by the athletic trainer are critical in the optimal management of catastrophic conditions.

A basic premise must be formed at this point and adhered to at all times:

> All unconscious athletes should be managed as if a fracture or dislocation of the cervical spine exists until the presence of these injuries can be definitively ruled out.

On-field head and neck injuries are evaluated ideally by at least two certified athletic trainers. One athletic trainer must ensure stabilization and immobilization of the athlete's head by grasping the sides of the helmet and applying **in-line stabilization** on the cervical spine until pathology has been ruled out. A second athletic trainer performs the necessary palpation, sensory, and motor tests (Fig. 16–4). One member of the staff must act as the leader and direct the actions of all others at the injury scene. In situations when only one certified athletic trainer is present, other on-site personnel may be directed to assist in management of the athlete's condition. Prior discussion and practice are compulsory to ensure orderly and precise action by the support staff.

Athlete's Position

The initial assessment of an on-field head and neck injury may be further complicated by the position in which the athlete is found. A supine athlete is in the optimal alignment for subsequent evaluation and management. When athletes are side-lying or prone, the evaluation is more difficult.

If, as determined in the next section, the athlete's vital signs are present, there is no need to move the athlete until a complete on-field evaluation is performed and the athlete's disposition determined. However, when an athlete is prone or side-lying, the absence of vital signs takes precedence over the possibility of a spinal fracture. The athlete must be rolled into the supine position in the safest manner possible. These procedures are discussed in On-Field Management of Head and Neck Injuries in this chapter.

Determination of Consciousness

When an athlete is "down" on the field or court, the athletic trainer's first priority is to establish the

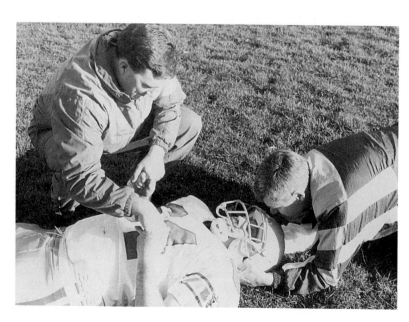

Figure 16–4. Head and neck trauma is best managed by two responders. One athletic trainer stabilizes the head while the second performs evaluative techniques.

athlete's level of consciousness. A moving and speaking athlete establishes that the ABCs are present and functioning. Even under these circumstances, however, a cervical fracture should be suspected and the athlete's vital signs regularly monitored. Once at the scene of a possible head or neck injury, the athletic trainer should stabilize and immobilize the athlete's head by grasping the sides of the helmet or head and applying in-line stabilization on the cervical spine until pathology to the spine has been ruled out (as described in the previous section).

- **Level of consciousness:** While moving toward the scene of the injury the athletic trainer should note whether the athlete is moving. Once at the scene, an attempt should be made to communicate with the athlete. If verbal communication fails, the athlete's responsiveness to painful stimuli should be checked. This is performed by applying pressure to the lunula of a fingernail, applying pressure to the orbit just below the medial eyebrow, rubbing the sternum, or pinching the cheek (Fig. 16–5).

- **Primary survey:** If the athlete is unconscious or unable to communicate, the athlete's ABCs should be checked. The athletic trainer should look, listen, and feel for breathing (Fig. 16–6). If breathing is absent, a modified jaw thrust is used to open the airway. In the event that no carotid or radial pulse is found, someone should be sent to summon advanced medical assistance and cardiopulmonary resuscitation should be started. The On-Field Management section of this chapter contains further discussion of this topic.

- **Secondary survey:** Although the suspicion of brain or cervical spine trauma takes precedence, the examiner must not overlook the possibility of other trauma to the body once the athlete's condition has been stabilized. The extremities and torso should be inspected for bleeding or indications of fractures and/or dislocations.

The following components of an assessment of a head-injured or neck-injured athlete assume a sideline evaluation is being conducted. A descriptive on-field management procedure is detailed later in this chapter.

History

The history-taking process of a head-injured athlete not only determines the injury mechanism but also assesses the athlete's level of brain function. Much of this portion of the evaluation is initially conducted when the athlete is on the field and then repeated at regular intervals on the sideline. In the event that the athlete becomes unconscious, the clinician should proceed to the inspection phase of the evaluation while continuing to monitor the vital signs. Throughout the evaluation, the athlete must be questioned and observed for the presence of subtle signs and symptoms indicating a head injury (Table 16–2).

- **Location of symptoms:** The athlete should be questioned regarding the location and type of pain or other symptoms experienced following the injury. In many instances the athlete volunteers this information before being asked.
  - **Cervical pain:** The most significant finding during this portion of the examination is cervical pain or muscle spasm. The significance of this finding is magnified when it is accompanied by pain, numbness, or burning, which may or may not radiate into the extremities.
  - **Head pain:** Diffuse headaches are a common complaint following brain trauma. Localized pain can indicate a contusion, skull fracture, or intracranial hemorrhage.

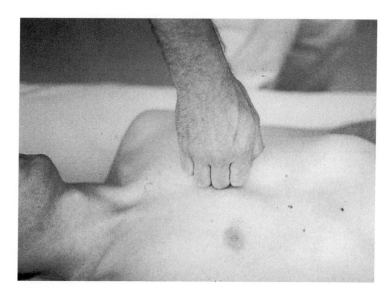

Figure 16–5. Attempting to elicit a pain response from an athlete. This test is performed by squeezing the athlete's fingernail, pinching the athlete, or applying pressure with a knuckle to the athlete's sternum.

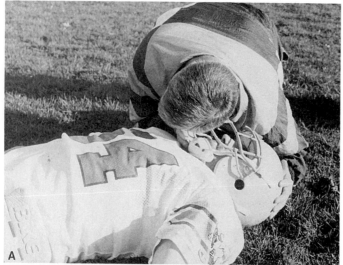

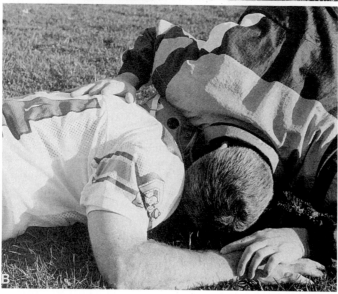

Figure 16–6. Establishing the presence of an open airway, breathing, and circulation. (*A*) Supine athlete. (*B*) Prone athlete.

- **Mechanism of head injuries:** The type of injury inflicted to the head and cervical spine is somewhat dependent on the nature of the force delivered (Fig. 16–7). This information may be obtained by someone who witnessed the injury if the athlete is unconscious or groggy.

Table 16–2. Signs and Symptoms of a Head or Neck Injury To Observe for Throughout the Evaluation

Blurred vision
Confusion
Disorientation
Dizziness
Headache
Incoordination
Nausea
Nystagmus
Tinnitus

○ **Coup:** A coup injury results when a relatively stationary skull is hit by an object traveling at a high velocity (e.g., being struck in the head with a baseball). This type of mechanism typically results in trauma on the side that was struck.

○ **Contrecoup:** When the skull is moving at a relatively high velocity and is suddenly stopped, such as when falling and striking the head on the floor, the fluid within the skull fails to decrease the brain's momentum proportional to that of the skull, causing the brain to strike the skull on the side opposite the impact. This mechanism includes forces that are transmitted up the length of the spinal column, such as when falling and landing on the buttocks.

○ **Repeated subconcussive forces:** Athletes receiving repeated nontraumatic blows to the head (e.g., boxing, heading a soccerball) have a higher degree of degenerative changes within the CNS.[6] When the athlete remains exposed to

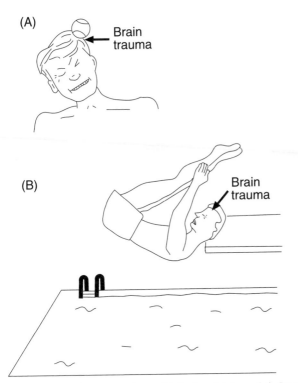

Figure 16–7. Mechanisms of an athletic head injury. (*A*) Coup mechanism caused by a moving object striking the head, resulting in brain trauma on the side of the impact. (*B*) Contrecoup mechanism caused by a moving head striking a stationary object. Trauma occurs to the brain on the opposite side of the impact as it rebounds off the skull.

this type of trauma, electroencephalographic (EEG) activity is disrupted and neuropsychological impairment results.

- **Mechanism cervical spine injuries:** Most of the forces directed toward the cervical spine are capable of being dissipated by the energy-absorbing properties of the cervical musculature and intervertebral disks through controlling spinal motion.[7] The most common mechanisms of injury to the cervical spine involve hyperflexion, hyperextension, or lateral bending and may be accompanied by a rotational component.

Flexion of the cervical spine is the mechanism most likely to produce catastrophic injury.[7–11] As the crown of the head makes contact, the cervical spine and skull flexes. Once the neck is flexed to approximately 30 degrees, the cervical spine's lordotic curve is lost (Fig. 16–8). In this position the effectiveness of the cervical spine's energy-dissipating mechanism is rendered ineffective, thus transmitting forces directly to the cervical vertebrae, creating an **axial load** through the vertical axis of the segmented columns (Fig. 16–9).

- **Loss of consciousness:** This portion of the history-taking process is closely related to the determination of the athlete's memory status. The responses given by the athlete immediately after the

injury should be recorded for future comparison. The athlete should be questioned regarding a momentary loss of consciousness following the impact ("Do you remember being hit?"). The athlete may also describe "seeing stars" or "blacking out" at the time of the impact, both of which indicate transitory unconsciousness.

- **Prior history of concussion:** Although the timing of the question may not be appropriate immediately following the injury, at some point the athlete must be questioned regarding the number of prior instances of head-related trauma. This information should also be obtainable in the athlete's medical file.

- **Complaints of weakness:** A general malaise is to be expected following a cerebral concussion. Reports of muscular weakness in one or more extremities is a more serious finding, possibly indicating trauma to the brain, spinal cord, or one or more spinal nerve roots.

Inspection

If the athlete is wearing protective headgear at the onset of the inspection process, a decision must be made regarding whether and when to remove it. The helmet should not be removed if there is any lingering suspicion of a cervical spine fracture or dislocation. Much of the inspection and palpation process can be performed with the helmet still in place.

Bony Structures

- **Position of the head:** The examiner should observe the way in which the athlete's head is positioned. Normally the head should be upright in all planes, although the face may have a normal downward attitude. A laterally flexed and rotated skull that is accompanied by muscle spasm on the side opposite that of the tilt is indicative of a dislocation of a cervical vertebra.

- **Cervical vertebrae:** Viewing the athlete from behind, the examiner observes the alignment of the spinous processes. A vertebra that is obviously malaligned (rotated or displaced anteriorly or posteriorly) can signify a vertebral dislocation. If this finding is consistent with the findings of pain, neurological impairment in the upper extremity, and tenderness during palpation, the cervical spine must be immobilized and the athlete transported to a hospital by ambulance.

- **Mastoid process: Battle's sign,** ecchymosis over the mastoid process, is indicative of a basilar skull fracture.

- **Skull and scalp:** The athlete's skull and scalp should be inspected for the presence of bleeding, swelling, or other deformities.

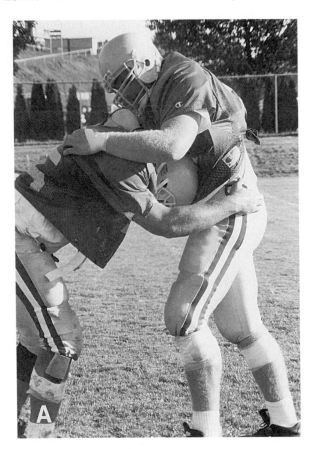

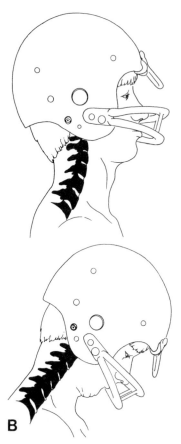

Figure 16–8. Making contact with the crown of the helmet results in axial loading, compressing the cervical vertebrae (From Torg,[8] with permission).

Eyes

- **General:** The general attitude of the athlete's eyes should be noted. A dazed, distant appearance is commonly attributable to mental confusion and disruption of cerebral function.

- **Nystagmus:** While observing both of the athlete's eyes simultaneously, the clinician should note the presence of involuntary cyclical movement, or nystagmus. This clinical sign, although it may normally occur in the athlete, is indicative of pressure on the eyes' motor nerves or disruption of the inner ear.

- **Pupil size:** Equality of the size of the athlete's pupils should be noted. A unilaterally dilated pupil is indicative of intracranial hemorrhage placing pressure on cranial nerve III. Some athletes may normally display unequal pupil sizes, **anisocoria** (Fig. 16–10). Although this condition is benign, its presence should be detected during the preparticipation physical examination and noted in the athlete's medical file to avoid confusion during the evaluation of a head injury.

Nose and Ears

Blood or other fluid leaking from the nose or ear should be checked for CSF in its content. A sample of the drainage is collected by allowing it to be absorbed in a piece of sterile gauze. If CSF is contained within the fluid, a pale yellow halo will form around the sample of the gauze.

Bleeding from the ears, even in the absence of CSF in the fluid, can indicate a skull fracture. Bleeding from the nose may represent either a nasal fracture or a skull fracture. Ecchymosis under the eyes, "raccoon eyes," may occur not only after a nasal fracture, but also after a skull fracture (the suspicion of a skull fracture is increased when "raccoon eyes" are present).

Palpation

Palpation should not be performed over areas of obvious deformity, or suspected fracture, especially in the cervical spine and skull. Placing too much pressure on these structures can cause the bony fragment to displace, possibly resulting in catastrophic consequences.

Bony Structures

- **Spinous processes:** The athlete is positioned sitting on the bench and leaning slightly forward. Standing behind the athlete, the examiner di-

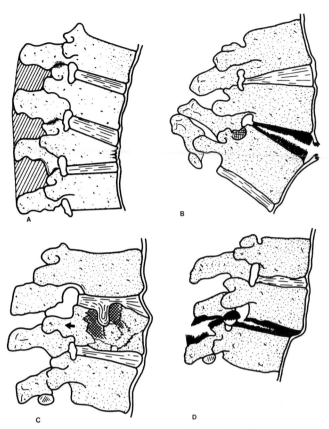

Figure 16-9. Mechanisms of cervical spine injuries and the resulting trauma. (*A*) Flexion mechanism resulting in compression of the vertebral body; (*B*) extension mechanism resulting in tearing of the anterior longitudinal ligament and intervertebral disk; (*C*) compression mechanism resulting in a posterior burst of the bone; (*D*) flexion and rotation injury resulting in a dislocation of the cervical vertebrae. (From Mueller, FO, and Ryan, AJ,[11a] p 204, with permission.)

rectly palpates the spinous processes of C7, C6, and C5 (Fig. 16-11). At approximately the C5 level the spinous processes become less defined. The examiner continues to palpate the area of the spinous processes of C4 and C3, noting for tenderness or crepitus.

• **Transverse processes:** Although the transverse processes of C2 are the only ones that are directly palpable (approximately two fingers' widths below the mastoid process), the areas over the transverse processes of the remaining cervical vertebrae are palpated.

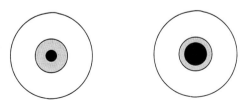

Figure 16-10. Anisocoria, unequal pupil size. This condition may result from pressure on cranial nerve III or it may be congenital.

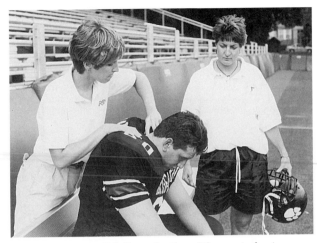

Figure 16-11. Sideline palpation of the cervical spine.

• **Skull:** The examiner begins palpation of the skull at the inion, the occipital bone's posterior process. Palpation is continued anteriorly toward the face, palpating the temporal bones and their mastoid processes, and the sphenoid, zygomatic, parietal, and frontal bones (see Fig. 16-1).

Soft Tissue

• **Musculature:** To identify muscular spasm, the trapezius and sternocleidomastoid muscles should be palpated. In addition to the muscle's reaction to a strain, spasm may result from insult to a cervical nerve root or may reflect the body's protective response to a cervical fracture or dislocation.

• **Throat:** The complete palpation of the anterior throat may be warranted to rule out trauma to the larynx, trachea, or hyoid bone.

Functional Tests

The goal of the functional testing of a head-injured or neck-injured athlete is to assess the status of the CNS. This portion of the examination is initiated when the athlete's airway, breathing, circulation, and level of consciousness are examined. This section of the chapter assumes that the athlete is conscious and capable of responding to the functional tasks presented. The cervical spine must be assessed first to rule out bone or joint dysfunction.

Memory

One of the most obvious dysfunctions following brain trauma is the athlete's loss of memory. The inability to recall events prior to the onset of the injury is termed **retrograde amnesia**. When the athlete cannot remember events following the onset of injury it is termed **anterograde amnesia** or posttraumatic amnesia (Fig. 16-12).

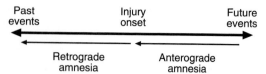

Figure 16–12. Types of amnesia. Loss of memory from onset backward in time is known as retrograde amnesia. Loss of memory following the onset of the injury is anterograde amnesia.

• **Retrograde amnesia:** Retrograde amnesia is the most common form of memory loss resulting from athletic-related head trauma. This dysfunction may be as subtle as not remembering the impact causing the trauma or as severe as a total disorientation regarding time, person, and place. The severity of retrograde amnesia is based on how far back in time the memory is distorted, following a set of questions ordered from the most recent event and progressing backward in time. The same set of questions should be repeated to determine whether the athlete's memory is returning, deteriorating, or remaining the same. Further deterioration of the memory, or acutely profound memory loss that does not return in a matter of minutes, warrants the immediate termination of the evaluation and transportation to an emergency facility.

Determination of Retrograde Amnesia

Position of athlete	On-field: In the athlete's current position (see instructions regarding moving the athlete). Sideline: Standing, sitting, or lying down.
Position of examiner	In a position to hear the athlete's response.
Evaluative procedure	The athlete is asked a series of questions beginning with the time of the injury. Each successive question progresses backward in time as described by the following set of questions: What happened? What play were you running? (or other applicable question regarding the athlete's activity at the time of injury) Where are you? Who am I? Who are you playing? What quarter is it? (or, what time is it?) What did you have for a pregame meal? (or, what did you have to eat for lunch?) What is your name?
Positive test results	The athlete has difficulty remembering, or cannot remember, events occurring before the injury.
Implications	Retrograde amnesia, the severity of which is based on the relative amount of memory loss suffered by the athlete. Not remembering events from the day before is more significant than not remembering what play was being run.
Comments	The examiner should record the athlete's response and verify the answers with the athlete's teammates or coach.

• **Anterograde amnesia:** Although significant retrograde amnesia is a cause of concern, fading or fogging memory identifies a progressive deterioration of the athlete's cerebral function. The athlete should be questioned regarding the sequence of events following the injury:

○ How did you get to the sidelines?
○ Who has spoken to you since?
○ Do you remember my asking you those questions before?

The athlete's anterograde memory can be partially determined by the ability to remember a list of items. After a period of time has passed (e.g., after being allowed to shower) the athlete is asked to recite this list to the examiner. The inability to do so may indicate pressure within the cranium caused by hemorrhage (see top of page 487).

Cognitive Function

Trauma to the cerebrum can result in unusual communication between the athlete and the examiner. This can manifest itself through unusual behavior, irrational thinking, and apparent mental disability or personality changes.

Determination of Anterograde Amnesia

Position of athlete	On the sideline or in athletic training room.
Position of examiner	In a position to hear the athlete's response.

Evaluative procedure	The athlete is given a list of four unrelated items with instructions to memorize them, for example:
	  Hubcap
	  Film
	  Dog tags
	  Ivy
	The list is immediately repeated by the athlete to ensure that it has been memorized.
	After a period of time the athlete is asked to repeat the list to the examiner.

Positive test results	The inability to completely recite the list.
Implications	Anterograde amnesia, possibly the result of intracranial bleeding.

- **Behavior:** The athlete's behavior, attitude, and demeanor may become altered after brain trauma. This may take the form of violent, irrational behavior, inappropriate behavior, and belligerence. Following a head injury the athlete may verbally and/or physically lash out at those attempting to assist.

- **Analytical skills:** The athlete's analytical skills can be determined through the use of simple math skills (e.g., "What is 100 minus 7?").

- **Information processing:** The athlete's ability to process the information and assimilate facts should be noted. Confusion regarding relatively simple directions, such as "Sit on the bench," indicates profound cognitive dysfunction.

Balance and Coordination

Following a head injury, the athlete's balance and coordination may be hindered secondary to trauma involving the cerebellum or the inner ear. A profound loss of muscular coordination, ataxia, may be obvious as the athlete attempts to perform even simple tasks.

- **Romberg's test:** Romberg's test is the classic technique used to determine the athlete's level of balance and coordination (Fig. 16–13). Note that there are variations of this test, but the underlying goal of each variant is to determine the athlete's ability to maintain an erect posture.

Romberg's Test (Fig. 16–13)

Position of athlete	Standing with the feet shoulder-width apart.
Position of examiner	Standing lateral to the athlete, ready to support the athlete as needed.
Evaluative procedure	The athlete shuts the eyes, abducts the arms to 90° with the elbows extended. The athlete tilts the head backward and lifts one foot off the ground while attempting to maintain balance. If this portion of the examination is adequately completed, the athlete is asked to touch the index finger to the nose (the eyes remain closed).
Positive test results	The athlete displays gross unsteadiness.
Implications	Lack of balance and/or coordination indicating cerebellular dysfunction.

- **Heel-toe walk:** Resembling a field sobriety test, the heel-toe walk assesses the athlete's ability to maintain balance (Fig. 16–14).

Heel-Toe Walk (Fig. 16–14)

Position of athlete	Standing with the feet straddling a straight line (e.g., sideline).
Position of examiner	Beside the athlete ready to provide support.
Evaluative procedure	The athlete walks heel-to-toe along the straight line for approximately 10 yd. The athlete returns to the starting position by walking backward.
Positive test results	The athlete is unable to maintain a steady balance.
Implications	Cerebral or inner ear dysfunction that inhibits balance.

Monitoring Vital Signs

Techniques for determining the vital signs are described in Chapter 10. The following are qualitative parameters that are relevant following a head or neck injury.

- **Respiration:** In addition to the number of breaths per minute, the quality of the respirations should be determined:

Type	Characteristics	Implications
Apneustic	Prolonged inspirations that are unrelieved by attempts to exhale.	Trauma to the pons.
Biot's	Periods of **apnea** followed by hyperapnea.	Increased intracranial pressure.
Cheyne-Stokes	Periods of apnea followed by breaths of increasing depth and frequency.	Frontal lobe or brain stem trauma.
Slow	Respiration consisting of fewer than 12 breaths per minute.	CNS disruption.
Thoracic	Respiration in which the diaphragm is inactive and breathing occurs only through expansion of the chest. Normal abdominal movement is absent.	Disruption of the phrenic nerve or its nerve roots.

- **Pulse:** The athlete's pulse rate and quality must be monitored in regular intervals until the possibility of brain or spinal injury has been ruled out.

Pulse abnormalities attributed to these conditions include:

Type	Characteristics	Implications
Accelerated	Pulse >150 beats per minute (bpm) (>170 bpm usually has fatal results).	Pressure on the base of the brain; shock.
Bounding	Pulse that quickly reaches a higher intensity than normal, then quickly disappears.	Ventricular systole and reduced peripheral pressure.
Deficit	Pulse in which the number of beats counted at the radial pulse is less than that counted over the heart itself.	Cardiac arrhythmia.
High-tension	Pulse in which the force of the beat is relatively increased as noted by the amount of force required to arrest the pulse.	Cerebral trauma.
Low-tension	Short, fast, faint pulse having a rapid decline.	Heart failure; shock.

Apnea: The temporary cessation of breathing.

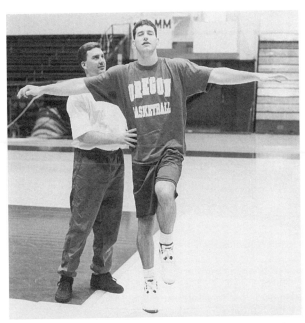

Figure 16–13. Romberg's test to determine the athlete's balance and coordination. Note that this test has many variations.

- **Blood pressure:** Blood pressure readings should be taken concurrently or immediately after each pulse measurement. These measurements should be recorded and repeated at regular intervals. Increased blood pressure indicates severe intracranial hemorrhage.

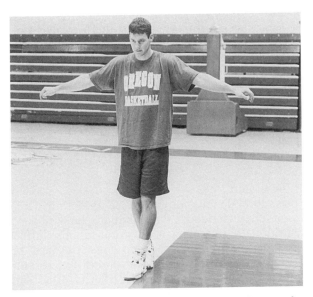

Figure 16–14. Heel-toe walk to test the athlete's balance and coordination.

Neurological Tests

Twelve pairs of **cranial nerves** (CNs), identified by Roman numerals (CN I to CN XII), arise from the brain and transmit both sensory and motor impulses (Table 16–3). The *ganglia* of the sensory component are located outside the CNS, whereas the ganglia of the motor nerves are located within the CNS. Increased intracranial pressure results in impairment of the motor component of the cranial nerves involved but leaves their sensory component intact.

Cranial Nerve Function

An assessment of the cranial nerves should be conducted immediately following the injury and repeated in 15- to 20-minute intervals until the severity of the head injury has been determined. As noted previously, accumulation of blood within the cranium places pressure on the cranial nerves, impairing their function. Information regarding the loss of many of these functions, such as vision, smell, and taste, are volunteered by the athlete. The following tests are ordered by the affected organ rather than by the cranial nerves themselves.

- **Eyes:** The athlete's **vision** (CN II) is assessed using a Snellen's chart (see Fig. 14–5) or by asking the athlete to read an object of reasonable size for the athlete's normal vision, such as the amount of time remaining on the scoreboard. With the use of a penlight, the pupil's **reaction to light** (CN III) should be determined by covering one of the athlete's eyes and briefly shining the light into the opposite pupil. Normally, the pupil should constrict when the light strikes it and dilate when the light is removed. Using a penlight, finger, or other object held approximately 2 ft from the athlete's nose, the equality of **eye movement** (CNs II, IV, and VI) is determined by moving the object up, down, left, right, and finally, inward toward the athlete's nose.
  Diplopia experienced by the athlete may be indicative of cerebral dysfunction, pressure on CN III, IV, or VI causing spasm of the eye's extrinsic muscles, or a fracture of the eye's orbit. Any double vision that does not rapidly subside indicates the immediate need for advanced medical assistance.
- **Face:** The athlete is asked to raise the eyebrows and forehead, smile, and frown (CN VII); clench the jaw (CN V); swallow (CNs IX and X), and stick out the tongue (CN XII).
- **Ears:** The functions of CN VIII include hearing, in which any disruption should be apparent. Tinnitus, which is determined in the history-taking

---

Ganglion (nerve) (pl. ***ganglia***): A collection of nerve cell bodies housed in the central or peripheral nervous system.

Table 16–3. Cranial Nerve Function

Number	Name	Type	Function
I	Olfactory	Sensory	Smell.
II	Optic	Sensory	Vision.
III	Oculomotor	Motor	Affects pupillary reaction/size. Raises upper eyelid. Adducts eye and rolls eye downward.
IV	Trochlear	Motor	Rolls eye upward.
V	Trigeminal	Mixed	Motor: muscles of mastication. Sensation: nose, forehead, temple, scalp, lips, tongue, and lower jaw.
VI	Abducens	Motor	Moves eye laterally.
VII	Facial	Mixed	Motor: muscles of expression. Sensory: taste.
VIII	Vestibulocochlear	Sensory	Equilibrium. Hearing.
IX	Glossopharyngeal	Mixed	Motor: pharyngeal muscles. Sensory: taste.
X	Vagus	Mixed	Motor: muscles of pharynx and larynx. Sensory: gag reflex.
XI	Accessory	Motor	Trapezius and sternocleidomastoid muscles.
XII	Hypoglossal	Motor	Allows tongue movement.

portion of the examination, demonstrates possible malfunctions of CN VIII. The athlete's balance and equilibrium can be assessed through the use of Romberg's test.

• **Shoulders and neck: If the presence of a cervical injury has been ruled out,** manual resistance against neck extension (see Fig. 9–25), neck rotation (see Fig. 9–27), and shoulder shrugs (see Fig. 11–37) is used to determine the integrity of CN XI.

Spinal Nerve Roots

A complete neurological evaluation is required for any athlete suspected of suffering brain or spinal trauma. When the athlete is on the sideline or in the athletic training room, a complete upper- and lower-quarter neurological screen should be performed to test for normal sensory, motor, and reflex functions (see Chapter 9). The neurological tests to be performed while the athlete is on the field or court are less nerve root–specific and are explained in the On-Field Management Section of this chapter.

Pathologies and Related Special Tests

Organized football has a fatality rate of 3 deaths per 100,000 participants, with the majority of these fatalities being attributed to head or cervical spine trauma.[12] However, head and neck trauma can, and does, occur in sports other than football. Emergency preparedness should not be limited to the sport of football but, rather, should encompass all of the institution's athletic programs.

The ability to correctly identify and manage these conditions in a timely, safe, and efficient manner is a determining factor related to the successful management of a potentially catastrophic injury. Prudent decision making should be used in the determination of the athlete's status and disposition. More so than any other type of injury described in this text, a consistent standardized plan of action must be implemented immediately in the management of these conditions.

Head Trauma

Protective headgear has greatly reduced the number and severity of brain injuries in sports mandating their use. Furthermore, the incidence of skull fractures and skin lacerations in areas directly protected by the helmet has virtually been eliminated. The progressive nature of many of the symptoms of head injuries requires that athletes who have been released in apparently "good health" be given instructions on signs and symptoms to look for. These instructions should also be communicated to the athlete's parents, roommate, or spouse (see Home Instructions).

Concussion

A cerebral concussion is defined as a clinical syndrome characterized by immediate but transient posttraumatic impairment of neural function affecting equilibrium and disrupting consciousness due to brain stem involvement.[13] Several different rating scales are used to quantify the severity of concussions, ranging from 3- to 15-point scales. This text uses the 3-point scale recommended by the American Medical Association for the classification of athletic-related head injuries (Table 16–4).[14]

Contrecoup mechanisms are most commonly associated with the onset of injury, and the blow tends to be delivered over the occipital region. The

Table 16-4. Classification of Athletic-Related Concussions

Signs and Symptoms	Concussion Classification		
	Grade I	Grade II	Grade III
Loss of consciousness	None or transitory.	<5 min.	>5 min.
Memory loss	None or transient retrograde amnesia.	Retrograde amnesia; memory may return.	Sustained retrograde amnesia. Anterograde is possible with intracranial hemorrhage.
	None to slight mental confusion.	Slight to moderate mental confusion.	Severe mental confusion.
Motor ability	No loss of coordination.	Noticeable loss of coordination.	Profound loss of coordination.
Dizziness	Transient.	Moderate.	Obvious motor impairment.
Tinnitus	None.	Possible/transitory.	Prolonged.
Recovery	Rapid.	Slow.	Delayed.

Table 16-5. Evaluative Findings of a Cerebral Concussion

Examination Segment	Clinical Findings
History	Onset: Acute. Nature of pain: Headache, ringing in the ears, blurred vision, dizziness, unconsciousness. Mechanism: Blow to the skull or spinal column transmitting an injurious force to the brain.
Inspection	Eyes: Generally may appear glazed or dazed. Pupil sizes should be equal; a unilaterally dilated pupil may indicate pressure on CN III. Nystagmus may indicate pressure on the cranial nerves or dysfunction within the inner ear. Nose and ears: Fluid draining from the nose and ears should be checked for the presence of cerebrospinal fluid (see page 495). General: The entire skull should be inspected for secondary bleeding or contusions. The area over the mastoid process and the area beneath the eyes should be checked for ecchymosis, indicating a skull fracture.
Palpation	If the athlete was not wearing a helmet at the time of injury, the skull should be palpated to determine areas of point tenderness, possibly indicating the presence of a skull fracture.
Functional tests	Memory: Transient retrograde amnesia of the events leading up to the injury. An increased scope of memory loss is indicative of a severe concussion. The presence of anterograde amnesia warrants the immediate referral to a physician. Cognitive function: The athlete may display confused, violent, or aggressive behavior and may have diminished analytical function. Balance and coordination: These are diminished immediately after the injury but should return rapidly. Eyes: Blurred vision and unequal pupil size are present.
Ligamentous tests	Not applicable.
Neurological tests	Cranial nerve check, sensory testing, motor testing.
Special tests	Pulse, blood pressure, and respiration should be monitored. Retrograde amnesia test and anterograde amnesia test should be repeated at regular intervals. Romberg's test and heel-toe walk (balance and coordination) should be performed. Cerebral function tests (e.g., 100 minus 7) should be given.
Comments	The possibility of a cervical spine fracture must be assumed until such an injury can be ruled out. When the severity of the injury is in doubt, the athlete is referred to a physician for further evaluation. Athletes who are unconscious for a measurable period of time should be cleared by a physician before returning to competition. An athlete with a history of multiple head trauma or having symptoms following little or no physical trauma should always be referred for further assessment by a physician (see Postconcussional Syndrome and Second Impact Syndrome).

signs and symptoms range from little or no loss of consciousness and memory to profound loss of all cerebral functions (Table 16–5). Low-grade concussions are marked by the transitory loss of consciousness in a duration measured in seconds. Athletes who are unconscious for more than 30 seconds must be removed from competition and immediately referred to a physician. Other symptoms associated with concussions include dizziness, tinnitus, nausea, memory loss, and motor impairment, with

Table 16–6. Dysfunction Guide for Evaluating the Extent of Cerebral Concussions

Function	Slight	Severe	Comments
Consciousness	Unconscious for <15 sec.	Unconscious for >30 sec. Associated convulsion.	Deep unconsciousness lasting 15 to 30 sec may also be classified as severe, especially when accompanied by other severe ratings.
Memory	Athlete initially does not remember the immediate events leading to the trauma.	**Retrograde amnesia:** The athlete does not remember events prior to the mechanism of injury. **Anterograde amnesia:** The athlete does not remember events following the injury.	Transitory loss of memory of the injurious contact is to be expected and is often associated with a brief loss of consciousness (the athlete reports "seeing stars" or "blacking out").
Cognitive function	Slight transient mental confusion ("What happened?").	The athlete is disoriented to person, place, and/or time. The athlete displays violent, aggressive, and otherwise inappropriate behavior or language. The athlete cannot process information "normally."	These traits may be expected immediately after the injury. Their presence is labeled severe when they are prolonged.
Balance/ coordination	Slight unsteadiness or unsteadiness that rapidly subsides.	Profound disruption of the athlete's balance and coordination exists. The athlete is unable to walk without assistance and has difficulty performing basic manual skills.	These functions are based not only on the results of Romberg's test and the heel-toe walk but also on general observation of the athlete.
Tinnitus	None or transitory.	Prolonged tinnitus is described or worsens with time.	Ringing in the ears may be described immediately after the blow but should subside with time.
Pupil size	Equal. Both pupils are responsive to light.	Dilated pupil that is unresponsive to light.	Indicative of increased intracranial pressure on CN III. Unequal pupil size (anisocoria) may be normally present in the athlete.
Nystagmus	Absent.	Present.	Indicative of increased intracranial pressure or inner ear dysfunction. This may be normally present in the athlete.
Vision	Normal or initially "blurry," which quickly subsides.	Persistent blurred or double vision.	The athlete's normal vision should be taken into account (i.e., if the athlete wears glasses).
Nausea	None or slight.	Vomiting.	Cumulative effect.
Pulse	Within normal limits, possibly decreasing with rest.	Abnormally increasing or decreasing.	Indicative of intracranial hematoma.
Blood pressure	Within normal limits.	Rapidly rising or falling.	Indicative of intracranial hematoma.
Respirations	Normal.	Abnormal.	See Functional Testing section of this chapter.

the symptoms occurring along a continuum ranging from no disruption to total disruption. Severe cases may also be marked by convulsions, vomiting, and loss of bowel and bladder control.

To determine the extent of the injury, the findings of a cerebral concussion evaluation should be compared with the dysfunction guide in Table 16–6. In addition to unconsciousness, one or more findings within the "severe" classification warrant the athlete's being removed from competition and referred to a physician.

Determining the time for the safe return to play following a head injury is a major concern of medical personnel. As noted in the following sections, some severe head injuries may not produce significant signs or symptoms for some time following the actual trauma. This fact alone suggests that it is better to err on the side of caution. An athlete who sustains a mild concussion may be allowed to return to participation once all the signs and symptoms have cleared. Those athletes sustaining a moderate or severe concussion should not return to competition for several days, weeks, or months after the injury. Table 16–7 presents the recommended time to return to competition following cerebral concussions, assuming that all of the athlete's symptoms have cleared. This is ultimately the physician's decision. Advanced imaging techniques such as MRIs and CT scans can be used to help make a sound decision as to whether an athlete should return to competition or continue to be held out.[15]

Repeated head trauma can produce cumulative degenerative effects on brain function. Athletes with a history of multiple concussions can display the signs and symptoms of a current concussion in the absence of a recent history of head trauma.[16] Additionally, a concussion may produce lingering effects, be magnified by subsequent concussions, or mask underlying brain trauma.

Postconcussional Syndrome

Athletes suffering a cerebral concussion may describe a number of cognitive impairments for some time following the injury.[17] This syndrome is characterized by decreased attention span, trouble concentrating, impaired memory, and irritability. Exercise may cause headaches, dizziness, and premature fatigue. These symptoms may require that the athlete be evaluated by a neurosurgeon and may preclude a return to activity.

Second Impact Syndrome

Multiple concussions or other types of head injuries occurring within a relatively short time frame can produce catastrophic results.[18] The second impact may be relatively minor and not delivered directly to the athlete's head, consisting of a contrecoup mechanism of injury to the brain.[19] Initially following the injury the athlete may display no signs or symptoms of the disaster that may occur within the next 30 seconds.

The second trauma is thought to disrupt the autoregulation of the brain's blood supply, resulting in vasodilation and the subsequent engorgement of the intracranial vasculature.[20] The increased blood flow and vascular expanse increase the intracranial pressure and quickly disrupt the brain stem's normal function. Outward signs of spinal and cranial nerve involvement occur within 2 minutes of the trauma.

Initially the athlete may display the signs and symptoms of a grade I concussion but quickly collapses in a semicomatose state. Pressure on the cranial nerves results in rapidly dilating pupils that are unresponsive to light and the loss of eye motion. As the pressure continues to build, the athlete displays signs of respiratory distress secondary to disruption of the phrenic nerve.

Intervention must be swift and concise. The physician, paramedic, or other qualified personnel should intubate the athlete and may induce hyperventilation to facilitate vasoconstriction secondary to decreased carbon dioxide in the bloodstream. Even in the best-case scenarios, second impact syndrome has a 50 percent mortality rate.[19] This severity emphasizes the importance of preventing this

Table 16–7. Guidelines for Returning to Play Following a Cerebral Concussion

	1st Concussion	2nd Concussion	3rd Concussion
Grade 1 (mild)	May return to play if asymptomatic.	Return to play in 2 wk if the athlete is asymptomatic during the second week.	Terminate season; may return to play the following season if asymptomatic.
Grade 2 (moderate)	Return to play after being asymptomatic for 1 wk.	Minimum of 1 mo; may return to play then if asymptomatic for 1 wk; consider terminating season.	Terminate season; may return to play the following season if asymptomatic.
Grade 3 (severe)	Minimum of 1 mo; may then return to play if asymptomatic for 1 wk.	Terminate season; may return to play the following season if asymptomatic. Consider terminating career.	Career in contact sports is terminated.

Adapted from Cantu,[17] p 327.

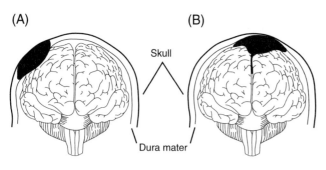

Figure 16–15. Intracranial hemorrhage. (*A*) Epidural hematoma, arterial bleeding between the skull and dura mater. (*B*) Subdural hematoma, venous bleeding between the dura mater and brain. Note that the meningeal spaces have been enlarged for clarity.

occurrence by prohibiting athletes from returning to athletic competition until all symptoms of a cerebral concussion have subsided and a physician has cleared the athlete's return to activity.

Intracranial Hematoma

Rupture of the blood vessels supplying the brain results in an intracranial hematoma, named relative to the meninges (Fig. 16–15). Subsequent hematoma formation within the enclosed space (the cranium) places pressure on the brain. The length of time until the onset of symptoms varies, depending on the type of bleeding involved (arterial or venous) and the location relative to the dura mater (above or below it).

Epidural Hematoma

Arterial bleeding between the dura mater and the skull results in the rapid formation of an epidural hematoma, with the onset of symptoms occurring within hours following the initial injury. The mechanism of this injury is that of a concussion, a blow to the head that jars the brain. Because of the con-

Table 16–8. Progression of Symptoms Associated With an Epidural Hematoma

- Athlete is unconscious or has other signs of a concussion (these are not prerequisite findings).
- Athlete has a period of very lucid consciousness, perhaps eliminating the suspicion of a serious concussion.
- Athlete appears to become disoriented, confused, and drowsy.
- Athlete complains of a headache that increases in intensity with time.
- Athlete manifests cranial nerve disruption.
- Athlete falls into a coma.
- If untreated, death or permanent brain damage occurs.

cussive mechanism, the athlete may be briefly unconscious and may show the signs and symptoms of mild concussion, although these are not prerequisite symptoms. These symptoms quickly subside and the athlete progresses through a very **lucid** period (Table 16–8).

As the size of the hematoma increases, the athlete's condition worsens at a rate proportional to the amount of intracranial bleeding. The athlete becomes disoriented, displays abnormal behavior, and complains of, or displays, drowsiness. A headache of increasing intensity may be reported, indicating pressure on the periosteum of the skull or an insult to the dura mater. Continued expansion of the hematoma results in outward symptoms via the cranial nerves, with a unilaterally dilated pupil being the most common sign.

Subdural Hematoma

Hematoma formation between the brain and dura mater usually involves venous bleeding. This type of injury accounts for the majority of deaths resulting from head injuries. Because venous bleeding occurs at a lower pressure than arterial bleeding, and because the blood collects within the fissures and sulci, the symptoms occur hours, days, or even weeks after the initial trauma. Acute subdural hematomas become symptomatic within 48 hr, whereas chronic hematomas may not manifest symptoms until 30 days following the trauma.[21]

Subdural hematomas may be classified as simple or complex. No direct cerebral damage is associated with a subdural hematoma. Complex subdural hematomas are characterized by contusions of the brain's surface and associated cerebral swelling.

Initially following the injury, the athlete is very lucid, even to the point of not displaying any of the signs or symptoms of a cerebral concussion. As the blood accumulates within the brain, the athlete begins to develop headaches, accompanied by a clouding of consciousness. Further hematoma formation results in the impairment of cognitive, behavioral, and motor ability, and signs of cranial nerve dysfunction may be noted. The potentially long duration between the trauma and the onset of symptoms illustrates the need for home instructions identifying the latent signs and symptoms of head injuries.

Skull Fractures

The prevalence of skull fractures is much higher in athletes who are not wearing headgear than in those who are. However, skull fractures can still occur in a head that is protected, especially in the bones around the helmet's periphery. Skull fractures are typically classified as **linear, comminuted,** or **depressed** (Fig. 16–16). Linear fractures, referred

Lucid: Pertaining to the state of mental clarity.

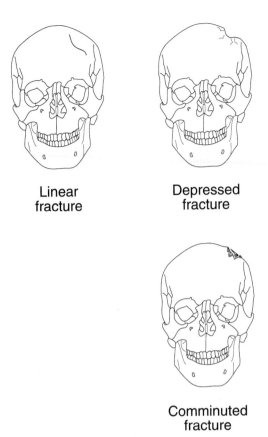

Linear fracture

Depressed fracture

Comminuted fracture

Figure 16–16. Types of skull fractures: linear, depressed, and comminuted.

to as hairline fractures in long bones, are caused by a blunt impact to the cranium, and the subsequent swelling causes the loss of the skull's rounded contour in the traumatized area. Comminuted skull fractures result in the skull's fragmenting. A slight depression is noted during gentle palpation of the fractured area. If the blunt force is of enough intensity or fails to become deflected by the round shape of the skull, a depressed fracture can occur. The skull's indentation is obvious on gross inspection. Additional concern is focused around the possibility of the fractured pieces of bone lacerating the meninges and brain.

Although depressed skull fractures are often obvious during inspection, linear and comminuted fractures are less evident. The traumatic impact often results in a laceration of the overlying skin. Although the bleeding must be controlled, no material or object should be inserted into the laceration or possible fracture site. Fractures of the ethmoid or temporal bones may result in the leakage of CSF from the nose or ears or in bleeding from the ears. (A discussion on determining the presence of CSF in fluids leaking from the nose or ears is presented in the Inspection section of this chapter.) With time, ecchymosis may accumulate beneath the eyes and over the mastoid process (Table 16–9). In addition to these symptoms, the athlete may also describe the signs and symptoms of a concussion caused by the blow to the skull.

Table 16–9. Evaluative Findings of a Skull Fracture

Examination Segment	Clinical Findings	
History	Onset:	Acute.
	Location of pain:	Pain over the point of impact. A headache may be described secondary to the trauma.
	Mechanism:	Blunt trauma to the head; either the skull being struck by a moving object or the skull striking a stationary object.
Inspection	Bleeding may occur secondary to the blow causing the fracture. Ecchymosis under the eyes ("raccoon eyes") and over the mastoid process (Battle's sign) may be noted. The rounded contour of the skull over the impacted area may be lost.	
Palpation	Crepitus may be felt over the fracture site. Palpation should not be performed over areas of obvious fracture.	
Functional tests	Not applicable.	
Ligamentous tests	Not applicable.	
Neurological tests	Same as for evaluation of a cerebral concussion.	
Special tests	Not applicable.	
Comments	The presence of a cervical fracture or dislocation must be ruled out. No object should be inserted into the site of a laceration. A cerebral concussion may also be associated with this injury. Athletes suspected of suffering from a skull fracture should be immediately referred to a physician.	

Cervical Spine Trauma

The advent of protective football helmets made the use of the head an attractive weapon for blockers, tacklers, and ball carriers. The resulting axial load on the cervical spine caused a high rate of cervical fractures and dislocations, many producing catastrophic results. During the 1976 season, the National Collegiate Athletic Association (NCAA) and the National Federation of State High School Associations (NFHSA) adopted rules outlawing contact with opposing players using the top (crown) of the helmet, a rule change that drastically reduced the incidence of cervical injury in football.[7] Despite this ruling, reviews of game films estimate that spearing still occurs in 19 percent of football plays, most of which go unpenalized.[11]

Spinal cord function is inhibited by one of two mechanisms: (1) impingement or laceration secondary to bony displacement and (2) compression secondary to hemorrhage, edema, and ischemia of the cord.[22] Although the effects of pressure placed on the spinal cord, with no death of its cells, are often transitory and reversible, actual trauma to the spinal cord itself is rarely reversible and results in permanent disability.

It is a false assumption that all athletes suffering from bony cervical trauma remain on the field. In fact, an athlete suffering a cervical fracture or dislocation may walk off under his or her own power. With this in mind, any complaints of pain in the cervical spine, with or without symptoms radiating into the extremities, should always be thought of as catastrophic until otherwise ruled out. Torg[23] has categorized risk groups, based on underlying trauma, as to their conditions predisposing the athlete to further cervical trauma (Table 16–10).

Trauma to the spinal cord above the C4 level has a high probability of death owing to disruption of the function of the brain stem or the phrenic nerve.

Trauma to the spinal cord anywhere along its length can result in the permanent loss of function of the nerves distal to the traumatized area.

The anatomy of the cervical spine is covered in Chapter 9. Prior to proceeding with this portion of the chapter, readers should take a moment to refresh their memory as to the important structures and anatomical relationships of this body area. Likewise, Chapter 9 also discusses injuries to the brachial plexus.

Cervical Fracture or Dislocation

The signs and symptoms of a cervical fracture and those of a dislocation are quite similar, and these two conditions often occur concurrently (Fig. 16–17). Cervical fractures in and of themselves do not cause spinal cord trauma. Rather, spinal cord trauma secondary to vertebral fractures results when a bony fragment lacerates the cord, swelling compresses the cord, ischemia affects the cord's cells, or the vertebra shifts, narrowing the spinal canal.

Cervical dislocations represent a much more serious direct threat to the spinal cord. Most often affecting the lower cervical vertebrae (C4 to C6) when the neck is forced into flexion and rotation, the superior articular facet passes over the inferior facet. The resulting dislocation decreases the diameter of the spinal canal, often compressing the cord.

Trauma to the cervical spine itself is identified by pain along its posterior and lateral structures and possible spasm of the surrounding muscles. If there is associated damage to the spinal cord or if displaced bone or swelling is compressing the cord, symptoms are manifested in the involved nerve distributions and in those nerves located distal to the site of the insult. Typically, these symptoms involve pain, burning, or numbness radiating into the extremities (Table 16–11).

Table 16–10. Risk Factors of Predisposing Conditions Resulting in Permanent Disability

Minimal Risk	Moderate Risk	Extreme Risk
Asymptomatic bone spurs.	Acute lateral disk herniation.	Acute large central disk herniation.
Brachial plexus neurapraxia.	Cervical radiculopathy–radial spur.	Cervical cord anomaly.
Certain healed facet fractures.	Facet fractures.	Occipitocervical dislocation.
Healed disk herniation.	Lateral mass fractures.	Odontoid fracture.
Healed lamina fracture.	Nondisplaced healed ring of C1 fracture.	Ruptured C1-C2 transverse ligament.
Healed spinous process fracture.	Nondisplaced odontoid fractures.	Stenosis of the cervical canal.
		Total ligamentous disruption of the lower cervical spine.
		Unstable fracture-dislocation.
		Unstable *Jefferson's fracture*.

Adapted from Torg.[23]

Jefferson's fracture: A fracture of a circular bone in two places; similar to breaking a doughnut in half.

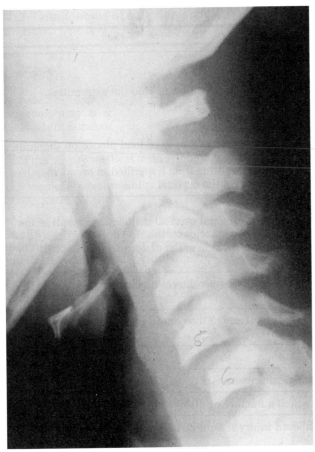

Figure 16–17. Fracture-dislocation of the C6 vertebra. Note the posterior displacement of the vertebral body relative to C5 and the fracture of the C6 spinous process.

The signs and symptoms of a stretch or pinch of the brachial plexus can mimic many of those of a spinal cord injury. The primary differences are found in the relatively rapid fading of symptoms associated with brachial plexus trauma and the fact that the symptoms most often occur unilaterally.

Transient Quadriplegia

Blows to the head that force the cervical spine into hyperextension, hyperflexion, or produce an axial load may result in transient quadriplegia, a body-wide state of decreased or absent sensory and motor function.[24-26] This results from neurapraxia of the cervical spinal cord and typically occurs secondary to stenosis of the spinal foramen (especially at the C3-C4 level), congenital fusion of the cervical canal, or cervical instability. The narrowing of the space through which the spinal cord passes predisposes it to compressive and contusive forces.

Initially, athletes suffering from transient quadriplegia display all the signs and symptoms of a catastrophic cervical injury. Symptoms range from sensory dysfunction to burning pain, numbness, or tingling in the upper and lower extremities. Likewise, upper and lower extremity motor function is inhibited, ranging from muscular weakness to complete paralysis. However, these symptoms clear within 15 min to 48 hr.

The definitive diagnosis of transient quadriplegia is made through imaging and electrophysiologic testing. X-ray examination is used to rule out fractures or congenital abnormalities of the cervical spine, and CT scans are used to gain a better definition of the cervical bony anatomy. The integrity of the spinal cord and its roots is determined through the use of MRIs, *electromyelograms*, and nerve conduction velocity testing.

ON-FIELD EVALUATION AND MANAGEMENT OF HEAD AND NECK INJURIES

The athletic trainer's decisions during a crisis situation are key to the proper management of head and neck trauma. No matter how unlikely these scenarios seem, students must realize that they do occur and, although generally attributed to football, head and neck injuries are possible in all sports. Sports that may be considered at high risk for causing head and neck injuries include but are not limited to baseball, diving, field hockey, football, gymnastics, hockey, lacrosse, rugby, soccer, softball, and wrestling.

It is the medical staff's responsibility to have a preplanned course of action that has been discussed and approved by the athletic training staff, physician, emergency medical service (EMS), and administration (Table 16–12).[27] Before each season's start, these procedures must be reviewed by the involved parties, with each understanding not only his or her own roles but also those of the others. Furthermore, the techniques discussed in this text must be reviewed and rehearsed until each member is comfortable performing the techniques described. The procedures described in this section assume that more than one responder knowledgeable of the plan is present.

Because of the importance of not unnecessarily moving a spine-injured athlete and the potentially catastrophic ramifications of doing so, an athletic trainer should conduct a meeting with each team, instructing the athletes not to help injured players to their feet. In too many instances these well-intentioned actions have resulted in an athlete's death or permanent paralysis.

Electromyelogram: The recording of the electrical activity within a muscle.

Spine Boarding the Athlete

In-line stabilization is maintained throughout these procedures until the athlete's skull is securely affixed to the spine board. These procedures should be discussed and practiced with the emergency medical squad.

Stabilizing the Cervical Spine

The cervical spine is best stabilized through the use of a semirigid collar, such as a Philadelphia collar (see Fig. 15–31). These devices are most easily applied when the athlete is not wearing shoulder pads or a helmet. Other types of collars can be used for stabilization when the helmet and shoulder pads are still in place.

After separating the two halves of the collar the posterior shell is compressed and slid behind the cervical spine, taking care to prevent spinal movement. This section should fit snugly beneath the athlete's occipital and mastoid processes. The anterior shell is fitted so that it envelops the athlete's chin. Most models have an opening on the sternal pad that allows access to the trachea in the event that a tracheotomy must be performed.

Supine Athlete

Spine boarding is best accomplished with a minimum of four people: the person who has been applying in-line stabilization (referred to as the leader) and a minimum of three people controlling the athlete's torso (Fig. 16–28). A fifth person may be recruited to manipulate the spine board. The leader maintains in-line stabilization throughout the roll and subsequent stabilization of the athlete on the spine board and is responsible for instructing and guiding the remaining personnel in the sequence to be performed.

The process of spine boarding a supine athlete involves rolling the athlete to the side, sliding the board under the athlete, and then positioning the athlete on the board.

- **Align athlete:** Before the athlete is placed on the board, the extremities must be aligned with the body. The arm on the side toward which the athlete is to be rolled is abducted to 180 degrees.

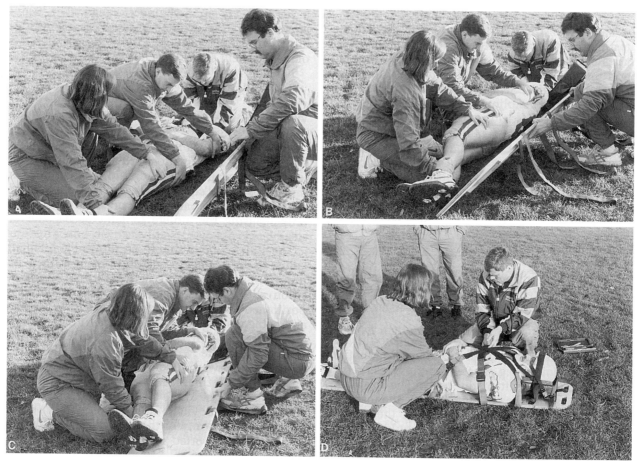

Figure 16–28. Spine boarding a supine athlete; see text for details.

- **Position personnel:** When the minimum of three torso personnel is used, one is positioned at the athlete's shoulders, one at the hips, and one along the legs. The hands should be spaced along the athlete, gripping underneath the athlete. Tall, heavy, or large athletes may require more personnel in order to be moved safely.

- **Roll to side:** On the leader's instructions, the athlete is rolled 90 degrees. The following command is used: "On the count of three we will roll the athlete toward you. Start and stop on my command. Ready? One, two, three, roll." It is the torso personnels' responsibility to maintain axial alignment of the spinal column by staying with the leader's pace.

- **Slide spine board:** If a single person is given the responsibility of manipulating the spine board, it should be slid so that it is flat on the ground and resting against the athlete. The board is positioned longitudinally so that the head of the spine board is matched with the athlete's head. If the torso personnel must position the spine board, the individual at the athlete's hips should be given the responsibility of manipulating the board.

- **Return athlete:** Once the leader is satisfied with the board's position relative to the athlete, he or she gives the command, "On the count of three we will roll the athlete on the board. Start and stop on my command. Ready? One, two, three, roll." Again, it is the torso personnel who are responsible for meeting the pace of the leader. Minor adjustments may be needed once the athlete is positioned on the board.

- **Secure athlete:** Once the athlete is properly positioned on the spine board, the torso is secured, using the strapping techniques applicable to the equipment being used. The cervical spine must be affixed, using the equipment supplied by the ambulance company or using commercially available equipment. If the athlete's helmet is left on, the head may be secured to the board by tape.

Prone Athlete

Prone athletes who are breathing but unconscious may be rolled onto the spine board in a safer and more orderly manner than that described under the on-field management of an unconscious athlete who is not breathing. The basic procedures are the same as those described for spine boarding a supine athlete, but the athlete must be rolled 180 degrees, rather than 90 degrees (Fig. 16–29). The person who is providing in-line stabilization to the cervical spine is again the operation's leader. A minimum of three additional people is necessary for this procedure to be safely performed. A fourth additional person is recommended to manipulate the spine board.

- **Align athlete:** Before the athlete is placed on the board, the extremities are aligned with the body. The arm on the side toward which the athlete is to be rolled is abducted to 180 degrees.

- **Position personnel:** When the minimum of three torso personnel is used, one is positioned at the athlete's shoulders, one at the hips, and one along the legs. The hands should be spaced along the athlete, gripping underneath the athlete. Tall, heavy, or large athletes may require more personnel in order to be moved safely.

- **Roll to side:** On the leader's instructions, the athlete is rolled 90 degrees. The command is given: "On the count of three we will roll the athlete toward you. Start and stop on my command. Ready? One, two, three, roll." Just as for the supine scenario, it is the torso personnels' responsibility to maintain axial alignment of the spinal column by staying with the leader's pace.

- **Slide spine board:** If a single person is given the responsibility of manipulating the spine board, it should be slid so that it is flat on the ground and resting against the athlete. The board is positioned longitudinally so that the head of the spine board is matched with the athlete's head. If the torso personnel must position the spine board, the individual at the athlete's hips should be given the responsibility of manipulating the board.

- **Return athlete:** Once the leader is satisfied with the board's position relative to the athlete, he or she gives the command, "On the count of three we will roll the athlete on the board. Start and stop on my command. Ready? One, two, three, roll." The torso personnel are responsible for meeting the pace of the leader. Minor adjustments may be needed once the athlete is positioned on the board.

- **Secure athlete:** The athlete is secured on the spine board as described in the previous section.

HOME INSTRUCTIONS

Because of the delayed onset of symptoms associated with intracranial hemorrhage, there is always the potential for a more serious condition to develop. The attending physician, in some cases, may elect to admit the athlete to the hospital for observation. In other cases the athlete is allowed to return home.

It is good practice to inform the athlete's parents or roommates of the delayed progression of the signs and symptoms of head injuries and to alert them to the appropriate course of action. A good method of doing this is through the use of a business card–sized instruction booklet. A list of emergency numbers (e.g., athletic trainer, physician, emergency room) is printed on the front cover. The card then opens to display a list of signs and symp-

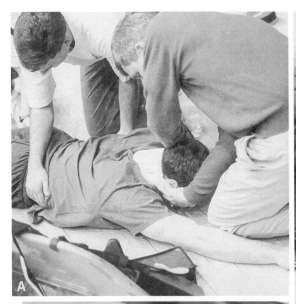

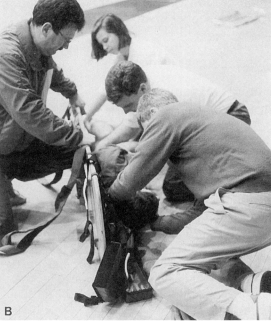

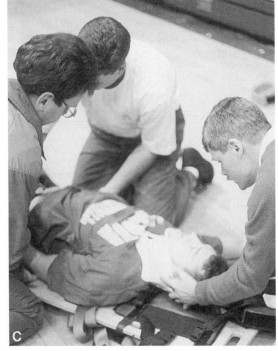

Figure 16–29. Spine boarding a prone athlete; see text for details. Note the cross-armed position of the leader applying in-line stabilization.

toms to alert the individual to a deteriorating condition (Fig. 16–30).

Behavioral changes, forgetfulness, confusion, anger, aggression, and malaise are the most outward signs. Additionally, the athlete may describe nausea, vomiting, a headache with increasing severity, and a loss of appetite. Although these symptoms may be caused by other conditions, their presence following a head injury may be cause for concern. The onset of any of the other signs and symptoms of a cerebral injury may also indicate a severe head injury (see Table 16–4 and Table 16–7).

Permission to take aspirin or other pain-relieving medication must be given by the physician. Many

of these medications, as well as alcoholic drinks, tend to thin the blood and inhibit the clotting mechanism, potentially increasing the rate of intracranial bleeding. Prohibiting sleep following a concussion is largely founded in fiction rather than fact. Although it is necessary to keep the athlete conscious immediately following the injury, sleep should, and must, be permitted at night. If enough doubt surrounds the athlete's condition to prohibit sleep, the physician will admit the athlete to the hospital for observation.

The medical staff or emergency room personnel should be immediately contacted if any of the latent signs or symptoms of intracranial hemorrhage are manifested.

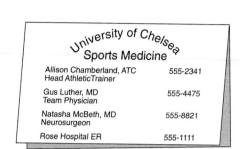

Head Injury Check List

Significant blows to the head must be treated with caution. Many of the signs and symptoms of brain trauma may not occur for some time following the injury. If you experience any of the following conditions, or if any questions arise concerning your condition, contact one of the emergency numbers printed on the reverse side of this card:

- Nausea and/or vomiting
- Ringing in the ears
- Blurred or double vision
- Persistent, intense headache or a headache that worsens in intensity
- Confusion or irritability
- Forgetfulness
- Difficulty breathing
- Irregular heartbeat
- Muscle weakness

You have a follow-up appointment on:_____

at:_____ am / pm.

Figure 16–30. Business card method of communicating home instructions to a head-injured athlete.

REFERENCES

1. Zemper, ED: Cerebral concussion rates in various brands of football helmets. Athletic Training: Journal of the National Athletic Trainers Association, 24:133, 1989.
2. Zemper, ED: Analysis of cerebral concussion frequency with the most commonly used models of football helmets. Journal of Athletic Training, 29:44, 1994.
3. McWhorter, JM: Concussions and intracranial injuries in athletics. Athletic Training: Journal of the National Athletic Trainers Association, 25:129, 1990.
4. Nelson, WE: Athletic head injuries. Athletic Training: Journal of the National Athletic Trainers Association,19:95, 1984.
5. Heck, JF, et al: Minimizing liability risks of head and neck injuries in football. Journal of Athletic Training, 29:128, 1994.
6. Tysvaer, AT, and Lochen, EA: Soccer injuries to the brain. A neuropsychologic study of former soccer players. Am J Sports Med 19:56, 1991.
7. Torg, JS: Epidemiology, biomechanics, and prevention of cervical spine trauma resulting from athletics and recreational activities. Operative Techniques in Sports Medicine 1:159, 1993.
8. Torg, JS: The epidemiologic, biomechanical, and cinematographic analysis of football induced cervical spine trauma. Athletic Training: Journal of the National Athletic Trainers Association, 25:147, 1990.
9. Otis, JS, Burstein, AH, and Torg, JS: Mechanisms and pathomechanics of athletic injuries to the cervical spine. In Torg, JS (ed): Athletic Injuries to the Head, Neck, and Face (ed 2). Mosby-Year Book, St Louis, 1991, p 438.
10. Torg, JS, et al: The epidemiologic, pathologic, biomechanical, and cinematographic analysis of football-induced cervical spine trauma. Am J Sports Med 18:50, 1990.
11. Heck, JF: The incidence of spearing by high school football carriers and thier tacklers. Journal of Athletic Training, 27:120, 1992.
11a. Mueller, FO, and Ryan, AJ: Prevention of Athletic Injuries: The Role of the Sports Medicine Team. FA Davis, Philadelphia, 1991.
12. Buckley, WE: Concussion injury in college football. An eight-year overview. Athletic Training: Journal of the National Athletic Trainers Association, 21:207, 1986.
13. Report of the Ad Hoc Committee to Study Head Injury Nomenclature: Proceedings of the Congress of Neurological Surgeons in 1964. Clin Neurosurg 12:386, 1966.
14. American Medical Association on the medical aspects of sports.
15. Hayes, RG, and Nagle, CE: Diagnostic imaging of intracranial trauma. The Physician and Sportsmedicine 18:69, 1990.
16. Maroon, JC: Assessing closed head injuries. The Physician and Sportsmedicine 20:37, 1992.
17. Cantu, RC: Criteria for return to competition after a closed head injury. In Torg, JS (ed): Athletic Injuries to the Head, Neck, and Face, ed 2. Mosby-Year Book, St Louis, 1991, p 326.
18. Schneider, RC: Head and Neck Injuries in Football: Mechanisms, treatment, and prevention. Williams & Wilkins, Baltimore, 1973.
19. Cantu, RC: Emergencies in sports. Second impact syndrome: Immediate management. The Physician and Sportsmedicine 20:55, 1992.
20. Sanders, RI, and Harbaugh, RE: The second impact in catastrophic contact: Sports head trauma. JAMA 252:538, 1984.
21. White, RJ: Subarachnoid hemorrhage: The lethal intracranial explosion. Emerg Med Clin North Am May:74, 1994.
22. Bailes, JE: Management of cervical spine sports injuries. Athletic Training: Journal of the National Athletic Trainers Association, 25:156, 1990.
23. Torg, JS: Criteria for return to collision activities after cervical spine injury. Operative Techniques in Sports Medicine 1:236, 1993.
24. Scher, AT: Spinal cord concussion in rugby players. Am J Sports Med 18:50, 1990.
25. Jordan, BD, et al: How to evaluate transient quadriparesis. The Physician and Sportsmedicine 20:83, 1992.
26. Torg, JS: Cervical spine stenosis with cord neurapraxia and transient quadriplegia. Athletic Training: Journal of the National Athletic Trainers Association, 25:156, 1990.
27. Harris, AJ: Disaster plan—a part of the game plan? Athletic Training: Journal of the National Athletic Trainers Association, 23:59, 1988.
28. Nelson, WE, et al: Athletic head injuries. Athletic Training: Journal of the National Athletic Trainers Association,19:95, 1984.
29. Putman, LA: Alternative methods for football helmet face mask removal. Journal of Athletic Training, 2:170, 1992.
30. Feld, F: Management of the critically injured football players. Journal of Athletic Training, 28:206, 1993.
31. Denegar, CR, and Saliba, E: On the field management of the potentially cervical spine injured football player. Athletic Training: Journal of the National Athletic Trainers Association, 24:108, 1989.
32. Bensen, MT (ed): 1994–95 NCAA Sports Medicine Handbook. National Collegiate Athletic Association, Overland Park, KS, 1994, p 65.
33. Sheehy, SB: Spinal cord and neck trauma. In Sheehy, SB: Mosby's Manual of Emergency Care, ed 3. CV Mosby, St Louis, 1990, p 400.
34. Pofeta, LM, and Paris, P: Emergencies in sports. Managing airway obstruction. The Physician and Sportsmedicine 19:35, 1991.
35. Caroline, N: Emergency Care in the Streets, ed 3. Little, Brown, Boston, 1983.Association, 25:147, 1990.

17

Environmental Injury

Environmental injuries are not limited to temperature extremes nor to outdoor activities. Gaining or losing heat from and to the external environment can occur gradually or suddenly. The body can adapt to exercise in most of the environmental extremes seen in athletics. Except for accidental exposure to very hot or very cold temperatures, environmental injuries are completely preventable.

CLINICAL ANATOMY

Regulation of the body's core temperature occurs primarily in the hypothalamus, although other centers are involved as well. Normally, the body temperature is higher than that of the surrounding environment and the core temperature is greater than that of the skin and extremities. As used in this text, the term "core temperature" is used to describe the actual temperature within the viscera.

Just as a furnace receives input from a thermostat, the hypothalamus receives input from thermoreceptors located in the skin, spinal cord, abdomen, and brain. In response to significant increases or decreases in the core temperature, the hypothalamus shunts blood toward or away from the skin. Additional temperature regulatory responses include increasing mechanical and chemical heat production when the core temperature drops too low or increasing sweating when the core temperature rises too high (Fig. 17–1).

Mechanisms of Heat Transfer

Heat exchange to and from the body occurs through radiation, conduction and convection, and evaporation. Each of these mechanisms relies on a temperature gradient between the body and the surrounding environment. The greater this difference, the greater the magnitude and rate of the exchange to and from the body.

Radiation

All objects emit heat in the form of infrared radiation. Normally, this exchange occurs in the form of the body losing heat into the environment. How-ever, when the body is placed in an exceedingly warm environment, such as on a hot, humid day or while sitting in a sauna or practicing in a wrestling room, the body gains heat through radiation.

Conduction and Convection

The body can gain or lose heat when it is in contact with an object having a temperature warmer or cooler than itself (the use of a hot pack or ice pack are examples of the body gaining or losing heat through **conduction**). Because the air contains molecules, the body can directly exchange heat with the atmosphere through conduction. The efficiency of this mechanism in still-standing air is quite poor. Circulating the air across the body greatly enhances the cooling process through the means of **convection**. The use of a room fan is an example of convective cooling.

Although conduction and convection most commonly occur with the air, it should be noted that with competing swimmers, water is the environmental medium through which most heat is lost. This explains why the temperature of competitive swimming pools is kept relatively low.

Evaporation

The evaporation of water from the skin carries heat with it, cooling the skin and subsequently lowering the core temperature. During athletic competition the body depends primarily on evaporation for heat loss. In response to exercise, the body's perspiration rate increases, covering the body with fluids to be evaporated.

Other Mechanisms

Heat is lost from the body through several other mechanisms, many of which are inconsequential or impractical during athletic competition. Respiration is the most common and applicable of these methods. As the air passes into the lungs, it travels through warm, moist passages, humidifying it. During expiration, water and heat are lost. Voiding the body through urination, defecation, or vomiting also transfers heat from the body. However, these mechanisms also serve to dehydrate the body.

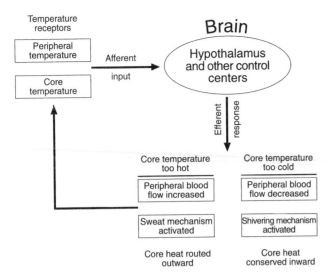

Figure 17–1. Schematic of the body's thermoregulatory system. Thermoreceptors in the extremities, skin, and within the viscera monitor the body's temperature. High temperatures result in increased peripheral blood flow and activate the sweating mechanism to route the heat away from the core. Cold core temperatures activate a mechanism that conserves the core temperature.

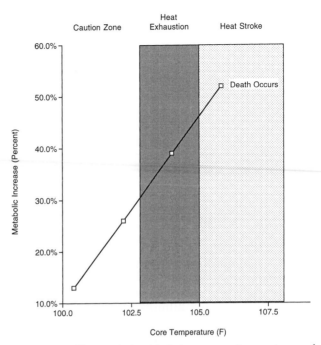

Figure 17–2. Linear relationship between core temperature and metabolism.

Blood Flow and Heat Exchange

The body responds to a hot, humid environment by increasing the blood flow to the extremities and subcutaneous vessels. The vessels in the skin dilate, allowing a large amount of blood to carry heat away from the core to be released into the environment by one of the previously discussed methods of heat transfer.

The total volume of the body's blood vessels is approximately four times greater than the heart's pumping capacity.[1] This disparity is compensated for by the body's routing more blood to the areas demanding oxygen and decreasing the supply to areas having a lesser demand. The body tissue constantly receiving the highest priority for oxygen is the brain.

During exercise a worsening cycle occurs when the body's core temperature begins to rise above normal. Increased core temperature caused by exercise increases systemic metabolism, which, in turn, further increases the core temperature. As the core temperature rises above 104.0°F, a linear relationship between the core temperature and metabolic demands is developed (Fig. 17–2).[2] Once the body's internal temperature reaches 107.6°F, the cardiovascular system can no longer meet the metabolic oxygen demand necessary to sustain life.

The brain is constantly monitoring the oxygen requirements of the exercising muscles, internal organs, and brain, making the adjustments necessary to maintain the viability of each while also keeping the core temperature within acceptable limits. Blood flow to the working muscles is increased, decreasing the supply of oxygen available to the other areas of the body. When this exertion occurs in a hot or humid environment, blood flow is further increased to the cutaneous vessels to cool the core temperature. This rerouted blood draws more blood from the viscera and the brain, causing its internal temperature to increase. Additionally, the increased metabolism associated with both the temperature rise and the exercising muscles further increases the temperature.

Sweating reduces the body's internal temperature by carrying heat outward, where it can evaporate into the atmosphere. The inherent efficiency in this process lies in the fact that water conducts heat 25 times more rapidly than air.[3] Unfortunately, the sweating process is also self-depleting.

Sweat is not pure water. When this fluid leaves the body it also carries with it electrolytes, namely sodium (salt) and potassium. The body's ability to efficiently sustain prolonged activity is directly related to the replacement of both water and electrolytes. When water is not replaced the efficiency of the cooling mechanism is impaired. The plasma volume is reduced, decreasing blood pressure, causing the heart to work harder to deliver the needed blood to those areas requiring it. When the electrolytes are not replaced, metabolic efficiency is hindered.

Heat Conservation

Just as the excessive gain of heat is counterproductive to the body, so is the excessive loss of heat. The body conserves heat by essentially reversing the process used to rid heat from the body. Blood is routed away from the superficial vessels and the skin, maintaining the core temperature inward. When the temperature drops below 86°F, the muscle tone increases and, eventually, shivering begins. The metabolism associated with these muscle contractions serves as a source of heat to rewarm the core. Chronic or prolonged exposure to a cold environment results in **chemical thermogenesis**, a process in which epinephrine is secreted into the bloodstream, increasing the metabolism of nonmuscular cells.[4]

Influence of Ambient Environment

The term "heat injury" is probably a misnomer because its onset is more directly related to the *relative humidity (RH)* than to the actual temperature of the air. Until the ambient air temperature exceeds 95°F or the relative humidity reaches 75 percent, sweating and evaporation account for virtually all of the heat dissipation from the core.[5] For every increase of 5°F, the percentage at which relative humidity raises the risk of injury is decreased by 10 percent (i.e., at 70°F the humidity danger zone is 80 percent RH; at 90°F the danger zone is 50 percent RH). Once the relative humidity reaches 100 percent and the air temperature reaches that of the skin, the body can no longer lose heat into the environment.[6] The resulting core temperature can increase to fatally high levels.

Acclimatization

Physiological systems can adapt to exercise in hot, humid environments through improved efficiency of the metabolic and cooling processes. Acclimatization is achieved by gradually exposing the exercising athlete to the environmental condition over a period of several days to weeks, depending on the magnitude of the environmental change.

The process of making the body a more efficient machine involves the modification of four individual components.[3] Increased stores of *adenosine triphosphate (ATP)* in skeletal and cardiac muscle, through increased glycogen stores, provide a more immediate energy source. The heart's efficiency is improved by increasing the cardiac output and stroke volume, allowing the heart to deliver more blood to the working muscles at a lower pulse rate. The improved efficiency of cardiac and skeletal muscle contraction results in decreased metabolic heat production. The body's sweat threshold temperature is lowered and the volume of sweat is increased, enhancing the rapid removal of heat from the body and preventing the core temperature from reaching the danger zone. Improved renal function results in a decreased level of salt being lost in the sweat, which, through osmotic properties, retains extracellular fluids and plasma volume.

EVALUATION OF ENVIRONMENTAL INJURY

The evaluative process of environmental injuries requires not only a knowledge of the athlete's symptoms but also the knowledge of the environmental conditions and factors that may predispose the athlete to injury arising from these conditions. A paradox occurs in that the same information used to evaluate the injury is also used to prevent the injury. Because of the relatively straightforward evaluation of these conditions, the format of the evaluative process has been altered from those presented in previous chapters.

History

• **Environmental conditions:** The magnitude of environmental extremes decreases the duration of exposure required for the onset of symptoms. Heat exposure is compounded by humidity and cold exposure by wind. These conditions, which are discussed in the Pathologies and Related Special Tests section of this chapter, should be known prior to competition or practice and influence whether or not the activity will be (or should be) held or modified.

• **Weight loss:** Recent weight loss can predispose the athlete to environmental injury, especially when it is caused through water loss. The use of weight charts can identify those individuals who are predisposed to heat injury secondary to water loss (see Prevention of Heat Injuries).

• **Recent history of illness:** Water and electrolyte loss is increased in the presence of illness, especially when it involves vomiting and/or diarrhea. Other illnesses increase the body's metabolic demands and decrease the body's resistance to stress by increasing the core temperature.

• **Nutrition:** Athletes who are dieting or simply have poor nutritional habits can be predisposed to environmental injury. Decreased intake of fluids and electrolytes decrease the plasma volume and can inhibit the metabolism necessary for athletic activity. High-protein diets can decrease the athlete's ability to cope with cold environments.

Relative humidity: The ratio between the amount of water vapor in the air and the actual amount of water the air could potentially hold based on the current temperature.

Adenosine triphosphate (ATP): An energy-yielding enzyme used during muscular contractions.

• **Other complaints:** Athletes suffering from heat injury may become confused and aggressive, often reporting a concurrent headache. Athletes suffering from water depletion are very thirsty, although this trait is not present with electrolyte depletion. Athletes suffering from cold injuries express a desire to warm up or, in extreme cases, to sleep.

• **Conditioning level:** Athletes who are poorly conditioned or are not acclimated are susceptible to heat injury. Proper conditioning assists the athlete in adapting to both hot and cold environments.

• **Body build:** Large muscle mass predisposes an athlete to heat injury secondary to increased metabolism.

Inspection

• **Skin:** The color of the athlete's skin provides evidence of the underlying condition. Minor heat-related injuries result in a pale texture to the skin whereas heat stroke, a medical emergency, often results in dark or red skin. In the majority of athletic-related heat injuries, the athlete sweats profusely. Cold injury causes the skin to have a waxy appearance that is red in minor cases or pale in more severe cases.

• **Muscle tone:** As the core temperature increases, the muscle tone decreases somewhat to reduce the amount of metabolic heat produced and assist in routing the heat outward to the skin. The exception to this is heat cramps. The body responds to a cold environment by increasing muscle tone by shivering.

• **Pupils:** Exposure to extreme heat or cold results in pupillary dilation and decreased responsiveness to light, an indication of decreased brain function.

Palpation

• **Skin temperature:** During heat exhaustion, the athlete's skin feels cool and clammy to the touch; during heat stroke it feels hot. Cold exposure results in decreased skin temperature.

Functional Tests

• **Pulse:** Heat injuries result in tachycardia in response to meet the body's demand for oxygen. Cooling of the core temperature causes the heart rate to become slow and weak.

• **Blood pressure:** During heat exhaustion and hypothermia, the blood pressure decreases and may result in syncope. Heat stroke causes an increase in the blood pressure.

• **Respiration:** Paralleling the findings of the heart rate, heat exposure increases the respiratory rate whereas cold exposure causes it to slow.

• **Mental state:** Prolonged increases or decreases of the intracranial temperature result in an alteration of the brain's cognitive function. Increased temperature results in dizziness, confusion, violent behavior, and unconsciousness. Cooling of the brain causes the athlete to become drowsy, eventually drifting into unconsciousness.

Pathologies and Related Special Tests

The delineation between heat and cold injuries is obvious. What is more difficult, however, is the delineation between the various types and severity of heat and cold injuries. The importance of prevention of environmental injuries has been emphasized throughout this chapter. Injuries from exposure to hot or cold environments are preventable, unlike the relatively unpreventable nature of the other injuries described in this text.

Heat Injuries

The effects of participating in a hot, humid environment, collectively referred to as **hyperthermia**, range from the relatively minor symptoms associated with heat cramps and heat exhaustion to the potentially fatal effects of heat stroke. Unfortunately, these are not progressive conditions. An athlete may collapse from heat stroke without displaying the signs and symptoms of the less serious conditions. Table 17–1, which presents the signs and symptoms associated with the various types of heat injuries, may be used to compare each.

The onset of heat-related injuries is directly related to the environment in which the athlete is participating and is based on the relationship between air temperature and humidity. The onset of heat injury is not limited to the summer or outdoor activities. Hot, humid gymnasiums, wrestling rooms, or even swimming pools can be the site of heat injuries. Despite the varying times and locations in which heat injuries can occur, they are all preventable through adequate rehydration and conditioning of the athlete.

Heat Cramps
Heat cramps are easily recognized by the spasm or cramping of skeletal muscle, most often affecting the lower extremity muscles. The underlying cause of heat cramps is debatable, but most often the loss of electrolytes secondary to excessive sweating is implicated.[5] Unconditioned athletes or otherwise conditioned athletes who are not acclimated to participating in a hot, humid environment are most susceptible to heat cramps. These conditions increase the athlete's sweating rate and volume, rapidly depleting the body of electrolytes.

Heat Syncope
A fainting spell caused by hot, humid environments, heat syncope is sometimes included as a symptom of heat exhaustion. Unlike fainting caused

Table 17–1. Evaluative Findings of Heat Illness

Evaluative Finding	Heat Cramps	Heat Syncope	Heat Exhaustion	Heat Stroke
Core temperature*	WNL†	WNL	103°F or above	105°F or above
Skin color and temperature	WNL	WNL	Cool Pale	Hot Red
Sweating	Moderate	WNL	Profuse	Heavy Possibly failing sweat mechanism
Pulse	WNL	Rapid and weak	Rapid and weak	Tachycardia
Blood pressure	WNL	A sudden, imperceptible drop in blood pressure, which rapidly returns to normal	Low	High
Respiration	WNL	WNL	Hyperventilation	Rapid
Mental state	WNL	Dizziness Fainting	Dizziness Fatigue Slight confusion	Confusion Violent behavior Unconsciousness
Other findings	Cramping in one or more muscle groups, usually affecting the lower extremity		Headache Nausea Vomiting Thirst	Headache Nausea Vomiting Dilated pupils
				Decerebrate posture

*As determined by the rectal temperature.
†Within normal limits for an exercising athlete.

by heat exhaustion, the unconsciousness or dizziness associated with syncope occurs in the absence of an elevated core temperature and is not related to the depletion of fluids or electrolytes.[1,3] Vascular shunting routes the blood outward to the skin and extremities to lower the core temperature. This sudden shift causes cardiac filling pressure and stroke volume to rapidly decline, decreasing cardiac output and blood pressure, depriving the brain of oxygen. Syncope can also have a metabolic, neurological, or cardiovascular origin or can be the result of a drug reaction. These issues are discussed in Chapter 18.

Heat Exhaustion

Heat exhaustion is characterized by sudden, extreme fatigue as the body is attempting to supply blood to the skin, to exercising muscles, and to the brain. Unlike with heat stroke, with heat exhaustion the hypothalamus is still functioning properly. The physiological effects of heat exhaustion can be traced to salt depletion or water depletion.[1] When these events are accompanied by profuse sweating and when fluids and electrolytes are not replaced, the body's volume of circulating fluid is depleted.

Sweating, vomiting, diarrhea, and excessive urination without substantial rehydration result in water depletion from the body, predisposing the athlete to heat stroke. Excessive loss of salt from the body causes a loss of extracellular fluid, reducing the plasma volume and subsequently reducing cardiac output and decreasing blood pressure. Severe cases of salt depletion result in peripheral vascular collapse, presenting the signs and symptoms of

traumatic shock. The presence or absence of thirst is a way of determining whether a heat illness is caused by water deprivation or salt deprivation. Athletes who are water depleted describe thirst, whereas salt-depleted athletes have no such craving. Heat exhaustion caused by salt depletion is not resolved by the ingestion of plain water. Most athletic-related cases of heat exhaustion are caused by water depletion, but the two commonly occur in conjunction with each other.

Athletes suffering from heat exhaustion have a rectal temperature above 103°F and present with profuse sweating, causing the skin to feel cool and clammy. In response to cardiovascular demands, pulse and respiration are rapid, but the loss of fluids causes the pulse to feel weak and reduces the blood pressure. The athlete may complain of a headache and appears fatigued and confused.

Heat Stroke

A medical emergency, heat stroke represents the failure and subsequent shutdown of the body's thermoregulatory system and occurs when the body is unable to shed its excess heat into the environment, causing the core temperature to rise above 105°F. Following this shutdown, the core temperature continues to increase, placing the cells of the internal organs and, most importantly, the brain at risk. Subsequently, all of the body's systems begin to fail. If untreated, death can occur from heat stroke within 20 minutes.[6]

Heat stroke is classified as classic or exertional. **Classic heat stroke** most often affects infants and the elderly, occurring during a period when they are exposed to a hot environment and are unable to re-hydrate or cool themselves. These individuals are marked by the absence of sweat. This symptom is often, and incorrectly, correlated with **exertional heat stroke**, which most commonly affects athletes.[7]

Exertional heat stroke occurs within a matter of hours during exercise in a hot and humid environment. In this scenario, profuse sweating occurs and fluids are not replaced, depleting the body of water and electrolytes. *Most athletes suffering from exertional heat stroke are sweating.* Using the definition of classic heat stroke, athletes suffering from exertional heat stroke may be misevaluated because of the presence of sweating.

The athlete's probability of survival is directly related to the quick identification of heat stroke and the immediate initiation of treatment. The only practical difference between heat stroke and heat exhaustion that can be determined on the field is the athlete's mental state. Violent behavior followed by unconsciousness are characteristic traits of heat stroke. The athlete's skin may feel hot compared with the finding expected of heat exhaustion. As the athlete's brain function diminishes, the pupils become fixed and dilated and the athlete may assume a decerebrate posture. The attempt to maintain blood pressure may account for the incidence of liver and kidney failure associated with heat injuries.[1]

Prevention of Heat Injuries

Table 17–2 presents a list of steps to reduce the incidence of athletic heat injuries and a series of conditions that may reduce an athlete's ability to dissipate the heat. More detailed information on preventing heat injuries can be found in introductory athletic training texts.

Environmental heat conditions should be determined prior to and during outdoor athletic competition. Traditionally, this has been done with the use of a sling psychrometer, a device that determines relative humidity through the temperatures derived from a dry thermometer and a wet one. The wet bulb temperature alone is often sufficient information regarding the modification of activity. Whenever possible, practice should be suspended when the wet bulb temperature exceeds 82°F.[8] The temperature and humidity can also be obtained from local radio stations or dial-in weather services, although these reports may not accurately depict local weather conditions. High temperature and humidity require that the activity be modified accordingly (Table 17–3).

In regions in which the temperature is normally hot and humid, practices should be regularly scheduled to avoid the environmental dangers, although in many regions the summer months may be predominated by these conditions.[9] Altering the duration and intensity of the activity is also useful in preventing hyperthermia. Longer events performed at a slower pace have less risk of heat injury than do shorter, more intense activities held in the same environmental conditions.[10]

During two-a-day practices, the proportion of body weight lost because of dehydration can be calculated through the use of weight charts (Fig. 17–3). In this procedure, athletes record their weight before and after each practice, with the percentage of body weight lost determining the risk of complications caused by the heat. Athletes who lose 3 percent of their weight from the start of one practice to the start of the next should be continuously monitored during practice and required to consume water frequently. Athletes displaying a 5 percent weight loss should be prohibited from practice. Those having a 7 percent drop are in extreme danger and should be withheld from participation until the weight loss is reduced to 3 percent.

Athletes should be allowed unlimited access to water before and during competition and practice and be encouraged to consume it even if they are not thirsty. The use of electrolyte drinks is also effective in reducing the number of heat-related problems experienced by athletes, thus improving performance. However, water is still an essential factor in preventing and recovering from heat injuries.

Gear made of substances that completely isolate the body from the external environment, such as neoprene or rubber, creates an internal environment with a temperature equal to or greater than the core temperature. Subsequent sweating raises the relative humidity within this suit to levels nearing 100 percent, actually predisposing the athlete to heat injury.

Last, athletes should report to practice physically fit and acclimated to the environment in which they will be competing. Athletes who have trained in a cool, dry environment are still predisposed to heat injury when moving to hot, humid areas.

Table 17–2. Prevention of Heat Injury

Predisposing Conditions	Prevention of Heat Injury
Elderly and prepubescent athletes	Acclimatization
Athletes with thick muscle mass	Proper nutrition: fluids and electrolytes
Athletes with prior history of heat problems	Avoiding environmental extremes
Illness, especially in the presence of vomiting and diarrhea	Wearing appropriate clothing
Overweight athletes	Unlimited fluids during practice
Unconditioned athletes	Sufficient rest periods
Unacclimated athletes	Rehydration following exercise
Medications	
Amphetamines, other stimulants	
Anabolic steroids	
Diuretics and alcohol	

Table 17–3. Guidelines for Modification of Athletic Competition in Hot or Humid Environments

Dry-Bulb Temperature	Wet-Bulb Temperature	Humidity	Consequences
80° to 90°	68°	<70%	No extraordinary precautions are required for those athletes not showing predisposition to heat injury. Athletes who are predisposed (e.g., unconditioned, unacclimated, or losing more than 3% of body weight from water loss) require close observation.
80° to 90°	69° to 79°	>70%	Regular rest breaks are necessary. Loose, breathable clothing should be worn and wet uniforms regularly changed.
90° to 100°		<70%	
90° to 100° >100°	>80°	>70%	Practice should be shortened and modified. The use of protective equipment covering the body should be curtailed.
	>82°		Practice should be canceled.

Note: All temperatures are in degrees Fahrenheit.

Cold Injuries

Injury from cold exposure is often overlooked during athletic injury evaluation. Athletes who are competing outdoors in cold, damp environments are most predisposed to this condition. Indoor activities, except under the most bizarre circumstances, do not normally predispose the athlete to cold injury. An exception to this is prolonged activity in a very cold swimming pool.

Hypothermia

Systemic cooling of the body, hypothermia, results from exposure to cold, damp air or immersion in cold water. The onset of hypothermia is not limited to subfreezing conditions. The body's core temperature begins to drop when the ambient temperature is less than the body temperature and is influenced by other environmental conditions such as wind and water. Clothing that has become wet from rain, snow, perspiration, or other means conducts heat way from the core, increasing the risk of hypothermia.

Once the core temperature drops below 95°F, the first sign of hypothermia, shivering, appears, pro-

viding a short-term source of heat by increasing the body's metabolism. Impairment of the body's regulatory systems occurs when the core temperature drops below 94°F, predisposing the individual to cardiac irregularities and impairing the heart's responsiveness to treatment.[11,12] A decreased cardiac stroke volume and an increased blood viscosity reduce the amount of blood reaching the brain, resulting in impaired mental function.

Cooling of the brain stem depresses the respiratory rate, resulting in body-wide **anoxia**. Systemic metabolism decreases, resulting in decreased metabolic heat production and further lowering the core temperature. As the temperature continues to drop, kidney function is impaired, disrupting the body's electrolyte balance.[11]

A core temperature between 90°F and 94°F is classified as **mild hypothermia**. Initially the athlete complains of feeling cold, and the shivering response is initiated. Interest in the activity at hand wanes and is replaced by the desire to warm up. Signs of motor and mental impairment are indicated by decreased athletic performance. **Severe hypothermia**, a potentially fatal condition, results when the core temperature drops below 90°F. The athlete's desire to warm up is overridden by the desire to sleep, causing the athlete to appear uncoordinated and to slur the speech. An examination of the vital signs reveals decreased pulse, respiration, and blood pressure (Table 17–4).

Frostbite

Unlike hypothermia, frostbite occurs only when the body is exposed to subfreezing temperatures. In response to this environment, the body protects the integrity of the core temperature at the expense of blood flow to the extremities, with the toes and fingers being the most vulnerable sites. During compe-

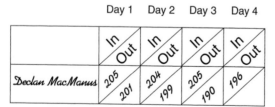

Figure 17–3. Weight chart. Each athlete weighs "in" prior to practice and weighs "out" afterward. In the example, the athlete should have been restricted from practice on day 4 because of a 5 percent loss of body weight.

Anoxia: The absence of oxygen in the blood or tissues.

Table 17–4. Evaluative Findings of Hypothermia

Onset	Gradual. A cold, damp, windy environment predisposes the athlete to hypothermia.
Pupils	Dilated in severe hypothermia.
Pulse	Slow and weak.
Blood pressure	Hypotension.
Respiration	Shallow and irregular.
Muscular function	Slight: Shivering. Mild: Motor impairment. Severe: Extreme motor impairment followed by muscle rigidity.
Mental status	This is reduced, according to the severity of hypothermia. The athlete's focus begins to drift from the task at hand. Mild: Desire to warm up. Severe: Desire to sleep.

tition the nose and cheeks are often uncovered, increasing the possibility of frostbite striking these areas. The freezing of the extracellular fluids results in **hypertonicity**, dehydrating the cells by drawing the fluids out from the cell membrane via osmosis, an event that is more damaging than the actual extracellular ice formation.[13] However, ice forming within the cell results in the permanent disruption of the cell membrane.

The magnitude and rate of nerve transmission is reduced when the nerves are cooled. This interruption makes the athlete initially unaware of the po-

tential damage to the skin. As the freezing progresses, the athlete experiences a cold, burning sensation that suddenly ceases and is replaced by a sensation of comfortable warmth, a warning sign of severe frostbite.

Unlike heat injuries, frostbite occurs through progressing degrees of severity, based on the depth of tissues affected, with one stage preceding the next. Superficial frostbite affects only the outermost layer of skin and initially appears with **hyperemia** and the development of edema within 3 hr. The superficial layer of skin **sloughs** within 1 wk following the injury.

Deep frostbite initially presents with the same signs and symptoms of superficial frostbite but involves the destruction of the full thickness of the skin. Blisters appear in 1 to 7 days. This tissue sloughs to expose a hard, black layer of tissue. Disruption of the blood supply to the affected body part and distal structures creates an environment that encourages the development of **gangrene**. The most severe cases of frostbite involve the total destruction of the tissues in the area, including bone.

Prevention of Cold Injuries

Common sense is the guide in preventing cold injuries. The environmental conditions are a combination of ambient air temperature and wind. **Wind chill** can quickly lower the air temperature equivalent to dangerously low levels capable of freezing the skin in a matter of minutes or even seconds (Table 17–5). In extremely cold tempera-

Table 17–5. Calculation of the Wind Chill Factor

Wind Speed (MPH)	Actual Thermometer Reading (°F)											
	50	40	30	20	10	0	−10	−20	−30	−40	−50	−60
	Wind Chill Factor (°F)											
Calm	50	40	30	20	10	0	−10	−20	−30	−40	−50	−60
5	48	37	27	16	6	−5	−15	−26	−36	−47	−57	−68
10	40	28	16	4	−9	−24	−33	−46	−58	−70	−83	−95
15	36	22	9	−5	−18	−32	−45	−58	−72	−85	−99	−112
20	32	18	4	−10	−25	−39	−53	−67	−82	−96	−110	−124
25	30	16	0	−15	−29	−44	−59	−74	−88	−104	−118	−133
30	28	13	−2	−18	−33	−48	−63	−79	−94	−109	−125	−140
35	27	11	−4	−20	−35	−51	−67	−82	−98	−113	−129	−145
40	26	10	−6	−21	−37	−53	−69	−85	−100	−116	−132	−148
	Little Danger			**Moderate Danger** Skin freezes within 1 min.			**Extreme Danger** Skin freezes within 1 min.					

Adapted from Sheehy, SB,[2] p 296.

Hypertonic: Having an increased osmotic pressure relative to the body's other fluids.
Hyperemia: A red discoloration of the skin caused by an increased capillary blood flow.
Slough: The peeling away of dead skin from living tissue.
Gangrene: The death of bony or soft tissue resulting from a decrease in, or loss of, blood supply to a body area.

tures, the athlete's skin should be covered as completely as possible and practical for the sport. Multiple layers of clothing provide better insulation from the external environment than a single layer (Table 17–6).

The athlete's diet may be a factor contributing to the onset or prevention of hypothermia.[14] High-protein diets should be avoided by individuals who face prolonged exposure to a subfreezing environment. Compared with diets high in carbohydrates or fats, those that are high in protein increase an individual's metabolic water requirements, thus decreasing the tolerance to cold.

MANAGEMENT OF ENVIRONMENTAL INJURIES

The premise for initial management of environmental injuries is to reverse the environmental extreme in which the athlete has been participating and return the core temperature to its normal range. A rapid response and transportation to a hospital is often necessary to keep the athlete alive, second only to quick recognition and intervening treatment.

Heat Injury

The management of all types of heat injuries require rehydrating the athlete with cool water. Electrolytes, especially salt, often need to be replaced, but the use of salt tablets should be avoided because of their potentially counterproductive effects.[5] Salt tablets delay gastric emptying and, if insufficient water is provided, fluids may be drawn from the extracellular space, causing further dehydration. Additionally, salt tablets are often poorly tolerated by the athlete, irritating the stomach lining and possibly resulting in nausea and vomiting. The use of commercial electrolyte drinks before, during, and after competition may be an effective method of reducing heat injuries, but drinking water should not be neglected.

Heat Cramps

Heat cramps are managed by controlling the symptoms and replacing fluids and electrolytes. While the athlete is on the field, the cramping muscle(s) should be stretched until the spasm subsides (Fig. 17–4). Once the athlete is returned to the sidelines, ice packs are applied to the involved area and the athlete's fluids and electrolytes replenished. The athlete may return to competition once the symptoms have cleared and the athlete has been rehydrated. These individuals should be frequently encouraged to consume fluids.

Heat Exhaustion and Heat Stroke

The treatment goals for athletes suffering from heat stroke or heat exhaustion are to reduce the core temperature and replace fluids and electrolytes. In each case **first aid cooling** must be initiated by moving the athlete from the hot environment to a shaded area or indoors, removing excess clothing, elevating the legs, and cooling the body through the use of ice packs, ice immersion, or fan-sprayed mist.

Heat exhaustion can be adequately managed by applying ice packs to the superficial arteries located at the lateral neck, axilla, groin, and the popliteal fossa (Fig. 17–5). Recently, a fan-sprayed mist has been used not only to treat but also to prevent heat injuries. These devices, often seen on football sidelines, spray a cool mist on the athlete to reduce the core temperature. A cold shower is also an efficient method of reducing the core temperature, but the

Table 17–6. National Collegiate Athletic Association's Recommended Guidelines for Reducing Cold Stress

Layering clothing	Several thin layers of clothing are best to retain body heat. Layers may be added or removed as needed.
Covering the head	As much as 50% of the body's heat is lost through the head.
Protecting the hands	The use of mittens rather than gloves is recommended to protect the fingers from frostbite.
Staying dry	Water increases the rate of heat loss from the body. Rather than wearing clothes made of cotton, wearing those made of polypropylene, wool, or other material that wicks moisture away from the skin is recommended.
Staying hydrated	Fluids are needed to maintain the body's core temperature and are as important in preventing cold injuries as heat injuries.
Warming up thoroughly	A thorough warm-up is required before competition to elevate the core temperature.
Warming incoming air	The use of a scarf or mask across the mouth warms incoming air.
Avoiding alcohol, nicotine, and other drugs	These agents cause vasoconstriction or vasodilation of the superficial blood vessels, hindering regulation of the core temperature.
Never training alone	An injury that prevents the athlete from walking may be catastrophic in cold climates.

Adapted from Benson, MT (ed),[14a] pp 35–36.

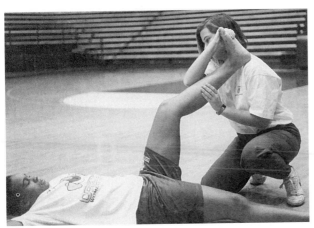

Figure 17–4. Treatment of heat cramp spasms by stretching the involved muscle group.

athlete should not be permitted to enter the shower unescorted.

Although ice packs may be used during the treatment of heat stroke, the ideal method of management of this condition involves immersing the athlete in cold water.[8] A shallow animal watering trough or child's swimming pool filled with water and ice can be used for this purpose, but the use of deep whirlpools should be avoided because of the inherent risk of the athlete drowning.

If the athlete is conscious and cooperative, copious amounts of fluids should be administered. In extreme cases of heat stroke the physician orders ***Ringer's lactate*** to be administered intravenously. If the athlete's symptoms do not subside or if heat stroke is suspected, the athlete must be immediately transported to the hospital because of the potentially fatal consequences.

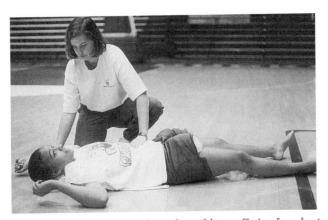

Figure 17–5. Emergency cooling of an athlete suffering from heat injury. Packing the areas in which arteries are relatively subcutaneous, the popliteal fossa, femoral triangle, axilla, and neck, serves to cool the core temperature.

Cold Injuries

As with heat injuries, the management of cold injuries involves removing the athlete from the insulting environment. In this case the athlete must be placed in a warm, dry environment, allowing the body to return to its normal temperature.

Hypothermia

After the athlete has been placed in a warm environment, the wet clothing should be removed and the body dried. The athlete should then be dressed in dry clothing or wrapped in a blanket.

Techniques to rapidly rewarm the body, such as immersion in a hot bath, must be avoided. Rapid rewarming dilates the peripheral vessels, causing lactic acid to be routed to the core. This leads to rebound hypothermia, which can cause a further decrease in core temperature secondary to hypotension and ventricular fibrillation.[12] Athletes should not be allowed to sleep, as doing so decreases metabolism and delays rewarming of the core. Warm drinks are not effective in raising the core temperature, and the use of alcoholic drinks must be avoided. The core may be quickly and safely rewarmed by the athlete's breathing the mist of a humidifier or other source of hot, moist air.[15]

Frostbite

Initially, frostbite can be limited by the athlete's keeping the affected body part moving, increasing the amount of metabolic heat production. When the athlete is still in the cold environment, frostbite of the fingers can be treated by the athlete's tucking the fingers in the axilla or crotch.[16] Once off the field, mild frostbite can be treated by immersing the body part in a warm (104°F to 110°F) bath. The affected area should never be rubbed, nor should snow be applied.

More significant frostbite should not be thawed if the risk of refreezing exists. Once the frozen part thaws, the athlete must not be allowed to walk on or use the affected part. If the athlete is still in the cold environment, steps should be taken to prevent hypothermia. Athletes suspected of suffering from frostbite must be immediately referred to a hospital so that a definitive diagnosis may be made and proper treatment initiated.

REFERENCES

1. Hubbard, RW, and Armstrong, LE: Hyperthermia: New thoughts on an old problem. The Physician and Sportsmedicine 17:97, 1989.

Ringer's lactate: A salt-based solution that is administered intravenously as a replacement for lost electrolytes.

2. Sheehy, SB: Environmental emergencies. In Sheehy, SB: Mosby's Manual of Emergency Care, ed 3. CV Mosby, St Louis, 1990, p 300.

3. Davidson, M: Heat illness in athletics. Athletic Training: Journal of the National Athletic Trainers Association, 20:96, 1985.

4. Spence, AP, and Mason, EB: Metabolism, nutrition, and temperature regulation. In Spence, AP, and Mason, EB: Human Anatomy and Physiology, ed 3. Benjamin/Cummings, Menlo Park, CA, 1987, p 754.

5. Birrer, RB: Heat stroke. Don't wait for the classic signs. Emerg Med Clin North Am July:43, 1994.

6. Murphy, RJ: Heat illness in the athlete. Athletic Training: Journal of the National Athletic Trainers Association, 19:166, 1984.

7. Roberts, WO: Emergencies in sports. Managing heat stroke: On-site cooling. The Physician and Sportsmedicine 20:17, 1992.

8. American College of Sports Medicine: Position stand on prevention of thermal injuries during distance running. Med Sci Sports Exerc 16:ix, 1984.

9. Francis, K, Feinstein, R, and Brasher, J: Optimal practice times for the reduction of the risk of heat illness during fall football practice in the southeastern United States. Athletic Training: Journal of the National Athletic Trainers Association, 26:76, 1991.

10. Noakes, TD, et al: Metabolic rate, not percent dehydration, predicts rectal temperatures in marathon runners. Med Sci Sports Exerc 23:443, 1991.

11. Nelson, WE-Gieck, JH, and Kolb, P: Treatment and prevention of hypothermia and frostbite. Athletic Training: Journal of the National Athletic Trainers Association, 18:330, 1983.

12. Robinson, WA: Emergencies in sports. Competing with the cold. Part II: Hypothermia. The Physician and Sportsmedicine 20:61, 1992.

13. Frey, C: Frostbitten feet. Steps to treatment and prevention. The Physician and Sportsmedicine 20:67, 1992.

14. Askew, EW: Nutrition for a cold environment. The Physician and Sportsmedicine 17:77, 1989.

14a. Benson, MT (ed): 1994−95 NCAA Sports Medicine Handbook. National Collegiate Athletic Association, Overland Park, KS, 1994.

15. Bowman, WD: Outdoor emergency care: Comprehensive first aid of nonurban settings. National Ski Patrol System, Lakewood, CO, 1988, p 291.

16. Steele, P: Management of frostbite. The Physician and Sportsmedicine 17:135, 1989.

18

Cardiopulmonary Conditions

Respiratory and cardiovascular injuries and illnesses are relatively rare in the athletic population. However, the occurrence of fatal episodes attracts a great deal of attention, especially when young, seemingly healthy individuals are stricken. The athletic trainer must be aware of the subtle early signs and symptoms, which may normally go unnoticed, but are vitally important to recognize to avert disaster. Once an episode occurs, a swift but thorough evaluation and response must be made, as the athlete's life is in immediate danger.

Although many athletic trainers and team physicians may never be faced with a life and death situation involving an athlete's cardiopulmonary system, it is certain that they are managing the medical care of athletes with pre-existing cardiac conditions.[1] The athletic trainer is increasingly challenged by athletes, young and old, who would have been withheld from exercise and competition in years past. These advances include college students participating in intercollegiate athletics following a heart transplantation.[2] The medical community has embraced exercise as a vital component of prevention and rehabilitation of these conditions.

All coaches, facilities coordinators, and other individuals who supervise athletic activities should maintain certification in cardiopulmonary resuscitation (CPR). In addition to standard CPR certification, athletic trainers should explore the feasibility of additional certification as an emergency medical technician (EMT) or paramedic.

CLINICAL ANATOMY

The heart and major vessels of the cardiovascular system lie within the mediastinum, between the lungs, from the first rib superiorly to the diaphragm inferiorly. The heart is lined by the fibrous and serous pericardium. The **fibrous pericardium** is the tough fibrous outer layer supporting the inner pericardial layer and the heart. The **serous pericardium** is further divided into a **parietal layer** lining the fibrous pericardium and a **visceral layer** that sits tightly against the heart. The serous pericardium allows the heart to move freely within the chest and buffers forces to the heart.

The heart is a four-chambered muscular pump delivering oxygenated blood to the tissues of the body. In the bloodstream, oxygen is exchanged for carbon dioxide, which is then returned to the lungs, where it is subsequently exhaled. The rate at which the heart beats is normally based on the metabolic needs of the body. The heart rate should increase to meet the metabolic demands of an exercising athlete.

The contraction of the cardiac musculature is controlled by an electrical system within the walls of the heart's chambers. This system allows for the synchronous contraction of the atria and ventricles, ensuring a smooth flow of blood through the cardiovascular system. Any disruption of the normal pattern of the electrical stimulus can cause failure of any of the body's systems, leading to death.

The **right atrium** of the heart receives deoxygenated blood from the head, neck, and upper extremities by way of the **superior vena cava**. The **inferior vena cava** delivers the deoxygenated blood from the trunk and lower extremities. As the right atrium contracts, the blood passes through the **tricuspid valve** and into the **right ventricle**. Contraction of the right ventricle causes the blood to pass through the **semilunar valves** into the **pulmonary arteries** and to the lungs, where it is oxygenated.

The newly oxygenated blood returns via the **pulmonary veins** into the **left atrium**. From the left atrium the blood is passed through the **mitral valve** into the **left ventricle** before it is distributed to the body. The left ventricle contains the greatest amount of cardiac muscle, as it must provide the force needed to propel the blood throughout the body. As the ventricles contract, the blood is pushed out the **semilunar valves** and into the **aorta**.

The valves of the heart all function as one-way valves (Fig. 18–1). The **tricuspid** and **mitral valves** are held tightly shut against the back flow of blood by the **chordinae tendinae** that are attached to **papillary muscles**. The muscles and tendon mechanically prevent the valve from opening in the wrong direction. The semilunar valves contain no papillary muscles, relying on their mechanical shape to prevent reflux of blood. The semilunar valves are tented and the back flow of blood causes the valves

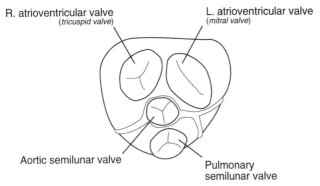

Figure 18–1. Valves controlling blood that is entering and exiting the heart.

to form pockets that fill and shut tightly together. Normally the heart makes "lubb" and "dupp" sounds as the valves open and close, respectively. Any reflux of blood through a faulty or leaking valve causes a decrease in the heart's ability to efficiently deliver the needed metabolites to the tissues of the body and alters the characteristic heart sounds (Table 18–1).

EVALUATION OF CARDIOPULMONARY INJURIES

Evaluation of cardiopulmonary injury and illness must be accomplished quickly and efficiently. Often the evaluation must be halted and management of the problem initiated before the examiner has a full understanding of the cause of the athlete's condition. Once the athlete is recognized as suffering from cardiopulmonary distress, the proper lifesaving techniques must be the first priority.

This chapter covers the evaluation of cardiac conditions as well as nontraumatic pulmonary injuries. The evaluation of traumatic pulmonary injuries such as pneumothorax and airway obstruction is covered in Chapter 10.

History

Athletes who suffer catastrophic cardiovascular injuries usually have some unrecognized or unreported history of previous symptoms. Careful preparticipation screening may help to increase the awareness of symptoms, yet many other symptoms may go unrecognized. Table 18–2 describes the pertinent information that should be obtained and recorded in the athlete's medical file and subsequently used to assist in identifying athletes who are potentially high-risk candidates for cardiopulmonary distress.[3]

Unfortunately, if the cardiopulmonary illness or injury is not recognized early, the results can be catastrophic. Sudden death can occur from a variety of cardiopulmonary conditions in athletes of all ages. Even when the signs and symptoms are quickly recognized, the athlete's life often cannot be saved without the use of advanced life support measures, which are not standard equipment at the site of competition. Any report of symptoms, either related or unrelated to physical activity, warrants the referral of the athlete for a complete evaluation by a physician (Table 18–3).

Location of the Pain

Cardiac dysfunction results in intense pain, tightness, or squeezing in the center of the chest. Other signs of ischemia to the cardiac tissues are manifested as referred pain into the right shoulder, arm, jaw, or epigastric area (see Fig. 10–16).

Pulmonary problems include difficulty with respiration and/or wheezing. The difficulty in breathing may cause the athlete to panic. These symptoms may be painful secondary to pulmonary obstruction, but typically these problems are recognized by the shear labor required as the athlete attempts to breathe. Excruciating, deep chest pain that develops in the mid and upper back is the most distinctive early sign of developing an aortic aneurysm, the typical cause of death in the athlete with **Marfan syndrome**.[4,5]

Onset

Cardiopulmonary illness in the athletic population is usually congenital or acquired gradually over time. These causes are usually manifested as previously unrecognized conditions that result in an acute climax of cardiopulmonary distress.

Table 18–1. Heart Sounds

Sound	Status	Interpretation
"Lubb"	Normal systolic	Ventricular contraction; synchronous with the carotid pulse
"Dupp"	Normal diastolic	Closing of the aortic and pulmonary valves
Soft, blowing "lubb"	Abnormal systolic	Associated with anemia or other changes in blood constituents
Loud, booming "lubb"	Abnormal systolic	Aneurysm
Sloshing "dupp"	Abnormal diastolic	Incomplete closing of the valves; blood is heard regurgitating backward
Friction sound	Abnormal	Inflammation of the heart's pericardial lining; pericarditis

Table 18–2. Cardiopulmonary Checklist for the Athlete's Medical File

Family History	Personal History	General	Orthopedic
Episodes of syncope, dyspnea, or chest pain Premature atherosclerosis Seizures Sudden death of a family member, especially at a young age	Episodes of syncope, dyspnea, or chest pain Premature atherosclerosis Seizures	Height Weight Vital signs Heart examination Lung examination Dislocation of the optic lens	Elongated appendages Unsteady or irregular gait Abnormal joint laxity Pes planus Club-shaped fingernails

Mechanism

The mechanisms of cardiopulmonary problems are not fully understood, but a strong link exists between the onset of these problems and a family history of these conditions. The most common underlying condition leading to the onset of cardiac problems in middle-aged and older athletes is **atherosclerosis** of the cardiac arteries, leading to ischemia in the cardiac tissues. The mechanism for atherosclerosis is not fully understood but is associated with several risk factors including smoking, hypertension, decreased activity, obesity, high cholesterol levels, and even normal progressive changes due to aging.

Pulmonary diseases once precluded a person from participating in sports, but with the advent of improved medications and treatment techniques, patients with pulmonary conditions such as **cystic fibrosis** and asthma are now participating in organized sports. Although the direct mechanism for pulmonary problems in athletes is the actual obstruction of the airway owing to mucus build-up or bronchospasm, underlying contributing causes are now being studied.

The incidence of **exercise-induced asthma** is seemingly on the rise. One explanation of the increasing frequency is that the increasingly poor air quality, especially in urban areas, triggers bronchospasm. Another school of thought relates increased cases of exercise-induced asthma to an increasing number of participants in athletic activities. As these people become involved in exercise, the mechanism for triggering their asthma is induced. In an effort to determine causes of exercise-induced asthma, especially those leading to fatalities among athletes, the National Athletic Asthma Registry has been established at the Temple University Hospital in Philadelphia.

Symptoms

Along with the intense chest pain and pressure associated with the ischemia of the cardiac musculature, the athlete may complain of dizziness, nausea, vomiting, and feeling faint. Although profuse sweating is a typical sign of cardiac arrest, this sign is often difficult to assess in an athlete who has been performing vigorous physical activity. Other symptoms of cardiac disorders that may be reported by the athlete are shortness of breath, lightheadedness, and fatigue. Disorders of the heart's electrical system may cause the sensation of the heart skipping beats or racing abnormally fast. Syncope, a sudden transient loss of consciousness, is often related to a cardiac **arrhythmia** and often occurs with previously mentioned symptoms of cardiac distress.

Complaints related to pulmonary problems include chest congestion, fatigue, and minor difficulty in breathing prior to the onset of the traumatic respiratory problem. Otherwise, the athlete exhibits labored breathing, characterized by a quick wheezing breathing pattern, often accompanied by unusual sounds.

Table 18–3. Signs and Symptoms of Cardiopulmonary Conditions

Cardiovascular	Both	Pulmonary
Panic Dizziness Nausea Vomiting Sweating Decreased blood pressure Distended jugular vein Pallor Clutching at chest Shoulder pain Epigastric pain	Chest pain Faintness Respiratory distress	Congestion Fatigue Anxiety Tingling in fingers and toes Spasm in fingers and toes Periorbital numbness Bending over

Atherosclerosis: The build-up of fatty tissues on the inner arterial walls.
Cystic fibrosis: A respiratory disease state in which the lungs produce too much mucus.
Arrhythmia: Loss of the normal heart rhythm; an irregular heart rate.

Prior Symptoms

Any previous episodes of symptoms associated with cardiopulmonary abnormalities recognized by the athlete should be noted and recorded in the athlete's medical record. Often athletes are reluctant to report a previous history of cardiopulmonary difficulties for fear of being disqualified from competition. Any individual with a history of cardiopulmonary symptoms should be examined by a physician before being allowed to participate, as this history may be the only finding before sudden death.

Inspection and Palpation

The athlete suffering from cardiopulmonary problems should be inspected even while being questioned about his or her complaints. In the case of the unconscious athlete, the examiner must always follow standard first-responder procedures, checking the airway, breathing, and circulation prior to any other assessment. In either case, the examiner must be prepared to perform lifesaving procedures if the athlete's condition warrants this. The examiner must use prudent decision making in a quick, precise fashion if the athlete is to have an optimal chance of survival.

Because the athlete with a cardiopulmonary condition must be assessed quickly, the inspection and pertinent palpation that goes along with the inspection are covered together, just as they are carried out together during this type of evaluation.

The Unconscious Athlete

- **Airway:** The first area to be inspected in the unconscious athlete is the integrity of the airway. Prior to checking the airway, however, the cervical spine should be stabilized in a neutral position if there is any possibility of head or neck injury (see Chapter 16). If the athlete is wearing a mouthpiece, it must be removed. The examiner should listen and feel for air being expired and observe for the rise and fall of the chest (see Fig. 16–6).

- **Breathing:** From the position used to inspect for a functional airway, the examiner assesses the breathing pattern and rate. A rate of fewer than 10 or greater than 30 breaths per minute requires assisted ventilation by properly trained personnel.[6] A labored, quick breathing pattern (dyspnea) is usually associated with some type of airway obstruction. Athletes with underlying pulmonary disease such as asthma or cystic fibrosis have labored breathing owing to obstruction from excessive mucus formation or bronchospasm. Athletes suffering from cardiac conditions may have difficulty breathing because of pain, but breathing is usually not as labored in these athletes as it is in those with pulmonary disorders.

- **Circulation:** The status of the circulation and thus the heart is assessed primarily by taking the pulse. While checking the airway and breathing the examiner palpates for the carotid pulse. The method for palpating this pulse and the assessment of the findings are found in Chapter 10.

Immediate activation of an emergency medical system is necessitated in the management of an unconscious athlete with suspected cardiopulmonary distress.

Conscious Athlete

- **Position of the athlete:** The athlete with cardiac problems will most likely be clutching the chest and may be bent over in pain. The athlete with a pulmonary problem may be bent over with hands on the knees so that the secondary muscles of respiration may be used to aid breathing. By putting the hands in a closed chain position, the sternocleidomastoid and pectoral muscles can aid in expanding the chest wall. In labored breathing these muscles may be observed to be contracting forcefully. The athlete may recruit the secondary muscles of respiration by sitting with the elbows on the knees and the head hanging between the legs.

- **Skin color:** The color of the athlete's skin is normally flushed immediately after exercise. Cardiopulmonary distress results in pale or ashen skin. First appearing in the lips, the discoloration progresses to cyanosis as the skin's tissues are deprived of oxygen. An unexpected change in skin tone from that normally associated with exercise should be a "red flag" for the examiner.

- **Airway:** The fact that an athlete is conscious does not rule out an airway obstruction, but the athlete's ability to speak indicates a clear airway. It should be established that the athlete has not swallowed any part of the mouthpiece, food, or other material, by direct inspection and by asking the athlete if he or she has swallowed anything.

- **Breathing:** The breathing pattern should be established for the conscious athlete suspected of having a cardiopulmonary problem. The method of establishing the rate and pattern of respiration is covered in Chapter 10.

- **Circulation:** While it is obvious that the conscious athlete's heart is beating, circulation must be assessed for rate and quality at the carotid pulse, as outlined in Chapter 10. The pulse should be frequently monitored and should return to normal levels within 5 minutes following cessation of the activity. If the pulse rate stays elevated, this may be indicative of underlying cardiac pathology.

- **Sweating:** Anyone suffering from cardiac problems sweats profusely; however, the athlete involved in vigorous physical activity sweats as a normal occurrence. In the absence of physical activity, complaints of chest pain and profuse sweating are classic symptoms of cardiac distress.

- **Responsiveness:** In general, the athlete suffering from a cardiac condition becomes lethargic and weak. Many conditions of the heart decrease left ventricular outflow, resulting in a decreased cardiac output.[7] The athlete may also suffer from syncope, the causes of which are discussed later in this chapter.

- **Nausea and vomiting:** Acute myocardial infarction often brings about nausea and vomiting.[8]

During assessment of a conscious athlete with symptoms of cardiopulmonary distress, deterioration in the condition of the vital signs warrants immediate activation of an emergency medical system.

Functional Tests

The special tests for cardiopulmonary distress are limited by the expertise of the athletic trainer. Once it has been determined that the athlete is in acute distress, the athletic trainer becomes the provider of basic life support until assistance arrives.

The athlete's airway, breathing, and circulation must be established and appropriate actions taken if any or all of these functions are missing. Otherwise, the athlete's pulse, blood pressure, and respiration must be continuously monitored and recorded.

Pathologies and Related Special Tests

Unfortunately, many of the conditions predisposing athletes to cardiopulmonary distress go unnoticed or unreported until an acute attack occurs. Early identification and intervention provide the best opportunity for athletes suffering from cardiopulmonary conditions to safely participate in athletics as well as perform the activities of daily living.

Syncope

Depending on its underlying cause, syncope can be an ominous sign of underlying cardiac abnormality, a symptom of heat illness, or simply a benign occurrence.[9,10] Syncope may not be initially reported by the athlete but should always be considered a sign warranting further assessment by a physician, particularly when it occurs during activity, or **exertional syncope.** The five potential mechanisms of this event, shown in Table 18–4, are common in athletes during practice and competition, and once the cause of the episode is determined, appropriate management and, possibly, prevention are indicated.

Hypertrophic Cardiomyopathy

Sudden death is a rare occurrence among athletes.[11] When an apparently healthy, active, and vibrant athlete is stricken, the results are especially devastating. The most common cause of sudden death in the young athlete is hypertrophic cardiomyopathy, a condition that may not display any physical signs or symptoms until an autopsy is performed.[12,13]

Hypertrophic cardiomyopathy is a condition in which the heart's muscles enlarge but the heart's chambers remain the same size. Although this condition most often afflicts the left ventricle and interventricular septum, the left atrium and right ventricle may also be involved.[14] The enlarged muscles place an increased amount of force on an unchanged volume (the blood contained within the

Table 18–4. Causes of Syncope in Athletes

	Vasovagal Reactions	Decreased Blood Volume	Metabolic Conditions	Cardiac Disorders	Drug Reactions
Cause	Venous dilation, increased vagal tone, and bradycardia following an anxiety-provoking event	Dehydration and electrolyte imbalance as in: Heat illness Vomiting Diarrhea Prolonged fasting Hemorrhage	Hypoglycemia associated with diabetes	Arrhythmias associated with hypertrophic cardiomyopathy, atherosclerosis, or anomalous coronary arteries	Stimulant abuse; may masquerade as arrhythmia, dehydration, or vasovagal reactions
Signs and symptoms	Lightheadedness Dizziness Profuse sweating Nausea	Lightheadedness Dizziness Nausea Visual disturbances	Fatigue Headache Profuse sweating Trembling Slurred speech Poor coordination	Palpitations Irregular heartbeat	As associated with arrhythmia, dehydration, or vasovagal reactions

chambers), increasing the pressure on the inter-ventricular septum and aorta. Acute failure may produce syncope, cardiac arrhythmia, or, in the most profound cases, a rupture of the septum or aorta, resulting in death.

Although the ability to evaluate and successfully treat the athlete who has suffered an acute episode is limited, the athletic trainer should be aware of the evaluative findings and predisposing factors leading to it.[15] The strongest indicator of an athlete's predisposition to sudden death is a family history of cardiovascular-related sudden death. The preparticipation examination's medical history questionnaire must be able to identify any history of cardiac-related sudden death:

Has any family member suffered a heart attack or other heart condition?	Yes	No

Any "yes" answer indicates that the athlete should be examined and subsequently cleared for participation by a cardiologist.

A significant heart murmur or characteristics of Marfan syndrome may also be present. In many cases of sudden death the occurrence of arrhythmias has been previously documented in the athlete's history.[5,12,16] Associated congenital anomalous coronary circulation may also be discovered following the sudden death of a young athlete.[17]

Acutely, the athlete may experience excessive fatigue, exertional syncope, dyspnea, or the sensation of arrhythmias while exercising (Table 18–5). The symptoms of hypertrophic cardiomyopathy are more likely to occur during exercise than during rest.[16] Occasionally, these episodes occur following bouts of vigorous activity or during stoppage in play.[17]

Definitive diagnosis of this condition is complex because of the varying presence and inconsistent reporting of significant symptoms, extensive range of testing procedures, and their subsequent interpretation by cardiologists. The 16th Bethesda Conference on cardiovascular abnormalities established guidelines for competition eligibility that are often used when safe participation decisions must be made by a physician (Table 18–6).[18] Athletes displaying any of the preceding symptoms should be referred to a physician for a complete medical work-up.

Myocardial Infarction

Athletes suffering a myocardial infarction or heart attack during exercise have a better chance of survival than those collapsing from hypertrophic cardiomyopathy. The onset of myocardial infarction is caused by blockage of the heart's coronary arteries, causing a depletion of oxygen to the cardiac muscle, eventually resulting in necrosis.

The athletic trainer must be aware of the *prodromal* symptoms in athletes who are at risk of a heart attack so that they can be referred and screened for coronary disease. Also, the athletic trainer should be aware of the signs and symptoms of an acute myocardial infarction. Quick recognition of an acute attack and a rapid response provides the athlete with a better chance of survival. Once a living heart attack victim enters a hospital, the chance of survival rises 50 percent.

Table 18–5. Evaluative Findings of Hypertrophic Cardiomyopathy

Examination Segment	Clinical Findings	
History	Onset:	Congenital or acquired.
	Location of pain:	Pain does not occur until an acute attack; then it resembles that of a myocardial infarction.
	Mechanism:	Hypertrophy of the heart's chambers, especially the left ventricle, increasing pressure on the interventricular septum and aorta.
	Risk factors:	Family history of cardiac sudden death.
		Significant heart murmur or arrhythmia.
		Marfan syndrome.
		Anomalous coronary circulation.
Inspection	Fatigue and exertional syncope are present.	
Palpation	Arrhythmia is experienced during exercise.	
Special tests	Complete cardiovascular examination: electrocardiogram, ultrasound imaging, and so on.	
Comments	Symptoms are more likely to occur during exercise than at rest.	

Prodromal: Pertaining to the interval between the initial disease rate and the onset of outward symptoms.

Table 18–6. Recommendations for Eligibility for Exercise in Athletes with Cardiovascular Disease

---

Conditions Contraindicating Vigorous Exercise
  Acute myocarditis
  Congenital coronary artery anomalies
  Congestive heart failure
  Hypertrophic cardiomyopathy
  Left ventricle hypertrophy (*idiopathic*)
  Marfan syndrome
  Pulmonary hypertension
  Right ventricular cardiomyopathy
  Uncontrolled arrhythmias or valvular heart disease

Conditions Requiring Modified Activity and/or Continuous Monitoring
  Uncontrolled hypertension
  Uncontrolled atrial arrhythmias
  Aortic insufficiency
  Mitral stenosis
  Mitral regurgitation

The athlete usually has had some previous symptoms including chest pain, fatigue, and syncope. A strong family history of heart disease, hypertension, **hypercholesterolemia**, a history of smoking, excessive body weight, or a previous history of coronary artery disease are all considered risk factors for heart attack.

Individuals suffering a myocardial infarction complain of intense pain in the chest, often radiating to the jaw, right shoulder, and arm. A typical finding of myocardial infarction is profuse sweating, but this may be an unreliable finding in an athlete involved in vigorous physical activity. The lips and fingernails may appear cyanotic. Nausea and/or vomiting may be experienced. The pulse may be abnormally high and irregular for some time after exercise has been discontinued, and respirations may be quick and shallow. Evaluation of the blood pressure reveals hypotension, as the ailing heart is not able to produce sufficient output.

The symptoms presented in Table 18–7 indicate the need to immediately transport the athlete for further assessment and treatment, as these symptoms may become progressively more severe and result in death quite rapidly.

Arrhythmias

Arrhythmias, irregular heart rhythms, can be relatively common in the athletic population. Although many of the causes of arrhythmia are benign or can be controlled through the use of medications, other causes are potentially fatal. Any arrhythmia reported by the athlete or discovered during a physical examination should be further evaluated by a cardiologist to prescribe the appropriate management and determine the athlete's ability to safely participate in athletics.

Table 18–7. Evaluative Findings of a Myocardial Infarction (Heart Attack)

Examination Segment	Clinical Findings	
History	Onset:	Acute.
	Location of pain:	Intense chest pain, possibly radiating to the jaw, right shoulder, and arm.
	Mechanism:	Ischemia of the cardiac muscles.
	Risk factors:	Family history of cardiac disease.
		Hypertension.
		High blood cholesterol level.
		Overweight/obesity.
		Smoking.
		Known atherosclerosis.
Inspection	The athlete is sweating profusely. Cyanosis is present. Nausea and vomiting may occur. Shallow, rapid respirations are present.	
Palpation	Rapid, irregular pulse is found.	
Special tests	Blood pressure testing reveals hypotension.	
Comments	The emergency medical squad should be summoned. The athlete should be treated for shock. The symptoms should continue to be monitored. If cardiac arrest occurs, CPR should be initiated.	

Idiopathic: Of unknown cause.
Hypercholesterolemia: A high blood cholesterol level caused by a high intake of saturated fats.

As described in Chapter 10, cardiac contusions or violent chest compression may also disrupt the athlete's normal heart rhythm.

Bradycardia

Bradycardia, a heart rate below 60 beats per minute, is common in highly trained athletes and is often termed "athlete's heart." This condition was once considered pathological and recommendations were made for the individual to cease activity. However, it has been recognized that the decreased heart rate is associated with enhanced cardiovascular function.[19]

Occasionally athletes with a slow heart rate may experience syncope, especially when at rest. Normal sinus tachycardia takes over during exercise, decreasing or eliminating the manifestation of symptoms of bradycardia.[20,21] Any athlete with unexplainable bouts of syncope at rest and bradycardia should be examined by a physician to rule out significant cardiac implications.

Tachycardia

Tachycardia, an increased heart rate, can be characterized as a normal response to a stressful circumstance. Other causes of tachycardia can result in sudden death. Clinically, athletes with tachycardia may become excessively fatigued, describe exertional syncope, and experience a sensation of the heart's "racing." Evaluation of the pulse can reveal sustained heart rates in excess of 200 beats per minute. The inefficient action of the heart results in a decreased blood pressure.

An athlete suspected to be suffering from tachycardia and presenting with a normal **sinus rhythm** should be withheld from activity and referred for further evaluation by a physician. Sustained tachycardia indicates that the athlete should be transported to a medical facility by trained personnel, as this condition can degenerate into ventricular fibrillation and result in sudden death.

Marfan Syndrome

Unlike those with other cardiac disorders, athletes with Marfan syndrome exhibit certain signs during physical inspection. Classic physical findings of individuals suffering Marfan syndrome are an arm span greater than the person's height and elongated metacarpal and metatarsal bones, causing the hands and feet to appear disproportionately large.[22] Overall, there may be laxity throughout all the athlete's joints. Kyphoscoliosis may be noted in the athlete's thoracic spine. Steinberg's thumb, in which the athlete is able to oppose the thumb beyond the ulnar border of the hand, is also a significant musculoskeletal determinant of Marfan syndrome.[5,23]

Although Marfan syndrome is a disease of the body's connective tissue, failure of the cardiac system usually leads to the death of the athlete. In this syndrome, the connective tissue providing strength to the aorta is decreased, leading to weakness of this tissue. Even when the syndrome is recognized and the athlete is removed from strenuous activity, the athlete can suffer aortic aneurysms leading to immediate death.[24,25]

While usually asymptomatic during exercise, Marfan syndrome can be detected during the athlete's physical examination (Table 18–8). The typical first finding leading to the diagnosis is that of a dislocated lens in the eye.[26] This finding, in con-

Table 18–8. Evaluative Findings of Marfan Syndrome

Examination Segment	Clinical Findings	
History	Onset:	Congenital.
	Location of pain:	The athlete may offer no complaints of cardiac disorder and have no previous history of problems.
	Mechanism:	Congenital, deteriorating disease state.
Inspection	Tall individuals whose arm span is greater than their height typify those with this syndrome. Elongation of the metacarpals and metatarsals is present. Kyphoscoliosis is noted. Dislocated lenses of the eye may be found.	
Ligamentous tests	Multijoint laxity.	
Special tests	Cardiac examination reveals multivalvular disease and an abnormal aorta.	
Comments	Definitive diagnosis of Marfan syndrome is made by a physician.	

Sinus rhythm: An irregular heartbeat characterized by an increased rate during inspiration and a decreased rate during expiration.

junction with the physical appearance findings, warrants a full cardiac examination.

Cardiac testing may produce various abnormalities, with the most common an abnormal aorta and multivalvular deformities, leading to prolapse of the valves and aortic valve regurgitation.[5,25] The decreased amount of connective tissue in the aortic wall leaves it prone to rupture during the extreme pressures it faces as blood is pumped from the left ventricle. Aortic root dilation is a prominent abnormality that eventually leads to aortic dissecting aneurysm.[4] Signs of an aneurysm are the most common finding on echocardiography. Regardless, the recommendation for these athletes concerning future participation is complete cessation of their physical activity.

Hypertension

High blood pressure is the most common cardiovascular abnormality affecting athletes and is more prevalent in the African-American population than in other races.[27] Increased peripheral vascular resistance to blood flow, secondary to vasoconstriction, increases the pressure required to force blood through the vessels.

Although systolic pressures greater than 140 mm Hg and diastolic pressures greater than 90 mm Hg are the clinical benchmarks for hypertension, the athlete's average blood pressure should be compared with the normative data reflecting the athlete's gender, age, height, and weight. The average of repeated readings is required because of the variables influencing blood pressure, including the possible anxiety associated with the procedure itself.

Once the presence of hypertension has been established, its cause must be identified so that appropriate intervention can take place. Unregulated hypertension can result in myocardial infarction, stroke, kidney failure, and disturbances in vision. Most athletes with controlled hypertension can safely participate in athletics, assuming that no associated organ damage has occurred. Athletes with unregulated hypertension should be limited to low-intensity activities and be closely monitored.

The Asthmatic Athlete

Asthma is caused by a narrowing of the bronchial tree, resulting in difficulty breathing. This narrowing results from an increase in mucosal secretions, bronchospasm, or both. Persons with asthma can be divided into two groups, determined by the predisposing cause of the condition. **Extrinsic asthma** is caused by **allergens** such as hay fever, insect stings, pollen, animal **dander**, or foods. The cause of **intrinsic asthma** is less well defined, but the most common type in athletes is **exercise-induced asthma**.

Asthma is characterized by dry wheezing during respiration, an event that may be frightening to the athlete as well as to bystanders (Table 18–9). During an episode the athlete experiences tightness in the chest during inspiration but tends to have greater difficulty during expiration. If a partial obstruction occurs high in the airway, as with laryngeal injury, there tends to be more difficulty with inspiration than with expiration. It is not uncommon for the asthmatic athlete to experience repeated dry coughing during the asthma attack.

Athletes with extrinsic asthma have attacks precipitated by contact with one of the allergens. Intrinsic exercise-induced asthma is most commonly caused by exercise in a cold, dry climate, as the cool air triggers the bronchospasm. Athletes with exercise-induced asthma usually have fewer symptoms during activities with brief periods of intense work, with exercise in a relatively warm, humid en-

Table 18–9. Evaluative Findings of an Asthma Attack

Examination Segment	Clinical Findings	
History	Onset:	The disease itself is congenital or acquired. The attacks are acute.
	Location of pain:	In the chest. Breathing is difficult, more so during expiration than inspiration.
	Mechanism:	Bronchospasm due to allergens (extrinsic) or cold, dry air during exercise (intrinsic).
Inspection	Wheezing occurs with respiration. Repetitive dry coughing is present.	
Comments	Many asthma attacks can be quickly controlled through the use of an inhaler.	

Allergen: A substance that, when contacting the body's tissues, results in a state of sensitivity.
Dander: Small scales from animal hair or feathers causing an allergic reaction in some individuals.

vironment, and with improvement in their aerobic condition.

Individuals with asthma often have knowledge of their condition prior to participating in organized sports. It is not unusual for high school athletes to use preparticipation medication or carry inhalers to control asthma attacks. This is important information for the athletic trainer to include in the athlete's medical record, and it may necessitate carrying medication for the athlete in case of emergency.

Hyperventilation

Conditions such as asthma, *metabolic acidosis, pulmonary edema*, or anxiety can increase the minute volume ventilation rate by increasing the athlete's respiratory rate. Subsequently, the body's oxygen and carbon dioxide levels are skewed by decreasing the level of carbon dioxide and increasing the level of oxygen. This imbalance results in dizziness, tracheal spasm, an increased heart rate, and, eventually, fainting. Once the oxygen and carbon dioxide levels are stabilized, the symptoms quickly subside.

ON-FIELD MANAGEMENT OF CARDIOPULMONARY ILLNESS

The most important aspects of the management of any suspected cardiopulmonary injury or illness are the basic ABCs of first aid. The examiner must establish that the athlete has an *a*irway, that *b*reathing is occurring, and that *c*irculation is present. Unfortunately for some of these athletes, such as those suffering from hypertrophic cardiomyopathy, illnesses that are not identified before participation may be fatal despite the most heroic lifesaving measures.

For other cardiac conditions in which the presence of breathing and a pulse has been established, the most important task of the athletic trainer is to initiate the emergency management system. Beyond this the athletic trainer must take control of the situation and keep the athlete, and those around the athlete, as calm as possible. The vital signs should be continually monitored and documented until assistance arrives.

Asthma

Athletes with asthma can usually manage their own condition and may or may not require the athletic trainer's assistance. Proper management of these conditions includes having the athletes' medications on hand, marked as belonging to them, and quickly making it available to them. These athletes are usually well versed and capable of dispensing their own medication but should be assisted as needed.

Under ideal circumstances, athletes suffering from asthma have previously been identified and are carrying an inhaler. In these circumstances the athletic trainer should assist the athlete by ensuring that he or she is using the inhaler and is moved to the sideline until the breathing becomes controlled.

If the athlete does not have an inhaler available, the situation must be managed as a pulmonary emergency. Because the primary problem is in exhaling rather than inhaling, the athlete should attempt to perform controlled diaphragmatic breathing, using the abdominal muscles to slowly, yet

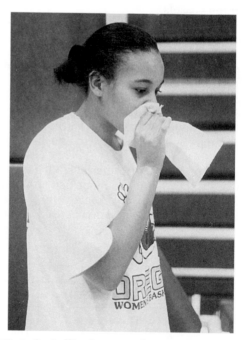

Figure 18–2. Controlling hyperventilation. Breathing into a paper bag recirculates carbon dioxide in the respiratory system and re-establishes the body's oxygen–carbon dioxide balance.

Metabolic acidosis: Decreased blood pH caused by an increase in blood acids or a decrease in blood bases.
Pulmonary edema: Swelling of the lung and its tissues.

forcefully, push the air from the lungs. Placing the athlete in a sitting position so that the arms are resting on the knees assists in expiration.

Typically, the athlete suffering from an exercise-induced asthma attack experiences the symptoms approximately 10 minutes after beginning exercise. Managed with inhalers and cessation of exercise, the athlete's symptoms usually cease after 30 minutes. In some cases the symptoms worsen before they clear.[28] More than half of athletes with exercise-induced asthma experience a **refractory period** following asthma attacks. During this 2-hr period, the athlete seems resistant to a recurrence of the symptoms while performing similar activities.[29]

Hyperventilation

Hyperventilating athletes can be managed by controlling the rate at which carbon dioxide is lost from the body. The traditional method involved having the athlete breathe into a paper bag (*not* a plastic bag) held tightly around the mouth and nose (Fig. 18–2). An alternative method involves having the athlete breathe through only one nostril by holding the opposite nostril closed.

REFERENCES

1. Mangus, BC, and Finnecy, T: A pilot study of cardiac disorders in division I athletes. Athletic Training: Journal of the National Athletic Trainers Association, 25:237, 1990.
2. Finnecy, T, and Mangus, BC: Athletic participation after cardiac transplantation: A case study. Athletic Training: Journal of the National Athletic Trainers Association, 19:224, 1989.
3. Smith, AN, and Bell, GW: Hypertrophic cardiomyopathy and its inherent danger in athletics. Athletic Training: Journal of the National Athletic Trainers Association, 26:319, 1991.
4. Ballenger, M: Dissecting aneurysms. Emergency Magazine 17:25, 1985.
5. Maron, BJ, Epstein, SE, and Roberts, WC: Causes of sudden death in competitive athletes. J Am Coll Cardiol 7:204, 1986.
6. Feld, F: Management of the critically injured football player. Journal of Athletic Training, 28:206, 1993.
7. Cecil, LF: Cecil's Essentials of Medicine. WB Saunders, Philadelphia, 1986.
8. Erkkinen, JF: Nausea and vomiting. In Greene, HL, Glassock, RJ, and Kelley, MA (ed): Introduction to Clinical Medicine. BC Decker, Philadelphia, 1991, p 283.
9. Hargarten, K: Emergencies in sports: Syncope in athletes. Life-threatening or benign? The Physician and Sportsmedicine 19:33, 1991.
10. Hargarten, KM: Syncope. Finding the cause in active people. The Physician and Sportsmedicine 20:123, 1992.
11. Amsterdam, EA, Laslett, L, and Holly, R: Exercise and sudden death. Cardiol Clin 5:337, 1987.
12. Maron, BJ, et al: Sudden death in young athletes. Circulation 62:218, 1980.
13. Maron, BJ, Roberts, WC, and Epstein, SC: Sudden death in hypertrophic cardiomyopathy. Circulation 65:1388, 1982.
14. Van Camp, SP: Exercise-related sudden death: risks and causes. The Physician and Sportsmedicine 16:96, 1988.
15. Pipe, AL, Chan, K, and Rippe, JM: A case conference. Asymptomatic heart murmur in a professional football player. The Physician and Sportsmedicine 16:53, 1988.
16. Burke, AP, et al: Sports-related and non-sports-related sudden cardiac death in young adults. Am Heart J 121:568, 1991.
17. Thomas, RJ, and Cantwell, JD: Case Reports. Sudden death during basketball games. The Physician and Sportsmedicine 18:75, 1990.
18. Munnings, F: The death of Hank Gathers: A legacy of confusion. The Physician and Sportsmedicine 18:97, 1990.
19. Alpert, JS, et al: Athletic heart syndrome. The Physician and Sportsmedicine 17:103, 1989.
20. Lichtman, J, et al: Electrocardiogram of the athlete. Arch Intern Med 132:763, 1973.
21. Northcote, RJ, et al: Is severe bradycardia in veteran athletes an indication for a permanent pacemaker? British Medical Journal 298:231, 1989.
22. Gocke, TV: Case report: Marfan's syndrome. Athletic Training: Journal of the National Athletic Trainers Association, 21:341, 1986.
23. McKusick, V: Heritable Disorders of Connective Tissue, ed 4. CV Mosby, St Louis, 1972.
24. Anderson, RE, and Pratt-Thomas, HR: Marfan's syndrome. Am Heart J 46:911, 1953.
25. Pan, CC, et al: Echocardiographic abnormalities in families of patients with Marfan's syndrome. J Am Coll Cardiol 6:1016, 1985.
26. Allen, RA, et al: Ocular manifestation of Marfan syndrome. Transactions of the American Academy of Oplthalmology/Otolaryngology 71:18, 1967.
27. Strong, WB, and Steed, D: Cardiovascular evaluation of the young athlete. Pediatr Clin North Am 29:1325, 1982.
28. McFadden, ER: Exercise-induced asthma. Assessment of current etiologic concepts. Chest 91:151, 1987.
29. Schoeffel, RE: et al: Multiple exercise and histamine challenges in asthmatic patients. Thorax 35:164, 1989.

Appendix
Reflex Testing

Deep tendon reflexes are elicited with a threshold response following a quick stretch of the muscle tendon that causes a reflexive muscular contraction. The procedure involves tapping the tendon with a reflex hammer with just enough force to elicit the response. Practice is required to develop the right "touch" to elicit a reflex response; the amount of pressure required varies from reflex to reflex and from person to person. Gaining a reflex response is somewhat eased by the athlete's slightly tensing the muscle.

Reflexes must be checked bilaterally with the limb held at approximately the same position with equal amounts of muscular tension. The reflex can be graded on a four-point scale:

0 No reflex elicited
1 Reflex elicited with reinforcement
2 Normal reflex
3 Hyperresponsive reflex

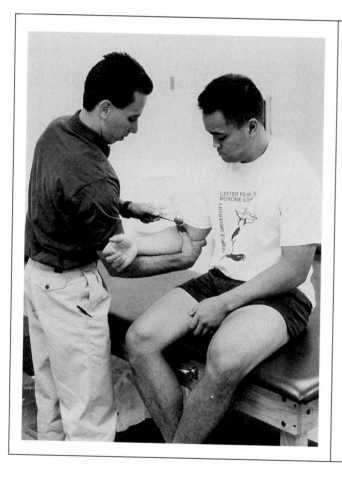

Nerve root:	C5.
Muscle:	Biceps brachii.
Position of the athlete:	Seated.
Position of the examiner:	Standing to the side of the athlete with the forearm cradled in one arm. The thumb is placed over the tendon.
Evaluative procedure:	The thumb is tapped with the reflex hammer.

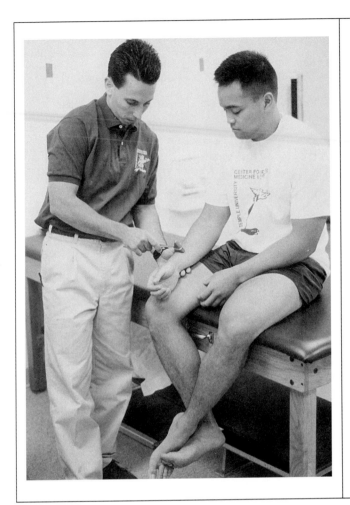

Nerve root:	C6.
Muscle:	Brachioradialis reflex.
Position of the athlete:	Seated.
Position of the examiner:	Cradling the arm of the athlete.
Evaluative procedure:	The distal portion of the brachioradialis tendon is tapped with the reflex hammer. The proximal tendon may be substituted.

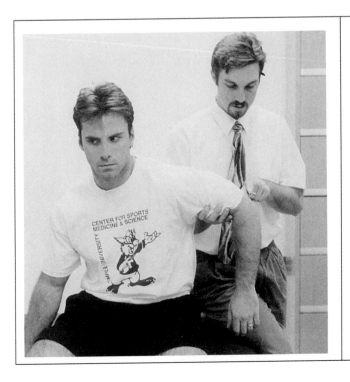

Nerve root:	C7.
Muscle:	Triceps brachii.
Position of the athlete:	Seated.
Position of the examiner:	Supporting the athlete's shoulder abducted to 90° and the elbow flexed to 90°.
Evaluative procedure:	The distal triceps brachii tendon is tapped with the reflex hammer.

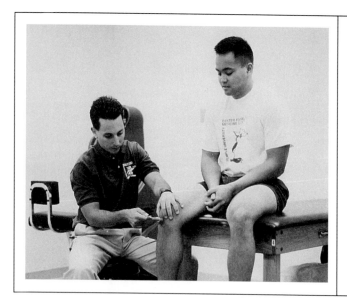

Nerve root:	L4.
Muscle:	Patellar tendon (quadriceps femoris).
Position of the athlete:	Sitting with the knees flexed over the end of the table.
Position of the examiner:	Standing to the side of the athlete.
Evaluative procedure:	The patellar tendon is tapped with the reflex hammer.

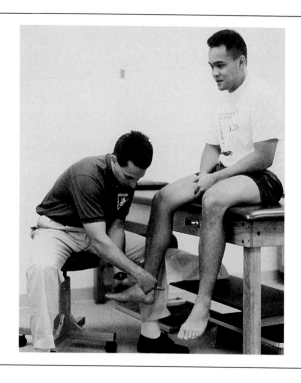

Nerve root:	S1.
Muscle:	Achilles tendon (triceps surae muscle group).
Position of the athlete:	Sitting with the knees flexed over the edge of the table.
Position of the examiner:	Seated in front of the athlete, supporting the foot in its neutral position.
Evaluative procedure:	The Achilles tendon is tapped with a reflex hammer.

Glossary

Abduction: Lateral movement of a body part away from the midline of the body.

Accessory motion: Motion that accompanies active movement and is necessary for normal motion but cannot be voluntarily isolated.

Accessory navicular: An abnormal osseous outgrowth on the navicular of the foot.

Active range of motion: Movement through the range of motion produced by muscle contractions.

Activities of daily living (ADLs): The skills and motions required for independence in the day-to-day activities of life.

Adduction: Medial movement of a body part toward the midline of the body.

Adenosine triphosphate (ATP): An energy-yielding enzyme used during muscular contractions.

Allergen: A substance that, when contacting the body's tissues, results in a state of sensitivity.

Amenorrhea: Absence of the menstrual period.

Anatomical position: The position the body assumes when standing upright with the feet and palms pointing naturally forward.

Anisocoria: Unequal pupil sizes; may be a benign congenital condition or may occur secondary to brain trauma.

Anoxia: The absence of oxygen in the blood or tissues.

Antagonistic: In the opposite direction of movement (e.g., the antagonistic motion of extension is flexion).

Antalgic: Having a pain-relieving quality; analgesic.

Anteversion: A forward bending or angulation of a bone or organ.

Aperture: An opening into bony spaces or soft tissue canals.

Apnea: The temporary cessation of breathing.

Apophysitis: Inflammation of a bone's growth plate.

Apprehension response: The display of anxiety, pain, or withdrawal of the body part secondary to the fear of a joint's being forced into dislocation.

AROM: Active range of motion.

Arrhythmia: Loss of the normal heart rhythm; an irregular heart rate.

Asymptomatic: Without symptoms.

Ataxia: A loss of muscular coordination indicating brain trauma.

Atherosclerosis: The build-up of fatty tissues on the inner arterial walls.

Athletic trainer: An individual who is skilled in the prevention, evaluation, treatment, and rehabilitation of athletic injuries.

Atrophy: A wasting or decrease in the size of a muscle or organ.

Auscultation: The act of listening to bodily sounds.

Avascular necrosis: Death of cells secondary to lack of an adequate blood supply.

Avulsion: The tearing away of tissue.

Axonotmesis: A disruption of a nerve's axon and myelin sheath while the epineurium remains intact.

Ballotable patella: Floating of the patella caused by capsular swelling.

Baseline measurements: The initial physical findings, usually performed while the athlete is in a healthy state.

Battle's sign: Ecchymosis collection over the mastoid process indicative of a skull fracture.

Beevor's sign: Movement of the umbilicus as the athlete performs a half sit-up, indicating interrupted innervation of the abdominal muscles.

Bell's palsy: Inhibition of the facial nerve secondary to trauma or disease, resulting in flaccidity of the facial muscles. In individuals suffering from Bell's palsy the face on the involved side appears elongated.

Biohazard: A substance that is toxic to humans, animals, or the environment.

Biomechanics: The effect of muscular forces, joint axes, and resistance on the quality and quantity of human movement.

Bipartite: Referring to the pathological condition of a bone's being in two separate parts.

Bleb: A large, loose blood vessel having the potential to rupture.

Bolster: A support used to maintain the position of a body part.

Bone scan: The use of injected radioactive material, which is absorbed by bones undergoing remodeling, to enable these areas to be visible on x-ray examination.

Boutonnière deformity: A contracture of the finger marked by extension of the metacarpophalangeal and distal interphalangeal joint and flexion of the proximal interphalangeal joint.

Brachial plexus: A network of nerves arising from the cervical spine that supplies the upper extremity.

Bradycardia: A slow heart rate, generally accepted to be below 60 beats per minute.

Break pressure: See break test.

Break test: An isometric contraction against manual resistance provided by the examiner; used to determine the athlete's ability to generate a static force within a muscle or muscle group.

Bunion: Inflammation of the bursa overlying the medial aspect of the first metatarsophalangeal joint.

Bursa (pl. **bursae**)**:** A fluid-filled sac that decreases friction between adjoining soft tissues or between soft tissue and bones.

Calcific tendinitis: Formation of calcium within a tendon.

Camel sign: Sign indicated when the patella and patellar tendon appear as a double hump, revealing a high-riding patella (patella alta).

Capsular pattern: A line of decreased motion associated with injury of a joint's capsular tissue. Capsular patterns are specific to each joint.

Cardinal planes: Imaginary lines dividing the body into upper and lower (transverse plane), anterior and posterior (frontal plane), and left and right (sagittal plane) relative to the anatomical position.

Carotid sinus: An area near the common carotid artery that, when stimulated, results in vasodilation and a lowering of the heart rate. When this occurs suddenly, unconsciousness may result.

Carrying angle: The angle assumed in the frontal plane by the humerus and ulna when the arm is at rest.

Cartilaginous joint: A relatively immobile joint in which two bones are fused by cartilage.

Catastrophic injury: An injury that causes permanent disability or death.

Cauda equina syndrome: A lesion affecting the cauda equina (the terminal portion of the spinal cord and its distal nerve roots) that may be indicated by bowel or bladder signs.

Cerumen: A reddish-brown wax formed in the auditory meatus.

Chemosis: Swelling of the conjunctiva around the cornea.

Cholecystitis: Inflammation of the gallbladder.

Chondroblast: A cell that forms cartilage.

Ciliary gland: A form of sweat gland on the eyelid.

Clarke's sign: A grinding sensation occurring when a downward force is applied to the patella while the quadricep is isometrically contracted, indicating the presence of chondromalacia.

Claudication: Intermittent lameness and limping.

Clawhand: Hand positioning characterized by hyperextension of the proximal phalanges and flexion of the middle and distal phalanges resulting from trauma to the median and ulnar nerves.

Claw toes: Toes characterized by hyperextension of the metatarsophalangeal joint and flexion of the proximal and distal interphalangeal joints.

Closed chain exercise: See closed kinetic chain.

Closed kinetic chain: Motion that occurs when the distal portion of the extremity is weight bearing or otherwise fixed.

Closed-packed position: The point in a joint's range of motion at which its bones are maximally congruent; the most stable position of a joint.

Collision sports: Individual or team sports relying on the physical dominance of one athlete over another. By their nature, these sports mandate violent physical contact.

Compressive force: A force applied along the length of a structure, causing the tissues to approximate one another.

Computed tomography: Imaging of a cross section of tissue by a computer-enhanced x-ray image (CT scan).

Concurrent: Occurring at the same time.

Congenital: A condition existing at or before birth.

Contact sports: Individual or team sports in which contact between two players, although not an integral part of the game, is unavoidable.

Contractile tissue: Tissue that is capable of shortening and subsequently elongating; muscular tissue.

Contracture: A pathological shortening of muscular fibers inhibiting the lengthening of the muscle.

Contraindication: Procedure that may prove harmful given the athlete's current condition.

Contralateral: Pertaining to the opposite side of the body or the opposite extremity.

Contrast imaging: The use of a dye to enhance x-ray images.

Contrecoup: Injury on the side opposite that of the impact.

Converge: Two or more units joining to form a single structure.

Corticosteroid: A substance that permits many biochemical reactions to proceed at their optimal rate (e.g., tissue healing).

Coup: Injury on the side of the impact.

Coxa valga: Medial angulation of the knees ("knock knees").

Coxa vara: Lateral angulation of the knees ("bow legs").

Crepitus: Repeated crackling sensations or sound emanating from a joint or tissue.

CT scan: See computed tomography.

Cyanotic: Dark blue or purple tint to the skin and mucous membranes caused by a decreased oxygen supply.

Cystic fibrosis: A respiratory disease state in which the lungs produce too much mucus.

Dander: Small scales from animal hair or feathers causing an allergic reaction in some individuals.

Deep tendon reflexes: An involuntary muscle contraction caused by a reflex arc in the spinal cord, initiated by the stretching of receptors within a tendon.

Definitive diagnosis: The final determination as to the type and extent of an injury or illness, with all other possible causes being ruled out. Only physicians can make a definitive diagnosis.

Defibrillation: The process of returning a normal heartbeat.

Dental caries: A destructive disease of the teeth; cavities.

Dermatome: An area of skin innervated by a single nerve root.

Diaphysis: The shaft of a long bone.

Diffuse: Scattered; widespread.

Diplopia: Double vision.

Dislocation: The displacement of the articular surfaces of two joints.

Disposition: The immediate and long-term management of an injury or illness.

Distal: Away from the midline of the body moving toward the periphery; the opposite of proximal.

Diverge: To split.

Dorsal: Referring to the posterior aspect of the hand and forearm relative to the anatomical position, and to the superior portion of the foot and toes.

Dorsiflexion: Flexion of the ankle; pulling the foot and toes toward the tibia.

Dynamic overload: Injury to the muscle as it generates more forces than it is capable of withstanding.

Dysmenorrhea: Pain during menstruation.

Dyspnea: Air hunger marked by labored or difficult breathing; may be a normal occurrence after exertion or an abnormal occurrence indicating cardiac or respiratory distress.

Dystrophy: The progressive deterioration of muscle.

Eccentric muscle contraction: A contraction in which the elongation of the muscle is voluntarily controlled. Lowering a weight is an example of an eccentric contraction.

Ecchymosis: A blue or purple area of skin caused by the movement of blood into the skin.

Ectopic pregnancy: The formation of a fetus outside of the uterine cavity.

Electrolyte: Ionized salts including sodium, potassium, and chlorine in blood, tissue fluid, and cells.

Electromyelogram: The recording of the electrical activity within a muscle.

Emergency medical technician: A health care professional versed in the emergency and immediate care of injury and illness.

Emmetropia: Normal visual acuity in terms of the point at which light focuses on the retina.

End-feel: The specific quality of movement felt by an examiner moving a joint to the end of its range of motion.

End-point: The quality and quantity of a ligament's ability to limit movement.

Endodontics: The field of dentistry specializing in the management of injuries and diseases affecting the pulp of a tooth.

Enophthalmos: The inferior displacement of the eye, indicating a ruptured globe or orbital fracture.

Epineurium: Connective tissue containing blood vessels surrounding the trunk of a nerve, binding it together.

Epiphyseal line: The area of growth found between the diaphysis and epiphysis in immature long bones.

Epistaxis: A nosebleed.

Etiology: The cause of a disease (also the study of the causes of disease).

Eversion: The movement of the plantar aspect of the calcaneus away from the midline of the body.

Exercise-induced asthma: Bronchospasm caused by exercise in a cold, dry climate.

Exophthalmos: The anterior bulging of the eye, indicating a ruptured globe or orbital fracture.

Exostosis: An abnormal growth of bone in an area in which excessive stress has been applied.

Extension: The act of straightening a joint, increasing its angle.

Extensor mechanism: The mechanism formed by the quadriceps and patellofemoral joint that is responsible for causing extension of the lower leg at the knee joint.

Extracapsular: Outside of the joint capsule.

Extravasate: Fluid escaping from vessels into the surrounding tissue.

Extrinsic: Arising from outside of the body or away from the body part being described.

Facet: A small, smooth, articular surface on a bone.

Facet joint: An articulation of the facets between each contiguous pair of vertebrae in the spinal column.

False joint: Abnormal movement along the length of a bone caused by a fracture or incomplete fusion.

Fascia: A fibrous membrane that supports and separates muscles and unites the skin with the underlying tissues.

Fine motor control: Specific control of the muscles allowing for completion of small, delicate tasks.

Flexible collodion: A mixture of ether, alcohol, cellulose, and camphor, which dries to form a firm protective layer.

Flexion: The act of bending a joint, decreasing its angle.

Foramen (Pl. **Foramina**): An opening in a bone or organ through which other structures pass.

Force couple: Coordination between dynamic and static contractions of opposing muscle groups to perform a movement of a joint.

Forefoot valgus: Eversion of the forefoot relative to the hindfoot.

Forefoot varus: Inversion of the forefoot relative to the hindfoot.

Forefoot: The area of the foot formed by the metatarsals and the phalanges.

Fossa: A depression on a bone.

Freedom of movement: The number of cardinal planes in which a joint allows motion.

Frog-eyed patellae: Patellae that ride superiorly and laterally relative to their normal position.

Frontal plane: A vertical plane passing through the

body, dividing it into anterior and posterior portions.

Functional tests, sport-specific: The use of activities and motions that closely represent the athlete's sport and position to assess a body part's readiness to return to competition.

Functional tests: Assessment of the athlete's ability to move a body part actively, passively, and against resistance. Also encompasses the normal activity of the internal and sensory organs.

Gait: The sequential movements of the spine, pelvis, knee, ankle, and foot when walking or running.

Ganglion (nerve) (pl. ganglia): A collection of nerve cell bodies housed in the central or peripheral nervous system.

Ganglion cyst: A collection of fluids collecting within the tendons of the wrist or ankle.

Gangrene: The death of bony or soft tissue resulting from a decrease in, or loss of, blood supply to a body area.

Genu valgum: The femur and tibia are angled inward.

Genu varum: The femur and tibia are angled outward.

Gingivitis: Inflammation of the gums.

Gonad: An organ producing gender-based reproductive cells; the ovaries or testicles.

Goniometer: A device used to measure the motion, in degrees, that a joint is capable of producing around its axis.

Gout: A form of acute arthritis marked by inflammation and pain in the distal joints.

Graft: An organ or tissue used for transplantation. In an allograft, tissue is received from the same species. In an autograft, tissue is transplanted from within the same individual.

Gross deformity: An abnormality that is visible to the unaided eye.

Growth plate: The area of bone growth in skeletally immature athletes; the epiphyseal plate.

Guarding: Voluntarily or involuntarily assuming a posture to protect an injured body area, often through muscular spasm.

Hallux rigidus: Decreased mobility of the first metatarsophalangeal joint; also referred to as hallux limitus.

Hallux valgus: Excessive valgus deformity of the first metatarsophalangeal joint.

Hammer toes: Toes characterized by hyperextension of the metatarsophalangeal joint and the distal interphalangeal joints and flexion of the proximal interphalangeal joint.

Heel spur: An abnormal bony outgrowth on the calcaneus.

Hemarthrosis: Blood within a joint cavity.

Hematoma: A collection of clotted blood within a confined space (*hemat,* blood; *toma,* tumor).

Hematuria: Blood in the urine.

Hemothorax: Blood in the pleural cavity.

Hepatitis B virus (HBV): A virus resulting in inflammation of the liver. Following a 2- to 6-week incubation period symptoms develop, including gastrointestinal and respiratory disturbances, jaundice, enlarged liver, muscle pain, and weight loss.

Herniation: The protrusion of a tissue through the wall that normally contains it.

Hill-Sachs lesion: An articular cartilage defect on the posterior aspect of the humeral head caused by the impact of the humeral head following an anterior glenohumeral dislocation.

Hindfoot: Area of the foot formed by the talus and calcaneus.

Hindfoot valgus: Eversion of the calcaneus relative to the tibia.

Hindfoot varus: Inversion of the calcaneus relative to the tibia.

History: An account, analysis, and recording of events prior to the onset of an injury or illness.

Homans' sign: Pain arising from simultaneous passive ankle dorsiflexion and squeezing of the calf, indicating deep vein thrombosis.

Hook-lying: Lying supine with the hips and knees flexed.

Human immunodeficiency virus (HIV): The virus that causes acquired immune deficiency syndrome (AIDS).

Hyaline cartilage: Cartilage found on the articular surface of bones. It is especially suited to withstand compressive and shearing forces.

Hypercholesterolemia: A high blood cholesterol level caused by a high intake of saturated fats.

Hyperemia: A red discoloration of the skin caused by an increased capillary blood flow.

Hyperhidrosis: Excessive or profuse sweating.

Hypermetropia: Farsightedness occurring when light rays come into focus at a point behind the retina.

Hyperreflexia: Increased action of the reflexes.

Hyperthermia: Increased core temperature.

Hypertonic: Having an increased osmotic pressure relative to the body's other fluids.

Hypertrophy: The increase in the cross-sectional size of a muscle, bone, or organ.

Hyporeflexia: A diminished or absent reflex response.

Hypothermia: Decreased core temperature.

Hysteria: An increased or heightened state of panic.

Idiopathic: Of unknown cause.

Incontinence: A loss of bowel and/or bladder control.

Injected: Congested with blood or other fluids forced into an area.

Insidious: Of gradual onset; with respect to symptoms of an injury or disease having no apparent cause.

Inspection: To visually examine the results of a disease or injury.

Instability: The inability of a joint to function under normal functional stresses.

Interosseous: Between two bones.

Intrathecal: Within the spinal canal.

Intrinsic: Arising from within the body or within the body part being described.

Inversion: The movement of the plantar aspect of the calcaneus toward the midline of the body.

Ionizing radiation: Electromagnetic energy that causes the release of an atom's protons, electrons, or neutrons. Ionizing radiation is potentially hazardous to human tissue.

Ipsilateral: Pertaining to the same side of the body.

Ischemia: Decrease in local blood flow secondary to the obstruction of the blood vessels.

Isokinetic dynamometer: A device that quantitatively measures muscular strength through a preset speed of movement.

-itis: Suffix indicating the inflammatory state of particular tissues (e.g., tendinitis, bursitis).

Jefferson's fracture: A fracture of a circular bone in two places; similar to breaking a doughnut in half.

Jersey finger: The inability to flex the distal interphalangeal joint secondary to an avulsion or rupture of the flexor digitorum longus tendon.

Joint reaction forces: Forces that are transmitted through a joint's articular surfaces.

Joint stability: The integrity of a joint when it is placed under a functional load.

Keloid: Hypertrophic scar formation secondary to excessive collagen.

Kehr's sign: Pain referred to the upper left shoulder following spleen trauma.

Kidney stones: A crystal mass formed in the kidney that is passed through the urinary tract.

Kienböck's disease: Osteochondritis or slow degeneration of the lunate bone.

Kyphosis: An abnormal posterior convexity of the spinal column, especially in the thoracic region.

Labrum: A dense, fibrous connective tissue that deepens the socket associated with ball-and-socket joints.

Laxity: The amount of movement allowed by a joint's capsule and/or ligaments.

Legg-Calvé-Perthes disease: Avascular necrosis occurring in children age 3 to 12 years, causing osteochondritis of the proximal femoral epiphysis.

Long bone: A bone possessing a base, shaft, and head.

Lower motor neuron lesion: A spinal cord lesion resulting in decreased reflexes, flaccid paralysis, and atrophy.

Lower quarter screen: Assessment of the neurological status of the peripheral nervous system of the lower extremities through the evaluation of sensation, motor function, and deep tendon reflexes.

Lucid: Pertaining to the state of mental clarity.

Lumbarization: Condition in which the first sacral vertebra fails to unite with the remainder of the sacrum.

Lupus: A systemic disease affecting the internal organs, skin, and musculoskeletal system.

Lymph nodes: Nodules located in the cervical, axillary, and inguinal regions, producing white blood cells and filtering bacteria from the bloodstream. Lymph nodes become enlarged secondary to an infection.

Macrotrauma: A single force resulting in trauma to the body's tissues.

Malingering: Faking or exaggerating the symptoms of an injury or illness.

Mallet finger: Inability to extend the distal interphalangeal joint secondary to an avulsion of the extensor tendon.

Malocclusion: A deviation in the normal alignment of two opposable tissues (e.g., the mandible and maxilla).

Manual muscle testing: A specific procedure used to evaluate the functional status of a muscle's innervation and contractile tissues.

March fracture: A stress fracture of the second, third, or fourth metatarsal. Named because of the high incidence of this condition in foot soldiers.

Marfan syndrome: A hereditary condition of the connective tissue, bones, muscles, and ligaments. Over time, this condition results in degeneration of brain function and in cardiac failure.

Mastication: The chewing of food.

McKenzie exercises: A protocol of exercises used during the treatment and rehabilitation of spinal lesions, involving flexion and extension, for strengthening the lumbar spine. These exercises are named for their developer, Robin McKenzie, an Australian physiotherapist.

Mechanism: A physical or biological process through which an injury or illness is produced.

Median: Along the body's midline.

Menstruation: The period of bleeding during the menstrual cycle.

Metabolic acidosis: Decreased blood pH caused by an increase in blood acids or a decrease in blood bases.

Microtrauma: Small, repetitive injurious forces.

Midfoot: Area of the foot formed by the navicular, three cuneiforms, and cuboid.

Mononucleosis: A disease state caused by an abnormally high number of mononuclear leukocytes in the bloodstream.

Morton's toe: A foot type characterized by the second toe's extending past the great toe.

Motor neurons: Those neurons that send signals from the central nervous system to the muscular system.

Movie sign: Pain arising in the patellofemoral joint caused by prolonged knee flexion, such as when sitting, indicating bursitis or other inflammatory condition.

Muscle guarding: See guarding.

Musculotendinous unit: The group formed by a muscle and its tendons.

Myelin sheath: A fatty-based lining of the axon of myelinated nerve fibers.

Myopia: Nearsightedness, occurring when light rays come into focus in front of the retina.

Myositis ossificans (traumatica): Formation of bone within the connective fascia and intramuscular extensions of a muscle. This condition most commonly affects large muscle masses and results secondary to a contusion.

Necrosis: The death of one or more cells.

Nélaton's line: An imaginary line drawn from the anterior superior iliac spine to the ischial tuberosity. Coxa valga should be suspected if the greater trochanter is located above this line.

Neurapraxia: Loss of function of a peripheral nerve without degenerative changes; occurs secondary to stretching of the nerve, epineurium, and myelin sheath.

Neuroma: A tumor or abnormal growth within the nerve, resulting in hypersensitivity.

Neurotmesis: A complete disruption of a nerve.

Neurovascular: Pertaining to a bundle formed by nerves, arteries, and veins.

Noncontractile tissue: Ligamentous and capsular tissue surrounding a joint.

Nonunion fracture: A fracture that fails to spontaneously heal within the normal time frame for the involved bone.

Normative data: Normal ranges of data collected for comparison during the evaluation of an athlete. Athletes have norms different from the general population on most measures.

Nystagmus: Rhythmical oscillation of the eyeballs. This condition may be either congenital or the result of a traumatic injury.

Objective data: Finite measures that are readily reproducible regardless of the individual collecting the information.

Occlusion: The process of closing or being closed.

OCD: See osteochondral defect.

Open chain exercise: See open kinetic chain.

Open kinetic chain: Motion that occurs when the distal portion of the extremity is non–weight bearing.

Open-packed position: The joint position at which its bones are maximally incongruent.

Ophthalmologist: A medical doctor specializing in injury, diseases, and abnormalities of the eye.

Opposition: A combined movement that allows the thumb to touch each of the four fingers.

Osteoarthritis: Inflammation and eventual degeneration of a joint's articular surface caused by injury or excessive forces transmitted through the joint.

Osteoblasts: Cells concerned with the formation of new bone.

Osteochondral defect (OCD): Disruption of a bone's articular cartilage secondary to a fracture or degenerative softening.

Osteochondritis dissecans: Wearing away, delamination, of the chondral surface and the subchondral bone.

Osteoclasts: Cells that absorb and remove unwanted bone.

Osteoporosis: Decreased bone density common in postmenopausal women.

Overpressure: A force that attempts to move a joint beyond its normal range of motion.

Overuse syndrome: Injury caused by accumulated microtraumatic stress placed on a structure or body area.

Painful arc: An area within a joint's range of motion that causes pain, representing compression, impingement, or abrasion of the underlying tissues.

Pallor: Lack of color in the skin.

Palpation: Assessment of injuries and illness through touching and feeling the body.

Parasympathetic nervous system: A series of specific effects controlled by the brain regulating smooth muscle contractions, slowing the heart rate, and constricting the pupil.

Paresthesia: The sensation of numbness or tingling, often described as a "pins and needles" sensation, caused by peripheral nerve lesions.

Passive range of motion: Movement of a joint through the range of motion by means other than a muscle contraction; used to assess the range of motion available to a joint and to establish the quality of the end-point.

Patella alta: A patella having an abnormally high position relative to the joint line of the knee.

Patella baja: A patella having an abnormally low position relative to the joint line of the knee.

Patency: The state of being freely open.

Pathology: A condition produced by an injury or disease.

Pathomechanics: Abnormal motion and forces produced by the body, most often occurring secondary to trauma.

Pelvic inflammatory disease: An infection of the vagina that spreads to the cervix, uterus, fallopian tubes, and broad ligaments.

Pericarditis: Inflammation of the exterior lining of the heart; marked by fever, chest pain, and an irregular pulse.

Periorbital: Pertaining to the area around the eye, including the eyebrow and contiguous portion of the nose, cheek, and temple.

Periosteum: A fibrous membrane containing blood vessels covering the shafts of long bones.

Peripheral vascular disease (PVD): A syndrome involving an insufficiency of arteries and/or veins in maintaining proper circulation.

Peristalsis: A progressive smooth muscle contraction producing a wavelike motion that moves matter through the intestines.

Pes cavus: A condition characterized by an increased height of the foot's medial longitudinal arch.

Pes planus: A condition characterized by the flattening of the foot's medial longitudinal arch.

Pes planus, rigid: Pes planus that is present while the foot is both weight bearing and non–weight bearing.

Pes planus, supple: Pes planus that is present only while the foot is weight bearing. The medial longitudinal arch is present when the foot is non–weight bearing.

Photophobia: The eye's intolerance to light.

Physical therapist: A health care professional versed in the rehabilitation of disease and injury through physical means.

Physician: A health care professional versed in the evaluation, diagnosis, and management of disease and illness through the art of medicine and surgery.

Piano key sign: A rebounding or bobbing of the distal clavicle when pressure is applied, caused by a sprain of the acromioclavicular ligament.

Pilonidal cyst: An infection over the posterior aspect of the median sacral crests resulting in severe pain and disability.

Plane of the scapula: The alignment assumed by the glenoid fossa when the scapula is resting in the anatomical position on the torso.

Plane synovial joint: A synovial joint formed by the gliding between two or more bones.

Plantarflexion: Extension of the ankle; pointing the foot and toes.

Plica: A thickening or fold in the joint capsule.

Pneumothorax: Air pockets forming within the pleural cavity.

Postpartum: Following childbirth.

Posttraumatic amnesia: The loss of memory from the time of trauma onward, also known as anterograde amnesia.

Postconcussional syndrome: A progressive deterioration of cognitive function following repeated brain trauma.

Preiser's disease: Osteoporosis of the scaphoid resulting from a fracture or repeated trauma.

Priapism: Spontaneous penile erection indicating a thoracic or cervical spinal cord lesion.

Prodromal: Pertaining to the interval between the initial disease state and the onset of outward symptoms.

Prognosis: The course a disease or injury is expected to take.

PROM: Passive range of motion.

Pronation (foot and ankle): The combined motion produced by calcaneal eversion, foot abduction, and ankle dorsiflexion.

Pronation (forearm): Movement at the radioulnar joints allowing for the palm to be turned downward.

Proprioception: The athlete's ability to sense the position of one or more joints.

Protraction (scapular): Movement of the vertebral borders of the scapula away from the spinal column.

Proximal: Near the midline of the body; the opposite of distal.

Pulmonary edema: Swelling of the lung and its tissues.

Pump bumps: Exostosis on the posterior aspect of the calcaneus owing to excessive external pressure and/or friction.

Pus: Normally a yellow fluid containing leukocytes escaping from an infected area.

Q angle: The angle formed by the pull of the quadriceps muscle on the patella and the patellar tendon's insertion on the tibia.

Raccoon eyes: Ecchymosis formation beneath the eyes secondary to a skull or nasal fracture.

Radial deviation: Movement of the hand toward the radial (thumb) side.

Radiculopathy: Any disease condition affecting the spinal nerve roots.

Radionuclide: An atom that, when disintegrating, emits electromagnetic radiation.

Ramus: A division of a forked structure.

Raynaud's phenomenon: A reaction to cold consisting of bouts of pallor and cyanosis, causing exaggerated vasomotor responses.

Referred pain: Pain at a site other than the actual location of trauma. Referred pain tends to be projected outward from the torso and distally along the extremities.

Reflex inhibition: The inability of a muscle to actively contract secondary to sensory impulses.

Relative humidity: The ratio between the amount of water vapor in the air and the actual amount of water the air can potentially hold based on the current temperature.

Reposition: The return motion from opposition.

Resisted range of motion: The determination of a muscle or muscle group's ability to produce tension; may be performed dynamically through the range of motion or statically in the form of a break test.

Resonant: Producing a vibrating sound on percussion.

Retinaculum: A ligamentous tissue serving as a restraining band to hold other tissues in place.

Retraction (scapular): Movement of the scapular vertebral borders toward the spinal column.

Rheumatoid arthritis: Degeneration of a joint's articular surface caused by an immunologic reaction of the body.

Rigidity: A pathological loss of a joint's motion or a soft tissue's elasticity.

Ringer's lactate: A salt-based solution that is administered intravenously as a replacement for lost electrolytes.

Role delineation: The determination of the tasks and functions particular to a profession.

RROM: Resisted range of motion.

Sacralization: Fusion of the first lumbar vertebra to the sacrum.

Sagittal plane: A vertical plane passing through the body, dividing it into left and right sides.

Scapular tipping: The inferior angle of the scapula moving away from the thorax while its superior border moves toward the thorax.

Scapular winging: The vertebral border of the scapula lifting away from the thorax.

Screw home mechanism: External rotation of the tibia during the terminal range of knee extension.

Sebaceous gland: Oil-secreting gland of the skin.

Sensation: The ability of the athlete to perceive sensory stimuli such as touch discrimination or temperature.

Sequestrated: Pertaining to a necrotic fragment of tissue that has become separated from the surrounding tissue.

Sesamoid bone: A bone that lies within a tendon.

Shear forces: Forces from opposing directions that are applied perpendicular to a structure's long axis.

Shoulder girdle: The functional structure of the shoulder formed by the scapulothoracic, acromioclavicular, and glenohumeral joints.

Sign: An observable condition that indicates the existence of a disease or injury. Signs are usually apparent during the inspection process.

Sinus rhythm: An irregular heartbeat characterized by an increased rate during inspiration and a decreased rate during expiration.

Sinus tarsi: A landmark, rather than a discrete anatomical structure, marked by a depression over the anterior lateral portion of the foot just distal to the lateral malleolus.

Sinus: A cavity within a bone.

Sinusitis: Inflammation of the nasal sinus.

Slipped capital femoris: Displacement of the femoral head relative to the femoral shaft; common in children age 10 to 15 years and especially prevalent in boys.

Slough: The peeling away of dead skin from the living tissue.

Soft tissue: Structures other than bone, including muscle, tendon, ligament, capsule, bursa, and skin.

Special tests: Particular stresses applied to the bone to exhibit the pathomechanics of a joint or structure.

Sports medicine: The application of medical and scientific knowledge to the prevention (including training methods and practices), care, and rehabilitation of injuries suffered by individuals participating in athletics.

Sprain: The stretching or tearing of ligamentous or capsular tissue.

Sputum: A substance formed by mucus, blood, or pus which is expelled by coughing or clearing the throat.

Squinting patellae: Patellae that are medially rotated.

Staphylococcal infection: An infection caused by the *Staphylococcus* bacteria.

Stenosis: Constriction of an opening or passage.

Step deformity (shoulder): A high-riding clavicle indicative of an acromioclavicular joint sprain or a fracture of the distal clavicle.

Step-off deformity (spine): A depressed spinous process caused by spondylolisthesis.

Strain: Injury to the musculotendinous unit resulting from excessive stretch or tension.

Stress fracture: A fracture caused by repetitive low-load forces to a bone.

Stridor: A harsh, high-pitched sound resembling blowing wind, experienced during respiration.

Subconjunctival hematoma: Leakage of the superficial blood vessels beneath the sclera.

Subluxation: The partial or incomplete dislocation of a joint usually transient in nature; the joint surfaces relocate as the forces causing the joint displacement are relieved.

Subtalar joint: The articulation between the superior surface of the calcaneus and the inferior portion of the talus, allowing 1 degree of freedom of movement: inversion and eversion.

Subungual hematoma: Collection of blood under a fingernail or toenail.

Sudden death: Unexpected and instantaneous death occurring within 1 hour of the onset of symptoms; most often used to describe death caused secondary to cardiac failure.

Sulcus: A groove or depression within a bone.

Supination (foot and ankle): The combined motion produced by calcaneal inversion, foot adduction, and ankle plantarflexion.

Supination (forearm): Movement at the radioulnar joints allowing for the palm to turn upward, as if holding a bowl of soup.

Sympathetic nervous system: The part of the central nervous system supplying the involuntary muscles.

Symptom: A condition not visually apparent to the examiner, indicating the existence of a disease or injury. Symptoms are usually obtained during the history-taking process.

Syncope: Fainting caused by a transient loss of oxygen supply to the brain.

Syndesmosis joint: A relatively immobile joint in which two bones are bound together by ligaments.

Synovial hinge joint: A joint separated by a space filled with synovial fluid.

Synovial membrane: The membrane lining a fluid-filled joint.

Systematic: Orderly, based on a specific sequence of events.

Tarsal coalition: A bony, fibrous, or cartilaginous union between two or more tarsal bones.

Tensile force: Force applied along the fibers of a tissue. Excessive tensile forces cause a tearing of the tissues as they are stretched beyond their normal length.

Theater sign: See movie sign.

Thrombophlebitis: Inflammation of a vein and the subsequent formation of blood clots.

Tibial collateral ligament: The medial collateral ligament of the knee.

Tinel's sign: Distally radiating paresthesia caused by tapping over the site of a superficial nerve, indicating inflammation or irritation of the nerve.

Tinnitus: Ringing in the ears.

Tracer element: A substance that is introduced into the tissues to follow or trace an otherwise unidentifiable substance or event.

Tracheotomy: A method of delivering air to the lungs by incising the skin and trachea and inserting a tube to form an airway. This emergency technique is used only when the athlete's life is threatened by an immovable obstruction of the upper airway. Training is required to properly perform this technique.

Triage: The process of determining the priority of treatment.

Triceps surae muscle group: The muscle group formed by the gastrocnemius, soleus, and plantaris, sharing the common attachment of the Achilles tendon on the calcaneus.

Trigger point: A pathological condition characterized by a small, hypersensitive area located within muscles and fasciae.

Trophic: Pertaining to efferent nerves controlling the nourishment of the area they innervate.

Tubercle: A nodulelike projection off a bone, serving as an attachment site for muscles and ligaments; referred to as a tuberosity in the lower extremity.

Tuberosity: A nodulelike projection off a bone, serving as an attachment site for muscles and ligaments; referred to as a tubercle in the upper extremity.

Turf toe: The sprain and subsequent inflammation of the first metatarsophalangeal joint.

Ulnar deviation: Movement of the hand toward the ulnar side of the forearm.

Ultrasonic imaging: The use of sound waves above the range of human hearing to visualize the subcutaneous tissues.

Uniplanar: Occurring in only one of the cardinal planes.

Upper motor neuron lesion: A spinal cord lesion that results in paralysis, loss of voluntary movement, spasticity, sensory loss, and pathological reflexes.

Upper and lower quarter screens: Assessments of the neurological status of the peripheral nervous system of the upper and lower extremities, respectively, through the evaluation of sensation, motor function, and deep tendon reflexes.

Valgus force: A force applied toward the body's midline (medially).

Varus force: A force applied from the body's midline outward (laterally).

Vasoconstriction: A decrease in a vessel's diameter.

Vasodilation: An increase in a vessel's diameter.

Vasomotor: Pertaining to nerves controlling the muscles within the walls of blood vessels.

Visual acuity: The eyes' ability to see normally (i.e., 20/20 vision).

Volar: Referring to the palmar side of the hand and forearm.

Wallerian degeneration: Degeneration of a nerve's axon that has been severed from the body of the nerve.

Whorls: Swirl markings in the skin. Fingerprints are images formed by the whorls on the fingertips.

Index

Numbers followed by an "f" indicate figures; numbers followed by a "t" indicate tables.